Clinical Skills in Treating the Foot

For Churchill Livingstone:

Associate Editor: Robert Edwards
Project Manager: Yolanta Motylinska
Design: George Ajayi
Typesetting and Project Management: Helius

Clinical Skills in Treating the Foot

SECOND EDITION

Edited by

Warren A. Turner PhD BSc DpodM MChS
Assistant Director, School of Education, Health and Sciences, University of Derby, UK

Linda M. Merriman PhD MPhil DPodM MChS CertEd
Dean, School of Health and Social Sciences, Coventry University, UK

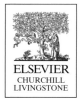

ELSEVIER
CHURCHILL
LIVINGSTONE

EDINBURGH   LONDON   NEW YORK   OXFORD   PHILADELPHIA   ST LOUIS   SYDNEY   TORONTO   2005

ELSEVIER
CHURCHILL
LIVINGSTONE

First published 1997
Second edition 2005
  Reprinted 2007

ISBN 978 0 443 07113 3

British Library Cataloguing in Publication Data
A catalogue record for this book is available from the British Library

Library of Congress Cataloging in Publication Data
A catalog record for this book is available from the Library of Congress

Notice
Knowledge and best practice in this field are constantly changing. As new research
and experience broaden our knowledge, changes in practice, treatment and drug
therapy may become necessary or appropriate. Readers are advised to check the most
current information provided (i) on procedures featured or (ii) by the manufacturer
of each product to be administered, to verify the recommended dose or formula, the
method and duration of administration, and contraindications. It is the responsibility
of the practitioner, relying on their own experience and knowledge of the patient,
to make diagnoses, to determine dosages and the best treatment for each individual
patient, and to take all appropriate safety precautions. To the fullest extent of the
law, neither the publisher nor the editors assume any liability for any injury
and/or damage.

The Publisher

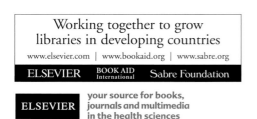

Working together to grow
libraries in developing countries

www.elsevier.com | www.bookaid.org | www.sabre.org

ELSEVIER   BOOK AID International   Sabre Foundation

ELSEVIER   your source for books,
journals and multimedia
in the health sciences
www.elsevierhealth.com

The
publisher's
policy is to use
**paper manufactured
from sustainable forests**

Printed in China

Contents

Contributors

Paul Beeson MSc BSc(Hons) DpodM MChS
Senior Lecturer in Podiatry, University College
Northampton, UK

Michael Curran Mphil BSc(Hons) MChS CertEd
Senior Lecturer in Podiatry, University College
Northampton, UK

Joy Dale
Lecturer in Podiatry, Directorate of Podiatry,
University of Salford, UK

Dr David Gerrett PhD MSc BPharm MRPharmS
Head of Pharmacy, School of Education, Health
& Sciences, University of Derby, UK

Dr Tim Kilmartin
Consultant Podiatrist, Ilkeston Community
Hospital, Ilkeston, Derbyshire, UK

Dr Marilyn Lord
Senior Lecturer, King's College Hospital,
London, UK

Dr Linda M. Merriman PhD Mphil DpodM
MChS CertEd
Dean, School of Health and Social Sciences,
University of Coventry, UK

Dr Robert S. Moore FFAEM
Consultant in Emergency Medicine, Countess of
Chester Hospital NHS Trust, Chester, UK

Patricia S. Nesbitt PGD(BioEng) PGC(Sports Pod)
DpodM MChS
Acting Head of Podiatry, University College
Northampton, UK

Terry O'Donnell MSc BA(Hons) PGCE
Senior lecturer in Sociology of Physical Activity,
Exercise and Health, Leeds Metropolitan
University , UK

Professor David Pratt PhD CSci MIPEM CPhys
MInstP SRCS ARCP
Lead Clinician, West Midlands Rehabilitation
Centre, Birmingham, UK

Trevor Prior
Consultant Podiatrc Surgeon, Homerton
University Hospital, London, UK

Dr Kate Springett PhD FChS DPodM
Head of Department of Allied Health
Professions, Canterbury Christchurch
University College, Canterbury, UK

Mr David R. Tollafield DPodM BSc(Hons) FCPodS
Consultant in Primary Care, Walsall Teaching
Trust, Manor Hospital, Walsall, UK

Dr Warren A. Turner PhD BSc DpodM MChS
Assistant Director of School of Education,
Health & Sciences, University of Derby, UK

Ben Yates MSc BSc(Hons) FCPod(S) DPodM
Podiatric Surgeon, Trauma and Orthopaedics,
Great Western Hospital, Swindon, UK

Preface

This second edition of *Clinical Skills in Treating the Foot* has been written as a companion volume to *Assessment of the Lower Limb*, 2nd edition. This volume focuses on the treatment of foot-related disorders.

This book has been written with the needs of a broad range of health professionals in mind. It has been designed to support anyone providing treatment for patients with foot disorders. Although primarily of interest to podiatrists and student podiatrists, the book should prove a useful reference for others involved in the provision of treatment of the foot.

The book is set out into three sections. Section 1, Essential Principles of Management, is concerned with the general principles of managing foot disorders, and the context in which treatment of the foot takes place. This includes chapters on treatment planning, evidence-based practice, governance and audit, clinical protocols, clinical emergencies and health promotion. These chapters provide a useful background to the provision of treatment of the foot. They will also assist clinicians with the development of strategies for planning, reviewing and evaluating the nature and appropriateness of their work with clients.

Section 2, Methods of Managing Foot Conditions, is concerned with the application of clinical therapeutics to foot disease, and includes chapters on operative techniques, surgery and the foot, pharmacology, physical therapies, mechanical therapies, chair-side devices, prescription devices, and footwear therapy. This section provides detailed information on the nature and application of therapeutic techniques.

Section 3, Managing Specific Client Groups, considers the particular needs of special groups and includes chapters on the adult foot, the child's foot, sports injuries, and the management of tissue viability. This section identifies the specialist areas of practice appropriate to these patient groups. As such, it provides an introduction to key specialist practice fields in the management of foot disease.

It is hoped that the use of case examples, illustrations and photographs throughout the text will assist readers in understanding the key principles involved in the provision of treatment of the foot.

Dr Warren A. Turner
Dr Linda M. Merriman

Acknowledgements

No volume such as this is the work of the editors or chapter authors alone. A significant number of other people have contributed to the development of this text, and to them we are very grateful. In particular, thanks are due to those who contributed as authors of chapters in the first edition of this book, whose work has provided the foundation for revision in this edition. Particular thanks go also to Prof. Robert Ashford, Steve Avil, Dr John Carpenter, Anne Marie Carr, John Colin Dagnall, Joy Dale, Richard Goslin, Allen Hinde, Dr Timothy Kilmartin, Cameron Kippen, Dr Marilyn Lord, Dr Jean Mooney, Trevor Prior, Keith Rome and Louise Stuart, all of whom made significant contributions to the first edition, which have been built on in this edition of the book.

Thanks to those who reviewed the content of chapters prior to submission, in particular thanks to Prof. Dawn Forman and Dr David Gerrett, for advising on chapter content. Thanks also for those who provided useful and constructive feedback on the first edition of this text.

Colleagues at Churchill Livingstone have been a source of immense support throughout this project, and have endured the work with calm grace and good patience. Thanks to Mary Emmerson Law, Dinah Thom and Jane Ward. Particular thanks to Robert Edwards, who has provided welcome support and encouragement throughout the preparation of the second edition of this book.

Essential principles of management

1

Treatment planning

Warren A. Turner
Linda M. Merriman

INTRODUCTION

Ineffective clinical interventions often arise from incorrect diagnosis, ineffectual planning of treatment or a combination of both. The formulation of clear treatment plans is crucial for the delivery of effective and efficient foot care. Effective treatment planning for patients with foot health problems can make a significant contribution to the health of communities.

Mobility, independence, symptom relief and quality of life can be significantly enhanced by effective provision of foot health services. Patients can be maintained for longer in their own communities, retaining their independence, maintaining activity levels and thereby reducing the load on acute or long-term hospital and care facilities.

Effective foot health provision is a highly cost-effective process but is reliant on the development of rational and appropriate treatment planning. This chapter explores who needs foot health treatment and how effective treatment planning can be enabled. The key components and processes involved in a treatment plan are identified.

WHO NEEDS TREATMENT FOR DISORDERS OF THE FOOT?

Decisions often have to be made regarding the provision of foot health services, particularly when such services are funded from limited public funds. How should resources for the management of foot problems be distributed?

Who has the greatest need? Who should receive publicly funded foot health care, and who can afford to pay for self-funded care?

The answers to questions such as these are often difficult to find. Commissioners of public health services rely on information from a variety of sources to make key decisions concerning service provision. These include:

- patient demand
- evidence base for clinical and cost effectiveness of the service
- competing demands for funding
- health outcome targets
- risk of not providing services
- which individuals/groups are most at risk/in need?
- historical levels of service provision
- levels of service provision in comparable communities
- epidemiological trends
- impact on other services.

As well as public health organizations being in a position to identify population or community needs for foot health provision, individuals are often involved in identification of need for care. Many authors have attempted to define the term need. Bradshaw (1972) identified four types of need (Table 1.1). Kemp & Winkler (1983) adapted the above classification of need and utilized the following classification in their survey of podiatric need:

- activated need: a requirement for foot care that is consciously recognized by the sufferer or a third party (demand); action is taken to meet the requirement
- felt need: a requirement for foot care that is consciously recognized by the sufferer or a third party but no action is taken to meet the requirement (potential demand)
- potential need: requirement for foot care that is not acknowledged by an individual yet a practitioner who undertook a clinical assessment of the individual would consider there was a need.

Two Department of Health (DoH) surveys concerning foot health needs have been undertaken (Clarke 1969, Cartwright & Henderson 1986). Both adopted similar methodologies and reported a high level of need that was not being met. Other needs-based surveys, although they adopted different methodologies, concurred with these findings (Kemp & Winkler 1983, Elton & Sanderson 1987, Wessex Feet 1988). More recently, a major study in Cambridge, UK has identified that a significant number of elderly people identified as being 'low risk' for serious foot disease have developed significant pathologies, including infection and ulceration within a short period of time (Campbell et al 2000). This study identified the greatest risk of serious pathology to be amongst those over 85 years of age and those who are unable to care for their feet themselves.

Research has shown that there are often differences between practitioners and the general public when assessing the level of need. Clarke (1969) commented that practitioners' estimates of unmet needs (or normative needs) exceeded not only people's demands for foot health services but also their perceived needs (felt needs that were not being met). A high percentage of the general public did not consider they were in 'need' of treatment despite practitioners arriving at a clinical decision that treatment was needed.

One interesting explanation for this phenomenon lies in research undertaken by Dunnell & Cartwright (1972). The authors asked 1400 adults about their general health: 28% said they were

Table 1.1 Types of need as identified by Bradshaw (1972)

Type of need	Description
Normative	Need defined by an expert
Felt	A want expressed by the patient or a third party
Expressed	A felt need which is turned into action (demand)
Comparative	Arrived at by studying the characteristics of people in receipt of a service and identifying those with similar characteristics, but not in receipt, as being in need

in excellent health, 39% good health, 24% fair health and 9% poor health. When those in 'good' or 'excellent' health were asked if they had experienced any health-related problems in the last few weeks, only 9% said they had not. The common symptoms reported were: 'headaches, skin disorders, accidents and trouble with feet and teeth'. It would appear that the participants accepted that 'trouble with feet' was 'part and parcel of life'.

Epidemiological studies have shown the level of foot health among the general public to be low. Minor foot and foot-related problems of the earlier years are often neglected but can, in some cases, lead to more serious health problems in middle and later years.

Need surveys are not always helpful in informing decisions about the allocation of resources. Manning & Ungerson (1990) believed that the incommensurability of different needs made distribution of resources according to need a poor guide to public policy. Factors other than the findings from need surveys should be used in arriving at decisions about the allocation of resources. These factors include:

- demographic trends
- waiting lists
- strategic plans of health commissioning agencies
- public expectations
- political pressure groups
- responsibility for health.

Manning & Ungerson (1990) raised the issue of who should be responsible for the nation's health. For example, who is responsible for the foot problems of the person born with spina bifida or the individual who contracts the acquired immunodeficiency syndrome: that particular individual, the family or the state?

Foot hygiene, routine nail care and well-fitting footwear should be the responsibility of each individual. The undertaking of these routine tasks can prevent a number of foot problems from arising and, as a result, reduce the need for foot health services. For a variety of reasons (e.g. poor eyesight and arthritis), some individuals may be unable to undertake these tasks them-

selves. In these instances, family, friends and the voluntary, private and statutory services have a role to play.

The annual sales of proprietary products for the self-treatment of some foot pathologies (e.g. corns and verrucae) lead one to assume that a large number of the general public are actively involved in treating their own foot problems. The overall philosophy of a good foot health service should be to promote informed self-care. As long as self-treatment is safe to use and will not lead to unnecessary complications, it can provide a useful adjunct to treatment provided by the health care practitioner.

Many practitioners are faced with long waiting lists and have to make daily decisions as to which patients are in the greatest need and should, therefore, receive treatment first. Various approaches have been used to prioritize need. Table 1.2 lists some conditions that may be considered appropriate for priority treatment because of the potential risk of deterioration where no treatment is made available.

Table 1.2   Features of presenting problems that require immediate attention

Feature	Associated signs and symptoms
Pain	Constant weight bearing and non-weight bearing
	Affects patient's normal daily activities
Infection	Raised temperature (pyrexia)
	Signs of acute inflammation
	Signs of spreading cellulites, lymphangitis, lymphadenitis
Ulceration	Loss of skin
	May or may not be painful
	May expose underlying tissue
Acute swelling	Unrelieved pain
	Very noticeable swelling
	May have associated signs of swelling
Abnormal skin changes	Distinct colour changes
	Discharge may be malodorous
	Itching
	Bleeding

WHAT IS 'TREATMENT'?

The *Oxford English Dictionary* defines 'treatment' as 'Management in the application of remedies; medical or surgical application or service'.

It is necessary to draw a distinction between 'treatment' and 'management'. Management is concerned with identifying those actions that should be taken to effect a change. Such management will often include actions that the patient or their carer(s) should take, actions that other health professionals should provide (e.g. following referral), and actions which the foot health professional should provide (e.g. specific treatments). A treatment plan, however, is simply a description of the medical and/or surgical modalities that will be applied to a particular patient. Therefore, a patient management plan is subtly different from a treatment plan. Whilst a treatment plan only specifies and describes actions that will be performed by an individual or group of health providers for a patient, a management plan is more wide ranging. This will often include details of recommended actions for the patient, carer and other health care and medical staff.

An example showing the distinction between a management plan and a treatment plan is provided in Case Study 1.1.

THE TREATMENT PLANNING PROCESS

The treatment planning process is informed by, and follows on from, thorough history taking and examination (primary patient assessment). A thorough assessment is essential in order to:

- identify the aetiology, e.g. trauma, pathogenic microorganisms
- identify any factors that may influence the choice of treatment, e.g. current drug therapy, patient's personal circumstances, vascular status

---

Case study 1.1

Jody is a 12-year-old schoolchild. She has developed a painful plantar wart on her right forefoot. She has tried home application of topical caustics, but these have not been able to resolve this lesion. Jody says that the lesion is getting larger, is spreading and is becoming more painful. It is affecting her ability to play games at school, and she has been banned from swimming and using the communal school showers. Jody becomes upset when her mother speaks about how Jody has been unable to join her friends in swimming sessions and in school games sessions.

Assessment of Jody's feet shows a large well-circumscribed verruca pedis lesion beneath the right first metatarsophalangeal joint. The lesion is extremely painful following application of lateral pressure.

The diagnosis of this condition is, therefore, a plantar verruca pedis lesion, based on history and clinical examination of the patient. The therapeutic objectives, agreed with the patient and her guardian, are:

1. To reduce pain and discomfort
2. To provide a cure of the condition and eradicate the verruca pedis lesion
3. To enable Jody to return to normal activity levels (including swimming and school games) and, therefore, improve her quality of life.

A management plan is agreed with the patient and her guardian, as follows:

1. Jody to use a file to reduce the hard skin overlying the verruca on a once daily basis
2. Jody and her guardian to attend the podiatry clinic once a week for laser therapy treatment
3. The podiatrist to apply laser therapy to the lesion each week
4. The podiatrist to monitor and review the outcomes of the therapy
5. Jody's parents to talk to the school regarding appropriateness of the ban on swimming.

A treatment plan is then prepared by the podiatrist as follows.

1. Weekly debridement of the lesion to capillary bleeding
2. Weekly application of laser therapy using 660 nm, 20 Hz, irradiation with an energy density of 10 J/cm for a 12 week period
3. Application of post-treatment sterile dressings
4. Advice concerning: filing of lesion, swimming and activity
5. Review of success at 12 weeks, consider cryosurgery or curettage in longer term.

- assess the extent of pathological changes to inform the prognosis
- establish a baseline in order to identify whether the condition is deteriorating or improving as a result of treatment
- note any previous treatments that have been used, together with an indication of their success or reasons for failure.

Information gained from the assessment should enable the practitioner to make a diagnosis and identify the underlying cause of the problem. Unfortunately, this is not always possible. In these instances, treatment has to focus on the management of the symptoms of the condition, for example pain control. Symptomatic relief may be all that can be achieved in certain cases.

All of the above information is used to inform the aims and outcomes of treatment and the selection of appropriate therapeutic modalities. The treatment planning process, however, does not end with the delivery of treatment. It is essential that practitioners evaluate the effects of their treatment in order to ensure that patients receive the most appropriate and effective treatment. It is often necessary, in the light of experience and with the passage of time, to review and update the initial assessment and diagnosis and make changes to the treatment plan. The treatment planning process should, therefore, form an uninterrupted loop, with each stage informing the next stage in the process (Fig. 1.1).

Principles underpinning treatment

The following principles should underpin any treatment plan.

- Practitioners should take into account patients' psychological, social and personal circumstances, as well as their medical status. A holistic approach should be adopted rather than one that focuses on a specific problem, such as a hammer toe.
- Practitioners should be careful not to belittle a patient's concerns, even when they may think these have little substance. The patient should always be listened to. Practitioners can often easily resolve these concerns by giving

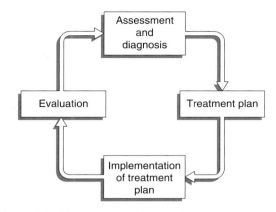

Figure 1.1 The treatment planning process.

appropriate information about the nature of the problem and self-help advice.

- Patients must give their informed consent to any treatment. It is important that patients are fully informed about their treatment in order that they can decide whether they wish to receive it and, if they do, which treatment they feel is appropriate for them.
- Practitioners have a duty of beneficence and non-maleficence. A patient's right to refuse treatment should be respected (see Ch. 3). Some practitioners have been accused of paternalism, that is, taking responsibility away from, and not involving, patients with their treatment.
- Treatment plans should be informed by findings from research and audit: evidence-based health care. It is the responsibility of all practitioners to review their practice continually and to ensure that the rationale for their clinical decisions is based on the best evidence available. Practitioners need to know how to evaluate available research evidence and use this evidence to inform their practices.
- A treatment plan involves a contract between the patient and the practitioner. Most treatment contracts are informal verbal agreements, but in some instances practitioners are using written contracts. The components of a treatment contract are outlined in Box 1.1. It is essential that the patient is fully informed about all aspects of the plan and is willing to actively participate with and undertake their part of the contract.

- Every effort should be made to reduce the likelihood of iatrogenic problems. These can occur as a side-effect of many forms of treatment. Practitioners should always inform the patient of the potential risks or side-effects associated with treatment.

Components of a treatment plan

A treatment plan involves the following:

- identification of the problem(s)
- the intended aims of treatment
- the outcome(s) of treatment
- details of the therapeutic interventions
- mechanisms for monitoring and evaluation.

Identification of the problem(s)

If a treatment plan is to be effective, the patient and practitioner must be in agreement about the need for treatment. It is important that both parties are aware of the purpose of treatment: in other words, why treatment is being provided. If patients present with more than one problem, these should be prioritized in order of need for treatment.

Intended aims of treatment

The ideal aim of any treatment should be to remove or reduce the effects of the cause of the problem. Unfortunately, this may not be possible. As already highlighted, in these instances, the practitioner's primary role is to achieve relief from symptoms. In many cases, this involves the relief of pain.

Box 1.1 Components of a treatment contract

1. Identification of the problem(s) that require therapeutic intervention.
2. The aims and outcomes of the proposed treatment.
3. The patient's participation in the treatment, e.g. self-help, change of footwear.
4. The practitioner's role in the treatment, e.g. type of treatment to be used and the frequency of visits.
5. How the outcomes of treatment will be reviewed.

Merriman (1993) identified a range of aims associated with the treatment of foot problems. These are summarized in Table 1.3.

Outcomes of treatment

It is also important that the patient is informed about the likely outcome of treatment. Four outcomes are associated with the treatment of foot-related problems.

Table 1.3 Aims of treatment

Aim	Commentary
Restore tissue viability	This primarily relates to situations where ulceration has occurred. The main aims of treatment are to promote healing and reduce excessive forces on the foot
Maintain tissue viability in those with at-risk feet	A number of systemic and local conditions can adversely affect the tissues of the lower limb. In these cases, the main aims of treatment are to prevent loss of tissue and infection and reduce excessive forces on the foot
Improve foot function and maintain tissue viability	Many patients present with painful secondary skin lesions resulting from abnormal foot function. These lesions, if not effectively treated, may progress to aseptic ulceration and subsequent infection. The aim of treatment in these instances is to improve foot function and thereby prevent loss of tissue viability
Improve foot function	Abnormal foot function may not always result in secondary skin lesions and adversely affect tissue viability. In these instances the aim of treatment is to reduce abnormal foot function
Prevention of abnormal foot function	This relates to preventive work, which is primarily, although not exclusively, carried out with children. For example, abnormal foot function can be avoided with appropriate advice and early intervention in patients involved in sporting activities

Cure The complete resolution of the problem. This is usually dependent upon the identification and removal of the underlying cause. For example, a painful, vascular corn on the dorsum of a hammer toe may be cured through an arthrodesis to straighten the toe and reduce the enlarged proximal interphalangeal joint.

Rehabilitation A noticeable improvement in the problem but not complete resolution. In this situation, it is likely that the symptoms can be satisfactorily addressed but it is not possible to eradicate the underlying cause completely. For example, a neuropathic ulcer can be resolved with the aid of operative skills, chemical therapy and appropriate orthotic devices. However, it is not possible to resolve the problem completely because of its underlying systemic nature, although the possibility of reoccurrence may be reduced by education and self-help as well as by routine monitoring and review.

Palliation Prevents a deterioration in the symptoms but does not lead to a noticeable improvement or reduction in symptoms. For example, it may be possible to keep a patient suffering from peripheral vascular disease comfortable with the use of pain-relieving drugs, but because of the underlying disease process, the condition cannot be radically improved unless the patient receives surgical intervention such as an arterial bypass.

Prevention An important treatment outcome. Often this intervention takes the form of foot health education and promotion. For example, a patient known to be predisposed to chilblains can be given appropriate foot health advice, together with insulating insoles prior to the onset of cold weather.

It is important that the outcomes of treatment are realistic. Research has shown that patients prefer it when they are informed about their health problems and are given an accurate prognosis (Bostrom et al 1994).

Therapeutic interventions

An array of treatment modalities can be used to treat foot problems (Box 1.2). Most treatment plans encompass two or more of these modalities. Some modalities primarily lead to symptomatic relief whereas others attempt to reduce or remove the effects of the underlying cause.

Debridement and enucleation The use of debridement and enucleation leads to an immediate reduction of symptoms from skin lesions such as corns, calluses and blisters. However, this intervention rarely addresses the underlying aetiology.

Pharmacology In many instances, pharmacological management is aimed at treating the symptoms of the problem, e.g. anti-inflammatory drugs, analgesics. Antimicrobial drugs are the exception. These drugs aim to eradicate the underlying problem, be it bacterial, fungal or viral.

Mechanical Mechanical therapies encompass a broad spectrum of devices. They can be used not only to treat symptoms but also to address the underlying cause. For example, the insertion of a shock-absorbing insole may improve shock absorbency during gait and reduce discomfort in the knees and hips, whereas a splinting device can correct flexible soft tissue deformities.

Physical Heat, cold, massage and exercise are primarily used to reduce symptoms. However, in certain instances, physical therapies may remove the underlying cause, e.g. cryotherapy destroys viral wart tissue, and exercise may correct inefficient muscle action.

Surgical Surgical intervention can reduce symptoms and also remove or reduce the effects of the underlying cause. For example, the symptoms and broad forefoot appearance associated with hallux abductovalgus deformity can be addressed by surgery.

Box 1.2 Therapeutic modalities used in the treatment of foot problems

- Debridement and enucleation
- Pharmacology
- Mechanical
- Physical
- Surgical
- Advice
- Referral

Advice The role of the practitioner as an effective health educator has much to commend it. Advice should be an integral part of any treatment plan. It should include information about the cause of the problem, how to prevent the problem(s) from occurring or reoccurring and how the patient can self-treat the existing problem. Clinical consultations are an ideal situation in which to offer advice to the patient. As part of the consultation, interchange of information may be addressed, not only about the well-being of the feet but also about specific concerns relating to the general health of the patient. Chronic diseases, such as diabetes mellitus or arthritis, may not be preventable at this time, but by identifying their complications early, many of the problems associated with these conditions, such as functional disability, ambulatory dysfunction and pain, can be postponed. The role of health promotion and education in modifying the disease process is essential (see Chs 5 and 17).

Referral Sometimes it may be inappropriate for the practitioner to treat the patient, for example because of lack of equipment or experience. In these instances, it is important that the patient is referred to another practitioner. Any referral should always be accompanied by a written letter containing relevant details about the patient.

Monitoring and evaluation

Several mechanisms can be used to monitor the effects of and evaluate treatment.

• Record improvements/deteriorations from one treatment to the next using a progress chart (Fig. 1.2).
• Write up any treatment notes using the SOAP format (Weed 1970) (Table 1.4). This provides a forum, at each treatment, for the practitioner and patient to assess and review the effects of the previous treatment and update the assessment findings.
• Set a date to review the outcome of a course of treatment. The practitioner and patient identify a date when they will jointly review the outcomes and effectiveness of the course of treatment. This is helpful for conditions that are

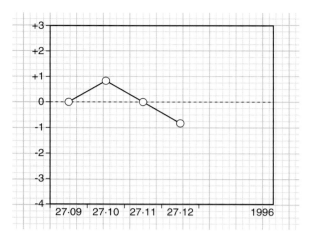

Figure 1.2 Treatment progress can be monitored with a progress chart.

known not to show immediate improvement after treatment. For example, it is not appropriate to judge the outcome of a course of ultrasound for the treatment of enthesopathy until the end of the course of therapy.

If treatment results in iatrogenic problems, fails to relieve symptoms or fails to reduce the effects of the underlying cause, the practitioner should always re-evaluate the situation. This involves reviewing and updating the assessment and diagnosis, and evaluating the suitability of the components of the current treatment plan.

Table 1.4 The SOAP format for monitoring and evaluating treatment

	Term	Description
S	Subjective	The patient's concerns
O	Objective	Signs and features of the condition. This involves undertaking a full or partial examination
A	Assessment	The practitioner's clinical impression in light of the subjective and objective findings
P	Plan	The sequential action which should be taken

THE MULTIDISCIPLINARY TEAM APPROACH

Increasingly, management of patients is proven to be more effective when this is the result of several health professionals working together to provide the patient with management strategies. The patient is at the centre of the process, and his/her views and wishes should be paramount when a multiprofessional management plan is developed.

Usually, one member of the multidisciplinary team will provide the majority of the care for a particular patient, with other members of the team providing supportive care. An example of this is in the management of diabetic foot ulceration. In this case, the podiatrist is the main provider of care to the patient, but additional support may be provided by the diabetologist, the diabetes specialist nurse, the GP, the dietician and others. Figure 1.3 illustrates the likely membership of the diabetes multidisciplinary team.

The case conference is a useful method for enhancing the delivery of care and facilitating multiprofessional involvement. A case conference is held as required and will involve the patient and/or their carers, and all members of the professional team providing support. In some cases, this may involve both health and social care professionals, and health providers from both primary and secondary care. The purpose of a case conference is for all involved in the delivery of care to agree on the most appropriate strategy for continuing care provision, and to ensure that all factors which may influence decisions are communicated across the team. They are also useful to ensure that the patient is kept fully informed and is able to influence key decisions concerning their treatment. Case conferences can result in an agreed action plan, set review criteria and assist with identifying resource requirements.

Key to the effectiveness of any multidisciplinary team is the availability of time, effective communication and organization. It is essential that all members of the team are aware of each other's role and the contribution each member can make. Multidisciplinary teams work best when the members of the team meet on a regular basis to plan and discuss issues. Working in close geographical proximity to each other is very helpful. The team should spend time together away from the patients. This helps the team to develop an understanding and appreciation of each member's role, as well as facilitating the development of sound and effective channels of communication

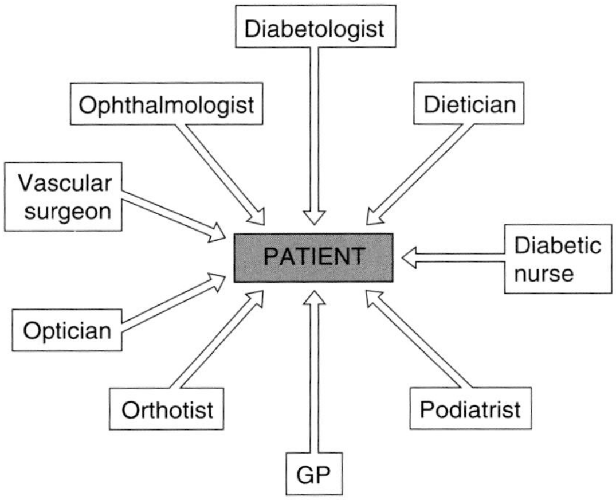

WHY DO TREATMENT PLANS FAIL?

All practitioners find themselves asking why a treatment plan has failed from time to time. A multitude of factors may be responsible for such failure. Lack of agreement between the practitioner and the patient about the purpose of the treatment plan is one obvious cause. For example, the practitioner may have failed to communicate to the patient the purpose of treatment and its likely effects. Conversely, the patient may have had unrealistic expectations of what the treatment would achieve.

In some instances, the assessment may have failed to reveal contraindications to treatment or, owing to lack of relevant information from the patient, may have led to the practitioner making an incorrect diagnosis. The choice of treatment

Figure 1.3 Members of the multidisciplinary team involved in the management of the diabetic foot.

modalities may have been incorrect; other alternative forms of treatment may have been more appropriate.

Many practitioners point to non-compliance as a prime cause for treatment failure. The issue of compliance has been mentioned as far back as c. 200 BC by Hippocrates in his work 'On decorum': 'Keep a watch also on the faults of the patients which often make them lie about the takings of things prescribed'. In essence, non-compliance is the patient's failure to fulfil the clinical prescription (Haynes et al 1979). Compliance may, therefore, be defined as one individual agreeing with, or consenting to, another's suggestions, and it will usually involve dominant and recessive roles.

A number of studies have been undertaken into patient compliance, and these have revealed relatively high non-compliance rates. For example, Ley (1988) found that between 10 and 25% of patients were admitted to hospital on account of non-compliance. Non-compliance or non-adherence is thought to result from the following factors (Harvey 1988):

- volitional: the individual makes a rational decision not to follow advice; this may be predicated by a number of factors, e.g. cost, perceived benefits
- accidental: the individual forgets or mis-understands the advice
- circumstantial: the individual may be involved in a range of situations that may affect following advice, e.g. painful side-effects, death in the family.

The process by which patients decide whether or not they wish to concur with advice is complex and is influenced by numerous internal and external factors. Patients will be influenced by a number of inherent factors, such as personality, affect, social and religious background, age and intelligence. Patients' perceptions of their illness and its prognosis, together with the presence or lack of symptoms, will modify their behaviour. A patient suffering from diabetes whose father died from the same disease may treat health more seriously than someone of good health with a minor ailment.

Patients' understanding of their illness and of medical advice can indirectly affect their compliance with treatment. Studies have shown that patients do not recall a large proportion of medical information given during consultations (Ley 1988). Ley (1988) also found that the provision of information in the form of leaflets was one of the factors that improved the amount of advice remembered and subsequently led to a good treatment outcome. Advice to patients may take many forms: details of dressing changes to be carried out, the application of proprietary medicaments, advice on purchasing footwear. The presentation of the information is very important. Short words, short sentences and logical progression are essential for clarity. Medical terminology and jargon are to be avoided or, if used, explained to the patient. The introduction of blank spaces on the leaflet, into which instructions specific to the individual patient are written, is a convenient way of overcoming this deficit.

Practitioners will also influence patients' decisions. Practitioners develop perceptions about their patients as soon as the patient enters the consulting room. This initial non-verbal assessment may influence or even prejudice how the practitioner approaches the consultation. Accurate assessment requires that the social distance between practitioner and patient is reduced (Plaja et al 1968) and that the barriers created by education, social class, occupational status and ethnicity are identified (Di Matteo & Di Nicola 1982).

Open communication between practitioner and patient is essential to developing a good rapport and mutual respect. Monitoring the patient's response to advice and information is essential. Svarstad (1976) reported that, if practitioners neglected to question their patients about compliance, they tended to conclude that the practitioner did not attach much importance to the regimen or did not believe in its efficacy.

Various factors can influence patient compliance. Compliance may be impaired if treatment shows no obvious improvement in symptoms or results, e.g. preventative measures such as diets. The success of treatment versus the resistance to the disease is another important factor. Other factors include:

- costs to the patient
- duration of the course of treatment
- complexity of the treatment process
- side-effects associated with the treatment
- inconvenience to the patient and disruption to the patient's daily living
- prior experiences of treatment which involved pain or were unsuccessful.

If a treatment's obvious effects are to improve symptoms, the patient is likely to respond in a positive manner. This carries a risk, as the patient may stop the treatment too early because of the initial rapid improvement.

Some health educators argue that emphasis should be placed on empowering patients to make decisions and choices about their health and treatment (Totnes 1992). In the past, the emphasis has been on practitioners directing and telling patients what was best for them. Empowerment is achieved when the practitioner works with the patient so that the patient, not the practitioner, identifies the patient's own needs. The practitioner's role is to facilitate, not direct, the patient to arrive at a decision. The practitioner has to accept that the patient's

informed choice regarding treatment may not be the one the practitioner would have chosen.

SUMMARY

It is the responsibility of all practitioners to inform and regularly update their clinical skills and knowledge. All treatment plans should take into account available evidence from research and audit. When designing and implementing a treatment plan, it is essential that the practitioner bases it on findings from a thorough assessment. The most effective treatment plans are those that have been agreed following the sharing of knowledge and opinions between health and social care professionals, and which have the wishes of the patient as paramount.

Once a treatment plan is implemented, it should be routinely evaluated in order to ensure that patients receive appropriate and effective treatment. The promotion of good foot health and the prevention of disease is as important as the treatment of foot problems. The overall philosophy of foot health services should be to promote informed self-care so that services can be focused on those patients who most require intervention.

REFERENCES

Bostrom J, Crawford-Swent C, Lazar N, Helmer D 1994 Learning needs of hospitalised and recently discharged patients. Patient Education and Counselling 23: 83–89
Bradshaw J 1972 The concept of social need. New Society 19: 640–643
Campbell J A, Bradley A, White D, Turner W, Luxton D E A 2000 Do 'low-risk' older people need podiatry care? Preliminary results of a follow-up study of discharged patients. British Journal of Podiatry 3: 39–45
Cartwright A, Henderson 1986 More trouble with feet: a survey of foot problems and chiropody needs of the elderly. DHSS, London
Clarke M 1969 Trouble with feet. Occasional papers on social administration, No. 29. Bell, London
Di Matteo M R, Di Nicola D D 1982 Achieving patient compliance: the psychology of the medical practitioner's role. Pergamon Press, New York
Dunnell K, Cartwright A 1972 Medicine takers, prescribers and hoarders. Routledge & Kegan Paul, London
Elton P, Sanderson S 1987 A chiropodial survey of elderly persons over sixty five years in the community. The

Chiropodist 42: 175–178
Harvey P 1988 Health psychology. Longman, New York
Haynes R B, Taylor D W, Sackett D L 1979 Compliance in health care. Johns Hopkins University Press, Baltimore, MD
Kemp J, Winkler J 1983 Problems afoot; need and efficiency in footcare. Disabled Living Foundation, London
Ley P 1988 Communicating with patients. Croom Helm, London
Manning N, Ungerson C 1990 Social policy review 1989–1990. Longman, London
Merriman L 1993 What is the purpose of chiropody services? Journal of British Podiatric Medicine 48: 121–124, 128
Plaja A O, Cohen L M, Samora J 1968 Communication between physicians and patients in outpatients clinics, social and cultural factors. Milbank Memorial Fund Quarterly 46: 161–214
Svarstad B 1976 Physician–patient communication and patient conformity with medical advice. In: Mecanie D (ed) The growth of bureaucratic medicine. Wiley, New York

Totnes K 1992 Empowerment and the promotion of health. Journal of the Institute of Health Education 30: 4

Weed L 1970 Medical records, medical education and patient care. The problem-orientated record as a basic tool. Year Book Medical Publishing, Chicago, IL

Wessex Feet 1985 A regional foot health survey. Wessex Regional Health Authority. The Chiropodist 43: 152–168

2

Evidence-based practice and clinical governance

*Warren A. Turner**

INTRODUCTION

Clinicians are in a relatively powerful position in terms of determining what will be done to a patient, at a given time, for a given problem. This significant responsibility places an obligation on the clinician to ensure that he/she is the right person to do the right thing, to the right patient, at the right time and in the right way. This is the fundamental basis of *clinical governance*. Essentially, clinical governance is about making sure that each patient is able to receive the most appropriate care for his or her requirements at the time. Clinical governance is defined and described in detail in the paper *A First Class Service* (Department of Health 1998).

Linked to clinical governance is the concept of *evidence-based practice*. As the term suggests, evidence-based practice is about making sure that any intervention provided for a patient is based on sound evidence and is indicated as the most appropriate intervention for the patient's needs.

This chapter explores further the notion of evidence-based practice and focuses on concepts of clinical governance and audit.

*Warren Turner acknowledges the contribution to the first edition of this chapter by David Tollafield and Robert Ashford.

DOING THE RIGHT THING

Historically, health professionals have based clinical decisions based on a number of key assumptions.

1. Unsystematic observations made on diagnosis, prognosis, investigative tests and treatments during the course of a clinical education and career are valid experiences for clinical decision making.

2. The knowledge that they have received a detailed clinical and theoretical training in a given field is a justification for clinical decision making.

3. A combination of both common sense and medical training is enough to enable a practitioner to evaluate new tests or treatments.

4. Guidelines for clinical practice can be determined from experience.

The above paradigm is challenged by contemporary approaches to decision making. The challenge proposes a paradigm shift towards a more empirical approach. Therefore, evidence-based practice may be based on assumptions that are more like the following.

1. An understanding of the conventions and rules of evidence is essential in order to interpret the literature correctly relating to causation, investigation, prognosis and therapeutic modalities.

2. A knowledge of the basic mechanisms of disease alone is not sufficient to enable safe and rational diagnosis and treatment.

3. Clinical experience and insight is essential for the development of effective practice. Systematic recording of observations and outcomes can aid confidence in approaches to diagnosis, prognosis and treatment.

Clinicians must, therefore, ensure that they possess the skills necessary to read and interpret relevant literature critically. Clinicians should not rely on personal experience alone but should be confident that most other clinicians faced with the same patient would agree with the proposed course of action. It is also important that clinicians are able to live with uncertainty, as there are many unproven interventions that are routinely used in the provision of clinical care of the foot.

Evidence-based practice demands a particular set of critical appraisal skills:

- clear identification of the presenting problem
- identifying the information needed to solve the problem
- conducting a search of the literature
- discussing with colleagues and other health professionals
- selecting the best of the evidence
- application of the rules of evidence to assess validity
- ability to communicate and justify intentions to treat
- ability to identify strengths and weaknesses of available options
- ability to extract the essential clinical message
- ability to apply this to the patient.

Evidence-based practice is, therefore, a means of checking that investigations and treatments offered to a patient are those that the best available evidence agrees as being the most appropriate at the time.

In practice, clinicians have a variety of sources of clinical evidence upon which to base practice decisions;

- professional journals
- evidence-based medicine web-sites (e.g. Bandolier)
- opinions of more experienced clinical colleagues
- conference abstracts
- patient testimony
- professional body guidelines and recommendations
- patient advocacy groups
- government bodies (e.g. NICE (National Institute for Clinical Excellence))
- local health provider protocols
- professional networks
- universities and research establishments.

It is important for all clinical professionals to keep their clinical skills up to date. Compulsory continuing professional development is often a requirement to remain registered or licensed to practice. Some professional and statutory bodies require their members to undergo regular specific, or core, training. This is often in areas such as basic life support, administration of anaesthesia and infection control.

Regular clinical updating can help to ensure that a clinician has the skills and knowledge needed for safe and effective practice.

Clinical audit

The continuous evaluation of treatment is incumbent upon all who practise in any medical health discipline. While the term 'audit' in general applies to 'accounting', in health circles it has been applied to collecting information about clinical activity in order to measure quality based on predetermined good standards.

The practitioner is required to collect data for a variety of reasons, one of which is for the purposes of an audit. In this chapter, the reasons why it is necessary to audit within the health arena are discussed, and the cyclical nature of audit is described to show its importance within schemes for managing the patient. The term 'outcome' is used a great deal in this chapter, as it is the end result of treatment that is most reported when evaluating the success or failure of a treatment plan. However, while the outcome is obviously of great importance, it should be made clear from the outset that carrying out an audit is more complex than merely looking at the end result. Within the context of an audit, the following questions are uppermost: *why, what, when, who and how to audit?*

Good clinical audit can assist rather than deter good codes of practice. Important goals for designing good codes include ensuring the accurate collection of meaningful data, choosing data that can be measured by recognized methods and ensuring that the data collected are repeatable and representative of the activity under analysis. How successful one is in accomplishing these goals will determine the real value behind any audit activity.

It is not possible to cover all that there is to know about audit in one chapter. While there are dedicated books that offer much greater detail, few books have been written solely with the practitioner in mind. Since the requirement for greater accountability within our clinical activities will undoubtedly grow, the practitioner should be mindful of changing trends. Therefore, in this chapter, the emphasis is placed on making the practitioner aware of the potential behind appropriate audit techniques. The measurement of outcome must look towards a number of common scientific methods, and these are considered briefly towards the end of the chapter.

The approach to audit preparation has been divided into three parts: lessons learned from an historical perspective, the purpose of clinical audit from the traditional viewpoint and analysing treatment in order to provide a method with which to carry out the clinical measurement of outcome.

HISTORICAL PERSPECTIVE

There has been a distinct lack of audit in past centuries in the area of health and treatment and few authors took account of bad practices. This omission has led to considerable bigotry amongst medical practitioners. Florence Nightingale, known for her opposition to the doctors of her time, reduced mortality to such an extent that her practices were adopted on a greater scale. She used a basic clinical audit that was concerned with daily outcome; this was simply recorded as 'relieved', 'unrelieved' or 'died'. She criticized the case records of that period (c. 1855) as having little value in assisting treatment and bearing a poor correlation with each patient's disorder. By instigating new nursing methods, her mortality figures showed that the death rate was reduced from 40% beforehand to 2% after implementing new techniques. Her figures also showed that the survival rate of patients wounded in battle improved significantly as the distance from hospital increased, because of the delay in encountering the conditions in hospital that actually promoted morbidity. Today, these facts are astounding – they seem so obvious that it is difficult to understand how they were not apparent at the time.

One reason for the lack of open practices in the 19th and early 20th centuries may have been that severe criticism or even penalties would have discredited those engaged in seemingly faulty practices.

A further illustration of the problems caused by an intransigent medical community is the case of Ernest Groves at the turn of the 18th century. He criticized the collection of clinical data as being inadequate. He argued that the information collected showed the 'best' results rather than the average results. From his evidence, he believed that records should be collected in a standard way in order to obtain the most authoritative information with no bias. In fact, what Groves was recommending was an Audit Commission of its time. However, not only did the medical profession fail to support any of his ideas, but the British Medical Journal deemed his paper to be unworthy of comment and 'stonewalled' him. This type of activity was not confined to Britain. In the USA, Ernest Codman received similar retribution following publication of his paper on the 'End result system'. He was forced to resign from the hospital staff for conduct unbecoming of a physician. Nowadays, he is considered to be the originator of modern health care quality assurance and the concept of medical staff accountability.

Mortality associated with surgery has played a disproportionate role in the history of medical audit. As medicine and the media have matured, events other than death from disease and medical practice have been notably reported, although not necessarily through audit. Pharmaceutical products undergo far more scrutiny than other treatment practices and have to conform to strict legal codes. The drug industry has only to recall media reporting – as witnessed by the response to the Distiller's drug thalidomide – in the 1960s. A drug designed for a different age group was given to pregnant women to help them with morning sickness. The effects on the developing fetus were not appreciated until many children were born with significant limb aberrations.

The changes advocated by Codman and Groves have taken considerable time to be adopted by the health care system worldwide. Indeed, even today, economic and political factors are the real reasons for changes in the current audit perspectives. The political concern about adverse public opinion has led to suppression of sensitive issues in hospitals. The public of today not only expects high standards but is rather intolerant of medical mistakes, no matter how minor.

Audit can offer some prediction of problems and can minimize many issues, by altering standards of care and practices, if implemented soon enough.

The *case conference* offers 'performance review' of medical and surgical management. This type of audit consists of case meetings, known as morbidity and mortality conferences, where doctors consider the effects of treatment in privacy and where notes are limited, if recorded at all. In this manner, doctors can discuss and share information honestly and learn from gaps in their knowledge. *Peer Review Organizations* (PROs) have been developed in order to ensure that cost containment and quality of care are fostered. This particular audit tool is used in the USA. Pro forma criteria are applied when reviewing case records. Senior doctors can investigate further any major deviations, and sanctions such as withholding payment can be imposed if the quality of care falls below a certain stated standard.

Cost containment is an issue that has gathered momentum and has accelerated the need for audit. The need for audit systems within the UK Health Service has instigated a series of reports and investigations into how to collect data, what data to collect and what to do with it. In 1979, the Merrison Report, supported by a Royal Commission, looked at how data were collected. In the conclusions, collected data were generally felt to be inaccurate, to be produced in the wrong form and to be gathered too late for any appropriate action to be taken. It is interesting to note that problems of information handling described by Nightingale in the 1850s and Groves in the early 1900s still existed in the 1970s. Korner set out in 1980 to identify and resolve some of the problems arising from poor information systems within the NHS.

Seven reports were published between 1982 and 1984, and these started to accelerate the move towards departmental computerization and the collection of numerous sets of data. However, the issues regarding analysing outcomes of treatment were not addressed by Korner (Pollock & Evans 1993).

The UK Department of Health and Social Security soon began to work on 'performance indicators'. By 1987, nine consultation papers looked at a wide range of services, including support services, and six areas of health – acute hospital services: support services, community services, services for the mentally ill, services for the elderly, and maternity and children's services. Performance indicators were used to set targets that could be measured and also targets against which comparisons could be made. For instance, in the acute services, numbers of operations for certain groups are now recorded, providing a regional picture of activity. The length of in-hospital stays versus day-case surgery patients is recorded, and the numbers of cancellations and cases per session are noted. The number of avoidable deaths, along with information on age, health and operation code, are also compiled.

Working Paper 6 of the *Working for patients* White Paper (Department of Health 1989) recommended that there should be 'an effective programme of audit [which] will help to provide the necessary reassurance to doctors, patients and managers that the best possible quality of care is being achieved within the resources available'. This recommendation made explicit a programme that promulgates the use of audit as a tool to achieve better levels of care.

This historical narrative gives some idea of how audit has arisen out of changing attitudes and practices. In the past, disease was identified as resulting from poor clinical practices, such as unsatisfactory standards of preparation and care of the patient. By the 1980s, surgeons started to fear contamination from the patient, as bloodborne diseases such as the human immunodeficiency and hepatitis viruses raised concern. These potentially fatal alterations in pathogenesis inflicted by cross-infection reversed the belief that patients alone were at risk. Despite modern medicine affording a high-quality state of care,

we are now increasingly vigilant when dealing with blood and body fluids. Such cross-infections from an inadvertent stab injury could prove fatal. Regular clinical audit and research of techniques offer a heightened state of awareness.

The quest to cut costs arising from needless waste and inexpeditious treatments has come about as a result of studying health practices in the last 20 years. Cost containment has been undertaken by administrative management and by independent bodies rather than by the medical professions.

Cost containment has been politically influenced by the need for accountability and for a form of acceptable practice that lives up to the expectations of an enlightened, better-educated society. 'Waiting times', 'politeness' and 'explanation' are among new standards being enforced upon clinical practice, even though many practitioners may well practise good interpersonal skills anyway.

THE PURPOSE OF CLINICAL AUDIT

This section provides an overview of the audit process, which should help the practitioner to appreciate the preparatory steps that are required when addressing clinical activity. In order to understand the stage that audit has now reached, it is necessary to consider first the traditional views of health care held by managers and hence these will be discussed.

The field of audit has developed a wide lexicon of terms; many of these will be explained in this section.

Terminology

Quality

Donebedian (1966) suggested that there are three components associated with the quality of health care: good technical care, interpersonal relationships and good amenities. The aims include effectiveness, efficiency, satisfaction and safety. In contrast, Maxwell (1984) identified six dimensions for health care quality, including, in addition to Donebedian's points above, relevance of care (to the whole community), fairness and social acceptability (Pollock & Evans 1993).

When considering quality, Pollock & Evans emphasized the difference between effectiveness and efficiency. *Effectiveness* implies that the correct steps are taken in providing treatment, while *efficiency* relates to the distribution of resources based on need. Of the other two aims, *satisfaction* relates to reaching a desired outcome from treatment and *safety* should include the avoidance of unnecessary problems arising from treatment.

Compassion plays a large role in a patient's perceived quality of care and, to the ill patient, is more important than knowledge of complicated results or impressive diagnostic tests.

Standards of care

Standards are usually set in terms of supplying products or delivering a service; both of these can be applied to health care. Setting standards is one thing, but monitoring and maintaining standards is rather more difficult. This is because specifying standards is demanding, requiring a high level of expertise that can be agreed and understood comprehensively (Ellis & Whittington 1993). Setting standards may be undertaken by a profession, a purchaser or an institution such as a hospital. Specification is more difficult because each standard has to be defined precisely to account for wide variations of a human, rather than an inorganic, nature. The person setting any standard must have a detailed knowledge of what is achievable. Manufacturers of machine-made items, by comparison, will have less trouble specifying the tolerance of products. For the purpose of applying quality assurance standards to the clinical setting, these terms will not be separated further, as many of the mechanisms are similar to audit.

Quality assurance

It is important to understand the difference between audit and quality assurance. Quality assurance sets standards and measures compliance. An audit does this too; however, an audit may also be undertaken to identify the standards themselves against which compliance might be measured, as well as looking at the structure, process and outcome that will assist in defining quality assurance.

Since the difference is subtle, consider, for illustrative purposes, the simple example of a product being manufactured to specific standards. In this case, defective items are removed if they fail to meet the required standard of manufacture either because of faulty finish or because of lack of intended function. This whole process could be audited, for example, to see if quality assurance methods were being appropriately applied to minimize customer complaints. The outcome might surmise that no faulty products produced would equate to no customer complaints. In reality, this might be hard to achieve and targets might be set to account for some faults arising. The audit could then be repeated to identify the number of adjusted faulty products expected to reach the shop or customer. Any lowering of the figure would be deemed to be unsatisfactory, and the structure and process of manufacture would have to be reviewed carefully to correct the problem.

Performance indicators

Performance indicators (PIs) were set for the purpose of resource efficiency measures. In fact, PIs are linked to quality assurance. As these have been highly confusing in the way that they have been used for internal and external comparisons, they have, not surprisingly, been avoided in the clinical field (Ellis & Whittington 1993).

PIs do not measure outcome. The Department of Health has used PIs in comparing the performance of one hospital with another; a common example uses waiting times for appointments and treatment. The standard initially set may require all hospitals to see new patients within a certain time. Having set this standard, performance is then measured against it. Differences in performance will show up between different hospital services. The reasons for such variations, however, are not explained by simply quoting performance-related figures alone. This lack of discrimination is a point of concern for health care professionals, who, although they may work hard, look less effective on paper. For example, one professional may be in high demand because of his or her success compared with a similar professional in another hospital or centre. The waiting time for the less-popular practitioner may look more attractive, creating an unfair bias in any such data collected. This emphasizes that the effectiveness (an outcome) is excluded from such a measurement.

Criteria and standards

Criteria and standards are defined by purchasers or managers of the service. It is important to note the difference between the two. Audit criteria are general statements about delivery of patient care. They focus on those aspects that can be used to assess the quality of such care. Criteria-based audit was carried out in the early to mid-1970s in the USA. This work resulted in audits being based on criteria against which actual practice was compared. From the criteria, standards applicable to the clinic can be developed (Table 2.1).

Why audit?

The broad aims of audit might be considered as:

- improving the quality of patient care
- utilizing resources efficiently
- providing an objective assessment of clinical activity
- enabling the practitioner to demonstrate quality of patient care
- reflecting on the effectiveness of care.

The purpose of audit is to gain information so that strengths and weaknesses can be identified. Once data have been collected, improvements in the organizational structure and process can be initiated (Tucker 1995). Changes in patient management need to be identified when clinical practice is at fault. Conversely, practice should be promoted where it has been shown to be beneficial. In health care, the *product* is the service provided to the patient, and this might be the

Table 2.1 Criteria and standards have different implications

Criteria	Standard
The notes of patients taking anticoagulant drugs should be clearly marked	The notes of all patients on anticoagulant drugs should be clearly marked, i.e. 100%
Patients should not be kept waiting for treatment more than 20 minutes	80% of patients should be expected to be seen in 20 minutes
Patients requiring nail surgery for onychocryptosis should receive an appointment within 3 days	60% of patients should be seen in less than 3 days

intended outcome for the health service. The outcome for the patient, however, is measured in terms of the improvement in their condition. A practitioner will view his or her outcome in a similar manner: the improvement of the patient's condition. Measurement of this outcome must be considered objectively. This will be considered below in the section on analysing treatment.

All health care individuals may believe that they are doing a good job. How does a practitioner know whether this is indeed the case? Such an assumption raises fundamental questions regarding national standards, the personalities of individuals involved, the types of training and education that practitioners have received, differences in treatment modalities, different local initiatives and available financial resources. Performance is based upon the expected standards set down by a profession, which, in turn, are underpinned by the accepted practice expected by 'society'.

The reasons why we want to audit are based on our acceptance that quality in health care depends upon many facets of our work. These facets require analysing as they have a direct bearing on how a health system can deliver efficient and effective care. Audit comprises the audit of patient care from records, moral and ethical issues of care, economic provision of care, educational responsibilities of care and psychological attitudes of care linked to the whole system of delivery.

Patient records

An audit should show that, in undertaking care, the patient has not been placed at unnecessary risk and that all appropriate investigations have been conducted with safety in mind. The process used in treating a patient should be clearly identified in the case records. A patient with an ankle fracture, for example, would require an X-ray scan to confirm the diagnosis and identify the best treatment. The use of X-ray reports should be identifiable in the records and it should have been undertaken at the appropriate time during the initial examination routine. Effectiveness can be assumed if no complications arise leading to symptomatic healing. Effectiveness can be further assumed where the patient with the ankle fracture returns to normal function within a reasonable period. This should include a full, unencumbered return to work, ability to walk as before without a limp, good ankle range of motion and freedom from pain. All these recorded results from treatment equate to the desired outcome. Failure to follow the appropriate process (e.g. if the correct diagnostic enquires are omitted) may lead to delays in normal return to daily routines; extending the time off work could have financial repercussions for the patient and for the hospital. Effectiveness can be observed within the case records provided that the method of recording is clear and unambiguous.

Any response to patients' needs and expectations forms the basis of 'patient satisfaction'. Clear ground rules exist as to how patients should be managed; a fair and sensitive approach with sufficient explanation will allow them to contribute to their own care plan. True satisfaction can only be reached when the patient and the practitioner agree that an effective change has occurred.

Moral and ethical reasons

Practitioners are responsible for recording and reporting information in an honest manner and in an accurate way; in this respect, they have a duty. Essential information should be passed on to colleagues where necessary to avoid ineffective management. Standards of expected behaviour can be identified again from case notes: by the care taken and the conformity to expected practice. Deviation from expected standards of documentation can place a 'legal emphasis' upon practice ethics. Drug reactions or complications from treatment hitherto unknown must be made known. The moral and ethical aspects of clinical activities form part of the overall picture of clinical audit but may not be isolated unless deviation from practice causes serious concern. The use of ethics committees in hospitals provides the correct network for practitioners to set up radical and less-accepted types of patient care.

Economic process

Poor structure and efficiency can lead to waste and elevated costs. Areas where waste and inefficiency are experienced are not restricted to the clinic alone but are also found in the administration and support services. Where the practitioner is reliant upon the activities of others and these activities are not carried out properly, the effects upon the service provided can be highly detrimental. The activities of the whole health unit should be monitored, although the specific areas where inefficiency is suspected to lie can be focused upon once they have been identified.

Educational reasons

The practitioner has a professional duty to remain up to date with developments. Altering clinical practice may be implemented by a case conference, publication or research projects. The principal purpose of the audit should be justified on the basis that the result could yield a helpful change in practice or, conversely, could support continuation of a particular practice. Furthermore, if certain standards are expected, the audit will check that such standards are being met.

Psychological reasons

The daily routine can be highly frustrating for the practitioner. Good psychological stability is essential in managing patients, to avoid transposing personal problems to the patient and thereby affecting rapport. A good working environment and administrative support are essential for good service delivery. An audit reviewing daily activities can increase motivation by reporting on achievements as well as problem areas. A change brought about as a result of an audit recommendation can further motivate a practitioner if the change leads to positive achievements. It is true, however, that the opposite effect can be created when changes are constantly stipulated. In these situations, one finds that no sooner has a method been employed than it is changed for a different set of practices. This can lead to disorientation. Achieving the correct balance is essential and important, because any deviation in care can affect colleagues and patients.

Summary

In conclusion, the reasons for audit are diverse but include general and practical reasons. Practitioners are not encouraged to audit every aspect of their practice at once. Auditing in health care not only accounts for patient management but also includes how the practitioner interfaces with the system of care.

What to audit?

Current convention is to use a framework based upon a model proposed by Donebedian (1966). Donebedian suggested that clinical practice could be classified into three discrete dimensions. They are discrete in terms of their individual characteristics but overlap when considered together in medical care. The three dimensions are:

- *structure*: asks where the service is provided, with what facilities the work is done and who has done it
- *process*: asks what is done and how it is done
- *outcome*: tells what has been done, how well it was done and what the effect has been.

When carrying out an audit, it is important that there is an agreed system by which a clinical activity will be examined. The activity should be well defined and the practitioner should be clear about what needs investigating. The *subject* of the proposed audit needs to be defined. Here are several examples that illustrate the point.

- *Why do clinics have so much out-of-date stock?* This refers to the subject of waste and efficiency.
- *Are diabetic patients seen frequently enough to promote the most efficient management of plantar metatarsal ulcers?* The subject is cost and relates to outcome.
- *Consider the diabetic patient ulcer protocol: do all GPs receive a treatment summary following each consultation?* The subject relates to professional ethics communication.
- *Does the complaints system function efficiently?* Again the subject is process orientated and is related to the effectiveness of clinical protocol.

The structure component relates to what goes on in the clinical setting and tends to be easier to pinpoint. The facility where treatment is delivered should be able to meet the needs being placed on it. For example, are there enough care assistants to manage basic foot care, thus releasing practitioners to attend high-risk categories? Are there sufficient examination rooms available to deal with a reasonable number of patients requiring a 3 hour session?

The process of delivery of care should be studied to ensure that the steps taken are in accordance with legal and medical ethics, that case records are up to date and legible, and that treatment plans have been considered and can be shown to be efficient and effective. Then, if the process is followed correctly, it usually follows that the outcome will be satisfactory (Donebedian 1988).

The outcome represents the effects of care on the health status of patients and populations. It is cheaper to audit process and structure than to audit outcome, because outcome depends on following the effects of treatment over a period of time. As a result, outcomes are slower to evaluate. Furthermore, measurement of outcome is complicated, and many of the designs and strategies used are flawed.

Criteria for audit

It has been found that if criteria are defined carefully, it should be possible to obtain an overview of current practice (see Table 2.1). The next step would be to agree with colleagues what standards should be applied to a specified practice. It is often the case that standards cannot be agreed until current practice has been analysed and assessed using clear criteria, and the results discussed.

The first attempt at auditing often highlights problems of particular interest. This enables explicit criteria to be clearly defined and standards to be set for the next time around. It is also important when setting criteria and standards not to be too complicated: they should be kept as simple as possible. It is essential that the practitioner collects information that is relevant; the parameters, as with research methods, must be laid down carefully before any data collection commences. A pilot study can provide information valuable to the design of criteria.

In conclusion, the practitioner will be more motivated when analysing the treatment system, the effects of treatment upon patients, the influence of new drugs on specific conditions, the ways to minimize the use of drugs, and the use of new equipment and procedures as a way to reduce treatment costs. The list is endless but one clearly needs to identify areas for analysis that are relevant to treatment delivery.

Standards of care

Standards can be measured. The first UK Patient's Charter is one example that lends itself to audit. The outcome of the Charter is that patient satisfaction should be reached over a number of stated objectives. Choice, access, information and waiting times are emphasized within statements about the seven basic rights and the nine charter standards. NHS health care delivery now has to embrace the Charter. However, while the outcome of an audit may imply that certain standards are indeed being met, the quality of treatment cannot be assumed to be high, since the Charter is based on quantity, for example time, numbers, cost.

When to audit?

If a clinical problem arises for which there is a simple explanation, then the use of an audit is inappropriate. Audits attempt to account for problems that are less obvious. Often, it is only once the audit procedure has begun that problems which exist begin to come into focus. In this way, a problem might be identified first, and then further study would be required to establish the cause of the problem. For example, a cyclical audit might throw up inefficiency recurring on a monthly or annual basis. Another audit would then be designed to establish where the inefficiency arises and how it might be avoided.

Continuous audit

Certain data need to be collected continuously, such as:

- patient numbers, for example, will fall into treatments performed
- numbers of patients discharged
- numbers of complaints/compliments
- specific treatment comparisons, e.g. number of laser treatments against cryotherapy.

The collection of data is important to make future judgements and predictions about a service. When a service is new and relatively unproven, then the managers of that service will need to ensure that their economic requirements are met to enable their service requirements to be met. An audit in these terms may need to be repeated so that the data can be used to indicate a trend. In this case, *structure* and *process* are the subjects of study. Estimates for increasing a clinical provision will depend upon the business plan of that department. Inadequate data will not help to create a strong case for the expansion of a service and will give rise to poor accountability and highlight poor clinical management. For example, a practitioner may become unmotivated when insufficient resources are allocated because a manager, through inadequate audit, has failed to identify the problem.

Sampled audit

An irregular or sampled audit is used to check that a process is being undertaken or that criteria reflecting standards of care are being adhered to. For example, a practitioner may wish to study the effect of a particular treatment if speculative evidence suggests that one type of treatment has risks that have not previously been suspected. In this case, the audit does not have to be repeated, and a single sampled audit may be all that is necessary. Conversely, a practitioner may only wish to undertake an audit occasionally to check changing trends.

A study examining discomfort from tourniquet pressure around the ankle during surgery was based on surgical procedures where a cuff was placed around the ankle to obtain haemostasis (Tollafield et al 1995). The practitioners wanted to know if an anaesthetic infiltrated above the cuff could extend the time of the operation by providing greater comfort. The results showed that a single nerve infiltration above the ankle was insufficient to extend comfort time around the ankle, although most patients were able to undergo surgery quite comfortably for 45–60 minutes using the technique without adverse effects. The *outcome* was measured in terms of effective reduction in discomfort. The evidence supported the use of the technique, providing an objective standard of care for patients undergoing treatment for specific periods of time. These types of clinical audit analysis can be found in most professional journals. The subject does not have to be a patient; for example, a new drug may be compared with an accepted older drug to decide if efficiency or cost might be improved for a specific treatment. While the study has a scientific basis in its design, it will also serve to provide information about the outcome in terms of treatment effectiveness.

Cyclical audit

The use of an occasional or cyclical audit can help the practitioner to monitor trends in practice on a regularly allotted basis, for example every 2, 3, 4 or 5 years. Cyclical audit is, there-fore, useful in deciding when to change a clinical practice by holding a significant review formally at predetermined points. Any changes that arise from evidence collected can be used to improve the effectiveness and efficiency of the service as well as to monitor many of the selected issues already described.

Duration of audit

Two clear objectives should be aimed for when setting a time scale for audit: sufficient data should be collected and a definite outcome should be established. Most audits are determined retrospectively but the concept of prospective design during planning will provide for a more robust analysis.

Collection size Audit is formed from raw data collected as counts or frequencies in occurrence. When should collection cease? The answer lies perhaps in having sufficient information to predict trends. If a small number of counts are to be made, then the selection should be as random as possible, with the choice of who to select being left to an independent person so as to avoid bias. On the one hand, a group of 50 patients should be small enough to count; on the other hand, 5000 patients may be accurately represented by a proportion, say 10% (500), if they are randomly selected.

Collection period A period of time is necessary to achieve the required amount of data. If the effects of treatment are to be recorded, sufficient time must be allowed to ensure that the problem does not recur and that side-effects do not arise from management. The period selected for review should ideally be such that some sustained, measurable improvement of the foot condition could reasonably be expected.

Some sensory loss is normally expected following hallux valgus surgery. Consequently, if an analysis is undertaken over an insufficient period, false-negative results might be obtained. Nerve regeneration can take 9 months; an audit completed after 3 months would probably be flawed if nerve regeneration was used as the main criteria for success.

Summary

In conclusion, the timing of audit is determined by the aims and objectives of the audit. The results obtained must be complete, the sample size must be large enough, and the period of time selected must consider interfering factors, particularly those associated with outcome, that may extend the study because of the need to wait for full patient recovery.

Who to audit?

In general, practitioners tend to audit *patient groups*. While the practitioner is most likely to want to study the patient, the patient is not, in fact, the only possible target of study. The 'provider' of the service, or even the 'purchaser', could be the target, depending upon the aims and objectives stated. (These latter terms have been included because they are used in the 1990 NHS reforms associated with Trust management. They refer to the body that delivers the service (provider) and the body that pays for the service (purchaser).) Using the model in Box 2.1, the audit comprised *three* subject groups: GPs (purchasers), patients and patient case records. Equally, the individual or group aspect of an analysis might be an activity, the function of a piece of equipment or the cost of using a particular pharmaceutical product. Some of these

issues are considered in Donebedian's terms in the 'Mechanics of audit' below.

In conclusion, the practitioner's needs may be different from those of managers or purchasers, although they are no less important than dealing with service delivery as an overall strategy in terms of who to audit. While managers will want to know that a process is being adhered to and that the outcome is the delivery of that service, the practitioner has the option to qualify or quantify treatment. This is one of the most recent developments in clinical work and the emphasis in the latter part of this chapter will be on treatment outcomes.

ANALYSING THE EFFECTS OF TREATMENT

How to audit

This is the *procedure* by which audit is undertaken.

Mechanics of audit

Audit questions can be framed in terms of structure, process and outcome. These components can be broken down so that the practitioner can better understand 'what' as well as 'who' to audit. Unfortunately, 'how' to audit is less clear, because the aforementioned terms tell us nothing

---

Box 2.1 Auditing three subject groups

Tollafield & Parmar (1994) undertook an audit on day-care foot surgery. This used the five questions outlined below and each was amplified as a summary.

WHY: the main objectives were to consider the efficiency of foot surgery as assessed by perceptions and attitudes of medical and lay individuals and to record patient outcomes.

WHAT: foot surgery was the subject selected. This had a very wide remit, encompassing a range of degrees of complexity of surgery.

WHEN: the time interval had been agreed.

WHO: this was a closed sample group in terms of patient selection. The patient group had all been referred to, or were already part of, a foot care service

HOW: the methodology was established by collecting data from GPs and patients through open and closed questionnaires. Records of the treatment were then compared with the responses provided by patients.

METHOD: forms were filled in by hand by a non-independent researcher and transferred to a mainframe computer for analysis by independent researcher.

about how to measure, how to record data, how to process data and how to present data. The audit procedure will need to encompass planning performance, and the measurement and review of clinical activities as suggested in the list below. The audit process may involve a number of stages (Fig. 2.1):

- initial stage
  - plan the study (audit)
  - collect the data
  - analyse the data
  - measure performance (outcome)
- repeat stage
  - set new criteria
  - measure performance again
  - improve practice
  - monitor changes and effectiveness
  - repeat cycle.

Research and audit   The most robust form of audit follows similar principles as those applied to research methodology. The overlap with research is evident, as the quality of the final analysis depends on there being an adequate number of samples. The design of an audit must be carefully thought out in advance to take account of the type of data needed at the end.

The results of audit and research may well be used differently, though each is designed to bring about a change. Both share a common goal in this respect and both may refute past attitudes about management of the patient in terms of effectiveness and efficiency. Research should be

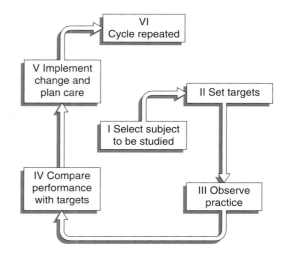

Figure 2.1   Full audit requires at least five stages. (Adapted from Lawrence et al 1994.)

performed under strict controls; audit has more flexibility but must be equally rigorous if the results are to be taken seriously.

Results should be considered carefully to reflect true change. For example, when introducing a new method into practice, critical analysis is important: a 50% response from a patient survey is inconclusive as the implication is that, while half may have been helped by the new method, half were not helped. Surveys use questionnaires, and a lack of response must always be assumed to be a response in the negative. Careful interpretation of results must be considered in audit as well as in research.

Table 2.2   Comparison between audit and research

Feature	Research	Audit
Purpose of study	Collects evidence to test a theory	Collects information to measure best practice
Data collection	Prospective	Retrospective
Scientific principles	Rigorous principles are repeatable	Uses audit principles, which may not be repeatable
Experiments	May involve humans	Never includes experiments on humans
Results	Factual and will accept or refute hypothesis	Decides whether standard of care has been met and indicates changes needed
Publication	Published	Internal use but may be circulated widely

Reproduced with permission from Bradshaw (1995).

Table 2.2 attempts to differentiate research from audit, but, in practice, the difference is small when applied to clinical outcome. The comparison in the table (Bradshaw 1995) has been adapted but generally attempts to show that there is a clear division between research and audit. There is an intrinsic flaw here, because there is no reason why research itself cannot be audited. The process of research is often more time consuming and resource intensive.

Data collection

The practitioner may elect to use an independent person to conduct an audit. This certainly offers less bias. Data can be collected from responses to a questionnaire or from direct measurement of a clinical activity. Some examples have already been provided under 'When to audit?'. The main terminology concerned with collecting data can be found in all basic statistics texts; however, it is essential that the part played by the data in measuring the outcome be understood. Such data are known as *nominal, ordinal* and *interval*.

Nominal data Nominal data involve a simple 'yes' or 'no' response, offering one of two choices. Patients can cope with this but often wish to expand their answer over and above what is effectively a closed response. Did an injection for pain help you: yes or no? The patient may believe that the pain was reduced initially and that as time passed this was less so, with an overall impression that some improvement had been experienced. In this case, the 'yes' response would be correct but unqualified.

Ordinal data Ordinal data are collected in the form of a scale derived from predetermined points of view: 'like' to 'dislike' may have varying strengths of expression with a 'no view', or 'cannot make mind up' type of conclusion as a middle of the road response. The Likert scale, as this is called, is used frequently for questionnaire or interview responses, as shown below. The response is marked, obviating the need for a full written statement, and forms another example of a closed response (Box 2.2).

Ordinal data collection along these lines is easy to carry out, can be computerized and the

---

Box 2.2 Likert scale-type questionnaire

Has the original complaint been made:

1. Much worse
2. Worse
3. The same
4. Better
5. Much better   1   2   3   4   5

---

results analysed relatively easily. Where a facility exists for direct input onto computer at the time of the patient interview, then collection allows rapid analysis. Two problems can arise. First, this type of data has no mathematical power. There is no way to say that a '1' response for one patient is the same as a '1' response for another. Indeed, a '1' and '2' could mean the same for two different patients; how much worse (or better) a patient feels cannot be ascertained from the analysis. Second, collection from a computer, while desirable, means that the patient does not have time to consider their response in privacy. The issue of whether to use anonymous data collection is considered later.

Interval data and ratio scales Interval data and ratio scales are considered the most ideal. Measurements that do not have a true zero, such as temperature, are interval scales. Those measurements with true zero points, such as weight, are ratio scales. Mathematically, these scales form more powerful data. Unlike ordinal data, interval and ratio scales have an infinite number of values. Metres can be subdivided into centimetres and then into millimetres. Smaller values can be measured in micrometres or angstroms. The difference between measurements collected can be compared and will offer more meaning. A reduction in pressure over a metatarsal head from 980 to 150 kPa by the use of an orthosis is a quantitative measurement with greater objectivity than if the patient were to express a nominal or ordinal response. A reduction of 830 kPa represents an 85% improvement. This expression has powerful implications in terms of statistical testing.

Data fall broadly into two categories: *parametric* and *non-parametric*. The former is considered to allow the most powerful statistical analysis.

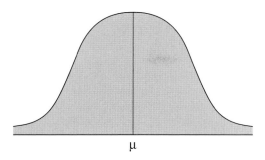

Figure 2.2 An example of parametric data reflected by a frequency curve with an ideal bell-shaped distribution. The centre point μ of a normal curve depends upon the value of the mean and the value of the standard deviation.

For the purpose of simple discussion, parametric data arise from samples that have a normal distribution, that is to say they fit the ideal shape of a frequency curve with a bell profile (Fig. 2.2). This form of data is predictable and has greatest frequency under the central part of the curve. Height in centimetres is a good example of parametric data, where the majority of people fall under the curve over a typical range depending upon sex, nationality and age. The ends of the curve never touch the x-axis and there is a very small percentage that falls outside the expected 'height'. The use of parametric data allows statements to be made about how likely data are to fall within bands known as standard deviations. The larger the value of standard deviation, the more distributed or spread out will be the data.

Data that fall outside normal distributions are, therefore, known as *non-parametric*. Unfortunately much of the clinical data collected falls into this latter category, making it more difficult to analyse statistically.

Questionnaires Questionnaires are a popular method of collecting clinical information from patients and practitioners. While they may seem simple, their implementation can create problems, and these will be discussed below. Reports from questionnaires should ideally show repeatability and offer the recipient a comprehensive summary of activity and outcome.

Fitzpatrick (1991) made a useful comparison between the collection of data via a self-completed questionnaire and collection via an interview. Table 2.3 emphasizes that no one method can preclude all the likely problems. An interview will ensure a 100% response from attendees but may not always achieve the honest or accurate response that a questionnaire filled out in the privacy of home might.

Questionnaires, especially when sent out by post, frequently fail to achieve high return rates. Hicks & Baker (1991) received responses to 76% (*n* = 226) of questionnaires when asking GPs to evaluate patient services. In another case, 48% (*n* = 478) of GPs returned questionnaires that contained six simple questions (Tagoe 1995). Tollafield & Parmar (1994) only received a 38% (*n* = 371) response from GPs to their questionnaire. The difference between these studies (which were unrelated) emphasizes the advantages of a simple over a more complex questionnaire. Hicks & Baker (1991) used a basic frame of 11 questions. The design was simple and relatively unambiguous, as shown in Box 2.3, using ratings alone rather than open or closed responses. By comparison, Tollafield & Parmar (1994) used 11 open and closed questions with a more complex design. Each of the three studies cited above used a postal survey.

The use of questionnaires often affects the quality of the information returned, and a compromise usually needs to be reached. For example, less-elaborate questionnaires may provide a higher return rate. The value of marketing

Table 2.3 Comparison between interview and self-questionnaires

Interview	Self-completed questionnaire
Sensitivity to the patient's concerns	Standardization of items
Flexibility in covering topics	No interviewer bias
Rapport	Anonymity
Clarification of ambiguities	Low cost of gathering data
Response adherence	No training needed
Ability to follow up questions	No immediate follow-up

Box 2.3 A simple questionnaire

Simple questionnaires (Hicks & Baker 1991) give little elaboration for each question posed, but the likely returns are higher than for ones with multiple domains. Clinical audit must strike a balance between having sufficient information and not having enough.

Quantity
1. Overprovided
2. Ample
3. Adequate
4. Inadequate
5. Grossly inadequate
6. Insufficient experience to offer an opinion

Quality
1. Excellent
2. Good
3. Adequate
4. Poor
5. Very poor

---

questionnaires is important; it is vital that the consumer does not consider the form to be yet another piece of paper!

In conclusion, questionnaire audits should be simple, they should be delivered and collected personally by an independent authority and they should have a layout that allows easy completion. These factors may motivate consumers to complete and return their questionnaires. Long and complex questionnaires have drawbacks unless conducted by personal interview.

Methods of measuring health and well-being

The best way to collect and evaluate data is to use conventional research methods. The practitioner should always be on the lookout for errors and other factors that could create bias, poor repeatability and poor validity.

Generic measurements Generic measurements apply to a wide group of practices based upon measuring health in terms of fitness. Fitness itself has a number of domains, ranging from physical to psychological well-being. Because the whole body may be involved with a disease process, isolating the foot can cause great difficulty when attempting to measure outcomes objectively, both before and after treatment.

In order to explain the concept of the generic measurement 'instrument', some examples are provided below with an accompanying discussion. Again we find that studies have mainly been carried out in the area of surgery, although the impact of disease on mobility has been studied extensively in physiotherapy and occupational therapy.

Health measures Anaesthetists use a system of grading patients suitable for induction anaesthesia on an ordinal basis, except that each patient is given a score. This is indivisible and runs from 1 to 5. The American Society of Anesthesiologists' (ASA) score of 1 infers that no organic, physiological, biochemical or psychiatric process exists. ASA 5 infers that the patient is moribund and not expected to survive.

QUALYS The quality-of-life index has been measured by workers such as Spitzer, Williams, Kind and Rosser to quantify disability and distress. When applied to cost in terms of how long a patient will live, and how much maintenance will cost for the period of treatment or benefit, the quality of life can be termed 'quality-adjusted life years' or 'Qualys'. Radford (cited in Pysent et al 1993) compared the cost of kidney therapy using cost per Qualy. A kidney transplant costed £1413 per Qualy, whereas haemodialysis costed £9075 per Qualy. The years gained per patient were calculated from an index. The cost of the treatment for the period expected was calculated as 6.1 years for haemodialysis and 7.4 years for kidney transplant. Dividing the total cost by the number of years produces the cost per Qualy.

Foot care has been studied by Bryan et al (1991). As they point out, Qualys have been considered largely in the area of 'high-tech' treatment (as above). When compared with repetitive maintenance care, as seen in the elderly domiciliary chiropody patient, the picture changes. Their figures were as follows: for haemodialysis in hospital, £19 129; for kidney transplant, £4099; for domiciliary chiropody, £229; and for in-clinic chiropody, £694. Chiropody is a low-cost service (prices based on 1989–90) and the gain from this type of care arises from preventing deterioration rather than from raising the health status of the patient.

As a measurement instrument, the Qualy can be easily misinterpreted. The application of this 'tool' has been in small populations. Differences arise between patients and workers as to how to interpret their health status, which means that any comparison is likely to have a poor correlation. The Qualy assessment assumes that every patient studied has an equal value for each year of life extended and it does not account for the differences of age. An older person may be regarded by society as having less worth than a younger person in terms of extension of quality of life. Of course, the converse may be true, but the point is that difficulties arise when false judgements are made. The fact that workers have very different attitudes to what constitutes health is well covered in the study of Bryan et al (1991). Wide variations existed in the responses of chiropody practitioners, who had more difficulty than nurses in assigning distress and disability ratings. This was put down to a lack of experience on the part of the chiropodists in using this type of assessment.

Health profiles A number of methods of measuring health have been developed for specific disabilities. In this case, the health status is considered rather than the quality of life. Practitioners should adopt a guarded approach to using such measurements.

First, the profile, which is constructed from a large number of patient responses based on simple life activities, must be applicable to the particular treatment being evaluated. Foot health, for example, may be determined by other systemic, physiological and psychological factors. The omission of one of these groups from the profile could invalidate the overall results and create false assumptions.

Consider the headings shown in Box 2.4, which are taken from the *Nottingham health profile* (NHP). Thirty-eight questions are grouped under six domains, although each domain is weighted differently. The practitioner needs to be clear on what aspect of health needs highlighting in such a study and in this respect the health profiles may be biased. Several other health profiles of this nature exist. The Arthritis Impact Measurement Scale (AIMS) includes

---

Box 2.4 The Nottingham profile

This is an example of a health profile. It attracts 38 questions in six domains:

- energy level
- pain
- emotional reaction
- sleep
- social isolation
- physical activities.

Domains may have different numbers of questions.

---

dexterity but also expands physical activities into nine domains. These include household, daily and social activities as measurements of incapacity against which improvement can be gauged. The Sickness Impact Profile (SIP) has 12 rather than six or nine domains, and in contrast with the previous measures has 130 questions as opposed to 45 for AIMS and 38 for NHP.

Second, when studying a new instrument, the repeatability factor should be investigated. Retest reliability coefficients can be measured for these profiles by repeating measurements between workers and comparing the results. A coefficient of 0.80 is promising, while less than 0.70 shows a weaker trend for repeatability. The values for the aforementioned health instruments are given in Table 2.4 (Pysent et al 1993).

Health profiles commonly use questionnaires. The results of repeatability testing show variations between each of the three examples given in the table. The use of an interviewer can make a difference: the SIP was measured at 0.97 with an interviewer but at 0.87 without. Health profiling can offer some elements of quality assurance, but the aim of the measurement should be

Table 2.4 Examples of reliability for three types of health profile

Health profile	Reliability
Nottingham health profile	0.87
Arthritis impact measurement scale	0.75–0.88
Sickness impact profile	0.97

Reproduced with permission from Pysent et al (1993).

decided before any recording commences. The real value of health profiling lies in what it can tell you about the effect of management.

Measurement of pain

Pain is a subjective response to physical stimuli and is complicated by emotional responses, which are less easy to predict. Pain is a useful outcome measure within the context of a clinical audit; it is also useful as an indicator of the effectiveness of treatment. Has pain been diminished as a result? The reduction of pain can be measured in many different ways, depending on the type of treatment: duration of resolution, side-effects (particularly from drugs), mobility improvement, emotional effects, changes in sleep patterns and the ability to use shoes that were previously abandoned.

Pain scales A nominal (binary) scale for pain of 'yes/no' can be used. This system offers a method of retrieving data quickly but will collect less-satisfactory detail about the effect of pain relief. The question posed may be asked in more than one way. In this case the likely accuracy will be greater and repeatability will be better, as ambiguity can be reduced.

Categorical scales can be used, where a score is attributed to a descriptor such as 'severe pain' or 'moderate pain'. It is interesting to note that the British National Formulary uses such descriptors for classifying analgesic strengths. Pain intensity or pain relief is measured using a number, for example 0 for 'no pain' and 3 for 'severe pain'. Good correlation has been shown between pain scores and pain intensity, offering a simple method for comparing intensity or relief of pain.

Visual analogue scales are favoured in many circles. The patient is asked to put a mark on a line (continuum), having first been told the extreme ranges. This barometer of pain intensity or relief can then be measured in millimetres using a ruler along the predetermined length of line selected (often 10 cm).

Pain charts such as the Oxford Pain Chart, the Burford Chart and the Evans Chart use category rating scales. The use of Likert scales can indicate the effectiveness of treatment within categories

such as poor, fair, good, very good and excellent. In one sense, the chart acts as a focused diary of pain intensity.

Pain questionnaires Questionnaires have been designed along the lines of the McGill Pain Questionnaire (MPQ). This design is similar to the methods seen previously in the NHP. The MPQ uses 102 pain descriptors, although a shortened version uses 78 questions. Patients with limited vocabularies and those classified as 'sick' respond less well than others. The time needed to prepare this type of measurement is lengthy compared with rating and analogue scales.

Physiological methods Physiological methods can be used to evaluate blood pressure, hormonal activity, respiratory levels and skin temperature. While useful for research, as a general form of audit these methods are less attractive. *Behavioural methods* require careful monitoring of a patient's physical changes. The method requires the practitioner to be available around the clock to assess food intake, alertness and facial responses such as distortion. However, different patients behave very differently, and the behavioural method system is, therefore, poor and insensitive as a measure.

Summary In conclusion, the weakness of using pain response alone affects the quality of measurement. The use of a broad range of factors, coupled with other aspects of the disease process or treatment such as healing and reduced doses of analgesics, is more helpful and offers greater sensitivity.

Measuring clinical outcome

Clinical activity measurement is today taken more seriously in health circles than it has been in the past, when many decisions were taken on the basis of empiricism. Pysent et al (1993) have criticized the lack of available methods for evaluating [orthopaedic] treatment. In point of fact it is not the shortage of methods alone but the specificity and reliability of such methods that lead to an unsuitable system of measurement. The majority of examples used in the latter part of this chapter have been taken from material in recent years.

When measurement forms part of the quantitative analysis, the assessment of outcomes becomes more robust. Once a reliable system has been found for analysing a particular pathology, providing that it is repeatable, valid and reproducible, then that system can be used as a measure of change. Several examples are given below that are specifically related to analysing the effect of treatment on the foot:

- assessment of deformity
- joint motion
- gait analysis.

Deformity In the foot, lesser toes, hallux, midfoot and hindfoot are the main focuses of problems. Kitoaka et al (1994) looked at a clinical rating system that used partial measurement with subjective features, as described in health profiles, but that focused on mobility. No useful repeatability study has been used to formalize the method, although the authors believe it to be a practical system that allows comparability of before and after treatment via a method of scoring. Moran & Claridge (1994) have used this method to show the changes in 12 patients following a particular surgery. The domains used in the study are shown in Table 2.5. An initial score indicates the extent of the problem, and the second, higher, score shows the average improvement made. The domains used are recognized criteria for identifying patient satisfaction; for example, patients regard an early return to wearing shoes after surgery as a recognizable improvement.

Joint motion Measuring joint motion suffers from the same problems as measuring deformity. In the case of joints, the excursion of motion is affected by temperature and synovial joint fluid viscosity. Variations in measurement may occur as a result of a practitioner's poor knowledge of anatomy, physiology and joint biomechanics. Relatively large joints of the foot, such as the subtalar and ankle joint, are complicated because their motion has no single dimension of movement. Inter- and intraclass correlation coefficients have been measured by Elveru (Pysent et al 1993) and are given in Table 2.6.

Sufficient care must be taken when interpreting quantitative data. If the technique can withstand scientific rigour, then as an audit tool it has great value. Measurement by goniometer provides a baseline value; if it is accurate, then the quantification of disability and improvement after treatment or otherwise may be recorded within the case records.

Gait analysis In recent years, the measuring instruments for foot contact pressures and forces have become more elaborate and more portable. Divided into ink mats, force and pressure platforms, as well as individual sensors used over specific points, these systems have been used to make comments about disability and altered contact phases during gait. Efficiency of oxygen uptake has been measured to assess energy consumption, although it has not been used for rou-

Table 2.5 Overall improvement can be expressed as a percentage average improvement, measured before and after operation (Moran & Claridge, 1994)

	Symptoms before	Symptoms after
Pain	7.2	27.2
Activity tolerance	10.6	14.1
Shoes	5.0	7.8
Cosmesis	2.2	4.4
Overall	4.1	8.8

Table 2.6 When using methods for evaluating change, the process should be repeatable. The inter- and intraobserver correlation coefficients indicate that the same observer is usually more reliable at repeating the measurement than different observers

Joint	Movement	Interobserver	Intraobserver
Ankle	Dorsiflexion	0.50	0.90
	Plantarflexion	0.72	0.86
Subtalar	Inversion	0.32	0.74
	Eversion	0.17	0.75

tine measurement. Most of these methods are too laborious for the everyday clinical situation and are more appropriate for academic research. Many workers have attempted to use gait analysis methods to measure the effect of orthoses and, therefore, the effects of treatment.

The common factor in each of the above cases is that the instrument of measurement is physical and needs calibrating to ensure repeatability. Errors arise from both instruments and patients, as well as from human handling (examiner). Any valuable conclusion must first include a statement of reliability, repeatability and validity; this is so important that it is worth repeating again and again. Unfortunately, some techniques still lack reliability or repeatability in measuring joint position, movement and ground–foot interface pressures, but improvements are encouraging.

EFFECTS OF MEASUREMENT ON TREATMENT POLICY FOR THE FUTURE

The development of research in health areas has affected the shape of outcomes dramatically, with many more practitioners now questioning the methods of assessment, the interpretation of results and the comparative effects of the different methods. The use of medication, orthoses and surgery is for the first time being questioned, where previously such treatment was accepted empirically. One of the major impacts of this work is directly related to cost of provision of treatment and the likely resources required.

Modern technology is constantly influencing the development of more rapid audit mechanisms. The use of pen-activated linked computers with interfacing microphones will allow medical records to be audited with ease and speed, will allow the generation of letters and will provide reasonable patient data security. Database analysis will provide rapid breakdown on treatment, drugs and complications. The link with clinical economics will drive the development of dedicated systems, which are currently being tested particularly in the North American Health Care system.

Presenting data

Case files are probably the commonest source of data in following treatment progress. Retrospective analysis is more frequently employed than prospective analysis. Loss of data is a significant problem leading to potentially incorrect conclusions. The use of computerized information or well-designed data books (similar to accounting books) can overcome this problem as long as they are kept up to date. Stamp pads designed to record simple data, such as foot lesions and vascular tree pressure indices, are helpful and easily identified within case records.

Practitioners should develop a system of summarizing information and recording improvement and deterioration in a systematic way at the end of each entry to allow for occasional audit. Clear writing and minimum use of abbreviations will greatly speed up the process of reviewing case records. A certain amount of standardization is recommended for such reviews to make comparison more informative.

Setting out the evidence

Tabulated results are valuable when presented with explanatory text. Each section of this text should be clearly marked and numbered, and it should have subsections. Consider Table 2.7, which shows how patients responded when questioned about returning to a service. The data were used in an internal report to show the percentage of patients prepared to return for day

Table 2.7 Auditing the same question: would patients be prepared to have surgery repeated in the same way again?

Year	Author(s)	Prepared to have surgery in the same way again (%)[a]
1991	Tibrewal & Foss	80
1987–91	Tollafield & Parmar	93
1993–94	Tollafield & Kilmartin	97

[a]The values in this table relate to different surgical centres and for Tollafield represent podiatry cases, and for Tibrewal represent orthopaedic cases.

surgery at three centres, having been sent a questionnaire 6 months or longer after the event.

Other forms of reporting may use data such as a research paper that can be published and cited. Sample sizes should be large enough and ideally include a control or comparison. Graphs, flow charts, histograms and pie charts are valuable tools for reporting trends for large data sets. Complicated statistics are undesirable as in many cases they are used inappropriately.

In conclusion, setting out internal and scientific audit reports requires clarity, with a sound structure that has a progressive and logical flow. The *objectives* should be stated, the *method* included and *results* brought together in tables or plots to highlight trends. The *conclusion* should be based upon the evidence presented without excessive elaboration. A *summary* is valuable, allowing the reader to scan the information quickly for relevance. Where audit requires a large amount of data collection, the report should have more than one section, allowing for unrelated information to be separated. The conclusion can then be used to bring all the sections together, if indeed there is a valid reason for doing this. Scientific audit may be more specific and require greater controls and analysis. Omitting the usual scientific principles and failing to use the style required will usually result in your paper being rejected.

SUMMARY

Evidence-based practice, clinical governance and audit are very large subjects and in a brief chapter many areas that would ideally be described in greater detail must be left to texts that are devoted solely to this subject. Emphasis has been placed here on applications within foot health care, with a bias towards measuring clinical outcomes.

The need to implement evidence-based and audit practices in the clinic is based upon many different requirements. Practitioners must take account of educational, legal, political, moral, ethical and research aspects in conducting their activities. Standards set for practice should ideally be underpinned by proving the effectiveness of treatment. Politics and economics drive medical audit today, leaving health care professionals to justify their selection of treatment.

Audit and clinical governance has come a long way since the days of Florence Nightingale and Ernest Codman, when medical dogma refused to recognize that old practices were outdated and ineffective.

REFERENCES

Bradshaw T W 1995 Clinical audit in theory and practice. British Journal of Podiatric Medicine 50: 3–5, 9

Bryan S, Parkin D, Donaldson C 1991 Chiropody and the Qualy; a case study in assigning categories of disability and distress to patients. Health Policy 18: 169–185

Department of Health 1989 NHS working for patients. CMNO 555. HMSO, London

Department of Health 1998 A first class service: quality in the new NHS. HMSO, London

Donebedian A 1966 Evaluating the quality of medical care. Millbank Memorial Fund Quarterly, Part 3: 166–206

Donebedian A 1988 The quality of care. How can it be assessed? Journal of the American Medical Association 260: 1743–1748

Ellis R, Whittington D 1993 Quality assurance in health care. A handbook. Edward Arnold, London, p 2–3

Fitzpatrick R 1991 Surveys of satisfaction: I Important general considerations. British Medical Journal 303: 887–889

Hicks N R, Baker I A 1991 A general practitioner's opinions of health services available to their patients. British Medical Journal 302: 991–993

Kitoaka H B, Alexander I J, Adelaar R S, Nunley J A,

Myerson M S, Sanders M 1994 Clincial rating systems for ankle–hindfoot, midfoot, hallux and lesser toes. Foot and Ankle International 15: 349–353

Lawrence M, Griew K, Derry J, Anderson J, Humphreys J 1994 Auditing audits: use and development of the Oxfordshire Medical Audit Advisory Group rating system. British Medical Journal 309: 513–516

Maxwell R J 1984 Quality assessment in health. British Medical Journal 228: 1470–1477

Moran M M, Claridge R J 1994 Chevron osteotomy for bunionette. Foot and Ankle International 15: 684–688

Pollock A, Evans M 1993 Surgical audit, 2nd edn. Butterworth–Heinemann, Oxford, p 25–27, 58–63

Pysent P, Fairbank J, Carr A 1993 Outcome measures in orthopaedics. Butterworth–Heinemann, Oxford

Tagoe M 1995 Patient satisfaction audit following podiatric surgery. In: Report of the Podiatry Association on podiatry and hospital foot services (Appendix B). Podiatry Association, London, p 18–22

Tibrewal S B, Foss M 1991 Day care surgery for the correction of hallux valgus. Health Trends 23(3): 117–119

Tollafield D R, Parmar D G 1994 Setting standards for day

care foot surgery. A quinquennial review. British Journal of Podiatric Medicine and Surgery 6: 7–20

Tollafield D R, Kilmartin T E, Holdcroft D J, Quinn G 1995 Measurement of ankle cuff discomfort in unsedated

patients undergoing day case foot surgery. Ambulatory Surgery 3: 91–96

Tucker P 1995 Clinical audit lectures. 20 Watling Street Rd, Preston, UK (personal correspondence)

FURTHER READING

ACCO 1990 Quality assurance. Instep 5–8

Ariori A R, Graham R B, Antony R J 1989 Results of a six month practice in podiatric day surgery in the NHS. Journal of the Podiatric Association April, 16

Ashcroft D J, Lavis G J, Russell L H 1979 Retrospective analysis of partial nail avulsions. The Chiropodist 34: 100–108

Beaton D 1990 Ingrowing toenails: a patient evaluation of phenolisation versus wedge excision. British Journal of Podiatric Medicine 45: 62

Bunbridge C A 1993 Survey of patient satisfaction with the quality of service provided by the West Berkshire Chiropody Department. British Journal of Podiatric Medicine 48: 46–48

Crombie I K 1992 Towards good audit. British Journal of Hospital Medicine 48: 182–185

Difford F 1990 Audit in person. British Medical Journal 300: 92–94

Duncan A 1980 Quality assurance: what now and where next? British Medical Journal 281: 300–302

Gaskell B 1989 Nail surgery: the patient's reaction. Enfield Health Authority Department of Chiropody. The Chiropodist 44: 174–176

Green Park Unit 1992 A guide to medical audit. Medical Audit Department, Musgrave Park Hospital, Northern Ireland

Griffiths C 1995 Clinical measurement. In: Merriman L M, Tollafield D R (eds) Assessment of the lower limb. Churchill Livingstone, Edinburgh

Helfand A E 1990 Guidelines for podiatric services in long-term care facilities. Journal of the American Podiatric Medical Association 80: 448–450

Helm P A 1981 Ingrowing toe nails. An evaluation of two treatments. British Medical Journal 283: 1125–1126

Jones O R, Christenson C J 1992 Podiatric utilization referral patterns at an army medical centre. Military Medicine 157: 7–10

Keefe M 1989 An audit of wart treatment in a Scottish dermatology department. British Journal of Podiatric Medicine 44: 271–274

Kilmartin T E, Barrington R L, Wallace W A 1992 The X-ray measurement of hallux valgus. An inter and intraobserver error study. The Foot 2: 7–11

Kind P, Rosser R, Williams A 1982 Valuation of quality of life: some pyschometric evidence. In: Jones-Lee M W (ed) The value of life and safety. North-Holland, Amsterdam

Kuwada G T 1991 Long-term evaluation of partial and total surgical and phenol matrixectomies. Journal of the American Podiatric Medical Association 81: 33–36

Mangan J L, Ashford R L, Murphy J S G, Beverland D E 1992 Waiting list initiatives: application to foot surgery. Medical Audit News 2: 44–45

Mangan J L, Ashford R L, Murphy J S G, Beverland D E 1992 A multidisciplinary approach to foot surgery waiting lists. The Foot 2: 29–33

McKee C M, Lauglo M, Lessof L 1989 Medical audit: a review. Journal of the Royal Society of Medicine 82: 474–478

Merriman L 1990 Manpower planning in chiropody: what is chiropody? British Journal of Podiatric Medicine 45: 179–182

Merriman L 1991 Manpower planning in chiropody treatment for life. British Journal of Podiatric Medicine 46: 36–40

Palmer B V, Jones 1979 Ingrowing toenails. The results of treatment. British Journal of Surgeons 66: 575–576

Society of Chiropodists 1991 Guidelines on standards of chiropody/podiatry practice. Society of Chiropodists, London

Spitzer W O 1987 State of science 1986: quality of life and functional status as target variables for research. Journal of Chronic Diseases 40: 465–471

Tollafield D R, Price M 1985 Hallux metatarsophalangeal joint survey related to postoperative surgery analysis. The Chiropodist 40: 283–288

University of Dundee 1992 Moving to audit. What every doctor needs to know about medical audit. University of Dundee Press, Dundee, UK

3

Clinical protocols

Linda M. Merriman
Joy Dale

INTRODUCTION

The first part of this chapter looks at the factors that influence how practitioners act and behave in clinical practice. This is followed by examination of four clinical protocols in which practitioners who are involved in the treatment of the foot need to be cognisant (Box 3.1).

A protocol states the course of action to be adopted by people working within a particular organization, profession or service. Clinical protocols are basically rules of how to proceed in certain situations. They provide health care practitioners with parameters in which to operate. The term 'code of practice' may be used synonymously with clinical protocols. A code comprises a set of laws or rules. Codes of practice may be formulated by statutory organizations, professional bodies, employers or voluntary organizations. They may cover a diverse range of issues or focus on a specific process or issue. For example, codes of practice related to the practitioner–patient relationship cover a broad range of issues, whereas a code of practice for the sterilization of instruments focuses on one specific issue. All codes of practice should be regularly reviewed and updated in the light of

---

Box 3.1 Clinical protocols
• Health and safety • Infection control • Liability insurance • Practitioner–patient relationship

current research in order to ensure the best delivery of clinical services.

WHAT INFLUENCES HOW A PRACTITIONER PRACTISES?

All health care practitioners are accountable:

- for their own individual actions
- for the care of other people
- to professional organizations
- to the general public.

When treating patients, practitioners must be aware of these obligations and responsibilities. In order to offer the best service to their patients and society in general, it is incumbent on practitioners to ensure that their practice is safe, does not put the patient at harm (i.e. is not maleficent) and is of benefit to the patient (i.e. is beneficent). Practitioners are accountable and responsible for their own actions, but in deciding how to act they will be influenced by the following:

- current legislation
- the codes of practice/conduct of professional organizations
- the codes of practice/conduct of employing organizations
- their own attitudes and beliefs.

All of the above influence the practitioner, but in some circumstances one may override the others (e.g. current legislation). Each of the above influences will be considered in turn.

Current legislation

Acts of Parliament and judicial decisions arising from what are commonly known as 'test cases' collectively impose legal responsibilities on practitioners. All practitioners should keep themselves informed about relevant Acts of Parliament that may affect their practice. Box 3.2 lists some of the Acts of Parliament that are relevant to health care practitioners involved in treating the foot. These Acts may be amended or replaced from time to time.

Box 3.2 Examples of relevant Acts of Parliament*

- Occupier's Liability Act 1957
- Health and Safety at Work Act 1974
- Data Protection Act 1974
- Reporting of Injuries, Diseases and Dangerous Occurrence Regulations 1985
- Consumer Protection Act 1987
- Ionizing Radiation (protection of persons undergoing medical examination or treatment) Regulations 1988
- Control of Substances Hazardous to Health (COSHH) 1988
- Pressure Systems and Transportable Gas Containers Regulations 1989
- Children's Act 1989
- Access to Health Records Act 1990
- Provision and Use of Work Equipment Regulations 1992
- Manual Handling Operations Regulations 1992
- Management of Health and Safety at Work Regulations 1992
- Personal Protective Equipment at Work Regulations 1992
- Electromagnetic Compatibility Regulations 1992

*Copies of these Acts/Regulations can be obtained from The Stationery Office.

Codes of practice/conduct of professional organizations

The practice of health care professions is influenced by statutory and professional bodies. There are specific statutory bodies responsible for most of the health care professions. For example, the statutory body for doctors is the General Medical Council, that for Allied Health Professions is the Health Professions Council, and that for nursing is the Nursing and Midwifery Council. The role of these statutory bodies varies but usually involves responsibility for initial education and issues related to practice and conduct. Chiefly, the statutory bodies are concerned with regulation of the professions to ensure that the public is protected from inappropriate practices and incompetent practitioners. Statutory bodies are responsible for maintaining registers of appropriately qualified individuals who are 'fit to practise'. They ensure ongoing fitness to practise of registrants through removal or suspension from the register of those found to be clinically incompetent, unfit to practise or having relevant criminal records. In addition, most statutory bodies also require registrants to demonstrate continued fitness to practise, by providing evidence of involvement in continuing professional development.

The practice of health practitioners, as well as being influenced by statutory bodies, is also affected by professional organizations. Most health professionals are members of one or more professional organizations, for example the British Medical Association (BMA), Royal College of Nurses (RCN) and the Society of Chiropodists & Podiatrists (SCP). These organizations have no statutory function; their role is to protect and promote the interests of their members. As part of this function, they produce their own codes of practice. The prime purposes of these codes are to:

- reassure the public that they can expect high standards of practice
- provide guidelines on best practice for members.

Codes of practice/conduct of employing organizations

The NHS is by far the largest employer of health care practitioners in the UK. It produces a range of codes of practice that influence the practice of its health care practitioners. For example, the NHS has a code of practice related to immunization of first-line practitioners for hepatitis B (HSG(93)40). The Patient's Charter (Department of Health 1991) is another example of a NHS code of practice. Initially, the Charter laid down standards for seven aspects of patient care; in April 1992 a further three were added (Box 3.3). Following the setting of these national standards, individual NHS Trusts and departments have published their own additional local standards.

A standard identifies the required level of practice. Clinical codes of practice are commonly expressed in terms of minimum standards. A minimum standard is the lowest acceptable level of practice necessary for the proper care of patients. Standards are arrived at from a number of sources, for example experts in the field,

---

Box 3.3 Patient Charter standards (Department of Health 1995)

- To receive health care on the basis of clinical need, regardless of ability to pay
- To be registered with a general practitioner (GP)
- To receive emergency medical care at any time, through the GP or the emergency ambulance service and the hospital accident and emergency department
- To be referred to a consultant acceptable to you when your GP thinks it necessary, and to be referred for a second opinion if you and your GP agree this is desirable
- To be given clear explanation of any treatment proposed, including any risk and any alternatives, before you decide whether you will agree to the treatment
- To have access to your health records and to know that those working for the NHS are under a legal duty to keep their contents confidential
- To choose whether or not you wish to take part in medical research or medical student training
- To be given detailed information on local health services, including quality standards and maximum waiting times
- To be guaranteed admission for treatment by a specific date no later than 2 years from the day when your consultant places you on a waiting list
- To have any complaint about NHS services – whoever provides them – investigated and to receive a full and prompt written reply from the chief executive or general manager

---

professional organizations, employers and special interest groups.

Individual attitudes and beliefs

We all have our own individual notions about what we consider to be right and wrong, about how we should treat other people and about what is fair and appropriate. These personal views are influenced by a range of circumstances: upbringing, schooling, religious beliefs and past experiences to name but a few. Sometimes there may be differences between our personal attitudes and beliefs and the law of the land or the codes of practice of the professional organizations of which we are members. In such instances, each individual practitioner must decide what he or she considers to be the most appropriate course of action. However, at all times the interests and needs of the patient should be paramount.

CLINICAL PROTOCOLS

Health and safety

Practitioners' responsibilities for health and safety are governed by the Health and Safety at Work Act (HSW) 1974 and associated Acts and Regulations. In January 1993, the Health and Safety Executive produced a code of practice for workplace health, safety and welfare (Health and Safety Executive 1993a). This code was in response to Section 16 (1) of the Health and Safety at Work Act 1974. Under this Act, responsibility for health and safety rests with the highest level of management but all individuals have a degree of responsibility for carrying out health and safety policies. Particular areas of responsibility may be designated to named individuals; for example the maintenance of clinical equipment may be the responsibility of a chief technician. However, the practitioner is ultimately responsible for the treatment a patient receives, and in the case of equipment the practitioner must be satisfied that it is safe to use at the point of contact.

For the practitioner involved with treating disorders of the foot, the following specific aspects of health and safety should be borne in mind. Some of these relate to specific Acts of Parliament, while others relate to a general consensus of what constitutes good practice:

- design of clinical areas
- safe use of equipment
- use of hazardous substances
- responsibilities of employers and employees
- health and safety risk assessment.

Design of clinical areas

The practitioner's involvement in the design of the treatment area is essential. The general layout of equipment should be decided upon during the initial planning stage. Early decisions prevent incorrect siting of integral fittings such as sinks and power points. Due consideration should be given to lighting, both natural and artificial. The position of light sources in relation to working surfaces is of particular importance.

The conversion of existing premises to provide suitable clinical accommodation can be problematic. Ornate ceilings, picture rails and skirting boards may be in keeping with the property but are not conducive to the creation of an ideal clinical treatment area. Advice from experts, such as architects and builders, can alleviate some of the difficulties. Discussion with colleagues who have experience of similar situations can prove invaluable.

Ease of access to clinical premises is of the utmost importance as patients may be disabled. In the UK, the Disability Discrimination Act (1995) aims to end the discrimination that people with disabilities face in employment, access to goods, facilities and services, and purchase of property or land. This includes the requirement that people providing services to the public must make 'reasonable' adjustments to ensure that the services are accessible by people with disabilities. Failure to do so can result in prosecution and large fines. Ground floor accommodation is therefore preferable unless a lift is available. Consideration should be given to the distance that patients need to walk or be transported from the entrance to the waiting area and then to the surgery.

Careful attention to planning of reception facilities and waiting areas pays dividends. Not only is it important to create a safe environment for patients, but attention should also be paid to ensuring that the reception area is welcoming. First impressions are important; hence the significance of welcoming reception facilities. Natural light and high ceilings provide a 'relaxing atmosphere' (Combs 1992). Adequate seating, particularly for the less agile, a children's play area and the availability of drinks are features appreciated by patients and, at the same time, ensure a safe and healthy environment. Clear signposting to treatment areas and facilities reduces patients' anxiety. It is often useful to involve representatives of users and potential users of the service in the planning of reception and waiting facilities.

A variety of patients' chairs are now on the market (Fig. 3.1). When selecting a chair, it is essential that the back rest is adjustable; chairs

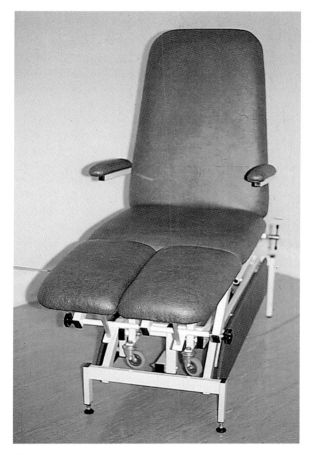

Figure 3.1 Flat-bed couch with adjustable back rest.

Examination lamps should be installed as additional lighting. These may be mounted on the wall or ceiling or may be fitted onto work units or mobile bases. The aim is to have a non-distorting, colour-corrected light source that can be focused on a particular site. To achieve this, lamps are extended by means of articulating arms. The length and range of movement of the arm should be assessed with regard to the position in which the lamp is to be mounted. Fluorescent tubes or incandescent lamps are most commonly used in routine clinical practice. The amount of heat generated by the lamp when in use is an important consideration. It is possible to purchase examination lamps that incorporate a magnifying glass; these lamps can be particularly helpful for observing skin changes and for operating.

Adequate storage space for supplies and portable equipment is of prime importance. A separate, lockable storeroom, adjacent to the treatment room, is desirable but not always possible. Storage racks and cupboards should be used efficiently. Labelling of cupboards with details of their contents is helpful, especially if other practitioners use the area. All drugs, needles and syringes must be stored in a locked cabinet. To promote compliance with this regulation, other items should not be stored in this space.

Safe use of equipment

All surgery equipment should be maintained as per the manufacturer's instructions. Servicing contracts with the manufacturer or specialist contractors ensure that maintenance procedures are not overlooked. Equipment that is to be repaired or serviced must be decontaminated first. For example, nail drill handpieces should be autoclaved and dust bags removed from drills. If adequate decontamination has not been carried out, the service engineers must be notified by appropriate labelling of the equipment.

The individual manufacturer's instructions for the use of specific equipment, such as cryosurgery and ultrasound equipment, must be followed and safety precautions must be strictly adhered to. For example, an exhaust hose to vent

with fully reclining back rests are essential for patient examination and the management of clinical emergencies. The height of the chair should also be adjustable; this facilitates easier access for the patient and provides a convenient working position for the practitioner, thus preventing known occupational hazards such as chronic back pain. The manufacturer's manual should be carefully studied to ensure safe usage.

The operating chair must be comfortable for the practitioner. The height of the chair and the position of the back rest should be adjustable. A five star base fitted with casters allows manoeuvrability and prevents tipping. The suitability of an operating chair should be assessed in combination with the patient's chair with which it is to be used.

noxious waste gas from cryotherapy systems should always be used (see Ch. 9).

The 'Memorandum of Guidance on the Electricity at Work Regulations' (Health and Safety Executive 1989) states the legal requirements for the maintenance of portable electrical equipment (including autoclaves). The user is charged with the responsibility for checking that equipment appears to be in a sound condition before use. The establishment of a system for the inspection and testing of equipment is also a requirement of these regulations. There continues to be significant improvements in the mechanical efficiency of nail drills. An effective dust extraction mechanism is a priority. Drills need to be robust to withstand heavy usage. This is particularly so in clinics used by several practitioners. The size and shape of the handpiece should be appropriate to the operator's hand. Adequate holders are needed to protect handpieces from damage when they are not in use. Autoclavable handpieces are essential. Drills may be fixed to work units by means of a bracket, positioned adjacent to an existing surface or used on a mobile base.

Certain equipment that may be used in diagnosing and treating foot problems, e.g. X-ray and laser equipment, is controlled by separate regulations. Advice on the safety aspects of these procedures may be obtained from authorities such as the National Radiological Protection Board.

Use of hazardous substances

The Control of Substances Hazardous to Health (COSHH) Regulations 1988 provides a framework for the protection of people against health risks from hazardous substances. In 1993, the Health and Safety Executive produced a useful step-by-step guide to COSHH regulations (Health and Safety Executive 1993b). Under the COSHH regulations, a risk assessment of all the substances encountered in practice must be made and any necessary action taken to reduce identified risks. Examples of hazardous substances used in the treatment of foot problems are strong acids and alkalis, solvents and adhesives.

Responsibilities of employers and employees

If five or more people are employed, the employer must have a written health and safety policy. In situations where complex procedures are undertaken, this policy should refer the reader to other, more specific health and safety documents. Codes of practice dealing with infection control and the use of orthotic laboratories are examples where specific documentation would be required. The law only requires safety policy statements to cover the health and safety of employees (Health and Safety Executive 1990a). However, it is recommended that a strategy for protecting other people (patients, visitors, cleaners, maintenance staff and contractors) who could be put at risk by activities undertaken during the course of practice be established.

Employers must ensure that employees are provided with adequate health and safety training, including refresher training. Changes made to existing policies must be made known to all employees. The implementation of safety policies should be closely monitored. Revision of policies is necessary from time to time in the light of experience or because of the introduction of new or altered practices. Health and safety regulations also apply to the self-employed. Practitioners who are self-employed have a duty to conduct their practices in such a manner so as to ensure, as far as is reasonably practical, that they and other persons who may be affected are not exposed to risks to their health and safety.

Infection control

Infection control is an integral part of good practice. The prime purpose of any infection control policy is to reduce the likelihood of cross-infection either between the practitioner and the patient or between patients. Practitioners involved in treating foot problems are, at times, likely to come into contact with the body fluids of their patients. Conversely, the patient may, under certain circumstances, come into contact with the body fluids of the practitioner (e.g. if a practitioner is cut with a scalpel). Of particular concern are the systemic infections transmitted by body fluids, human immunodeficiency virus (HIV) and hepatitis B virus (HBV). The other main risks of cross-infection are from localized infections of the feet involving bacteria, fungi or viruses. More recently, instrument-handling procedures need to take account of variant Creutzfeldt–Jakob disease and the possibility that contaminated surgical instruments could transmit the prions responsible for this disease from one patient to another.

In practice, there are many differences in the cross-infection procedures adopted by particular establishments or organizations; these differences do not usually present a problem. However, it is most important that each establishment/organization documents its infection control policy and that copies of this policy are available to all practitioners. An infection control policy should, as a minimum standard, encompass the following areas:

- routine clinical cleansing
- handwashing and use of gloves
- sterilization of instruments and dressings
- disposal of clinical waste
- spillages
- health of the practitioner.

Routine clinical cleansing

Cleaning of the clinical environment is essential to reduce the risk of cross-infection between patients and the personnel involved in the delivery of treatment. The cleaning of equipment and furnishings should be organized in terms of procedure, frequency of use and who is responsible. Cleaning procedures adopted must be justifiable. There is no evidence that the use of disinfectant solutions is of benefit in the cleaning of walls or floors (Maurer 1985, Ward 1990). Detergent solutions are adequate for most general cleaning. The effectiveness of cleaning depends to a large extent on the frictional scrubbing action that is applied to any surface. Walls need to be washed, at a minimum, every 3 months (unless splashing occurs). Floors require washing at least every day.

Infection control procedures are easier to undertake if units are of a simple design. The pristine condition of storage compartments is soon lost with continual usage. The whole unit must be easily cleaned. A durable and easily cleaned top surface of, for example, glass or stainless steel is necessary to isolate sterilized instruments. The unit should be mobile to allow easy access and to facilitate floor cleaning.

Durable floor covering is essential. Non-slip vinyl, extended to skirting level and with sealed seams, is a relatively safe option and can be easily cleaned. The choice of window blinds should also be influenced by ease of cleaning. Curtaining around changing cubicles should be washable and, in line with Department of Health regulations, fire-retardant. Worn furnishings, such as floor coverings, must be replaced before they become dangerous.

The safe removal of debris following each treatment has consistently been debated. Sweeping brushes disperse bacteria into the air (Babb 1963). Vacuum cleaners have been shown to have the same effect (Bate 1961). Wet-vacuum systems are acceptable but wet floors are hazardous. The solution lies in the collection of all debris at source (Fig 3.2). If reusable debris trays

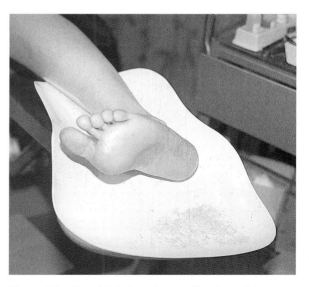

Figure 3.2 Foot debris tray shown without a moisture-proof cover (now recommended).

are used, they should be protected by a moisture-proof cover that is changed after every treatment.

Handwashing

Evidence strongly supports a causal relationship between handwashing and infection control (Larson 1988). The primary objective of clinical handwashing is to eliminate transient contaminants that have been acquired from patients or the environment and to reduce the resident flora of the skin to as low a level as possible. Transient contaminants are easily removed by thorough washing with soap and water. A vigorous scrub with a non-medicated soap for at least 10–15 seconds will reliably remove gross contamination (Knittle et al 1975). Antiseptic handwashing agents assist the removal of resident organisms. It is important that handwashing agents used for preoperative scrubbing have rapid and potent antimicrobial activity, that they be well tolerated and, ideally, that they exert a residual antibacterial effect for a prolonged period following the scrub (Maki 1989).

Many comparative studies of handwashing agents have been undertaken. Bendig (1991) concluded that a 4% chlorhexidine detergent solution was significantly more effective than 2% triclosan detergent solution. Cremieux et al (1989) found that the immediate efficacy of povidone–iodine and chlorhexidine were equivalent, but that the cumulative efficacy and remnant effects of chlorhexidine were higher than those of povidone–iodine. The properties of a handwashing agent should be evaluated in terms of expected usage.

Use of gloves

Protective gloves are now worn for all procedures that may involve exposure to blood, body fluids or other sources of infection. Non-sterile gloves are adequate for non-invasive work but sterile gloves must always be worn for any invasive procedure.

Practitioners often complain of the poor fit of non-sterile disposable gloves and resort to the use of sterile surgical gloves, which are much more expensive. The necessity to discard non-sterile gloves after each treatment is debatable (Baumann 1992). Provided that these gloves are not punctured, washing and disinfection may be adequate. To decontaminate gloves, washing with a hand-cleansing agent for 30 seconds is generally necessary (Douglas 1989). In practice, loose-fitting non-sterile gloves can be difficult to wash satisfactorily. Surgical gloves are damaged by frequent washing and become sticky through loss of talcum and/or starch on the surface (Mitchell et al 1983).

If gloves are to protect the practitioner and the patient against cross-infection, they must be used in the proper manner (Fig. 3.3). Handwashing is necessary before donning gloves and after their removal. When treatment is completed, immediate removal, in the case of an invasive procedure, or washing of gloves, in the case of a non-invasive procedure, is essential. To contain contaminants, gloves must be removed by turning them inside out.

The incidence of hand dermatitis and latex allergy is on the increase because of the wider and more frequent use of latex gloves in health care practice (Sharma 1991). Gloves can affect skin in different ways, for example hands may become dry and cracked or sweaty and swollen. Serious respiratory and generalized allergic responses to latex allergens have been observed. Severe allergic responses are not just confined to those with atopic tendencies but may also arise in relation to duration and frequency of contact. Therefore, the use of latex gloves is to be discouraged where alternatives (e.g. vinyl, nitrile) are available.

Instrument sterilization

Sterilization of instruments is an integral part of routine practice. Thorough cleaning of instruments prior to sterilization is essential. Blood and other adherent material will coagulate and become fixed on instruments as they pass through the heat sterilization cycle. Instruments should be cleaned in a dedicated sink using warm water and detergent. Robust, protective rubber gloves should be worn during this pro-

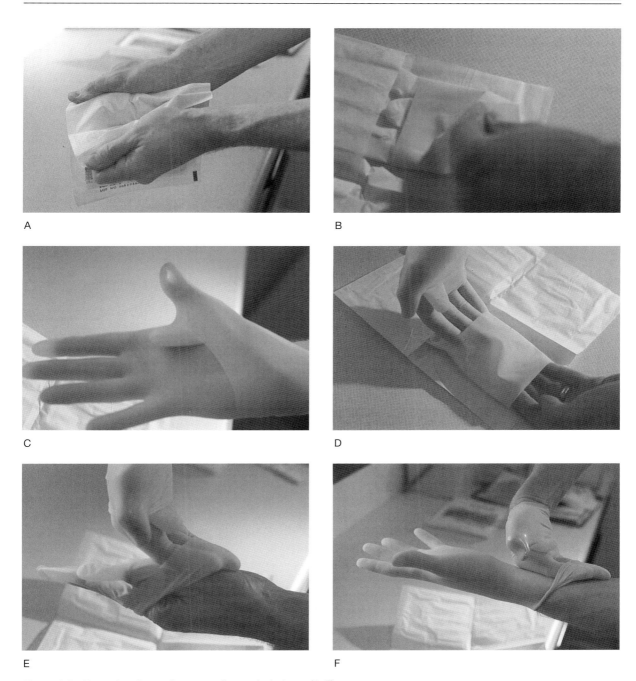

Figure 3.3 Procedure for putting on sterile surgical gloves (A–F).

cedure. A more convenient and efficient method is to use an ultrasonic cleaner (Fig. 3.4A). When washing instruments, excessive amounts of detergent or inadequate rinsing results in residues, which can subsequently damage the autoclave mechanisms.

Steam pressure autoclaves provide the most convenient and reliable method of achieving instrument sterilization (Fig. 3.4B). The cleaned instruments should be spaced out on the autoclave trays and closed instruments should be opened so that all surfaces will be exposed to steam during the sterilization process (Fig. 3.4C).

Prospective purchasers are strongly recommended to consider only models that comply with British Standard 3970 Part 4 'Specification for transportable steam sterilizers for unwrapped instruments and utensils' (see also Health and Safety Executive 1990b). The purchaser's choice of autoclave must be influenced first and fore-most by compliance with safety requirements. Autoclaves require commissioning before use, and operating instructions must be strictly adhered to. Steam sterilizers are pressure vessels and must comply with the 'Pressure systems and transportable gas container Regulations' (1989), whereby the user is required to have a suitable scheme for the periodic examination of the steril-izer. The insurers of premises on which auto-claves are being used must be notified.

Small steam sterilizers are generally consid-ered as being only suitable for the sterilization of unwrapped loads for immediate use (Department of Health 1990). In practice, there may be a short delay before instruments are

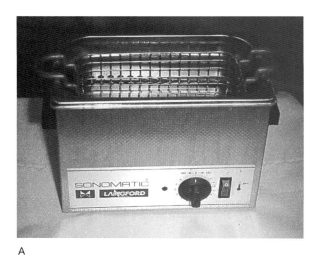

A

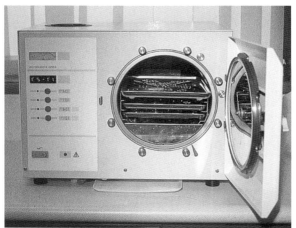

B

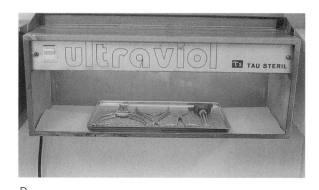

C

D

Figure 3.4 Procedure for the sterilization of instruments. A, Ultrasonic cleaner to ensure instruments are clean prior to autoclaving. B, Autoclave. C, Instruments should be spaced out and closed instruments should be opened prior to autoclaving. D, Storage of autoclaved instruments in the ultraviolet cabinet.

used. Contamination may then be minimized by placing the trays into an ultraviolet cabinet or by completely covering with sterile paper (British Medical Association 1989; Fig. 3.4D).

High-vacuum autoclaves are used to sterilize porous items, such as wrapped instruments, dressings and linen. In this type of autoclave, a vacuum is first created to enable the steam to penetrate the load more efficiently. At the end of the sterilization time, drying of the load occurs by means of the vacuum system. High-vacuum autoclaves are installed in central sterile supply departments (CSSDs) and hospital sterilizing units (HSDUs). Access to the services of a sterile supplies department is essential for all practitioners.

Regular maintenance and servicing of autoclaves is important. Daily checks to ensure that the autoclave reaches the appropriate temperature and pressure, and that these levels are maintained for the appropriate time, are necessary. A linked printer device can significantly enhance this vital quality-checking process. In addition to daily checks, autoclaves should be serviced at least annually with worn seals replaced, pressure and temperature validation and vessel pressure checks. These latter tests require specialist qualified servicing engineers to conduct, with the production of a report on the status of the autoclave and any action taken to maintain. A maintenance log should be maintained for each autoclave, providing details of all tests and maintenance performed.

Sterile packs

Costly sterilization processes will be negated if packs are wrongly stored or used. Packaging must not be damaged in any way if the contents are to remain sterile. Sterile products are marked with a 'use by' date after which their sterility cannot be guaranteed. Consequently, strict rotation of stock is necessary to avoid wastage. Contamination of the contents can occur if packs are incorrectly opened or misused. Paper autoclave bags should be opened by means of the side folds. Similarly, peelable wrapping must not be indiscriminately cut or torn open.

Single-use items

Instruments and equipment intended for single use (e.g. blades, needles and pipettes) must not be reused. Resterilization of these products is forbidden and failure to comply with this instruction invalidates the manufacturer's product liability. The practitioner then becomes liable if damage is caused to the patient as a result of using the recycled item. To prevent transmission of infection, the unused contents of single-dose containers and single-use packs should be discarded.

Disposal of clinical waste

Clinical waste generated in practice is segregated into two categories: sharps and non-sharps.

Immediate disposal of scalpel blades (sharps) is necessary on completion of treatment or if there is contamination with blood, pus or serum during treatment. Safe disposal of scalpel blades begins with careful removal of the blade from the handle. A specially designed instrument or other device gives some protection against injury (Fig. 3.5). Accidental injury caused by recapping hypodermic needles has been shown to be a common occupational hazard for hospital staff (Neuberger et al 1984). The practice of resheathing needles is generally prohibited. Dental needles are an exception, and the use of a finger guard or other safety device is necessary when

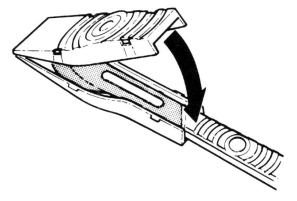

Figure 3.5 Example of a device for the safe removal of scalpel blades.

resheathing. Approved sharps containers are manufactured to Department of Health specification TSS/S/30.015. Blades, needles, syringes, glass and all other sharps are safely disposed of in these containers (Fig. 3.6).

Other clinical waste generated during patient treatment includes human tissue, soiled dressings, swabs and other contaminated material. Appropriately labelled, heavy-duty yellow plastic bags are mandatory for the storage and disposal of this type of waste. Double bagging is necessary if waste is known to be infected.

Waste awaiting collection must be stored safely in a lockable container. Responsibility for the safe disposal of clinical waste (including that generated during domiciliary treatments) ultimately rests with the practitioner (Department of the Environment 1991).

Spillages

Spillages should be dealt with immediately and in an appropriate way. Blood or other body fluid spillages should be disinfected with chlorine-releasing agents (i.e. 1% hypochlorite solution (10 000 ppm available chlorine) or chlorine-releasing granules before the area is cleared. Hypochlorites have antiviral properties and are active against HIV and HBV. Hypochlorites can damage fabrics and cause corrosion if used on metal surfaces. In these situations, 2% glutaraldehyde is a suitable alternative. Since medical history and examination cannot reliably identify all patients infected with HIV or other blood-borne pathogens, blood and body fluid precautions should be consistently used for all patients.

Health of the practitioner

As part of any infection control policy, it is incumbent on all practitioners to ensure that they do not act as sources of infection themselves. It is usual practice for all health practitioners to undergo occupational health screening and to show that they are up to date in their immunizations.

The NHS Management Executive (1993) 'Health service guidelines' requires that all practitioners who are at risk of acquiring HBV are immunized; this includes those practitioners who are at risk of coming into contact with blood or body fluids. Practitioners who do not respond to the vaccine must have routine blood checks to see if they are Be antigen (HBeAg)-positive carriers. Any practitioner who is a HBeAg-positive carrier should not perform exposure-prone procedures. Practitioners who are found to be HIV positive are advised to refrain from undertaking exposure-prone procedures, for example invasive surgery.

Liability insurance

Most health care practitioners take out professional insurance in order to provide third party cover in cases of negligence. Technically there is a difference between those practitioners who are employed and those who are self-employed and in private practice. Employers are liable for the actions of their employees who are acting in the course of their employment. This is known as

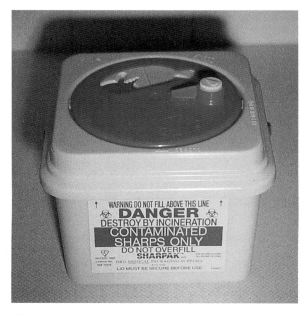

Figure 3.6   Disposal of 'sharps' into an appropriate container.

vicarious liability. The employer may also be liable, for example, by failing to set up proper working procedures or provide proper facilities for staff to do their jobs (employer negligence).

In cases of vicarious liability and negligence, it is usually the employer who pays compensation to the injured party. However, if the employee is not doing what he is employed to do, he is not protected vicariously. In this instance, the employer is likely to take counteraction and make a claim against the employee. It is because of this latter situation that many practitioners in employment elect to take up professional indemnity insurance.

Professional indemnity insurance is often included in annual subscriptions to a professional body. Practitioners should ensure that they are aware of any conditions applied by their indemnity insurance provider, including excess payments, requirements for registration, scope of practice, excluded practices, supervision requirements and any currency/CPD requirements.

If a practitioner is injured while treating patients in residential care or in their own homes, and is an employee, then the practitioner would be able to claim industrial injury benefit. Injuries resulting from the state of the premises visited are governed by the Occupiers Liability Act (1957). Unfortunately, problems may occur when attempting to gain compensation under this act. For example, the owner of a private house may not have insurance cover. If a motor vehicle is used in the course of professional practice, as in the case of domiciliary visiting or travelling between clinics, the motor insurance policy must be extended to include business usage.

In the case of a practitioner who operates a private practice, the Occupiers Liability Act (1957) imposes a duty on the practitioner to ensure that premises are safe for visitors (this includes patients). The Occupiers Liability Act (1984) extended this liability to trespassers (i.e. those who unlawfully enter premises). Public liability insurance cover may be obtained as part of a comprehensive policy, extension of a domestic policy (if the practice is part of domestic premises) or by a professional body's third party policy for members.

Practitioner–patient relationship

There are many aspects of the practitioner–patient relationship, most of which are beyond the remit of this chapter. For the purposes of this chapter the issues highlighted in Box 3.4 will be discussed.

Confidentiality

The relationship between the practitioner and the patient is a special one. Special relationships are those in which particular duties and obligations are owed and in which certain duties and obligations go beyond the scope of ordinary social conversation (Fromer 1981). The practitioner may be privy to personal, social and medical information about the patient and is, therefore, in a privileged position.

Most patients expect that the information they give will remain confidential and that they will certainly not read about it in the tabloid press the next day. Practitioners should note that, if they disclose confidential information, the burden of proof is upon the practitioner to prove it was morally justifiable (Beauchamp & Childress 1994).

It is quite legitimate for information about a patient to be shared between practitioners if it is deemed to be in the interests of the patient. In these circumstances, it is important to inform the patient of this prior to the information being passed on. The other instance where confidential information may be divulged is when a court of law requests the information or the patient has a notifiable disease.

In the majority of cases, it will be necessary for the practitioner to obtain proper consent from a patient in the form of a signed 'consent to disclosure' prior to providing details of confidential

Box 3.4 Practitioner–patient relationship

- Confidentiality
- Consent
- Complaints
- Negligence

patient records (or copies of the patient's record) to any third party. Those most often to request patient files include lawyers acting for the patient in a negligence case, and other health professionals. The patient or their proxy has a legal right of access to his/her clinical notes, and failure to provide authorized access can fall foul of the law.

Consent

When one discusses consent, a distinction needs to be made between 'informed' and 'educated' consent (Rumbold 1993). Informed consent refers to the information that a person receives, while educated consent relates to the ability of the patient to arrive at a reasoned decision based on that information. It is now generally accepted in health care practice that treatment should not be given without the patient's educated consent. This has not always been the case, and there are still those who consider that the practitioner has a right to undertake treatment that he or she thinks would be for the benefit of the patient. This is known as 'therapeutic privilege' and is still used when the patient is unable to give educated consent. An example of such a situation is when a patient is unconscious after a road traffic accident.

Before a patient gives educated consent, full details of the treatment, its indications, risks and contraindications, as well as details of alternative treatments, must be communicated to the patient. The patient has to be able to understand the nature of the information in order to make an educated decision. If a patient is considered unable to give educated consent, it is good practice to discuss the issue with the next of kin. In cases where patients consider they have been treated without their consent, they can claim assault and take out a criminal or civil case against the practitioner. It is then up to a court of law to decide whether there is a case.

With regard to children, it is customary practice that parents or guardians are informed of the procedure and their consent obtained. However, there is no law that states this must be so. Defining who is a child is not easy. In general, anyone who meets the criteria outlined below, whatever their age, can be deemed to be able to give consent to treatment:

- possesses a set of values and goals
- is able to communicate and understand information
- has the ability to reason and deliberate about one's choice (President's Commission 1982).

Consent is not binding; patients may withdraw their consent when they want. Patients' autonomy should be respected: all patients have the right to refuse treatment. Further information on medicolegal aspects of practice is covered in Chapter 4.

Complaints

From time to time, patient complaints may be made against an individual practitioner. Such complaints are usually about the manner in which the patient was treated or the actual treatment received.

At all times it is important that the practitioner acts in a manner to safeguard and promote the interests of the patient. If a patient wishes to make a formal complaint, this should be put in writing. The Patient's Charter (Department of Health 1995) specifies that every citizen has the right to 'have any complaint about NHS services (whoever provides them) investigated and to get a quick, full written reply from the relevant chief executive or general manager'. All NHS Trusts should have formal, documented policies and procedures related to the handling of complaints.

Staff training should be given on the implementation and operation of these policies and procedures. Similarly, sufficient information about making complaints should be publicized to patients, relatives, carers and the public. Complaints should be regarded in a positive light as they act as valuable feedback on the quality of services provided.

Patients who wish to make formal complaints about a practitioner in the private sector should be referred to the appropriate statutory and/or professional body.

Negligence

Negligence is considered to have occurred when the acceptable standards of care towards others are not met. These acceptable standards of care emanate from the customs, policies and practices of that profession. The dividing line between acceptable and unacceptable standards of care is often difficult to draw. Hence, cases of negligence are usually decided by courts of law and involve an array of 'expert' witnesses. Usually practitioners are judged to have been negligent when they knowingly did not observe acceptable standards or when they did not take into consideration known (usually cited in the literature) side-effects or other problems associated with a treatment.

With the advent of 'no win–no fee' type legal services, the number of initial claims against health providers is increasing. However, the number of cases that reach the courts are relatively few. Practitioners who are subject of negligence or other legal claims should avoid the temptation to respond directly to the patient or their legal representatives, instead referring all communications via the practitioner's profes-sional body or indemnity insurance provider. Failure to do so could result in the indemnity insurance provider refusing to meet any claims. Most negligence claims rely heavily on written records, including the patient's case notes. Therefore, it is essential that all practitioners maintain accurate, comprehensive, up to date and legible case notes for all patients.

SUMMARY

Health care practitioners are in a privileged position and should not abuse that privilege. At all times, the interests of the patient should be of paramount importance. All practitioners should practice within current legislation and observe codes of practice of appropriate bodies. Ovretveit (1992) believes that quality methods and philosophies, adapted to the special circumstances of the health services, will emerge as the most important response to health provision in the future. If practitioners adopt appropriate and effective protocols into their clinical practice, they should be in a position to offer their patients safe treatment and achieve high standards of care.

REFERENCES

Babb J R 1963 Cleaning of hospital floors with oiled mops. Journal of Hygiene 61: 393

Bate J G 1961 Bacteriological investigations of exhaust air from hospital vacuum cleaners. Lancet i: 159

Baumann M A 1992 Protective gloves. International Dental Journal 42: 170–180

Beauchamp T, Childress J 1994 Principles of biomedical ethics, 4th edn. Oxford University Press, New York, p 70

Bendig J W A 1991 Surgical hand disinfection: comparison of 4% chlorhexidine detergent solution and 2% triclosan detergent solution. Journal of Hospital Infection 15: 143–148

British Medical Association 1989 A code of practice for ster-ilisation of instruments and control of cross infection. British Medical Association, London

Combs R 1992 Clinic designed for two practices. Dental Economics 82: 51–54

Cremieux A, Reverdy M, Pons J et al 1989 Standardized method for evaluation of hand disinfection by surgical scrub formulations. Applied and environmental micro-biology 55: 2944–2948

Department of the Environment 1991 Waste management. The duty of care: a code of practice. HMSO, London

Department of Health 1990 A further evaluation of trans-portable steam sterilisers for unwrapped instruments and utensils. HEI No. 196. NHS Procurement Directorate, London

Department of Health 1991 The patient's charter. HMSO, London

Department of Health 1995 The patient's charter. HMSO, London

Disability Discrimination Act 1995. HMOS, London

Douglas C W I 1989 The use of various handwashing agents to decontaminate gloved hands. British Dental Journal 167: 62–65

Fromer M J 1981 Ethical issues in health care. Mosby, St Louis, MO

Health and Safety at Work Act 1974. HMSO, London

Health and Safety Executive 1988 Committee for Substances Hazardous to Health. HMSO, London

Health and Safety Executive 1989 Memorandum of guidance on the Electricity at Work regulations. HMSO, London

Health and Safety Executive 1990a Writing a safety policy statement: advice to employers HSC 6. HMSO, London

Health and Safety Executive 1990b Guidance note PM73: safety of autoclaves. HMSO: London

Health and Safety Executive 1993a Code of practice for workplace health, safety and welfare. HMSO, London

Health and Safety Executive 1993b COSHH. A step by step

guide. HMSO, London

Knittle M A, Eitzman D, Herman Baer M 1975 Role of hand contamination of personnel in the epidemiology of Gram-negative nosocomial infections. Journal of Paediatrics 86: 433

Larson E 1988 A causal link between handwashing and risk of infection? Examination of the evidence. Infection Control Hospital Epidemiology 9: 28–36

Maki D G 1989 The use of antiseptics for handwashing by medical personnel. Journal of Chemotherapy 1: 5–11

Maurer I M 1985 Hospital hygiene, 3rd edn. Edward Arnold, London

Mitchell R, Cumming C, MacLennan W, Ross P, Peuther J, Baxter A 1983 The use of operating gloves in dental practice. British Dental Journal 154: 372–374

Neuberger J S, Harris J, Kundin W, Bischane A, Chin T 1984 Incidence of needlestick injuries in hospital personnel: implications for prevention. American Journal of Infection Control 12: 171–176

NHS Management Executive 1993 Health service guidelines HSG(93)40. Department of Health, London

Occupiers Liability Act 1957. HMSO, London

Occupiers Liability Act 1984. HMSO, London

Ovretveit J 1992 Health service quality. An introduction to quality methods for health services. Blackwell Scientific, London

President's Commission for the study of ethical problems in medicine and biomedical and behavioral research 1982. Making health care decisions. US Government Printing Office, Washington, DC

Pressure Systems and Transportable Gas Container Regulations 1989. HMSO, London

Professions Supplementary to Medicine Act 1960. HMSO, London

Rumbold G 1993 Ethics in nursing practice. Ballière Tindall, London, p 94–99

Sharma S K 1991 Hand dermatitis from gloves. Occupation Environmental Medicine Reports 5: 45–48

Ward K 1990 Dirt in hospitals. All that glitters. Nursing Times 86: 32–34

FURTHER READING

Society of Chiropodists and Podiatrists 1992 Guidelines on Health and Safety at Work. Society of Chiropodists and Podiatrists, London

4

Clinical emergencies

Robert S. Moore

INTRODUCTION

All clinicians have a duty of care to their patients, and the patient has expectations of safety during treatment when attending a clinic for any kind of treatment. This applies to those visiting a GP, to individuals seeking dental treatment and to others undergoing major surgery. It should, therefore, equally apply to people seeking the services of a podiatrist. In any branch of medicine, complications can arise as a result of treatment. On occasion, these complications can be life threatening. Other crises can arise as a result of natural disease processes. It behoves the practitioner to be able to provide initial treatment for the patient until such time as further medical care becomes available. The main difficulty for those who are not routinely exposed to medical crises is one of recognition. Too often, individuals overreact to circumstances that are misconstrued as being life threatening but that often require simple, yet effective, measures to remedy.

The aim of this chapter is to highlight the nature of medical emergencies, to describe the pathological processes involved, to describe the common modes of presentation and to provide a framework on which to base early treatment. It will also provide the reader with information that should make provisional diagnosis more reliable.

THE NATURE OF MEDICAL EMERGENCIES

The definition of acute medical emergency is not as straightforward as it might at first seem.

Doctors tend to regard this status as being one where, without immediate treatment, there will be some irreversible pathological change. This may not necessarily imply loss of life. The difference comes in the time needed to take remedial action. Actions to save sight after a retinal detachment take on an urgency wherein treatment is likely to be necessary in a matter of some few hours, yet if a person suffers a cardiac arrest following myocardial infarction, treatment must be immediate.

Patients will also have their own idea of what constitutes an emergency. Pain is a common reason for attendance at accident and emergency departments, and urgent relief is sought and provided (Fig. 4.1). In these situations, though, it is frequently the case that there is no clinical 'emergency', that is, there is no immediate danger to life or limb. This difference in perception of the urgency of a situation often leads to difficulties in the busy accident and emergency department. Patients attend with a variety of painful conditions, and because of their pain, all are seeking rapid relief and treatment. However, some kind of sorting has to take place to identify those that require rapid intervention.

Triage is a concept that has been known since the period of the Napoleonic Wars. The majority of modern accident units now operate a system of early rapid assessment of all patients soon after arrival at the department (Fig. 4.2). This is normally performed by an experienced and adequately trained nurse. This nurse can identify patients who need rapid treatment and/or pain relief. Patients are prioritized and grouped into 'streams', each of which has a dedicated team of doctors and nurses. The various streams are described in Box 4.1. The outcome of treatment within the hospital environment for emergencies that arise within the community is frequently determined by the quality of prehospital care that is provided, and this is especially true in the case of resuscitation after witnessed cardiac arrest. Studies in the USA (Eisenberg et al 1979) have clearly indicated better outcomes for the management of cardiac arrest in areas where community programmes for the training of citizens in 'basic cardiac life support' have been implemented. Similar schemes in the UK have only been partially successful (Vincent et al 1984). The moral obligation on podiatrists and other health workers is clear. All should be capable of procedures that can hold a critical situation until such time as a higher level of expertise becomes available. However, this higher level of expertise is no longer confined to

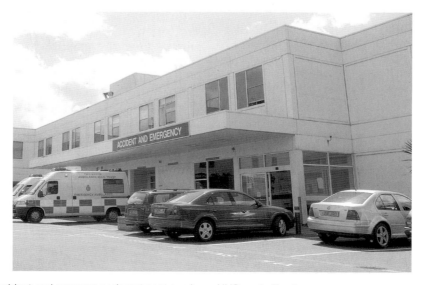

Figure 4.1 An accident and emergency department serving a NHS acute Trust.

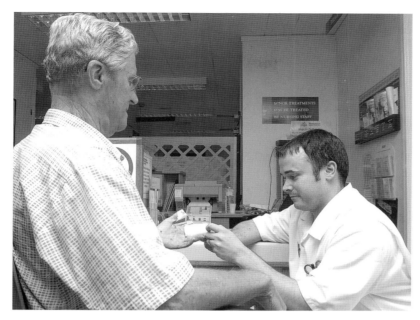

Figure 4.2 Early rapid assessment is crucial to determining treatment priority and moving the patient into the appropriate stream.

medical personnel. Ambulance crews who respond to initial calls are now commonly trained in advanced skills such as endotracheal intubation, defibrillation and intravenous cannulation. These 'paramedics' have undergone systematic training in the theoretical and practical aspects of emergency management at the scene of an incident. Furthermore, advances in

technology are allowing the extension of life-saving skills into groups formerly associated with first-aid practice only.

In summary, the management of any medical emergency requires a team of health care workers, as described in Box 4.2.

Medicolegal aspects of practice

In everyday practice, the most important factor to be considered after decisions have been taken regarding treatment is the question of consent. Without the consent of the patient, any act of

---

Box 4.1 Categorization of patients upon arrival at accident and emergency department

- **Minors:** patient has a non-life-threatening condition requiring simple investigation and treatment. This care can equally be provided by doctor or emergency nurse practitioner.
- **Assessment:** patient is more acutely ill or injured and will require more extensive investigation and observation. Typically the patient is being considered for hospital admission.
- **Resuscitation:** patient is acutely ill and is certain to be admitted. He/she may be in need of intensive support.
- **Children:** most departments make special arrangements for the care of children.

Box 4.2 Team of health care workers for the management of a medical emergency

- First responder: passer-by, friend, podiatrist, nurse, GP, etc.
- Primary care: paramedic, GP, hospital flying squad
- Secondary care: district general hospital/accident and emergency department
- Tertiary care: regional centre, e.g. burns unit.

surgical intervention can be construed as an assault upon the person, whether or not it might be in that person's best interests.

Consent can be implicit or explicit (Knight 1992, McClay 1996). Implicit consent is normally inferred from the cooperation of the patient by his attendance at the clinic or by his compliance during treatment. Explicit consent is necessary for more intimate examinations and surgical procedures. Explicit consent can be obtained verbally but requires a third party to act as a witness. Written consent provides a more secure form of record. In 1985, the concept of 'informed' consent was introduced, which established the need for practitioners to balance the major risks against the potential benefits entailed in a procedure, while still allowing them some discretion with regard to individual cases.

The Family Law Reform Act (1985) laid down that individuals of sound mind were able to give consent from the age of 16, although the advice from the courts concerning the rights of older children has been a little unclear since then. The Gillick case (1984) highlighted the need for parental involvement wherever possible in the management of young people. Parental consent can be overruled in special circumstances, where it is thought to be in the child's best interests. This may involve the child being effectively removed to a 'fit person' to allow, usually life-saving, treatment.

The ability to give consent implies a level of rationality and competence. Unconsciousness prevents this, and in these circumstances close relatives may be approached though legally they do not have the power to provide consent by proxy (Marquand 2000). If the situation is life threatening, treatment may be implemented on the assumption that the practitioner is acting in the best interests of the patient. Low intelligence does not affect the ability to give consent provided that the person retains the capacity to consent (i.e. he/she can appreciate the nature of the treatment, its rationale and its consequences). Patients detained under the Mental Health Act (1983) only forfeit their right of consent regarding their metal disorder but remain able to provide consent for other medical treatment,

provided they are deemed competent. Clearly, voluntary patients in a mental institution can give consent provided they have the capacity to comprehend the state of their own health.

CARDIOVASCULAR EMERGENCIES

All tissues of the body rely on an adequate cardiac output to maintain tissue oxygenation and to remove the products of local metabolism. If tissue perfusion is interrupted, then injury will follow. The period required for cell death is variable but is most acute in the brain, where hypoxic damage begins after only 4 minutes. Other sensitive areas include the kidney and the heart itself. The normal cardiac output in a resting adult is approximately 5 l/min. The ability of the heart to achieve this depends on three physiological variables.

- *Preload*. This describes the state of filling of the venous circulation and the filling pressure of the right ventricle. This can be assessed by taking measurements of the jugular venous pressure (JVP).
- *Afterload*. This refers to the resistance against which the heart has to pump. This reflects the tone of the arteriolar and capillary circulation, which, in turn, responds to changes in the sympathetic nervous system. Systemic blood pressure is an indirect measure of this.
- *Contractility of the myocardium*. This affects the force and efficiency of myocardial contraction and can be measured as the stroke volume.

Conditions such as myocardial infarction can lead to rapid alterations of these parameters and lead to reduction or loss of cardiac output, with serious consequences.

Cardiac arrest

Cardiac arrest will, if not recognized and treated immediately, lead rapidly to death. It is characterized by cardiac standstill detectable by the absence of the central pulses, rapid loss of consciousness and, within a few minutes, respiratory arrest. It is frequently associated with loss of sphincter control, manifest by gastric regurgitation and incontinence. It may arise as a result of a primary cardiac disturbance, such as acute myocardial infarction, or secondary to some other event such as asphyxia or massive haemorrhage. There are three recognized modes of cardiac arrest:

- *Ventricular fibrillation.* The fibres of the myocardium contract chaotically so that the pumping action of the heart is lost but there remains electrical activity detectable on an electrocardiograph (ECG). This electrical disturbance is potentially reversible, but only if treatment is delivered within a few minutes of onset.
- *Asystole.* There is no activity in the heart at all and no electrical activity is detected. This is rarely reversible and often follows on from prolonged ventricular fibrillation.
- *Pulseless electrical activity.* There is no activity within the heart but there is still electrical activity seen on an ECG. This condition is usually terminal, although, as it can follow certain physical derangements such as cardiac tamponade or massive haemorrhage, it is important for the clinician to look for an underlying cause.

The only effective treatment for cardiac arrest is defibrillation (Fig. 4.3). This technique has, in the past, been restricted to medical personnel, trained paramedics and some members of the nursing profession working in coronary care and intensive care units (ICUs). The introduction and wide acceptance of automated external defibrillators (Fig. 4.4) has significantly extended the availability of resources to diagnose and treat this condition. Guidelines for advanced cardiac life support were revised by the Resuscitation Council (UK) (2000) and the International Liaison Committee on Resuscitation. The importance of early treatment continues to be emphasized and there is encouragement for the professions allied to medicine to extend their training to facilitate a rapid response. If defibrillation is unavoidably delayed, the priority is to maintain some kind of rudimentary circulation to protect the brain. This is achieved by the basic life-support measures of maintaining a clear airway, ventilating the lungs and carrying out external cardiac compression (see Fig. 4.10, below). All first-aid courses teach these skills. Training in the full sequence of care is brought together in advanced life support

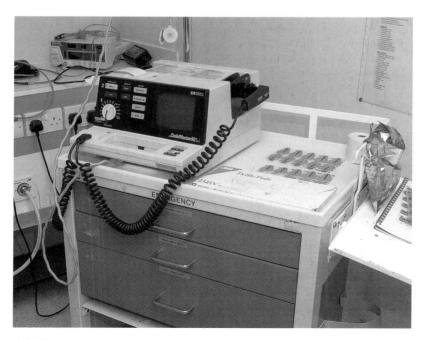

Figure 4.3 Manual defibrillator.

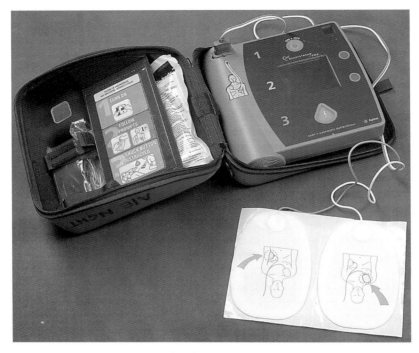

Figure 4.4   Portable automated external defibrillator (AED).

(ALS) and intermediate life support (ILS) courses in the UK and other countries.

Acute myocardial infarction

An estimated 300 000 people suffer a heart attack every year in the UK and about 140 000 die, many in the first hour after the onset of symptoms (British Heart Foundation Database 1999). Untreated, there is a 40–50% mortality within the first 2 hours of onset of symptoms (Fulton et al 1969). The primary disturbance is an interruption to the normal perfusion of the myocardium, leading to muscle necrosis and dysfunction. This change in perfusion can arise from a sudden vascular occlusion caused by thrombus formation in a coronary vessel or it can sometimes result from a spasm in the wall of an arteriole. The acute event may lead to ventricular fibrillation and other cardiac rhythm abnormalities. In other circumstances, the pump action of the heart may be impaired, leading to heart failure. The area around the dead (infracted) tissue is liable to be ischaemic and will lead to chest pain and rhythm disturbances. The pain is characteristically described as being retrosternal, tight and constricting, and frequently radiates into the left arm and up into the neck. It can sometimes be difficult for clinicians to distinguish this pain from that of oesophageal reflux or heartburn. Treatment depends upon early recognition and diagnosis. This allows the early administration of drugs that can reestablish vascular patency by breaking down the thrombus (thrombolysis). The first-line management comprises calling an ambulance to the scene, administering oxygen, sitting the patient up and giving a single tablet of *aspirin* if it is known that there is no contraindication. Aspirin in small doses reduces platelet adhesiveness and supports thrombolytic therapy. Adequate pain relief is usually only obtained by the use of morphine or one of its derivatives, although glyceryl trinitrate (GTN) may be of help.

Massive pulmonary embolism

A pulmonary embolism is an acute obstruction of the pulmonary circulation caused by a large blood clot impacting in the pulmonary artery. This clot usually develops in the peripheral venous circulation, most commonly in the pelvic bed or the lower limb. The clot then fragments and travels to the heart via the inferior vena cava. The primary event of deep venous thrombosis is associated with prolonged periods of bed rest or immobility, such as that encountered after major surgery. It is also linked to cigarette smoking and the use of oral contraceptives.

The mode of presentation is often identical to that of primary cardiac arrest, with severe central chest pain, sudden collapse, lack of pulse and loss of consciousness. However, there may be an antecedent history of chest pains caused by earlier minor emboli reaching the lungs. The patient may have a history of recent surgery. Electromechanical dissociation is more commonly encountered on ECG monitoring as the heart vainly attempts to beat against the obstruction. Treatment follows the guidelines for any cardiac arrest, but the results of treatment are poor. Success is more likely in centres equipped with access to thoracotomy and emergency cardiopulmonary bypass.

Massive haemorrhage

Haemorrhage refers to the extravasation of whole blood from the circulation. It can be described as internal (occult) or external (overt). External or overt haemorrhage refers to bleeding that is apparent, such as that from a laceration or nosebleed. Internal or occult bleeding can arise from injury to abdominal viscera or duodenal ulceration. When haemorrhage is severe, its recognition is crucial to the early and effective treatment of hypovolaemic shock.

Shock has been defined as 'inadequate perfusion of the tissues', but in all events leads to local hypoxia and cell death. Hypovolaemia is one cause of this state and its treatment is designed to minimize and reduce the duration of tissue hypoxia. The longer the duration of shock the more likely the chance that life-threatening complications will ensue. These complications range from early death to adult respiratory distress syndrome and acute renal failure.

The response of the body to haemorrhage is governed by activity within the sympathetic autonomic nervous system. These responses are at their most efficient in youth and become steadily attenuated with increasing age: hence the greater tolerance to haemorrhage in the young. The early response to haemorrhage comprises decreased activity in the baroceptors of the carotid sinus and aortic arch, which then causes a reflex increase in peripheral sympathetic tone. This clinically manifests as vasoconstriction in the skin and kidneys, with reduced urine output. This increase in peripheral vascular resistance helps to maintain blood pressure and perfusion to important areas. A further increase in sympathetic activity will raise the heart rate. These compensatory changes will usually be adequate for losses of up to 1 litre. When the loss exceeds this amount, or it has been incurred too quickly for the system to cope, then blood pressure will fall. If the fall is profound or prolonged, the problems mentioned above will appear. In particular, if haemorrhage is ongoing, then cerebral perfusion fails, leading to drowsiness, coma and death. This is likely with losses of 3 litres if not treated.

It is necessary to recognize life-threatening haemorrhage quickly and to replace fluid losses promptly. This will require early venous cannulation and transfusion. It is perhaps more important, in the first place, to attempt to arrest the bleeding, provided this can be achieved without delay. When the bleeding is from an open wound, haemostasis can usually be obtained by simple direct pressure over the wound via a simple dressing. This is aided by elevation of the injured part. This is particularly applicable to patients suffering heavy bleeding from rupture of a varicose vein at the ankle. In general, tourniquets are rarely necessary but, if applied, should be released every 20 minutes to prevent tissue ischaemia. When available, oxygen should be given to all patients sustaining a major haemorrhage. The presence of hypovolaemia related to haemorrhage has been recognized in recent years as being a leading cause of preventable death after trauma. The implementation of training in advanced trauma life support for clinicians has made significant progress in remedying this. Members of professions allied to medicine are also undergoing training.

RESPIRATORY EMERGENCIES

While the cardiovascular system provides a means of transport of metabolites around the body, the respiratory system is the means for exchange of oxygen and carbon dioxide with the atmosphere. There are a number of anatomical and physiological features that optimize this function. As with the cardiovascular system, if any of these features are suddenly impaired, pathological changes rapidly follow.

Physiology

The most obvious sign of life is breathing. This semiautomatic activity is necessary for ventilation of the lungs and renewal of the quality of alveolar air. It depends on a clear airway from the nasopharynx to the alveolus. It further depends upon an intact neuromuscular system connecting the respiratory centres of the brainstem to the intercostal muscles and diaphragm via the spinal cord. Finally, there is the need for structural integrity of the ribcage and pleural membranes, thereby allowing the mechanical effects of muscular contraction to be transferred to the lungs, enabling inflation and deflation.

Ventilation brings oxygen-rich air to the alveolus, but at this point the determining feature becomes the permeability of the capillary membranes to oxygen and carbon dioxide. This may be impaired by increased secretions, oedema or pathological processes that have caused scarring and thickening of the alveolar walls.

Pneumothorax

Lying between the lungs and the ribcage is the pleural space enclosed by the pleural membranes. This is usually only a potential space,

and the two layers of membrane are separated by a thin film of fluid. The pressure within this space is normally slightly negative with respect to atmospheric pressure, so that when the ribcage expands it indirectly exerts a bellows effect on the underlying lung, causing it to be inflated. If air should leak into this space, for example as a result of breakdown of a congenital bulla on the surface of the lung or a puncture trauma from a fractured rib, then the underlying lung will fall back from the ribcage and will not ventilate adequately. This will lead to poor oxygenation of the blood and systemic hypoxia. This condition is known as pneumothorax (Fig. 4.5). If it should happen that a one-way valve effect arises, whereby air can enter the pleural cavity but is trapped, then the intrapleural pressure will rise and quickly impair ventilation of the opposite lung and will later affect the venous return to the heart. This is a life-threatening emergency known as *tension pneumothorax* and has the capacity to cause death within minutes. It requires the rapid intervention of a clinician to allow escape of air to the exterior and reduce the intrathoracic pressure. This is achieved by aspiration of air from the intrapleural space or

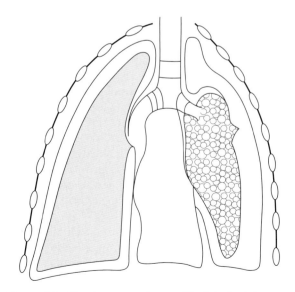

Figure 4.5 Simple pneumothorax with air in the left pleural space.

by placing a sterile plastic tube or chest drain through an intercostal space into the pleural cavity. This is then attached to a one-way valve system to prevent the return of air into the chest. Guidance on the method of choice has been issued by the British Thoracic Society (Miller and Harvey 1993).

Spontaneous pneumothorax commonly affects young healthy males but can arise in the elderly population as a complication of chronic obstructive airways disease. Traumatic pneumothorax can complicate almost any insult to the thorax, be it blunt or penetrating in origin. The common symptoms include unilateral chest pain that is worse on inspiration, shortness of breath and a history of a similar event. The patient, particularly if young, may be in little distress. In contrast, the patient with a tension pneumothorax will be extremely distressed by severe breathlessness, cyanosed with hypoxia and will rapidly lose consciousness unless treatment follows rapidly.

Asthma

Asthma is common, with a prevalence of between 1 and 40%, depending on geography. Evidence suggests that the true incidence is rising (Cochrane et al 1996). It is a condition characterized by a variable and intermittent degree of lower airway obstruction caused by narrowing of bronchioles. This narrowing can arise from smooth muscle hyperreactivity or from oedema of the mucosa. An acute attack commonly arises from a combination of the two. The characteristic symptom is breathlessness associated with an expiratory wheeze. Attacks may be spontaneous but frequently appear to be associated with upper respiratory tract viral infections. Other common associations are with exposure to allergens, such as grass pollen or animal hair, and with exercise. Asthma can vary in severity from a slight wheeze with nocturnal cough to a life-threatening situation where death may rapidly result without the highest standards of intensive care. A significant number of people still die each year from this ailment (1.5–3.0/10 000 per annum in the Western world

(Burney 1992) and guidelines have been revised for the medical management of this disease (British Guidelines on Asthma 1997).

The control of asthma is tailored according to the severity of symptoms in the individual. At one extreme, the patient may carry an aerosol inhaler containing a bronchodilator such as salbutamol or terbutaline (Fig. 4.6). This would be used only when symptomatic. If symptoms were more frequent, sodium chromoglycate might be added as a prophylactic agent. In the presence of recurrent wheeze, an inhaled steroid might also be indicated. When a severe attack intervenes, these drugs may be given in the nebulized state, providing a higher dose and a more reliable means of delivery. If this mode of treatment is implemented in the community and fails to lead to a rapid improvement, then the patient must be referred to hospital without delay. Asthma is unpredictable and dangerous, and medical advice must be sought whenever there is doubt about the severity of symptoms.

Obstructed airway

The airway is the area extending from the lips or nostrils to the alveoli. Obstruction of the airway will rapidly lead to hypoxia. In contrast to asthma, the wheeze that develops is generally inspiratory and is referred to as *stridor*. When stridor is acute, the patient will be distressed and there will be signs of rib recession and activity in the accessory muscles of respiration in the neck. Any object, if inhaled, can cause this. Commoner items include nuts, boiled sweets and, in children, marbles and similar trinkets. These may affect the normal healthy individual with normal reflexes, but in the individual whose consciousness is clouded by virtue of disease or drugs, the risk is higher because of attenuation of the normal protective cough reflexes. A common cause of respiratory obstruction in these circumstances is occlusion of the pharynx by the tongue dropping backwards through loss of muscular tone. Substances or items that may also be troublesome in these circumstances include broken or false teeth, food and vomit. In all circumstances, the need for early recognition

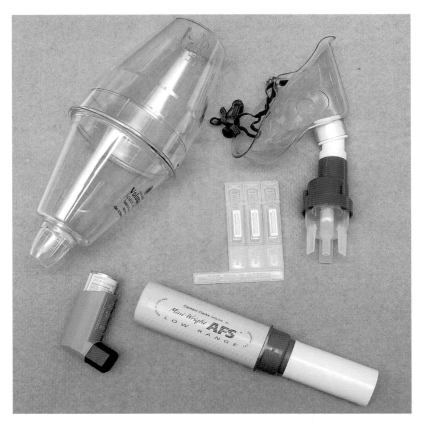

Figure 4.6 Therapeutic tools for asthma (anticlockwise from bottom right): peak flow meter, drugs and nebulizer mask, spacer and aerosol inhaler.

and relief must be emphasized. Simple remedies include safe positioning of the obtunded patient (Fig. 4.7), lifting the jaw to clear the tongue from the back of the pharynx and ensuring that there are no objects obstructing the back of the mouth. Surgical manoeuvres such as cricothyroidotomy are sometimes indicated in extreme circumstances in order to maintain an airway in life-threatening situations

NEUROLOGICAL EMERGENCIES

Epilepsy

Epilepsy is a term used to describe a wide spectrum of convulsive disorders that are either idiopathic or secondary to brain abnormalities such as a tumour or scarring following injury. Two common forms are grand mal and petit mal fits. The former is the classic tonic–clonic convulsion, in which the individual suddenly loses consciousness, sometimes after experiencing an 'aura', and collapses. There then follows a period of shaking of all the limbs before the patient relaxes into a period of stupor or unconsciousness (the post-ictal period) for a variable period. This kind of fit is a feature of local anaesthetic toxicity. If the period of convulsing is brief, then all that is required is to put the person into the recovery position (Fig. 4.8) and to remove sources of danger. If the fit has not stopped within 3–4 minutes, urgent treatment is required, and an ambulance must be called.

The other common kind of fit is called petit mal and is more common in the young. It takes

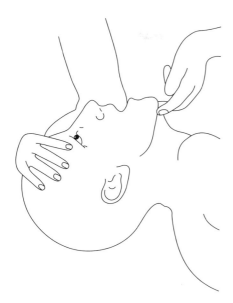

Figure 4.7   Maintaining the airway.

the form of brief 'absences' where the child suddenly appears to be daydreaming and then, just as suddenly, snaps out of it. It is rarely dangerous and, by virtue of its brief nature, often goes undiagnosed for some time.

Epilepsy can be well controlled by drugs such as phenytoin and carbamazepine, but prolonged fits require the parenteral administration of diazepam or lorazepam. With diazepam, the most rapid route of administration is intravenous, but it can also be given rectally to good effect in children. An intravenous dose of 5–10 mg is usually adequate for adults.

Subarachnoid haemorrhage

The meninges are a membranous covering of the brain and spinal cord that provide support and protection in addition to that afforded by the skull and spinal column. They are divided into three layers: the dura mater, which is a thick membrane lying immediately within the skull; the arachnoid mater, a thin membrane lining the dura; and the pia mater, which is very thin and fragile and adheres to the brain surface and spinal cord. Blood vessels supplying the underlying brain traverse the subarachnoid space on their way to the cortex. Occasionally, one of these vessels can rupture, causing a subarachnoid haemorrhage. This may be totally spontaneous, but frequently the site of rupture is a small area of dilatation of an arterial vessel known as a *berry aneurysm*. This is a developmental abnormality that may be asymptomatic until rupture. Another cause is the presence of an arteriovenous malformation.

The common mode of presentation is a sudden onset of severe headache associated with disturbed consciousness or confusion, nausea and vomiting, and visual disturbance. There is frequently a history of minor headaches in the weeks preceding a major incident, indicating earlier small bleeds. Unfortunately, these earlier episodes often go unheeded. Subarachnoid haemorrhage has a significant mortality and is no respector of age. Its frequently devastating effect on the brain can lead to rapid brain death in an otherwise healthy individual. Families of

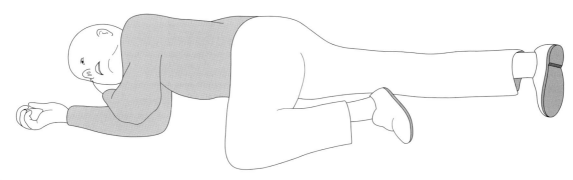

Figure 4.8   The recovery position.

the victims are frequently approached with regard to organ donation. Conversely, if the disorder is recognized early before severe brain injury has resulted, then neurosurgical intervention to clip off the offending vessel can be life saving.

Cerebrovascular accident

The term cerebrovascular accident (CVA) is a collective expression to describe injuries to the brain arising from an interruption to the normal blood supply of the brain substance. The term, therefore, includes subarachnoid haemorrhage, but it is normally used to describe incidents affecting the older generation. The popular term in the UK is 'stroke'. In older age groups, the development of cerebral ischaemia is a gradual process mediated by disease and degenerative changes such as atherosclerosis and atheroma. The damaged vessels are then more prone to occlusion by thrombus or to rupture. The incidence of cerebrovascular disease is 2/1000 per annum (Wade 1988) and is related to hypertension and cigarette smoking. Typically, in the elderly, stroke presents as an acute onset of weakness affecting one side of the body, with clouding of the conscious level and a variable degree of speech disturbance. The extent of brain injury determines the outcome and long-term morbidity. Early treatment consists of the administration of oxygen and care of the airways/breathing/circulation by resuscitation. In the longer term, the departments of physiotherapy, occupational therapy and speech therapy assume a high profile in rehabilitation.

On occasion, the classical symptoms of CVA may develop only to pass off again within a few hours. This syndrome is known as a transient ischaemic attack (TIA). These attacks may be frequent and may be the precursor to a complete CVA. At other times, TIA is an infrequent event that does not progress any further. Initial treatment comprises simple observation. Later, intervention may be considered with antiplatelet agents such as aspirin or dipyridamole, to lessen the risk of thrombotic episodes.

METABOLIC CRISES

Hypoglycaemia

Hypoglycaemia refers to the condition where the level of glucose in the bloodstream falls below normal levels. The normal blood glucose level is 2–8 mmol/l. The commonest cause for this abnormality is uncontrolled diabetes mellitus. The patient receiving regular insulin supplements may have injected too much insulin or may have missed a meal after a normal insulin dose. In either case, there is a relative excess of insulin, causing a fall in blood glucose. Other causes include the delayed hypoglycaemia associated with excessive alcohol consumption (this is particularly common in the young) and the rare hormone-secreting tumour insulinoma.

The early effects of hypoglycaemia result from dysfunction of the brain. Glucose is the only energy-supplying substrate for brain tissue and any lack rapidly leads to dysfunction. Signs and symptoms are similar to those of acute anxiety, with apprehension and agitation, tremor and clamminess. The patient will appear pale and becomes confused, and sometimes aggressive, before slipping into coma if treatment is not quickly given. Early treatment is reliant upon the administration of a carbohydrate load or simple glucose. If consciousness is lost, recovery usually follows the intravenous administration of 50% dextrose solution. Another remedy, sometimes carried by ambulance paramedics, is glucagon. This is a naturally occurring hormone that, following intramuscular injection, leads to rapid mobilization of glucose from the liver by stimulating breakdown of glycogen stores.

The need for rapid reversal of hypoglycaemia cannot be stressed too highly, as prolongation will lead to permanent brain injury.

Acute anaphylaxis

Acute anaphylaxis is a life-threatening emergency with a speed of onset of dramatic proportions. It follows the exposure of a susceptible individual to a substance or allergen that triggers a dramatic release of histamine from mast cells throughout the body. There is usually a history of previous exposure and similar, though often less-severe, reactions. Common allergens include drugs such as penicillin, some foodstuffs (e.g. nuts and strawberries), some vaccines (e.g. tetanus toxoid) and bee stings. Even a small exposure to allergen can lead to a severe reaction. The widespread release of histamine within the body leads to a catastrophic increase in capillary permeability and vascular dilatation. This is manifest as a dramatic fall in systemic blood pressure. Other more local effects of histamine release include widespread urticaria (hives), flushing of the skin and bronchospasm, causing breathlessness and wheeze.

Without prompt treatment the patient may quickly die. The first-line treatment consists of the intramuscular injection of epinephrine (adrenaline; 0.5 mg). It may also be given intravenously, but lower doses and more caution are required because of the high risk of cardiac arrhythmias. For this reason, epinephrine should only be administered intravenously in a hospital setting. Epinephrine should be followed by appropriate intravenous fluid replacement and the administration of antihistamines (chlorpheniramine) and steroids (hydrocortisone and/or prednisolone). Patients with life-threatening reactions frequently require management on an intensive care unit. Further guidance for first-responders is available from the Resuscitation Council of the UK (2002) and is described in Figure 4.9. A better method of management, however, is prevention. This can usually be secured by taking a full history before the administration of any new agents, particularly antibiotics. Appropriate alternatives can then be used in treatment. Some patients with a known susceptibility carry supplies of epinephrine (adrenaline) about their person for self-administration in the event of an emergency.

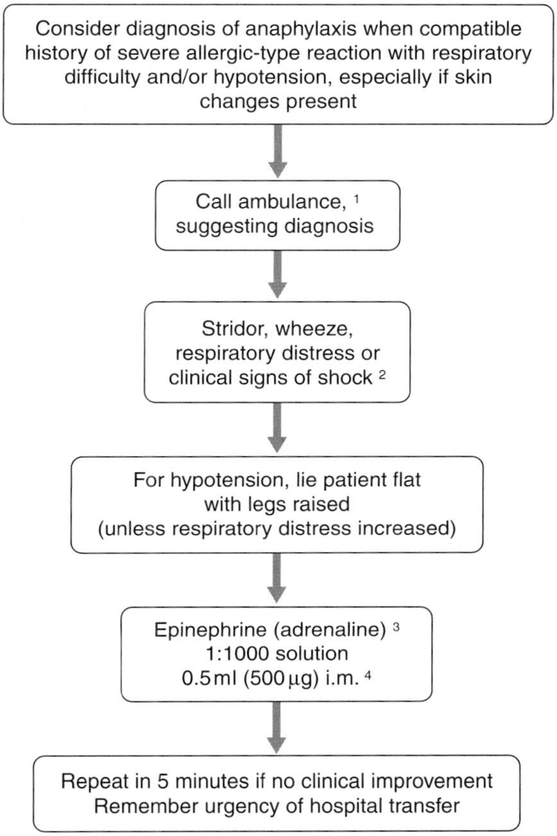

SOME SUBACUTE EMERGENCIES

Congestive heart failure

Congestive heart failure is a common condition in the elderly and is usually secondary to

Figure 4.9 Management of anaphylaxis for non-medical responders.

1. Ambulance will be equipped with oxygen, salbutamol and fluids, which may be used as adjunctive therapy.
2. If profound shock judged to be *immediately life threatening* give cardiopulmonary resuscitation (CPR)/advanced (cardiac) life support (ALS) if necessary.
3. Half doses of epinephrine (adrenaline) may be safer for patients taking amitriptyline, imipramine, or a beta blocker.
4. If adults are treated with an Epipen, the 300 mg dose will usually be sufficient. A second dose may be required, but this should be considered *only* if the patient's condition continues to deteriorate 5 minutes after the first dose. Remember the urgency of hospital transfer.

(Reproduced with permission of the Resuscitation Council (UK) 2002.)

ischaemic heart disease. It is characterized by a chronic failure of the right side of the heart, leading to fluid retention in the venous side of the circulation and in the pulmonary vasculature. This is manifest as breathlessness on exertion – or at rest in more serious cases – and oedema of dependent areas such as the ankles and sacrum. It may also be associated with angina. This complaint is usually treated with a combination of diuretics such as furosemide or amiloride, and digoxin (particularly if the heart rhythm is abnormal with atrial fibrillation). New drugs are becoming available to improve further the efficiency of the heart.

Unstable angina

Patients with angina frequently enter into a steady state whereby their angina is either infrequent or well controlled by medication. In these circumstances, episodes of chest pain follow patterns that depend upon factors such as exertion or stress, or they may simply be characterized by a certain frequency of attacks each week. This pattern implies that the quality of perfusion of the myocardium is also steady. If the pattern of pain changes so that episodes of pain are becoming more frequent or severe, the implication is that the coronary circulation is deteriorating. This situation may be the precursor to myocardial infarction. It is for this reason that a history of suddenly worsening angina is taken so seriously by medical staff and often leads to hospital admission for rest, risk assessment and a review of medication.

WHAT TO DO IF A PATIENT SUDDENLY LOSES CONSCIOUSNESS

Basic life support protocols have been developed (Fig. 4.10). First, the practitioner should ensure a safe environment for themselves and the patient.

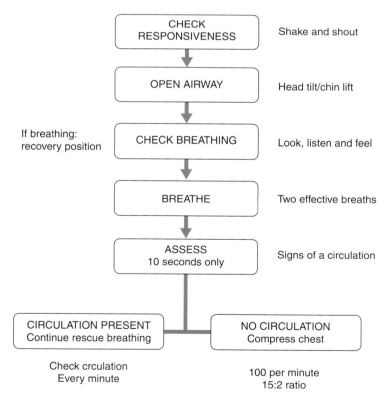

Figure 4.10 Basic life-support protocols. Send for help as soon as possible according to the guidelines. (Reproduced with permission of the Resuscitation Council (UK) 2000.)

1. Lie the patient supine
2. Check and, if necessary, clear the airway; remember dentures!
3. Check for breathing
4. Look for evidence of a circulation for up to 10 seconds (patient movements, coughs, etc.; only check for a pulse in the neck if you have been trained)
5. If your patient is breathing freely and has a good pulse, then there is no immediate danger; get help now. Put the patient in the recovery position
6. If either is absent, then start basic life support and seek help or call an ambulance urgently
7. In the midst of all this, keep a clear head and try to recall the events leading up to the collapse: this information will be invaluable to paramedics and clinicians involved in the treatment of your patient.

SUMMARY

From time to time, all health workers will be exposed to a medical emergency of some kind. Not all incidents that may be perceived as emergencies by non-medical staff will be seen as such by clinicians. In a podiatrist's clinic, where equipment and experience may not be suited to these events, the sense of urgency is evident nonetheless.

The key to sensible and safe management of all emergencies is to have a framework on which to base action. To preserve life, that framework is simply ABC: maintain *airway*, *breathing* and *circulation*. The rest can wait.

REFERENCES

British Heart Foundation Database 1999 National service framework for coronary heart disease. Ch 3 Heart attacks and other acute coronary syndromes. Online: http://www.doh.gov.uk/nsf/coronarych3.htm (accessed 11 July 2002)

British Mental Health Act 1983. HMSO, London

British Thoracic Society, National Asthma Campaign, Royal College of Physicians of London in association with the General Practitioner in Asthma Group, the British Association of Accident and Emergency Medicine, and the British Paediatric Respiratory Society and the Royal College of Paediatrics and Child Health 1997 British guidelines on asthma management: 1995 review and position statement. Thorax 52(suppl 1): S1–S20

Burney P G J 1992 Epidemiology. In: Clark T J H, Godfrey S, Lee T H (eds) Asthma, 3rd edn. Arnold, London

Cochrane G M, Jackson W F, Rees P J 1996 Epidemiology of asthma. In Cochrane G M, Jackson W F, Rees P J (eds) Asthma: current perspectives. Mosby-Wolfe, London, p 9–11

Eisenberg M S, Bergner L, Hallstrom A 1979 Cardiac resuscitation in the community. Journal of the American Medical Association 241: 1905–1907

Family Law Reform Act 1985. HMSO, London

Fulton M, Julian D G, Oliver M F 1969 Sudden death and myocardial infarction. Circulation 39: 182–191

Gillick (1984) QB 581, (1984) 1 AV ER 365; on appeal (1986)

AC112, (1985) 1 AV ER 533, CA: revised (1986) AC 112, (1985) 3 AV ER 402, 1–12

Knight B (ed) 1992 Legal aspects of medical practice. Churchill Livingstone, Edinburgh. p 39–47

Marquand P B 2000 Capacity to consent to or to refuse treatment. In: Marquand P B (ed) Introduction to medical law. Butterworth Heinemann, Oxford, p 27–38

McClay W D S 1996 Clinical forensic medicine, 2nd edn. Greenwich Medical Media, London, p 43–45

Miller A R, Harvey J E 1993 Guidelines for the management of spontaneous pneumothorax. British Medical Journal 307: 114–116

Resuscitation Council (UK) 2000 Basic life support resuscitation guidelines. Online: http://www.resus.org.uk/pages/bls.htm (accessed 10 July 2002)

Resuscitation Council (UK) 2002 The emergency medical treatment of anaphylactic reactions for first medical responders and for community nurses 2002. Online: http://www.resus.org.uk/pages/reaction.htm (accessed 10 July 2002)

Vincent R, Martin B, Williams G, Quinn E, Robertson G, Chamberlain D A 1984 A community training scheme in cardiopulmonary resuscitation. British Medical Journal 288: 617–620

Wade D 1988 Stroke: practical guides for general practice 4. Oxford University Press, Oxford

FURTHER READING

Colquhoun M C, Handley A J, Evans T R (eds) 1999 ABC of resuscitation, 4th edn. BMJ Books, London

Haslett C, Chilvers E R, Boon N A, Colledge N R, Hunter J A A (eds) 2002 Davidson's principles and practice of medicine 19th edn. Churchill Livingstone, Edinburgh

Health and Safety Executive 1997 First aid at work,

2nd edn. HMSO, London

Resuscitation Council (UK) Guidelines 2000. Online: http://www.resus.org.uk/pages/guide.htm (accessed 10 July 2002)

Yates D W, Redmond A D. 1999 Lecture notes on emergency medicine, 2nd edn. Blackwell Science, Oxford

5

Health and health promotion

Terry O'Donnell

INTRODUCTION

In the last quarter of the 20th century, not only has the range of approaches, activities and professional roles associated with health promotion made great progress but also the practice of health promotion takes place in a changing social world. Our understanding of the complex concept of health has been altered, particularly by a growing number of studies concerned with how health is understood and experienced at the everyday level. Users of health services have an increasingly consumerist orientation to health care and expect good-quality, tested services. More than this, 21st century consumers of health products and services expect to have choices, a say in how they are treated and monitoring and evaluation of the health commodities they consume. These expectations are increasingly recognized by health professionals, health service providers and commissioners, and by governments. Health promotion is now firmly established as an essential set of practices and is expected to be evidence based and open to scrutiny. Indeed, in the early years of the 21st century, many of the enterprises associated with health promotion are at the heart of public policies and government action. This is especially the case with the issue of tackling inequalities in health. Therefore, this chapter explores models and concepts of health, looks at the emerging concept and practices of health promotion and explores the issues facing 21st century podiatrists in relation to their involvement with promoting health as well as with preventing disease.

UNDERSTANDING HEALTH

Health is a complex and contested concept. In order to explore the various approaches to defining health and understanding different accounts of how health is enhanced and diminished, it is useful to begin with a short review of the development and impact of *biomedicine*.

The medical model of health

Biomedicine describes the dominant way of understanding disease and health within many countries of today's world. It emerged strongly in the 19th century in those countries that were the first to become modern, industrial societies. Biomedicine emphasizes explanations of disease in terms of biological factors and seeks to build its understanding from evidence derived from systematic processes of observation and experimentation. In other words, biomedicine is held to be based on scientific methods, which enables it to claim that its knowledge is valid and that those who are accredited practitioners may be considered to be experts in their fields. Nowadays, we increasingly recognize that all forms of scientific knowledge, including medicine, are produced in complex and dynamic ways and may be modified or even thoroughly changed in the light of new discoveries or new interpretations. As Karl Popper, one of the 20th century's most eminent philosophers of science, has established, the current scientific knowledge in any field is always *provisional* – it is the best we have for now (Popper 1959). However, although many aspects of our understanding of the nature of medical knowledge and practice are changing in the 21st century, we are still often influenced on a day-to-day basis by what has been termed the *medical model*. The medical model is mostly concerned with disease, which is thought of as biological malfunctioning in the organic machine that is the human body, resulting in specific pathologies (Barry and Yuill 2002). From this perspective, *health* is defined negatively and considered to be what we have in the absence of disease or disability.

The social model of health

The medical model may be contrasted with the social model, which argues that social conditions – such as socioeconomic status, unregulated water supplies, food markets dominated by heavily processed foods, stress – are fundamental causes of disease (Link and Phelan 1995). From the social model's perspective, health is more than the absence of ill-health. The first well-known effort to define a wider concept of health is that of the World Health Organization (WHO); in its founding Constitution, it defines health as 'a state of complete physical, social and mental wellbeing, not merely the absence of disease or infirmity' (WHO (1946) cited in Naidoo and Wills 2001). Many commentators have observed that this definition, while a step in the right direction, is somewhat overambitious (Downie et al 1992). Since then, the WHO has defined health as: '... the extent to which an individual or group is able, on the one hand, to realize aspirations and satisfy needs; and, on the other, to change or cope with the environment. Health is, therefore, seen as resource for everyday life, not the objective of living; it is a positive concept emphasizing social and personal resources, as well as physical capacities' (WHO 1984). This definition implies that there is a notion of a 'good life' that people should not only aspire to but also, in some measure, enjoy. It suggests the importance of people having some degree of control over their lives and that this entails not only personal life-skills but also having a reasonable share of social, economic and political resources. However, we must recognize that specifying the dimensions of a good life and quantifying appropriate shares of societal and global resources is complex and involves the making of value judgements. The medical and social models are compared in Box 5.1.

Socioeconomic factors and health

Figure 5.1 shows how individuals with their biological attributes fit into wider circles and environments, which all influence their experiences of health and disease. Our behaviours occur in social contexts and our lifestyle choices are constrained by both our material resources and the surrounding psychosocial pressures. Much of the 21st century literature on the determinants of health refers to proximal factors influencing health (those close to the individual) and distal factors (those found in local settings and the wider environments). This follows on from our developing understanding of how more distant mechanisms might impact on the health of individuals in clearly patterned ways.

The recently developed 'psychosocial perspective', for example, identifies three core assumptions (Elstad 1998):

- the distribution of psychological stress is an important determinant of health inequalities in present-day affluent societies
- psychological stress is strongly influenced by the quality of social and interpersonal relations
- social and interpersonal relations themselves are determined to a large extent by the magnitude of society's inequalities.

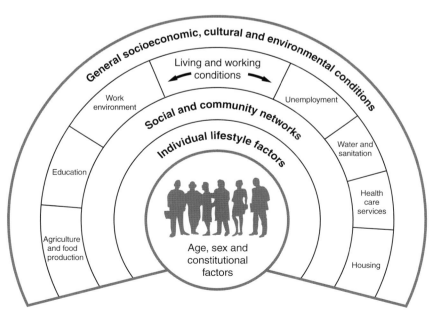

Figure 5.1   The main determinants of health (Acheson 1998, Figure 1).

Inequalities in health

Studies have found links between material deprivation and ill-health since the early 19th century, following the publication in 1842 of Chadwick's 'Report on the sanitary condition of the labouring population of Great Britain'. This showed that poverty, especially in the new industrial towns and cities, was inextricably tied up with high levels of infectious diseases, caused by insanitary living conditions such as contaminated water supplies and overcrowded housing rather than by the habits of the poor.

In 1980, the 'Inequalities in Health Report' (popularly known as the 'Black Report') showed clearly that the health gap between the richer and poorer sections of the population had widened between 1948 and the mid-1970s (Townsend et al 1988). With the exception of one cause of death (skin cancer), the economically deprived died in greater numbers at younger ages than the economically affluent. The Working Group producing this report analysed various mortality and morbidity data and argued that, while individual health-detracting behaviours were clearly involved, they had to be understood in the wider socioeconomic environment in which they were produced. Low and insecure incomes, unemployment and unstable employment, poor working conditions, poor housing in materially and culturally under-resourced neighbourhoods all contributed to lifestyles in which people were more likely to adopt health-damaging behaviours, such as smoking and nutritionally inadequate diets, than they were to find the personal resources needed to adopt and sustain healthy behaviours. The Black Report targeted many of its recommendations for change at the level of government policy on income distribution and taxation and income maintenance provisions for those not in paid employment because of retirement, sickness, disability or unemployment. The Black Report was neither welcomed nor implemented, even partially, by the Conservative administration to which it was presented in 1980 when its work was finished.

In spite of the response of the government of the day, the Black Report's influence was exten-sive and many research projects were subsequently established both to check that its findings were reliable and to develop further our understanding of the extent and nature of inequalities in health. An important ongoing study, the Longitudinal Study, has followed a sample of people drawn initially from the 1971 census and supplemented by samples of later births (Fox and Goldblatt 1982). This work has shown clearly that the extent and pattern of inequalities identified in the Black Report are real rather than being *artefacts* (that is they are not distortions inadvertently produced during the complex processes of analysing diverse statistical data). The 'Whitehall studies' have analysed the health of civil servants working in Whitehall from very senior civil servants to manual grade jobs such as messenger (Marmot et al 1991). They found that mortality rates increased and age of death decreased as we moved down the job grades. It was evident that the incidence of smoking was higher in the lower than in the higher grades; however, when the smoking variable was held constant, the mortality from coronary heart disease (CHD) was still significantly higher in the lower grades than in the higher grades. In 1988, the Health Education Council, as its last major public action before it was abolished and replaced by the Health Education Authority, published 'The Health Divide' in which Whitehead demonstrated that the widening health gap identified by the Black Report had actually widened further still during the 1980s. Nonetheless, when the UK's public health strategy 'The Health of the Nation' was launched in 1992, the White Paper made very scant reference to the existence of health inequalities (Department of Health (DoH) 1992). It referred to them as 'variations in health'. By the mid-1990s, there was a substantial evidence base to support the perspective that tackling inequalities in health meant tackling social inequalities, with the most recent evidence coming from the King's Fund, a charitable, independent foundation for research and policy analysis on health issues (Benzeval et al 1995). Such a view was deepened by Wilkinson's detailed analysis of mortality and morbidity data from several countries, in which he demonstrated that the widest gaps in health inequalities were to be found in those countries that had the widest gaps in incomes (Wilkinson 1996). He also showed that the countries with the largest gaps between the rich and poor tended to be the richest countries overall. This meant, for example, that the UK had a wider health inequality gap than Greece or Portugal. In 1995, the government did produce a document (DoH 1995), which called for:

- reducing the health gap
- health service purchasers to identify and tackle variations
- health service purchasers and trusts to monitor equity of access to services
- the DoH to work with other agencies to encourage health promoting social policies
- health variations to be a research priority.

By 1997, the Office for National Statistics had produced a Decennial Supplement containing detailed analyses of mortality differentials together with some exploration of morbidity and of wider perspectives on health inequalities (Drever and Whitehead 1997). In the same year, the Economic and Social Research Council (1997) launched a 5 year research programme into health variations, and the New Labour government, which took office in May 1997, set up an independent review of inequalities in health.

The Independent Inquiry into Inequalities in Health Report

The Independent Inquiry into Inequalities in Health was chaired by Sir Donald Acheson. It drew on peer review and scientific and expert evidence to review the evidence on health inequalities in England and Wales and published its report in the November of the following year (Acheson 1998). The report noted that, while average mortality has fallen in the last half-century, unacceptable health inequalities not only still existed but also have either widened in this period or remained the same. It stated that the weight of scientific evidence supported a socioeconomic explanation of health inequalities in which lifestyle and personal behaviours are

clearly located within the wider determinants of health (see Fig. 5.1). The report made 39 recommendations, many of them subdivided into further specifics, under the following headings: general; poverty, income tax and benefits; education; employment; housing and environment; mobility, transport and pollution; nutrition and the Common Agricultural Policy; mothers, children and families; young people and adults of working age; older people; ethnicity; gender; and the National Health Service (NHS). Of these, the report identified 'three areas which were regarded as crucial (Acheson 1998):

- all policies likely to have an impact on health should be evaluated in terms of their impact on health inequalities
- a high priority should be given to the health of families with children
- further steps should be taken to reduce income inequalities and improve the living standards of poor households.

The report also acknowledged that New Labour's emerging public health strategy, 'Our Healthier Nation' (OHN), aimed to reduce the health gap and improve the health of Britain's poorest. Overall, the Acheson Report presented a detailed account of the extent and nature of health inequalities in Britain near the beginning of a new millennium. The OHN White Paper represented the first time a government had fully acknowledging that health inequality runs throughout life (Box 5.2) and that government 'has a responsibility to address such deep-seated problems' (DoH 1999, Ch. 4, p 3). The OHN strategy is discussed in more detail later in this chapter.

Lay perceptions of health

We can add to our understanding of the concept of health by looking at lay people's meanings when they talk about health and ill-health. Studies show that lay people draw on both professional accounts of what is healthy and their own life experience. Furthermore, it is very common for people's health beliefs to be contradictory and inconsistent. This is not a measure

Box 5.2 Health inequality

- Life expectancy at birth for a boy is about 5 years less in the two lowest social classes than in the two highest: 70 and 75 years, respectively.
- Each of the main disease groups shows a wide health gap among men, with those in the highest two social classes experiencing lower mortality than men in the lowest two.
- Men aged between 20 and 64 years from the bottom social class are three times more likely to die from coronary heart disease and stroke than those in the top social class.
- Mortality from all major causes has been found to be consistently higher than average among unemployed men; unemployed women have higher mortality from coronary heart disease and suicide.
- Children from manual households are more likely to suffer from chronic sickness than children from non-manual households.
- Men in manual classes are approximately 40% more likely to report a long-standing illness that limits their activities than those in non-manual classes.
- Children from manual households are more likely to suffer from tooth decay than children from non-manual households.

From DoH (1999) Chapter 4, with permission.

of irrationality but is an indication of how ideas about health are socially constructed to reflect our gender, socioeconomic status, ethnicity, age status and the cultural biographies of both our times and our particular generation. While there may be a common core of ideas about what is involved in the subject of health, lay perceptions of health are various, complex and dynamic.

Concepts of health

The 'Health and Lifestyle Survey' was a major national sample study of 9003 people, both men and women, who were distributed across the adult age range from 18 years to 60 years and over. Comparisons between the sample and various sources of government population data show the sample to be a generally sound representation of the population of England, Wales and Scotland (Blaxter 1990). The study involved some physiological measurement of the members of the sample, but it was mainly based on asking questions using a self-completion ques-

tionnaire and a 1 hour interview, which used a mixture of precoded questions and open-ended questions. People's concepts of health were probed at the start of the interview before issues about their own health experience were discussed. Two groups of open-ended questions were used.

- Think of someone you know who is very healthy: Who are you thinking of? How old are they? What makes you call them healthy?
- At times people are healthier than at other times. What is it like when you are healthy?

The results showed that concepts of health contained several dimensions, differed between men and women, and changed over the life course. Women generally expanded more fully on the topic than men, and women of higher educational attainment, or higher occupational status, were most likely to hold multidimensional concepts of health. Differences were also evident according to whether the respondents were talking about themselves or about another person they considered to be healthy. For another person, they were more likely to emphasize leading a healthy life, never being ill and being physically fit. For themselves, they were more likely to emphasize being psychologically fit and being functionally able to do a lot. Interestingly, some respondents (15%) said that they could not think of anyone who was healthy and some (10%) said of themselves that they were unable to answer the question about what it was like when they felt healthy. Overall, a broad range of concepts relating to health was identified in the study (Box 5.3).

Health as self-control and health as release

Crawford (1993) interviewed people at length in their own homes to identify their views about health and the factors that influence health. He introduced himself as a person writing a book on how people think about health and he began each interview with the questions: Are you healthy? How do you know? The interviews covered such issues as perceived threats to health, environmental and lifestyle connections with health and individual moral responsibilities for health and ill-health. Two dominant concepts of health emerged from his analysis of the data gathered. Health was viewed as *self-control* or as *release*. Health as self-control laid emphasis on health as requiring effort, self-denial and will power. From this perspective, ill-health could be viewed as failure to follow the prescribed behaviours that were held to protect health and, as such, the concepts of blame and guilt were present. Health as release, by contrast, laid emphasis on enjoying lifestyles freely chosen and seeking pleasure and fulfilment. Crawford argued that not only are these opposing views of health in

---

Box 5.3 Health and lifestyle survey: broad categories of concepts of health

Health as not ill
Not having serious problems, not seeing the doctor.

Health despite disease
Having a diagnosed condition, such as diabetes or arthritis, but not feeling themselves to be ill.

Health as the 'healthy life'
Regularly engaging in healthy behaviours: for example jogging, healthy diet, not smoking.

Health as physical fitness
Prominent amongst younger respondents, especially men. Playing sports, having muscular strength or athletic capacities were all mentioned in this context.

Health as energy, vitality
Energy was the word used most frequently by women of all ages and older men to describe health; for younger men, it was a close second to 'fitness'. The concept seemed to cover both physical liveliness and psychosocial vitality.

Health as social relationships
Women were much more likely than men to refer to the importance of enjoying time spent with family and friends.

Health as function
The notion of being able to carry out daily tasks and chosen activities increased in importance with age. Some younger people said health was freedom.

Health as psychosocial wellbeing
Reference was made to such concepts as relaxation, fulfilment, spirituality, and happiness. It was used more by women than by men.

Health as a reserve
Essentially, a notion of some kind of inner resilience. Not greatly found in this study.

From Blaxter (1990), with permission.

---

tension within society generally, they may also be in opposition within individuals, who may struggle to achieve a balance between them. For example, we may subscribe to an ideal of the slim, toned and cared for body and engage for some of the time with healthy eating, follow physical activity guidelines and wear foot-friendly footwear. However, we may find it a struggle to be consistent, especially with those aspects that we do not much like. Additionally, we may find that these health-enhancing activities conflict directly with many of our ways of feeling good and enjoying ourselves, such as eating burger meals and chocolate, playing computer games and wearing footwear for our own purposes – being fashionable, rock climbing, dancing – without worrying about whether our feet are being damaged in the process. Indeed, as Crawford pointed out, whole industries produce a wide variety of goods and services that connect with one of these two concepts of health while conflicting with the other. More than this, our consumption choices and practices are key components of our self-identities in the 21st century. The lifestyles that many of us consider to be freely chosen are very much associated with the commodities we consume, and large amounts of money are spent in an effort to direct our choices. Many of us make judgements about our own moral worth and that of others on the basis of how healthy we consider our bodies to look and whether we think we are individually responsible for how they look. *Victim blaming* is an activity that is open to both lay people *and* health professionals and may itself be a health-detracting behaviour (Box 5.4).

FROM HEALTH EDUCATION TO HEALTH PROMOTION

The term 'health promotion' came into increasing usage in the 1980s, with the term 'health education' then being used to identify a variety of educational approaches that contribute to, but are one element of, health promotion. Prior to the 1980s, 'health education' was the term used to describe efforts to communicate with the public on health matters.

Box 5.4 Victim-blaming

Victim-blaming is a problem for several reasons:

- it fails to recognize that many of our choices are socially constrained
- it oversimplifies the pathways through which major diseases such as coronary heart disease, diabetes and cancers occur in particular individuals
- it may lead to low self-esteem, which can further detract from health
- it focuses selectively on some, but not all, health-damaging behaviours.

Traditional health education

We can trace the beginnings of the formal organization of health education in the UK to the formation in 1927 of the Central Council for Health Education. At this time, health education was considered to consist of using a variety of media to present health information and advice on behaviours that were understood to be either beneficial in terms of health or were to be avoided in order to prevent disease. It took another four decades before the Health Education Council (HEC) was set up in 1968 to develop a more extended approach to the use of educational strategies to prevent or reduce the incidence of disease. This organization was a good example of a quango (quasi-autonomous non-governmental organization), which meant that it was held to be independent of the government of the day while receiving most of its income from the state. The HEC established the occupation of health education officer, developed requirements for the education and training of this profession and worked to encourage health authorities to open health education departments as part of their NHS activities.

Government policies on prevention

The health care systems of the world's rich countries began to be increasingly concerned with preventing disease from the mid-1970s. There were two major factors underlying the emergence of this concern. First, these rich countries

had made an *epidemiological transition* in the first half of the 20th century. In the 19th and early 20th centuries, death had mostly been caused by infectious diseases such as respiratory tuberculosis and had affected infants, children and young adults as well as older people (McKeown 1976). By the mid-20th century, death was predominantly caused by the chronic degenerative diseases such as CHD and cancers and mostly occurred in mid to later life (Charlton & Murphy 1997). These diseases were increasingly understood to be both multifactorial in causation and closely associated with social conditions and lifestyles (Jacobson et al 1991). At the same time as the incidence and prevalence of degenerative diseases were rising, countries were finding that modern health care systems were becoming increasingly expensive (Allsop 1995). Therefore, cost containment of therapeutic health care services was the second key factor underlying the policy turn to prevention.

Canada was the first country to put a modern policy emphasis on preventing disease. 'A New Perspective on the Health of Canadians' report introduced the term *health promotion* and argued that improvements in the people's health would come from changing both personal lifestyle behaviours and aspects of the physical and social environments in which people live and work (Lalonde 1974). The report was very clear that only limited population health gains could be achieved by greater expenditure on technological medicine and hospital services directed at the sick. In the UK, the publication of a discussion document, 'Prevention and Health: Everybody's Business', in 1976 and a White Paper, 'Prevention and Health', in 1977 marked renewed government interest in adopting preventive strategies in the hope of improving the population's health. Both documents firmly located personal behaviours as the prime causes of ill-health and placed responsibility on individuals to achieve health improvements by changing unwise behaviour: 'Much ill-health in Britain today arises from over-indulgence and unwise behaviour ...' (DHSS 1976); 'people are encouraged to take more responsibility for their own health ... and to enable them to do so, there should be a greater flow of reliable information and advice' (DHSS 1977).

The White Paper drew on Caplan's work to identify three levels of prevention (DHSS 1977, Caplan 1969) (Box 5.5):

- primary prevention, which seeks to prevent the occurrence of disease
- secondary prevention, which seeks to detect disease early in its development
- tertiary prevention, which seeks to limit complications and disability arising from present disease.

By the late 1970s, the HEC was running large-scale mass media campaigns such as 'Look after yourself!' (LAY!) with the key goal of persuading the population to adopt healthier lifestyle behaviours such as not smoking, reducing dietary fat intake and taking exercise. Putting the onus on individuals had the advantages for governments of avoiding conflict with vested interests such as the tobacco industry and the dairy industry, and of being relatively cheap. Leaving the choice of taking action down to individuals also allowed governments both to refute charges of *paternalism* – that the government knows best and is telling people what to do – and, at the same time, to regard degenerative diseases as self-inflicted. This approach also worked with a medical model in that it took a largely negative approach to the idea of health: health is present in the absence of disease or disability.

Critical perspectives on traditional health education

The traditional health education that developed up to the 1980s has been widely criticized.

- It is considered to have opted to blame the individual victims of ill-health for their condition at the expense of engaging with the social conditions associated with the causation and distribution of disease (Naidoo 1986). There is strong evidence that the poorest die younger and in greater numbers from virtually all of the main contemporary causes of death (Townsend et al 1988, Acheson 1998).

> **Box 5.5** Examples of prevention in the NHS
>
> **Primary prevention**
> - immunization
> - fluoridation of water supplies
> - health visiting
> - health education.
>
> **Secondary prevention**
> - screening
> - periodic medical examinations.
>
> **Tertiary prevention**
> - treatment and rehabilitation.

- It is considered to use a *deficit* model of clients. People are thought of as lacking 'the facts' or are seen as 'ignorant' until 'given' education or information. This implies a *didactic* approach to education in which experts who have knowledge provide what *they* decide is the required amount of that knowledge for the client in the ways *they* consider best. Failure to acquire new knowledge in this manner may be attributed to one, or both, of poor communication skills on the part of the educator or some kind of learning disability on the part of the client. Clients who show evidence of acquiring and understanding knowledge, but who do not change in the desired ways, are likely to be viewed as *irrational* or labelled as *non-compliant* (Lutfey and Wishner 1999). These labels complete the cycle by confirming the deficiencies of the client as the problem.

- It is considered to have an oversimplified view that changes in knowledge and understanding would result in changes in behaviour. While mass media campaigns may put or keep an issue on a social agenda or may attract people's attention – especially, if like good advertising campaigns, they are amusing or in some way striking – they may not be very successful at doing more than simply raising awareness. The same applies to leaflets and information sheets. These media approaches may offer a means of supplying people with information and advice but they may be of limited help to people negotiating the complexities of changing behaviours in relation to the impact of such changes on self-identity and personal relationships on an everyday basis. An evaluation of the anti-heroin mass media campaigns of the 1980s ('Heroin screws you up') found a high level of awareness of the campaign but not the desired effect of making the use of heroin seem unattractive and undesirable to young people (DHSS 1987). Similarly, we know that the mass media campaigns of the late 1980s about the sexual transmission of HIV amongst heterosexual people provoked awareness, and sometimes concern and anxiety, yet they neither enabled people to deal with the practicalities of negotiating safer sex practices nor stopped them making their own risk assessments of the likely HIV status of prospective or current sexual partners (Lupton et al 1995).

The concept and scope of health promotion

The WHO played a leading role in opening up the field of action involved in the promoting of health to include, but also to go beyond, prevention and health education. In 1984, the WHO Regional Office for Europe established a new programme in Health Promotion. It defined health promotion in the following way: 'Health promotion is the process of enabling people to increase control over, and to improve, their health' (WHO 1984, p. 3). In the same discussion document, it proposed that five principles should inform the practice of health promotion (Box 5.6) and counselled against:

- inappropriately targeting individuals instead of tackling social and economic problems
- engaging in 'healthism': that is, treating health, especially physical health, as the most important goal in life.

Around this time, the WHO also developed targets for achieving 'Health for all' by the year 2000 (WHO 1985). Countries and their governments were asked to develop public health strategies that would enable them to achieve the targets relevant to them by the start of the new millennium. The targets were framed in terms of achieving reductions in mortality from specified causes such as CHD; achieving reductions in health-damaging behaviours such as smoking; achieving improvements to health-damaging

---

Box 5.6 Principles of health promotion

1. *Health promotion involves the population as a whole in the context of their everyday life, rather than focusing on people at risk for specific diseases.* It enables people to take control over and have responsibility for their health as an important component of everyday life, both as spontaneous and as organized action for health. This requires full and continuing access to information about health and how it might be sought by all the population, using, therefore, all dissemination methods available.

2. *Health promotion is directed towards action on the determinants or causes of health.* Health promotion, therefore, requires a close cooperation of sectors beyond health services, reflecting the diversity of conditions which influence health. Government, at both local and national levels, has a unique responsibility to act appropriately and in a timely way to ensure that the 'total' environment, which is beyond the control of individuals and groups, is conducive to health.

3. *Health promotion combines diverse, but complementary, methods or approaches*, including communication, education, legislation, fiscal measures, organizational change, community development and spontaneous local activities against health hazards.

4. *Health promotion aims particularly at effective and concrete public participation.* This focus requires the further development of problem-defining and decision-making lifeskills both individually and collectively.

5. While health promotion is basically an activity in the health and social fields, and not a medical service, *health professionals – particularly in primary health care – have an important role in nurturing and enabling health promotion.* Health professionals should work towards developing their special contributions in education and health advocacy.

From WHO Regional Office for Europe (1984), with permission.

environments and achieving gains in health equity by reducing health inequalities.

The Health of the Nation strategy

In the UK, this led to an explicit approach to base a national health strategy on WHO policy. The *Health of the Nation* (HOTN) White Paper laid out the government's approach to improving the population's health (DoH 1992). The strategy identified five key action areas – heart disease and strokes, cancers, mental illness, HIV and sexual health, and accidents – and set specific reductions in their incidence to be achieved within specified time periods. Additionally, the implementation of the policy identified two important components of achieving the goals of the strategy:

- 'health gains': which allowed a cost–benefits approach to evaluation
- 'healthy alliances': which allowed for a measurement of the extent of cross-departmental cooperation and collaboration with non-governmental agencies.

The HOTN was the central focus of public health in the UK from 1992 to 1997. An evaluation study of the strategy, commissioned by the new government in 1997, made a largely negative critique of the strategy (DoH 1998). It found the following:

- the HOTN was perceived as increasing overall prevention activity
- it was widely perceived to be dominated by a 'medically led', disease-oriented approach
- this concerned many and local authorities, especially, felt marginalized within it; furthermore, it peaked early in its life so that by 1997, 'its impact on local policy-making was negligible'.
- it did not seriously shape primary care activities or have much impact on the values and actions of health authorities.

The policy review identified several areas of learning that needed to be explicitly targeted within the forthcoming new public health strategy. Many of these had been first identified by the Ottawa Charter in 1986.

Impact of the Ottawa Charter

In 1986, the WHO called the first international conference on health promotion in Ottawa, Canada. The conference produced the Ottawa Charter that has been described as 'probably being the most important document in health promotion' (Naidoo and Wills 2001, p. 277) because it established five key elements of health promotion strategy. These are identified below, together with a review of how they now feature in UK public health:

- *Build healthy public policy.* All areas of public policy should be accountable for their impact on people's health (e.g. transport policy, incomes policy, farming policy). Lock described health impact assessment as 'a means of evidence based policy making for improvement in health. It is a combination of methods whose aim is to assess the health consequences to a population of a policy, project, or programme that does not necessarily have health as its primary objective' (Lock 2000, p. 1395). Public health policy for England as presented in 'Saving Lives: Our Healthier Nation' (OHN) endorsed the need to carry out health impact assessments of national and local policies (DoH 1999).
- *Create supportive environments.* Both physical and socioeconomic environments were included and the scale ranges from localities and workplaces to global extents (e.g. climate change). Specific places, such as schools, prisons, factories, call centres or neighbourhoods, are sometimes referred to in health promotion as settings, and specific health improvement projects may be funded for particular settings through such government initiatives as healthy living centres and health action zones (Box 5.7) to establish opportunities for physical activity and leisure activity.
- *Strengthen community action.* Communities include localities, such as a housing estate or village, and sections of the population, such as students or minority ethnic groups. Community development and empowerment of communities became central to much ground-level health promotion activity from the mid-1980s. OHN stressed a partnership of communities, individuals and government and outlines a range of

strategies to be developed within deprived communities in particular.

• *Develop personal skills*. Practitioners have widened the scope of health education from the early 1980s to go beyond changing and extending knowledge to also include the acquiring of a range of personal life skills. These are aimed at developing and maintaining high levels of self-esteem and self-efficacy. Personal skills include decision-making, assertiveness and becoming proactive in finding sources of knowledge and information. OHN referred to the establishment of NHS Direct, which includes an on-line health encyclopaedia as well as telephone contact.

• *Reorient health services*. This was a call for countries to ensure that their health care systems placed a focus on prevention and that funding be allocated to reflect the importance placed on strategies designed to obtain reductions in disease occurrence. Since its launch in 1998, the National Service Frameworks (NSFs) programme has sought to include identification of preventive strategies in the NSFs for specific conditions or population groups. The NSFs currently most relevant to podiatry practitioners are on:

- CHD (2000)
- older people (2001)
- diabetes (2001 and 2003)
- children (2004).

Additionally, current health policy has recognized the importance of actively seeking the full participatory involvement of patients in the management of chronic diseases (DoH 2001). The Expert Patient approach discusses diabetes as a case example of the approach in practice and reference is also made to arthritis. Both conditions figure largely in the case loads of NHS podiatry services. Recently, studies have shown increasing lay usage of internet sources to obtain knowledge and information about disease especially, and to facilitate self-organization by people with specific conditions (Hardey 1999).

Our Healthier Nation

OHN was the comprehensive public health strategy for England established by New Labour in 1999. It aimed to both improve health and to reduce the health inequalities gap, and, in so doing to prevent up to 300,000 premature deaths by the year 2010. Local areas were asked to assess and address local needs, especially in relation to cancer, CHD and stroke, accidents and mental health, and to ensure that they tackled local health inequalities. The strategy explicitly recognized that individual lifestyle decisions, which have an important effect on people's health, are often shaped by factors that lie outside of the individual's control, such as social exclusion. It therefore set up a 'three-way deal for health' involving individuals, communities and government (Box 5.8).

The Social Exclusion Unit (SEU) was set up in 1997 to work with departments across the whole of government. The Government has defined social exclusion as (Social Exclusion Unit 2001): 'A shorthand term for what can happen when people or areas suffer from a combination of

---

Box 5.7   Local initiatives

Health action zones (HAZs)
• HAZs were set up in areas of deprivation and poor health. There were 26 full HAZs covering some 13 million people in total. In addition, 10 Associated Health Action Zones (aHAZs) were set up in south-east England.
• HAZs were partnerships comprising NHS bodies, local authority bodies, community groups and bodies from the private and voluntary sectors. They represented a *whole systems approach* to achieving change for the better.
• HAZs were charged with improving the efficiency, effectiveness and responsiveness of services in their neighbourhoods and with developing trail-blazing ways to tackle inequalities in health.

Healthy living centres (HLCs)
• HLCs operated on lottery funding that is additional to government expenditure.
• HLCs targeted social disadvantage in areas and amongst groups of people.
• HLCs were project based, did not have to be a single 'centre' and there was no blueprint for projects, thus enabling a wide scope.
• Users and local communities had to be involved in both the design and the delivery of projects, which could include innovative health-screening programmes, personal skills development schemes or activities involving complementary therapies.

> **Box 5.8** A new contract for health: a three-way partnership between people, local communities and the government
>
> **Individuals**
> Individuals need to take responsibility for their own health. Better health information on the risks involved in a range of activities, practices and products – and the means of applying that information – is the bedrock on which improvements to the health of individuals will be made. However, better health opportunities and decisions are not easily available to everyone, so community action is important
>
> **Communities**
> Communities, working in partnership through local organizations, should deliver not only better information but also better services and better community-wide programmes. The roles of the NHS and of local authorities are crucial. They must become organizations for health improvement, as well as for health care and service provision. This joint responsibility is underlined by the new duty of partnership on NHS bodies and local government in the Health Act. All aspects of the way that the NHS works with other local bodies, from the reorganization of primary care services to the development of healthy neighbourhoods, from the NHS Direct phoneline to the creation of a new Health Development Agency, will be geared not just to treatment of illness but also to the prevention and early detection of ill-health. Many communities will be assisted by projects operating within health action zones or healthy living centres (see Box 5.7).
>
> **Government**
> Government will be creating the right conditions for individuals to make healthy decisions by using government policy to focus on the factors that increase the likelihood of poor health – poor housing, poverty, unemployment, crime, poor education and family breakdown. The Government is taking action to combat social exclusion, to make work pay, to support children and families and to promote community safety. Government will also take a powerful role in making clear the nature and scale of risks to health and, in some cases, will take protective action.
>
> From DoH (1999), with permission.

linked problems such as unemployment, poor skills, low incomes, poor housing, high crime, bad health and family breakdown.'

The SEU's work involves assessing the impact of public policies on the socially excluded, including the resource assumptions contained in departmental spending reviews and budget priorities. Through the OHN, health promotion and public health have been allocated extra funding through improved budgetary allocations and through additional funding sources such as the lottery.

Choosing Health

A new public health White Paper, 'Choosing Health: Making Healthier Choices Easier' (DH 2004) was published in November 2004. It seeks to build on OHN by using government action to make healthy choices more accessible for more people whilst encouraging individuals to make choices that will be better for their health. Tackling health inequalities remains central to public health concerns. The White Paper recognised that even in 2004, in some communities, the health gap between the top and the bottom was still increasing, whilst some neighbourhoods still had mortality rates as low as the national average had been in the 1950s.

Choosing Health was preceded by a detailed and critical review of prevention and public health activities in England in relation to their focus and cost-effectiveness. The Wanless Final Report (Wanless 2004) argued that government should seek active popular engagement with healthy lifestyles by setting achievable goals for national behaviour changes and being prepared to lead in shifting social norms towards healthier living. Previous targets for reducing smoking were criticized as being too low, whilst those for reducing obesity and physical inactivity were considered too high to be realistic in the short and medium term. Wanless also observed that, while evidence about the determinants of health and of health inequalities is good, we lack enough sound evidence about what actually works to reduce health inequalities and to increase health status overall. The White Paper's proposals were also informed by a detailed consultation with citizens, as well as with various experts and health professionals. Popular feedback stressed the importance of free personal choices in matters of lifestyle and health, but also identified the need for supportive frameworks to increase ability to act on personal choices, to ensure freedom from the damaging effects of others' choices and to enhance environments to make it more feasible to adopt and sustain healthy behaviours.

Tackling smoking, obesity, and physical inactivity are key concerns of the new public health strategy. They are considered in the context of everyday lives in the 21st century's consumer, but unequal, society and with specific focus on the needs of children and young people. Thus, as well as developing more direct support for individuals seeking to stop smoking, government will use legislation to ensure the provision of smoke-free environments in workplaces and public places, including restaurants and other licensed premises serving food, on a timetable covering 2006–2008. Local areas will be expected to achieve environmental improvements that will make physical activity, whether as play, active transport or recreational exercise, both safer and generally more attractive to local populations. Healthy food choices will be facilitated by seeking food industry changes to the composition of foods and to their market availability, as well as by more accessible nutritional information on foods. NHS accredited health trainers will support people to review their way of life, to identify possible changes and to make efforts to implement them.

Choosing Health describes its strategy as being the start, not the end, of a journey. Specific targets represent milestones against which progress may be assessed. Reaching these milestones involves critical and reflective application of various health promotion practices. Ways of working in health promotion are explored in the next section.

MAPPING APPROACHES TO HEALTH PROMOTION

Health promotion involves a wide diversity of practice and it is helpful to map models or core approaches in relation to their underlying perspectives on health, behaviour and change. Many analysts and practitioners have produced such maps and you may use textbooks such as those by Ewles and Simnett (1999) and Naidoo and Wills (2000) to explore some of these. Here we identify three broad categories of approaches

and, after introducing them, we look at their application to podiatry and the health of the foot and lower limb. The approaches we consider are:

- health risk advice strategies
- individual behaviour change strategies
- social change strategies.

Health risk advice

This entails providing information on health risks and ways of avoiding or managing them. It may include helping people to learn how to access a variety of sources of health risk advice for themselves, for example, through the Internet. Health risk advice may be provided in one-to-one sessions or small-group sessions by a variety of health professionals, both in primary- and secondary-care settings, and may involve the use of learning aids such as information sheets, leaflets and booklets. Mass media may also be used to offer health risk advice and, to date, these have included:

- campaigns using advertisements on hoardings, in newspapers and magazines, on television and in cinemas
- feature articles in various print media, including magazines and newspapers with free distributions
- soaps and other television programmes may play an active role from time to time in disseminating specific items of health risk advice.

Information on health risks may sometimes be a secondary element in materials being used for a different primary purpose. This can be the case with learning materials used within all levels of education institution from nursery to various adult educational settings. The HDA maintains some websites, such as Wired for Health, Mind, Body & Soul and LifeBytes, which engage directly with teaching and learning strategies used in schools (http://www.hda-online.org.uk).

In the 21st century, it is especially important that health risk advice provided by health professionals is considered to be valid in relation to contemporary validated evidence in the health field.

OHN argues that uncertainty in scientific knowledge should be shared rather than concealed and that the public should be involved in many risk deliberations. It must always be remembered that providing information is not the same thing as changing people's knowledge and understanding, and that changing knowledge is not the same thing as changing behaviours.

Individual behaviour change

Social cognition models, developed within social and health psychology, have sought, for many years, to predict and explain health behaviours. Some widely used models are:

- the Health Belief model
- the Theory of Planned Behaviour
- the Transtheoretical model.

These models, and related health behaviour research studies, are critically explored by Conner and Norman (1996). From the late 1990s, increasing emphasis has been placed on using social cognition models to design and implement intervention studies that explicitly look for modification of health behaviours. Rutter and Quine (2002) bring together a number of such studies where empirical work is advanced or has been completed. These include investigations of behaviour modification in relation to health-enhancing behaviours, such as reducing dietary fat intake, increasing intake of vitamin C, and reducing driving speeds, and in relation to the uptake of health screening behaviours and opportunities, such as breast self-examination and screening investigations for cervical and colorectal cancer. The studies help to identify where, and when, behaviour change interventions may be successful, but they also point out some of their limitations. Sustained behaviour change is more difficult to achieve than short-term change.

From the mid-1980s, the notion of empowerment has been an important concept in relation to seeking behaviour change by individuals and social groups. At an individual level, empowerment is taken to mean that people are more likely to act:

- when they feel that their actions may have an impact
- when they feel personally able to carry through and sustain any changes they, themselves, choose.

It is important that health professionals recognize that empowered individuals may make different behavioural choices from those advised in health risk advice. Such different choices might reflect different life priorities or constrained choices for action, rather than being the product of misunderstandings or simple disregard for expert advice. Empowerment is also important in relation to the social change approach to health promotion.

Social change

Social change refers to changes at levels beyond the immediate control of individuals ranging from neighbourhoods and communities to nation states and global organizations. Community development for health projects have existed for two to three decades, and have tended to draw, implicitly or explicitly, on the concept of empowerment as applied to people working with others (Amos 2002). As Rissell (1994) makes clear, 'empowerment' is difficult to define and may be used in a variety of senses. He cites a number of possible definitions, including (Rissell 1994, p. 41):

- a process through which people become strong enough to participate, share in the control of, and influence events and institutions affecting their lives
- the ability to act collectively to solve problems and influence important issues
- a social-action process that promotes participation of people, organizations and communities towards the goals of increased individual and community control, political efficacy, improved quality of life and social justice.

The WHO's advocacy of a settings approach to health promotion has encouraged international, national and local efforts to identify and act for change in a range of social contexts. These include the *Healthy Cities* initiative launched in 1986, which has had an impact in several countries, including the UK, the *Healthy Schools* programme (Beattie 2002) and the *Healthy College* project (O'Donnell and Gray 1993). OHN and associated strategies aimed at tackling health inequalities are explicitly seeking social change through collective action, and often involving public policy and governmental commitment. Both Health Action Zones and Health Living Centres offer scope for the development of local projects in which lay members of communities work together with a variety of professionals.

PODIATRY AND HEALTH PROMOTION

It is clear that podiatrists play key roles in both primary and secondary prevention of foot and lower limb conditions through educational and screening activities. Self-care by the users of podiatric services may be facilitated by both the acquisition of knowledge and by the development of confidence and competence in the necessary skills. This means that podiatrists are, or could be, involved in both health risk advice and individual behaviour change approaches to health promotion. User groups that may gain from podiatric health promotion include people with diabetes, children and people in later years. Clinic sessions provide many opportunities to offer health risk advice, listen to users' concerns and discuss issues.

A recent study found that podiatrists were interested in being involved in health promotion and considered it to be part of their professional role (O'Boyle et al 2000). However, they tended not to plan and prepare for it, and frequently did not record any such discussions in case notes, or include it explicitly within the treatment plan. The study also found that podiatrists felt inadequately trained for their health promotion role and felt that both pre- and post-registration education programmes did little to address this inadequacy. Many podiatrists felt that they were also handicapped by what they perceived to be a lack of resources, available time and management support. Somewhat worryingly, the study found that many podiatrists had very limited perceptions of the goals of health promotion in that they tended to describe health promotion in such terms as:

- saying what we think is best for patients
- fostering patient compliance
- changing patients' behaviour.

These are worrying because there is little evidence to suggest that the respondents in this study were aware of the complexities involved in changing health behaviours.

Whilst individual podiatrists may achieve a great deal through personal efforts to develop their health promotion role, it is likely that greater gains will be attained and sustained by:

- organized professional development in podiatric units
- review and development of podiatry education programmes
- planned involvement with health promotion in settings beyond the podiatry clinic.

Planned podiatric health promotion will entail the development and application of evaluation strategies, scrutiny of existing evidence and contribution to the extension of the evidence base of professional practice. In some instances, this may entail careful distinction between evidence-based professional knowledge and received, but unsupported by evidence, knowledge. For instance, it has been claimed that 'no epidemiological studies have evaluated the long-term effects on foot health associated with wearing high-heeled shoes' (Dawson et al 2002, p. 77). This study did not attempt to test hypotheses on the aetiology of foot problems as such. Rather it sought to relate the wearing of high heels over the life course with painful feet and abnormalities, such as calluses or corns, hallux deformities and hammer toes, in older women. The findings of the study did not support the widely held belief that wearing high heels is bad for feet. This is not to say that high heels do not harm feet, but that we do not, at present, have any evidence that they do. In a climate in which there is a growing public distrust of expert knowledge and of professionals' management of scientific uncertainty, it is important not to make unqualified or unvalidated claims in health risk advice. As Macintyre (2001) expressed it at a conference on *Evidence into Practice*, 'good intentions and received wisdom are not enough' in the practice of promoting health.

Case study: health-promoting podiatry and complications in diabetes

Primary prevention of foot complications in diabetes is associated with diabetes management: good blood-glucose control may help to reduce microvascular complications; and reducing cardiovascular risk factors may lower the susceptibility of the foot to ischaemia from macrovascular disease (Jeffcoate and Harding 2003). Good care of foot ulcers is a major element of secondary prevention of foot complications. Thus, people with diabetes who are at risk of foot complications in the short through to the long term, must try to maintain glycaemic control, carry out routine self-examination, perform regular foot care and obtain regular podiatry. Glycaemic control entails management of diet and any medication (tablets or insulin) prescribed for the condition. Both tobacco and alcohol consumption may influence metabolic balance, and, thus need to be managed; as does physical activity, which affects blood glucose concentrations (Gafvels and Lithner 1997). These are demanding activities which, together with a potentially stigmatizing sickness label, may impact not only on personal activities and lifestyles, but also on self-identity (Schur, et al 1999, Williams 2000). Furthermore, good glycaemic control may be difficult to maintain, sometimes even by the most assiduously compliant of patients, thus adding a sense of failure to the difficulties of coping with diabetes.

In a review of the research literature on non-compliant behaviour in diabetic patients, Lutfey and Wishner (1999) suggest that many studies take an approach that assumes 'compliance' and 'non-compliance' are fundamental qualities of individuals. Yet this assumption is not itself tested. Studies that focus on patient–practitioner interaction have shown that, while there have been many positive changes to improve communication of health risk advice to patients, there nonetheless remains an unchallenged assumption that patient behaviour must change to meet the needs of the medical system (Lutfey and Wishner 1999). Instead of 'compliance', Lutfey and Wishner argue for a concern with 'adherence', which they argue reduces the authoritative practitioner–submissive patient model and creates the space for a more collaborative relationship between the two parties in the determination of treatment goals. The importance of this shift from 'compliance' to 'adherence' is underlined by many studies investigating lay experiences of living with diabetes and coping with diabetes care (Campbell et al 2003). People with diabetes vary according to whether they:

- seek 'high' control of their condition by altering their management of it to fit the lifestyles they want to follow
- modify their lives to fit the condition, which they 'play down', and consider themselves to be healthy
- neither adjust their treatment to fit their lives nor accept the condition, but rather worry and agonize about their health (Kelleher 1988).

Patients were found to use concepts such as 'cheating' to describe their departures from medical advice or their recommended treatment plan, and a distinction could be made between those who did so with guilt and those who did so without guilt (Campbell et al 2003). The 'guilty cheaters' tended to have negative views of their condition and the limitations it imposed on their lifestyles, and sometimes escaped it by doing what they viewed as normal for non-diabetic patients. Those who cheated without guilt could be considered to 'cheat' *strategically*. They departed from 'medical advice in a thoughtful and intelligent way, in order to achieve a balance between the demands of the diabetes and the way the person wants to live their life' (Campbell et al 2003, p. 678). One study observed that 'patients are not passive recipients of medical advice. Rather they are active interpreters, and at times their interpretations lead them to quite different responses from those advocated by their doctors' (Murphy and Kinmouth 1995, p.191). In Wikblad's study, patients who were classed as having good metabolic control were also those most satisfied with their communication with health professionals. However, patients who were classed as poorly controlled said that they felt it necessary to hide their true behaviour in order to avoid negative responses from their practitioners (Wikblad 1991).

It follows from this discussion that health-promoting podiatry aimed at people with diabetes needs to be non-judgemental and open to patient–professional collaboration. Whilst patients may test out the validity of practitioners' advice against the reality of their own condition, they do still need both information and advice and opportunities to openly explore the disease management issues that concern *them*.

Conclusion

Health promotion is an expanding area of activity in a changing social world. People may often expect more from their health services and health professionals, while trusting them less. Lower apparent levels of trust combined with apparent ignoring of advice or non-adherence to treatment plans makes life difficult for health professionals. However, health professionals who engage thoughtfully and consistently with evidence-based health promotion practice can make significant contributions to both individual and population health gains.

SUMMARY

Basic ideas of health and health promotion have changed considerably since the 1970s. A medical model that is concerned with disease can be contrasted with a social model that considers the social conditions that may be causes of disease. Health promotion is increasingly seen as a way to reduce the load on the health services and to reduce inequalities in health and access to health provisions. It is now widely recognized that, whilst individual behaviour change is a very important element in improving health, such change will only happen if personally and freely chosen, and if facilitated by conducive environments and supported by adequate resources.

REFERENCES

Acheson D 1998 Independent inquiry into inequalities in health. HMSO, London. Available at: www.official-documents.co.uk/document/doh/ih/synopsis.htm (page 2 of 3)

Allsop J 1995 Health policy and the NHS: towards 2000, Longman, Harlow, UK

Amos M 2002 Community development. In: Adams L, Amos M, Munro J (eds) Promoting health: politics and practice. Sage, London

Barry A, Yuill C 2002 Understanding health. Sage, London

Beattie A 2002 Education for systems change: a key resource for radical action on health. In: Adams L, Amos M, Munro J (eds) Promoting health: politics and practice. Sage, London

Benzeval M, Judge K, Whitehead M (eds) 1995 Tackling inequalities in health: an agenda for action, King's Fund Institute, London

Blaxter M 1990 Health and lifestyles. London Routledge.

Campbell R, Pound P, Pope C, Britten N, Pill R, Morgan M, Donovan J 2003 Evaluating meta-ethnography: a synthesis of qualitative research on lay experiences of diabetes and diabetes care. Social Science and Medicine, 56: 671–684

Caplan G 1969 An approach to community mental health. Tavistock, London

Charlton J, Murphy M (eds) 1997 The health of adult Britain 1841–1994. (DS12 and DS13.) The Stationery Office, London

Conner M, Norman P (eds) 1996 Predicting health behaviour: research and practice with social cognition models. Open University Press, Buckingham, UK

Crawford R 1993 A cultural account of 'health': control, release and the social body. In: Beattie A, Gott M, Jones L, Sidell M (eds) Health and wellbeing: a reader. Macmillan, Basingstoke

Dawson J, Thorogood M, Marks S, Juszczak E, Dodd C, Lavis G, Fitzpatrick R 2002 The prevalence of foot problems in older women: a cause for concern. Journal of Public Health Medicine 24(2): 77–84

DH 2004 Choosing health: making healthier choices easier. The Stationery Office, London. Available at: http://www.dh.gov.uk/PublicationsAndStatistics/

Publications/PublicationsPolicyAndGuidance/ PublicationsPolicyAndGuidanceArticle/fs/ en?CONTENT_ID=4094550&chk=aN5Cor

DHSS 1976 Prevention and health: everybody's business. HMSO, London

DHSS 1977 Prevention and health. HMSO, London

DHSS 1987 Anti-heroin campaign: stage five research evaluation. HMSO, London

DoH 1992 The health of the nation: a strategy for health in England. HMSO, London

DoH 1995 Variations in health: what can the department of health and NHS do? Department of Health, London

DoH 1998 The health of the nation: a policy reassessed. The Stationery Office, London

DoH 1999 Saving lives: our healthier nation. The Stationery Office, London. Available at: http://www.archive.official-documents.co.uk/document/cm43/4386/4386.htm

DoH 2001 The expert patient: a new approach to chronic disease management for the 21st century. The Stationery Office, London

Downie R S, Fyfe C, Tannahill A 1992 Health promotion: models and values. Oxford University Press, Oxford

Drever F, Whitehead M 1997 Health inequalities decennial supplement series, DS15. The Stationery Office, London

Economic and Social Research Council 1997 Health variations programme: an outline of research awards. ESRC, London

Elstad J I 1998 The psycho-social perspective on social inequalities in health. Sociology of Health and Illness 20: 598–618 [Special issue on the sociology of health inequalities. See also a special issue of the Journal of Health Psychology (vol 2, issue 3) on health inequalities]

Ewles L, Simnett I 1999 Promoting health – a practical guide. Baillière Tindall, London

Fox A J, Goldblatt P 1982 Socio-demographic differentials in mortality: the OPCS longitudinal study. HMSO, London

Gafvels C, Lithner F 1997 Lifestyle as regards physical exercise, smoking and drinking, of adult insulin-treated diabetic people compared with non-diabetic controls. Scandinavian Journal of Social Medicine 25(3): 168–175

Hardey M 1999 Doctor in the house: the internet as a source of lay health knowledge and the challenge to expertise. Sociology of Health and Illness 21: 820–835

Jacobson B, Smith A, Whitehead M (eds) 1991 The nation's health: a strategy for the 1990s. King's Fund Institute, London

Jeffcoate W J, Harding K G 2003 Diabetic foot ulcers. Lancet 361: 1545–1551

Kelleher D 1988 Coming to terms with diabetes: coping strategies and non-compliance. In: Anderson R, Bury M (eds) Living with chronic illness. Unwin Hyman, London

Lalonde M 1974 A new perspective on the health of Canadians. Ministry of Supply and Services, Ottawa

Link B G, Phelan J 1995 Social conditions as fundamental causes of disease. Journal of Health and Social Behaviour Extra Issue: 80–94

Lock K 2000 Health impact assessment. Br Med J 320: 1395–1398

Lupton D, McCarthy S, Chapman S 1995 'Panic bodies': discourses on risk and HIV antibody testing. Sociology of Health and Illness 17: 89–108

Lutfey K E, Wishner W J 1999 Beyond 'compliance' is 'adherence': improving the prospects of diabetes care. Diabetes Care 22: 635–639

McKeown T 1976 The modern rise of population. Edward Arnold, London

Macintyre S 2001 Good intentions and received wisdom are not enough. Evidence into practice: challenges and opportunities for UK public health conference transcripts. Available at: http://www.hda-online.org.uk/ evidence/key.html#conf (accessed 21 March 2003)

Marmot M G, Smith G D, Stansfeld S et al 1991 Health inequalities among British civil servants: the Whitehall II study. Lancet 337, 1387–1393

Murphy E, Kinmouth A L 1995 No symptoms, no problem? Patients' understandings of non-insulin dependent diabetes. Family Practice 12(2): 184–192

Naidoo J 1986 Limits to individualism. In: Rodmell S, Watts A (eds) The politics of health education. RKP, London

Naidoo J, Wills J 2000 Health promotion – foundations for practice. Baillière Tindall, London

Naidoo J, Wills J 2001 Health promotion. In Naidoo J, Wills J (eds) Health studies: an introduction. Palgrave, Basingstoke

O'Boyle P E, Hodkinson F, Fleming P 2000 Health promotion in podiatry: podiatrists' perceptions and the implications for their professional practice. British Journal of Podiatry 3(1): 21–28

O'Donnell T, Gray G 1993 The health promoting college. Health Education Authority, London

Popper K 1959 The logic of scientific discovery. Harper and Row, New York

Rissell C 1994 Empowerment: the holy grail of health promotion? Health Promotion International 9(1): 39–47

Rutter D, Quine L (eds) 2002 Changing health behaviour. Open University Press, Buckingham

Schur H V, Gamsu D S, Barley V M 1999 The young person's perspective on living and coping with diabetes. Journal of Health Psychology 4(2): 223–236

Social Exclusion Unit 2001 Preventing social exclusion. The Social Exclusion Unit, London. http://www. socialexclusionunit.gov.uk/publications/reports/html/ pse/pse_html/summary.htm

Townsend P, Davidson N, Whitehead M 1988 Inequalities in health: the Black report and the health divide. Penguin, Harmondsworth

Wanless D 2004 Securing good health for the whole population – Final report. The Stationery Office, London. Available at: http://www.hm-treasury.gov.uk/ consultations_and_legislation/wanless/consult_ wanless04_final.cfm

WHO 1984 Health promotion: a discussion document on the concepts and principles. World Health Organization Regional Office for Europe, Copenhagen

WHO 1985 Targets for health for all. World Health Organization Regional Office for Europe, Copenhagen

Wikblad K F 1991 Patient perspectives of diabetes care and education. Journal of Advanced Nursing 16: 837–844

Wilkinson R 1996 Unhealthy societies: the afflictions of inequality. Routledge, London

Williams C 2000 Doing health, doing gender: teenagers, diabetes and asthma. Social Science and Medicine 50: 387–396

FURTHER READING

Links for many of the current reports referred to in the chapter are given below in the section on useful websites.

Useful textbooks

Ewles L, Simnett I 1999 Promoting health: a practical guide. Baillière Tindall, London

Jones L, Sidell M, Douglas J (eds) 2002 The challenge of promoting health: exploration and action. Palgrave, Basingstoke

Naidoo J, Wills J 1998 Practising health promotion: dilemmas and challenges. Baillière Tindall, London

Naidoo J, Wills J 2000 Health promotion: foundations for practice, Baillière Tindall, London

Oliver S, Peersman G (eds) 2001 Using research for effective health promotion. Open University Press, Buckingham

Rutter D, Quine L (eds) 2002 Changing health behaviour. Open University Press, Buckingham

Useful journals

Health Education Journal
Health Education Research: Theory and Practice
Health Promotion International

Useful websites

NHS
Department of Health
    http://www.doh.gov.uk
National Service Frameworks
    http://www.doh.gov.uk/nsf
The Expert Patient
    http://www.doh.gov.uk/healthinequalities/ep_report.pdf

Our Healthier Nation strategy
Our Healthier Nation
    http://www.ohn.gov.uk
Saving lives: our healthier nation (White Paper)
    http://www.archive.official-documents.co.uk/document/
    cm43/4386/4386.htm

Health action zones
    http://www.haznet.org.uk
Health Development Agency
    http://www.hda-online.org.uk
Healthy living centres
    http://www.doh.gov.uk/hlc/index.htm

Choosing Health: Making Healthier Choices Easier
http://www.dh.gov.uk/PublicationsAndStatistics/
    Publications/PublicationsPolicyAndGuidance/
    PublicationsPolicyAndGuidanceArticle/fs/
    en?CONTENT_ID=4094550&chk=aN5Cor

Health inequalities
Reducing health inequalities: an action report (DoH 1999)
    http://www.doh.gov.uk/pub/docs/doh/inequalities.pdf
Report of the Independent Inquiry into Inequalities in Health
    http://www.archive.official-documents.co.uk/document/
    doh/ih/ih.htm
Social exclusion unit
    http://www.socialexclusionunit.gov.uk/
Preventing social exclusion (Social exclusion unit report)
    http://www.socialexclusionunit.gov.uk/publications/
    reports/html/pse/pse_html/summary.htm
Tackling health inequalities: the results of the consultation exercise (DoH 2002)
    http://www.doh.gov.uk/pub/docs/doh/inequalities.pdf
Tackling health inequalities: summary of the 2002 cross-cutting review ((HM Treasury and DoH 2002)
    http://www.hm-treasury.gov.uk/media//EEDDE/
    Exec%20sum-Tackling%20Health.pdf

Non-governmental bodies
Diabetes UK
    http://www.diabetes.org.uk/
King's Fund
    http://www.kingsfund.org.uk

Methods of managing foot conditions

6

Operative techniques

David R. Tollafield
Linda M. Merriman

INTRODUCTION

This chapter concentrates on the operative techniques used to reduce or remove lesions affecting the skin and nails.

The term 'operative' suggests a requirement for surgical skills. Traditionally, routine skin care and surgery have been differentiated as requiring different skills. In reality, the skills used in both are derived from the same source. The way in which the scalpels are used may be different, but most of the techniques, invasive and otherwise, require the same considerations. The techniques often require adjunct therapies, details of which can be found in the relevant chapters, in order for the condition to be fully resolved. For example, enucleation of a corn may lead to an immediate reduction in the level of discomfort experienced by the patient, but if this improvement is to be maintained and the problem fully resolved, chemical and mechanical therapies, and in some cases physical therapies, may also be required. As with any therapy, the practitioner should always be mindful of the benefits and limitations. Box 6.1 summarizes the wide range of operative techniques associated with skin and nail lesions. There may be more than one approach to deal with any given problem.

OPERATIVE TREATMENT

Aims

The aims of carrying out operative techniques are:

- to provide an immediate reduction in the discomfort/pain

Box 6.1 Direct and indirect operating skills associated with cutaneous forms of treatment

Skin

Debridement (cutaneous skin)
- verruca
- fissure
- callus (tyloma)
- ulcer
- onychophosis

Enucleation
- corn (clavus) (Latin: heloma, H.)
  - hard (H. durum)
  - soft (H. molle)
  - vascular (H. vasculare)
  - intractable plantar keratoma (IPK)
  - seed corn (H. milliare)
  - subungual corn (H. subungualis)

Currettage (cutaneous)
- verrucae
- granuloma

Cautery (cutaneous and subcutaneous)
- thermal
  - heat
  - electrical
  - laser
  - cryotherapy (extreme cold below freezing): gases under pressure
- chemical
  - eschar-forming agents, e.g. silver nitrate: self-limiting
  - phenol: protein denatured
  - liquid nitrogen: cell destruction

Incisional (subcutaneous)
- stab: osteotripsy
- along a length linear or curved
- excisional skin biopsy (also punch)
- closing defects (multilobed/flaps)

Nails

Nail reduction (length and thickness)
- manual skills
  - long nails
  - onychomycosis
- power drill
  - onychauxis
  - onychogryphosis
  - onychomycosis

Nail ablation (whole or part of structure)
- onychocryptosis
- onychauxis
- onychogryphosis
- onychomycosis
- involuted (incurvated)

- to complement the use of other therapies as part of the management plan
- to prevent complications from arising as a result of non-treatment.

Operative techniques should be undertaken following patient assessment; this should include a full medical history. Once the likely cause of the problem has been established, a management plan should be implemented (Ch. 1).

Objectives

When carrying out operative treatment, a number of factors should be borne in mind. Techniques should be performed in a safe manner. The patient should not leave the clinic with more problems than when they entered. For example, if the patient's skin has been accidentally incised or abraded, appropriate measures should be taken to prevent infection developing. Particular attention should be paid to asepsis in high-risk groups. The objectives of operative treatment are the same for any patient situation where there is a risk involved. Techniques should be performed:

- in a safe manner
- with the minimum of discomfort to patients
- using appropriate motor processes
- within an acceptable period of time
- such that the outcome results in sufficient removal of the problem.

General considerations

Prior to discussing each technique in detail, the following areas will be considered:

- clinical procedure
- analgesia
- selection of instruments
- ergonomics
- time management.

Clinical procedure

When employing operative techniques, the patient is put at risk if a portal of entry results, whether inadvertently or as an intended outcome of the technique. It is essential, in this case, that a 'minimum touch' approach is used and attention is paid to the sterilization of instruments, the use of gloves and the postoperative care of any resulting portal of entry (i.e. with antisepsis and dressings; Ch. 3).

Analgesia

In general, most cutaneous techniques should not give rise to discomfort. Optimal skin tension will reduce unnecessary symptoms during debridement. Some patients may experience varying levels of pain, either as a result of a previous bad experience or because of low pain threshold; when this is identified, anaesthetic should be used, for example when enucleating a vascular corn with deep fibrosis. Some of the techniques discussed in this chapter should not be performed without the use of local anaesthesia.

The term 'analgesia' refers to an inability to feel pain and occurs without loss of consciousness (note that the terms 'anaesthesia' and 'analgesia' are often confused). Sensory loss associated with local anaesthetic (analgesic) has the advantage of allowing procedures involving incision to be undertaken painlessly. Most cutaneous procedures do not require local anaesthesia when the scalpel is used in the correct manner. Ethyl alcohol has the effect of cooling the skin and reducing sensation. This can be used in the form of a fine spray prior to infiltrating the skin with a hypodermic needle. Emla (Astra) is another useful agent, in cream form, which contains 2.5% lidocaine with 2.5% prilocaine. This is spread thickly onto the skin at least 2 hours before using a hypodermic infiltration. These agents add time to any procedure but are worth considering in children or very sensitive patients who become anxious.

Infiltration techniques are used to deposit the analgesic agent near a nerve. Regional anaesthesia is reserved for specific operative procedures, as described in Chapter 7, although infiltration may selectively prevent sensory information, allowing complete pain relief (analgesia). Long-acting anaesthetics such as bupivacaine (e.g. Marcain) provide a better analgesic effect. The addition of epinephrine (adrenaline) to all anaesthetics is highly beneficial and can extend the period of analgesia to as long as that obtained with Marcain, while maintaining a lower toxic dose in the tissues. Epinephrine (adrenaline) should be used cautiously around the toes as it has a vasoconstrictive effect.

Regional blocks (e.g. a common peroneal block) commonly affect both sensory and motor pathways, although direct infiltration into muscle will have a similar effect at the level of application. The patient should experience only a dull touch on the affected part when it is cut with a sharp instrument. Initially, temperature changes may be perceptible. A posterior tibial block will affect most of the plantar surface (Ch. 7). Direct infiltration can be beneficial when there is a disadvantage in producing more extensive anaesthesia.

Selection of instruments

There is a range of instruments at the practitioner's disposal (Fig. 6.1). It is essential that practitioners use the instrument that is most suitable for the technique they wish to undertake; no one blade should be used for all scalpel-based techniques. Some blades are more suited to enucleation, while others are more suited to debridement.

Use of instruments The techniques deployed to manipulate instruments physically will vary between practitioners. Tensing of muscles or the use of inappropriate muscles when holding instruments may result in premature fatigue. When reducing tissue by debridement, it is quite difficult to explain in words how much should be removed. The end result, however, should be that the patient's situation is improved compared with that prior to any form of management. The expert practitioner will be able to find a balance between over- and under-reduction. This kind of clinical judgement comes through practice and experience.

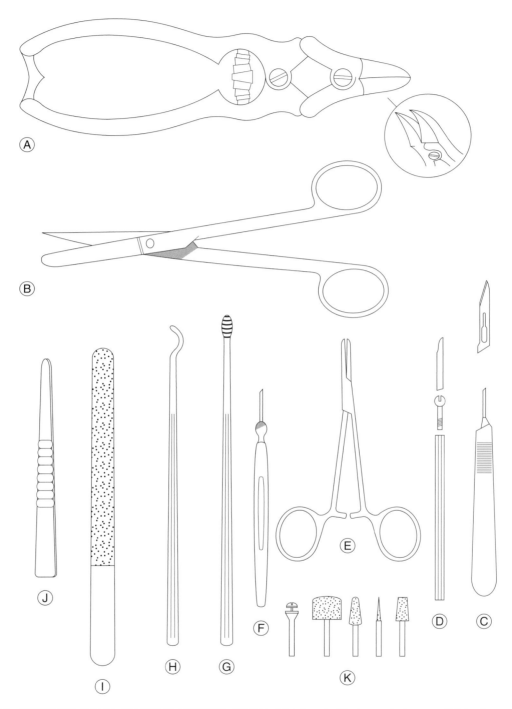

Figure 6.1 Instruments may be selected as preference dictates. A basic set of instruments for superficial cutaneous management is shown. A, nail nippers (cantilever style); B, dressing scissors; C, Baird–Parker handle 3; D, Beaver handle and blade 67; E, grasping forceps, e.g. Spencer–Wells or Halsteads; F, Baird–Parker handle 7; G, Blacks file; H, probe; I, rasp; J, forceps; K, burrs (various) and Moore's disc mandrill.

Ergonomics

When using the techniques outlined in this chapter, it is important for practitioners to consider their own working environment. For example, occupation-related problems such as back pain, eye strain and repetitive strain injury can result from inappropriate or incorrect seating positions.

Time management

Time is another significant factor in a busy routine clinic. A practitioner may have a very good technique and may achieve the aims outlined earlier, yet may take an inordinate amount of time to do this. Good time management is essential for efficient practice.

SUPERFICIAL TECHNIQUES USED ON SKIN

DEBRIDEMENT AND ENUCLEATION

Debridement is a French term used to denote the removal of unhealthy tissue (lesions). Lesions lending themselves to local debridement are listed in Box 6.1. The term 'enucleation' is used for this technique when referring specifically to corns.

Indications

The objective of debridement and enucleation is to reduce excessive keratinous tissue, which acts as an external pressure on the numerous nerve endings. In many cases, the effects of these techniques are short lived. The decision as to whether a lesion should or should not be debrided must be related to the sequence of the treatment plan. The long-term objective must be to provide minimal debridement, since the technique may, in fact, damage the tissues further.

Not all calluses need to be debrided. Calluses occur from a combination of excessive friction, shear and pressure on the skin. They are a normal reaction to excessive stresses on the skin (e.g. the hand of a manual worker usually exhibits thickened skin). In these instances, removal of the hard skin is not indicated. Corns need to be enucleated because they tend to be painful lesions and constitute the prime reason for the patient's appointment.

There are few contraindications to debridement and enucleation; those that do exist relate to disorders that affect tissue repair or are related to collagen defects. Patients with vascular impairment, insensate skin or connective tissue disorders, or patients undergoing chemotherapy, are particularly at risk from the complications that may arise from debridement and enucleation. The skin in these cases is easily traumatized and does not heal well. Another category of patient includes those suffering from bleeding diatheses. Patients with conditions such as absent clotting factors, vitamin deficiencies (vitamin C in particular) and fragility of blood vessels should be managed carefully.

Equipment

The scalpel is the most popular and common tool for debridement and enucleation. A nail drill fitted with an abrasive disc can also be used to debride thickened skin. There is a wide variety of differently sized and shaped scalpels and scalpel blades on the market. The 'Beaver' scalpel (Fig. 6.1D) is the one that most closely resembles the traditional solid scalpel, which was used prior to the advent of replaceable blades (Fig. 6.2). The advantage of the Beaver scalpel arises from the ability to fit different styles of 'mini-blade' onto one handle. In Figure 6.1D, only the 67 blade is shown; others do exist, such as blades 61–66, 68 and 69, which have chisel-shaped, pointed or hooked ends. Microblades are also available but they have less application in cutaneous debridement. Blades from the mini-blade system are screwed to a handle of the appropriate design to achieve a sufficient degree of stiffness; some scalpel handles are less suitable as they are more flexible.

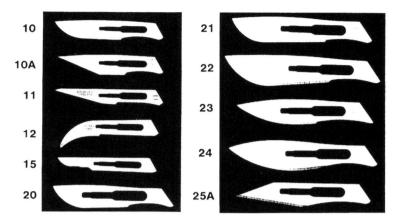

Figure 6.2 A wide range of detachable and sterile blades exists to fit the Baird–Parker (BP handle) systems. A number of variations can be found, such as the Martin and Nova patterns. All blades should be removed with blade removers. (Reproduced with permission from Bailey Instruments.)

Interlocking blades fitted to Baird–Parker (BP) handles (Figs 6.1C and 6.2), for example, have been known to snap when used on dense callosity. In these instances, the sterile disposable blade is dispensed onto the BP scalpel with the appropriate instrument, and removed with safety devices to prevent unnecessary laceration of the practitioner's fingers (Ch. 3).

Interestingly, American podiatrists use chisels, while in the UK, size 10, 11 and 15 blades are favoured. The 10 blade is a long, curved blade, while the 11 is a straight blade with a sharp point. Both the point and the straight edge are valuable in different situations. Both the 10 and the 11 blades are primarily used for debridement. In general, a large blade should be used on very thick plantar callus, and a smaller blade should be used on small lesions and lesions on the dorsum or apex of the toes.

For enucleation, a blade with a rounded end should be chosen, such as a size 15 blade. The rounded end of the instrument is used for enucleation (Figs 6.1D and 6.2 (blade 15)). After use on a patient, blades should be either discarded or sterilized. Inevitably, the lifespan of any autoclaved scalpel blade is limited, and only stainless steel blades can be adequately recycled. In either case, the scalpel handle must be autoclaved after each use.

Debridement techniques

Using a scalpel

Debridement is not a gross movement; the arm should remain as near to the side as possible. The area surrounding the tissue to be removed is held firmly between finger and thumb, as shown in Figure 6.3. Skin tension is important in preventing early blunting of the blade and in maintaining efficient cutting. Movement of the scalpel is achieved through a combination of thumb, forefinger and wrist action. The most common position in which to hold the scalpel is with the distal end between the thumb and forefinger and the proximal end in the cleft of the fourth and fifth fingers (Fig. 6.4). The practitioner should attempt to make controlled sliced cuts. This is achieved by angling the blade so that it is nearly parallel with the surface. The direction of movement will be dependent upon the site of the callus; usually a distal to proximal action is used.

The amount of pressure applied to the blade and the angle between the blade and the skin will affect the size of skin particles removed; small particles of the stratum corneum layer should be removed initially in order to judge the depth of reduction (Fig. 6.5). Deeper and more

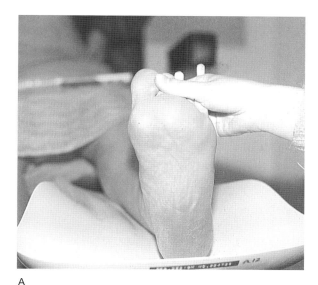

A

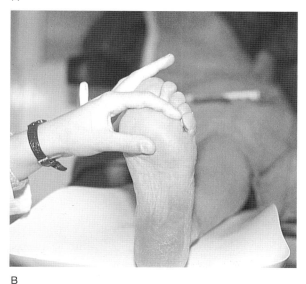

B

Figure 6.3   In each figure, a different method is shown to achieve skin tension, which contributes to effective use of the scalpel blade and prevents premature dulling of the edge.

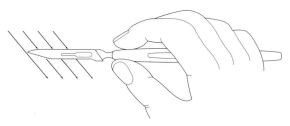

Figure 6.4   Position of the hand when using a scalpel to debride callosity. While the stroke is shown as diagonal to the skin surface, a combined downward stroke improves the cutting efficiency. An 11 blade is illustrated.

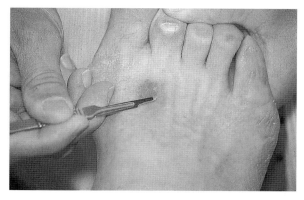

Figure 6.5   Positions for holding a scalpel. Sensitive areas require the practitioner to adopt a different position when holding the scalpel, e.g. debriding on the dorsum of the foot where the blade can inadvertently slip and slice the skin. The backward or reverse position shown offers good control with safety. A 15 blade is illustrated.

uneven thickened keratin can prove more difficult. In these cases, especially with uneven callus, an 'ecope' or 'scooping' action can be used. The ecope technique is effective for large areas of callosity complicated by deep furrows. The whole length of the 11 blade is used so that the wrist rotates the scalpel between two ridges.

A callosity comprises skin that has an excessive keratinous build-up and a yellow colour, as opposed to the pinkish colour of skin of normal thickness. Sometimes the skin may be macerated, which makes it look white. Alternative scalpel positions are adopted as necessary, particularly when working in sensitive areas.

Using a nail drill

The sanding disc attachment is fitted to the nail drill by way of a mandrill (see Fig. 6.1K). The disc is held parallel to the skin and is moved over the area of thickened skin to be reduced. The practitioner's thumb should be held against the skin to prevent any accidental slippage. A sanding disc is particularly useful where the skin is very dry or fissured, or where the state of the patient's skin is poor; in this case, a scalpel is not as useful because it can pull on delicate skin and, if there are fissures, may exacerbate the situation. The sanding disc can be applied gently to the area and does not result in further trauma. The area being sanded may become very warm as a result of the friction between the skin and the disc. Sanding discs should be discarded after use on each patient.

Enucleation techniques

For enucleation, the scalpel is best held between the finger and thumb, as if one is holding a pencil. Enucleating a corn requires the correct technique and much practice. It is very easy to leave much of the central core behind, causing pain soon after the patient has had treatment (see Fig. 6.6). It is essential that the overlying callus is debrided prior to enucleation. Failure to do this is one of the most common causes of poor enucleation, resulting in the practitioner enucleating overlying callus.

The term *enucleation* is perhaps a misnomer, as it implies complete removal. Because of this,

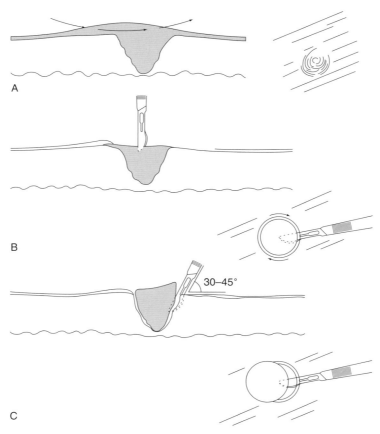

Figure 6.6 Enucleation technique. A, Debrided overlying callosity should be removed as shown to allow easier access to enucleate the corn. No attempt should be made to incise the lesion until the area has been well demarcated. B, Initially the corn should be incised vertically all the way around its perimeter. C, The blade (D15) should be angled at 45° and moved around the lesion. A grasping forceps may be useful to complete the manoeuvre.

'excision' will be used to mean complete removal and 'minute section' will be used for partial removal. With the excision approach, the whole of the corn is removed as one piece without puncturing the dermis, which would cause haemorrhage. The blade is held at an angle of 45° or more to the skin and is worked all the way around the juncture between the corn and normal skin. If the corn is large or if the site of the corn makes enucleation difficult, minute sections can be removed where the patient finds the procedure uncomfortable.

Ultimately, experienced practitioners use the technique they find most acceptable. Variations in the way the scalpel is held will depend upon the site of the lesion. Interdigital lesions are difficult to access, often leading to interdigital cleft injury. The most painful type of corn to enucleate is undoubtedly the intractable plantar keratoma.

Complications

The following problems may result from both debridement and enucleation:

- haemorrhage
- creation of a portal of entry
- over-reduction/overenucleation
- under-reduction/partial enucleation
- problems resulting from inappropriate technique.

Creation of a portal of entry   Creation of a portal of entry can be both avoidable and unavoidable. The pathological changes that result in callus and corn formation involve the proliferation of dermal papillae together with small capillary loops. Following debridement, these papillae can be easily damaged, resulting in bleeding. Once this has occurred, further debridement is masked by haemorrhage. Deep and direct pressure with gauze and using gloved hands may stem the flow. Chemical agents of choice can be selected, for example styptics or haemostatic dressings; current examples include ferric chloride (15%) aqueous, silver nitrate 20–40% (styptics) or Caltostat, to name but one of many dressings. These types of portal of entry are unavoidable.

Avoidable portals of entry can result from cutting the affected or adjacent unaffected skin either because of poor technique or because the patient suddenly moves. Appropriate aseptic measures should be adopted to dress the wound.

Over-reduction/overenucleation   If too much of the keratinous build-up is removed, the skin may feel very tender, especially on activity. A thin anti-friction pad, such as fleecy web or moleskin, can be applied to reduce any discomfort. If the over-reduction has been excessive, papillary haemorrhaging may occur, and in this case a dressing will be necessary.

Under-reduction/partial enucleation   Where insufficient keratinous material has been removed, the patient may continue to experience the same discomfort that was being experienced prior to treatment. An aseptic breakdown owing to the presence of bulky keratinous material may occur if this is unattended, especially in patients with poor skin quality or with areas experiencing higher pressures of load.

Problems resulting from inappropriate technique   The use of an unsuitable technique can result in an uneven finish, feathery appearance of the skin and practitioner fatigue. Attention should be paid to the following:

- maintenance of skin tension
- position of the practitioner
- use of muscles and resultant action
- position of the scalpel in relation to the skin
- sharpness of the blade.

Lack of skin tension results in the skin being pulled every time the scalpel blade is laid over the skin; this may lead to a feathery finish. Too much skin tension can give rise to patient discomfort, mask papillary bleeding and lead to practitioner fatigue. The position and action used by the practitioner can also lead to problems. Practitioners must ensure that they are not straining or using muscles that should not be used. A blunt blade will result in a feathery appearance to the skin, as the scalpel action will not cut all the way through it. A scalpel that is not held parallel to the skin will result in an uneven appearance when debriding. Failure to use the scalpel correctly when enucleating will produce an unsatisfactory result.

Special considerations

Site Lesions that require debriding and enucleating may occur on parts of the foot that are difficult to access (e.g. the heel and interdigital clefts). Practitioners should make use of aids, such as foot raisers, to access the heel, especially the posterior surface. It may be necessary to ask the patient to kneel on the chair with his back to you. With subungual corns and calluses, it is necessary to cut back the nail in order to expose the lesion prior to enucleation or debridement.

Excessive callus Some patients may suffer with extensive callosity. Such occurrences are rare but include conditions such as ichthyosis tylosis, where the callosity is present from heel to toes on the plantar surface. These patients may take up to an hour to debride effectively.

Complete excision of corns Corns can be extremely difficult to manage, even when a range of therapeutic techniques are available. Case study 6.1 illustrates this point, cautioning against the desire for complete removal of corns.

Neuropathic ulcers These require debridement of the keratinous edges in order to promote healing. Some authorities recommend extensive removal of the keratin in order to stimulate the formation of granulation tissue.

Verrucae Pathological changes that occur with verrucae bear similarities to changes in callosity, although verrucae have the distinction that they produce papillary haemorrhages.

Debridement of overlying callosity is usually indicated before chemical treatment.

Young patients Most patients will cooperate, but children can be wary, often because of fear of the scalpel. The scalpel is best left out of sight until needed.

Fidgety patients or patients with tremors Patients with tremors such as parkinsonism require the scalpel blade and operator almost to move with the tremor to achieve any reasonable result. Attempts can be made to occupy the attention of the fidgety patient by giving them a book to look at.

LANCING AND DRAINAGE

There are a number of lesions that can benefit from lancing and drainage. This technique is usually employed in acute situations before the condition has become chronic.

Equipment

The pointed end of an 11 blade is most commonly used. In the case of a *subungual haematoma*, a nail drill and a thin pointed burr are used.

Technique

A blister is usually lanced and drained; the use of two drainage points ensures better reduction of internal pressure than if one drain hole were used, with easier release of pressurized fluid. The epidermal tissue overlying the blister is usually left intact and a compressive dressing applied. Leaving the epidermal surface over the

---

Case study 6.1 Removal of callus

A 43-year-old white female nurse presented with a callus under her right foot that failed to resolve with debridement and insoles over a period of years. The patient requested excision, which was performed under regional ankle block. Reoccurrence took 8 weeks. Radiographs (with markers) revealed that the site of the corn did not lie beneath any bony prominence. Further surgery was performed using a skin flap to provide a fatty pad covering. The patient gained relief on the second occasion for 6 months, but the lesion returned even though functional orthoses with appropriate redistributive adaptations had been prescribed. Histopathology following both procedures excluded a foreign body or implantation cyst.

Conclusion: the replacement fat was reabsorbed and high shear forces stimulated further hyperkeratotic change. Further surgery has been ruled out because of poor prognosis.

site of the blister gives some protection to the underlying skin and is an attempt to avoid the risks of infection. A septic toe associated with a corn or blister is usually lanced by piercing the skin with the point of the 11 blade. The tip of the blade is placed at an acute angle to penetrate the epidermal surface. If appropriate, the area may then be debrided in order to encourage drainage and remove slough, which may impair healing. Particular attention should be paid to antisepsis when undertaking this technique.

Haematoma A subungual haematoma can give rise to excruciating pain on account of the build-up of pressure under the nail. Within 12 hours of the problem occurring, the fluid can be released by piercing the nail plate. A nail drill with a thin pointed burr is used. The point of the drill is held directly over the lesion and the nail is reduced until the underlying skin is reached, thus allowing the blood to escape. Before commencing this procedure, the practitioner should be certain of the diagnosis of haematoma, as other potentially more serious colour changes (e.g. malignant melanoma) can appear similar. Lancing or penetration of such lesions with a burr or scalpel would be extremely dangerous.

TECHNIQUES USED ON NAILS

NAIL CARE

Indications

Most people cut their own toenails; however, there are instances when it is either not possible or not appropriate for an individual to undertake this task. The following are examples of patients who may experience difficulty:

- cannot see clearly, e.g. with glaucoma
- cannot reach their feet, e.g. with arthritis
- cannot use instruments such as nail nippers
- have abnormal nails that are difficult to cut.

If toenails are not cut on a regular basis, a range of problems may result. Long toenails may

pierce the skin of adjacent toes, causing a portal of entry, which may result in infection and ulceration. Subungual ulceration may result from pressure caused by footwear pressing onto long nails. These complications are more prevalent in 'at-risk' patients.

In general, if patients have normal assessment findings, can see and reach their feet and can use a pair of nippers, then they should be able to undertake their own routine nail care. Diabetic patients, so long as they have a normal blood supply, normal sensation, no kidney disease, no eye problems and a stable blood glucose level, should also be encouraged to undertake their own routine nail care. Some of the general public, however, are not clear as to how this should be done. People often pick or poke down the sides of the nail, and, as a result, infections are easy to come by.

This section looks at how routine nail care should be undertaken for those who are unable to perform the task themselves and also indicates how the general public should perform this task.

Equipment

A pair of nail nippers and a file are the standard pieces of equipment. Nail nippers offer mechanical advantages over clippers. There are many types available on the market; cantilever styles are probably the most powerful, but can, in the wrong hands, cut through toes. Attention should be paid to the size of the nippers in relation to the size of the hand. Problems with tenosynovitis may result from the combination of a small hand and a large pair of nippers.

A practitioner may also wish to use a Blacks file, probe or scalpel where appropriate. All instruments should be sterilized between patients. In the case of self-care, instruments should be kept clean and washed after use in warm soapy water and dried thoroughly before use on another person.

Technique

An understanding of the anatomy of the nail apparatus, its relationship with the (distal) interphalangeal joint and the contribution made to nail growth by the nail bed, eponychium, hyponychium and sulcal edges is important. Nails should appear smooth – shape with a slight longitudinal and lateral curvature – dull, and have clean demarcations of the sulci. The nail plate is translucent but will appear pink because of the underlying nail bed. Contrary to common belief, nails should not be cut straight but marginally curved, depending upon the shape of the distal end of the toe. The nail should not be cut below the free edge. A nail should not be cut in one piece. It is easier, and preferable, to cut a nail in sections. After cutting, the nail should be filed over gently with a nail file, using a one-way action working from proximal to distal. There should be no rough or jagged edges to catch on hosiery, and the free edge of the nail should be visible. When you have completed the task, check between the digits to ensure that no pieces of nail are present. If left, these will pierce the skin and lead to an open wound. Unless the patient complains of discomfort, leave the sulci alone.

Complications

Problems may arise if one or more of the following has occurred:

- the skin surrounding the nail has been cut
- the skin of adjacent toes has been cut
- the nail has been cut below the free edge
- a piece of nail has damaged the practitioner's eye.

In the first two cases, appropriate dressing and, if necessary, antisepsis should be used. In the case of cutting below the free edge, long-term problems may result as the skin moulds around the short nail plate and the growing nail presses into surrounding skin. When cut, brittle or thickened nails can act as flying hazards. Eyes are often in danger, because of the position of the practitioner in relation to the patient's foot. Eye goggles can be used to reduce the likelihood of eye damage.

Special considerations

Thickened nails   Some nails may be thickened; the lesser fifth toes are the most likely, because of entrapment against the lateral side of shoes. Thickened nails can be reduced by debridement with a scalpel or by using a nail drill.

Nail tufts   Cutting nails may be hazardous when thick keratin and blood vessels become enmeshed as one, tethering down the nail plate, as in nail tufts or angiokeratoma (Fig. 6.7). Simple nail tufts have a blackened thrombosed appearance and usually arise as a result of previous trauma. Routine care and the use of silver nitrate to cauterize the blood vessels chemically can be helpful. However, this is only a superficial effect as the chemical lacks penetration. Serious problems may need to be excised.

Subungual exostoses   Subungual exostoses are not uncommon. The nail plate may be lifted at one end of the nail, so producing a thickened appearance. Lateral and medial oblique radiographs are the standard approach for differential diagnosis. Callosity and redness provide all the appearances of an expanding osteochondroma.

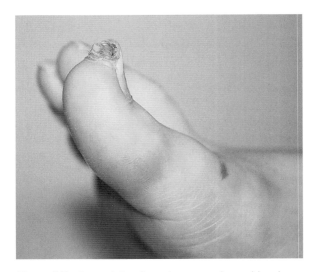

Figure 6.7   An angiokeratoma has caused a problem in trimming the nail. Careful nail management requires the nail to be thinned around the area. Cautery with hyfrecation may be offered, or silver nitrate to attempt to reduce the main vascular involvement. If management fails, surgical excision may be necessary.

Surgical excision is the treatment of choice (Fig. 6.8). Removal of part of the nail may be expedient but may only relieve the patient's discomfort for short periods. An exostectomy should be considered with a view to saving the nail.

Onychomycosis Nails with this condition vary in appearance and quality, ranging in cross-section from thin to thick and showing varying degrees of discoloration and separation from the nail bed. Some infections produce a brittle, honeycomb appearance in their late stages. Such nails can be removed or reduced so that they are thin enough to allow penetration of creams, ointments and lotions offering an antimycotic action. The nail can be reduced by using a scalpel or, preferably, a nail drill. Borotannic compounds tend to be inadequate in these cases, although they appear to slow fungal growth. The practitioner might also use clotrimazole, miconazole, amorolfine or tioconazole (Trosyl), all of which are painted onto the nail plate. These should be stopped if skin irritation occurs. Medications such as griseofulvin, terbinafine and ketoconazole can be taken systemically. There is recent evidence that shows that combinations of oral and systemic drugs (e.g. terbinafine oral tablets with amorolphine topical lacquer) obtain the best cure rates for onychomycosis.

Splits and furrows These are not very common. Median nail dystrophy has the appearance of a 'Christmas tree' rising in the centre of the nail plate. Reducing the asperitous surface so that it is level and smoother can be further assisted by covering with an occlusive cream. Creams might include Calmurid (urea-based) or a flexible collodion such as Opsite (Smith & Nephew).

Painful sulci from impacted skin debris Pain may arise from impacted skin debris (shed skin squames), in the sulci. A Blacks file or probe can be used to clear the groove. Prior to using these instruments, the debris can be softened. Shed skin squames will absorb water and swell, so any aqueous solution should assist in softening the debris. Hydrogen peroxide 10–20 vol applied to the sulci is particularly effective. A Blacks file or probe may be used to aid penetration of the hydrogen peroxide and to clear the sulci of debris. Both instruments should be used gently and carefully: if not, the patient may experience

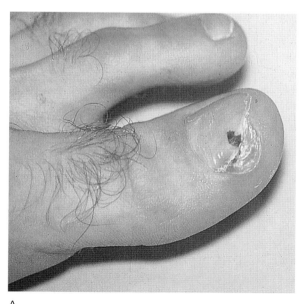

A

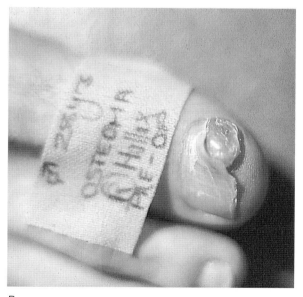

B

Figure 6.8 Two types of exostosis. A, Nail ablation (see later in this chapter) may be offered in mild nail elevation. B, Where there is a major nail deformity, the patient should have the bone excised with a view to allowing normal nail regrowth.

severe discomfort and the sulcus can be traumatized, resulting in a break in the skin. Postoperative emollient care is essential to ensure that there is not a repeat build-up of debris.

Painful sulci from onychophosis The epidermis can thicken along one or both sides of the nail sulcus, resulting in onychophosis. It is essential that the cause is established and an appropriate management plan implemented. Often the problem is lateral pressure from shoes or abnormal foot biomechanics. It may be necessary to cut back the nail in order to expose the lesion; in these instances the minimum amount of nail should be removed. This technique can be quite painful for the patient; local analgesia may have to be used. If a nail has to be cut back, it is essential that the sides are filed with a Blacks file in order to ensure that there are no roughened edges that could lead to further irritation of the sulcus. The callus should be debrided and the corns enucleated. Postoperatively, the sulci can be packed with cotton wool, foam or gauze. A pledget of cotton wool packed with tincture of benzoin (Friar's balsam), although dated, is a cheap and effective method. Other medications such as ichthammol and even clove oil have proven effective as conservative measures. Plastic sulcus gutters are more 'high-tech' but are probably no more effective. Repetitive sulcus pain should be treated by partial nail ablation.

Painful sulci from involuted nails This leads to discomfort as the nail irritates the sulcus. In these instances, clearing of the sulci, cutting back the nail and packing of the sulcus are all conservative methods that may be used. However, the deployment of these techniques may result in a vicious circle comprising repetitive conservative treatment, nail regrowth and pain. A partial or, if the nail is very deformed, total nail ablation may be the only way to resolve this problem.

NAIL DRILL

Indications

The nail drill can be used to reduce thickened and deformed nails and hyperkeratosis. Toenails are predisposed to thickening because of the prevalence of traumatic injuries to the foot and the trauma between the foot and shoe. Toenails may also thicken as a result of pathological conditions (e.g. psoriasis). Onychauxis (even thickening) or onychogryphosis (uneven thickening with deformity) may result. If left unattended, subungual ulceration or the piercing of adjacent skin may result.

Equipment

Nail drills can be powered by mains electricity or battery. Battery-powered drills are not as effective as the larger mains-powered drills. The drill can usually operate at variable speeds: 12 000 rpm is perhaps the most efficient. Care should be taken when selecting the speed as the nail plate can become uncomfortably hot if too high a speed is used or if the drill is used for a long period of time. Some nail drills include a fine water spray, these are particularly suited for use on nails requiring significant reduction. Water spray drills carry a reduced risk of burning the nail and surrounding tissues and do not require dust extraction as the nail dust and debris is dampened by the water spray and runs off the nail plate.

Drills without a water spray should be fitted with dust extraction to prevent occupation-related lung problems and reduce the problem of air-borne contamination arising from nail dust. The dust extraction bags should be changed regularly. Face masks are used by some practitioners in an attempt to reduce inhalation of nail dust, but the efficacy of these is not proven. Nail drills should be regularly maintained.

Burrs that fit into the drill handle come in many shapes and sizes, ranging from fine-pointed burrs, to release subungual haematomata, to broad-barrel burrs, to reduce nail thickness. The burrs are made from a range of materials, such as steel and diamond. The practitioner should equip the surgery with a selection of burrs (see Fig. 6.1). They should be sterilized between treatments. Ultrasonic cleansers can be used to dislodge debris from the burr prior to sterilization. Care must always be taken to use the correct size. A burr that is too small for the task will result in the drill having to be used for a longer period of time, causing warming of the nail. A burr that is too big may result in periungual damage.

Sanding discs can also be fitted, via an attachment, to nail drills. These discs are an abrasive piece of material, which is used to sand down hyperkeratosis, as discussed under debridement.

Burr technique

A one-way action should be used with a burr, working from the proximal to the distal end of the nail. The amount of pressure exerted onto the burr will affect the amount of nail reduced. Care should be taken not to apply too much pressure. The pressure should be kept constant, otherwise an uneven nail plate will result. In order to avoid the skin being caught by the burr, the adjacent skin may be masked by covering it with adhesive plaster cut to the shape of the surrounding skin. If the patient experiences discomfort, usually as a result of the nail becoming warm, stop the drill and spray the nail with an alcohol-based spray, returning once the nail has cooled down. It may be helpful to cut the length down and strip off the top layer of keratin with nippers prior to using the drill. In this way the plate is thinned, allowing for easier drilling.

Complications

The main complication from using the drill is the creation of a portal of entry via removal of too much skin or nail, or by catching adjacent skin. Appropriate antiseptic and dressing measures should be undertaken to prevent infection. Avoid using cotton wool around spinning burrs, as these can become entangled.

Special considerations

Subungual ulceration The practitioner must reduce any lytic (detached) parts of nail plate. A loose plate should be removed; nails that are lytic should be cut back as much as is allowed (Fig. 6.9). The ulcer heals with little assistance. Pain or infection should settle within a day or

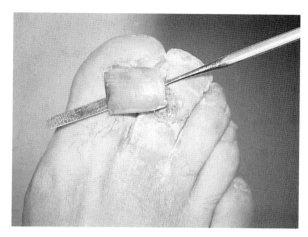

Figure 6.9 This patient presented with total lysis of the nail plate. This should be removed using local anaesthetic if attachment to the nail bed is still evident. All nails should be cut back as far as the nail is separated.

two in uncompromised patients. An antiseptic with sterile dressing should be applied.

NAIL SURGERY

NAIL ABLATION

Nail ablation techniques are indicated for a range of nail conditions:

- involution
- ingrowing toenail (onychocryptosis)
- abnormal structure and shape
- hypertrophy
- atrophy
- direct trauma
- minor exostosis
- soft tissue granulation
- onychomycosis
- subungual wart
- discoloration and lysis
- ungual fibromata
- subungual exostosis.

Involuted nails or ingrowing toenails, sometimes abbreviated to IGTN or o/c, are by far the most common reasons for performing nail surgery (Case study 6.2 and Fig. 6.10). *Ablation* means removal by surgery of a part, while *avulsion* suggests plucking out or tearing away. A range of ablation techniques may be performed on the nail. For the purposes of this chapter, these techniques will be divided into invasive and non-invasive. Non-invasive techniques relate to those procedures that do not cut into the skin and expose subdermal tissues. Using this approach, nail ablation techniques can be classified as follows:

- non-invasive
  - partial nail ablation
  - total nail ablation
- invasive
  - Winograd
  - Frost
  - Zadik
  - Syme's amputation.

The most common *non-invasive technique* is ablation with phenol. This is used in most of the cases that would benefit from removal of part or all of the nail. *Invasive techniques* for removing part of the nail are indicated when a large piece of periungual tissue needs to be removed in concert with the nail. Invasive techniques may not have the highest success rates, but the toe does heal faster than with non-invasive techniques. They are, therefore, useful for those patients who need to recover quickly and for those who, if they failed to heal, might be compromised. This latter group includes steroid users, diabetics and those likely to be oversensitive to chemical cautery.

Case study 6.2   An infected toe

A 47-year-old white female was treated by her GP for 6 months for an infected toe. Exuberant granulation was noted, which was subsequently excised. Closure could only be achieved once part of the distal phalanx had also been excised. At 6 months, excellent restoration of the toe was recorded despite loss of fat and bone (see Fig. 6.10A).

Conclusion: histopathology revealed multiple sinuses within a large granular nodule caused by abscess formation. Antibiotics had failed to reach the site and the patient would have been placed at risk from osteomyelitis if the lesion remained unattended.

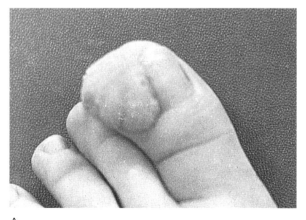

A

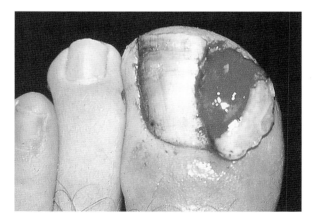

B

Figure 6.10   Ingrowing nail. A, Unsuccessful treatment of an ingrowing nail, which has formed abscesses. B, Common presentation of ingrowing nail or onychocryptosis, with exuberant hypergranulation.

Where possible, only part of the nail is removed in order to maintain the cosmetic appearance of the remaining part. Conditions such as involution and ingrowing toenails can be treated by this partial removal. In general, if more than 50% of the nail needs to be removed, a total nail ablation should be considered. The cosmetic appearance of the nail will be worse if only a small amount of nail is left. Some conditions, such as onychomycosis, discoloration and lysis, require the whole nail to be removed if treatment is to be successful.

Healthy vascular perfusion must be the most important criterion for any surgical technique. Presence of dorsalis pedis does not automatically suggest good perfusion to a toe; the posterior tibial artery is more important as it is the larger supplier of blood to the toes.

Non-invasive techniques can be performed in the presence of infection as long as the infection is restricted to the periungual tissues. When cellulitis is present, affecting more than the nail apparatus, a 1 week course of oral antibiotics is usually recommended prior to surgery. Non-invasive techniques can be undertaken in the second week, provided that the toe has responded to antibiosis. Healing will be more rapid once the source of infection is removed, particularly if drainage of the toe can be established.

Invasive techniques may also be performed in the presence of infection, but again with antibiotic cover. Incisional surgery will release pus that has been walled off. Deeper bone tissue must be protected. Local anaesthetics should not be infiltrated into infected tissue as this may result in the infection spreading. It is best to use proximal blocks wherever possible.

Malignancy

The nail plate should be examined for suspected subungual melanoma; these may take on the appearance of dark streaks. A specialist should be consulted prior to operating if a suspicious lesion around the nail plate is observed; biopsy is essential to confirm diagnosis. The prognosis and survival rates vary depending on speed of diagnosis, thickness of the lesion and the type of melanoma.

Radical excision is considered important around the boundary of the melanoma. Usually it is better for toes to be amputated, as grafting skin later can create difficulties with seeding.

Contraindications to nail surgery

The main reasons why invasive and non-invasive techniques may be contraindicated are:

- unsuitability for the administration of local analgesia
- poor healing post surgery
- bleeding disorders
- psychosocial problems resulting in poor aftercare or compliance
- severe uncontrolled organic disease.

Collagen disorders produce thin atrophic skin. In particular, scleroderma is contraindicated in order to avoid circulatory embarrassment. Active skin lesions such as psoriasis or eczema should also be avoided because of increased reactivity of the skin.

Peripheral vascular disease may be a reflection of other disease, of which diabetes is the most common. Failure to heal may give rise to secondary complications such as infection and gangrene. Patients undergoing chemotherapy or radiotherapy, or receiving high doses of steroids, are at risk. Failure to heal or produce a normal immunological response to infection may be very serious for at-risk patients.

Patients who are malnourished or who cannot attend to their own hygiene will be unsuitable. Patients who have suffered strokes or who have a mental disability should be judged on their individual merits. Patients with known violent tendencies tend to be unsuitable for local anaesthetics. Patients should not return home unaccompanied if attending for day surgery. Good support at home is needed for the immediate 24 hour period of postoperative recovery.

Patients with sickle cell anaemia (not the sickle cell trait) should not have tourniquets applied. Current medical convention is that patients with implants, Dacron bypass vessels and faulty heart valves must have prophylactic antibiotics.

Technique for nail surgery

Local anaesthetics

Nail ablation procedures affecting toes should be performed with good anaesthetic techniques (Fig. 6.11). The use of epinephrine (adrenaline) is considered to be contraindicated. The effects of vasoconstrictors in digital analgesia may not be as much of a problem as has previously been suggested, and this type of analgesia is commonly used by American podiatrists without detrimental ischaemia; nonetheless, excessive use of any injectable substance around the base of a digit (as in a ring block) may compress vessels. Common sense dictates the utmost caution with vasocon-strictors, although haemorrhage from granulation tissue is controlled with little risk to the patient if a vasoconstrictor is used as a hemiblock, thus dispelling some of the previous concerns about vasoconstrictors. Vascular risks probably increase with age, as digital vessels become less competent with degeneration of the vessel lumen; such findings have been observed when performing amputations without tourniquet.

Local anaesthesia with prilocaine (plain) 1–4% is adequate for most tasks, although many prefer lidocaine or mepivacaine. Most digits require no more than 2 ml, taking some 10–20 minutes to produce numbness for surgical ablation. Bupivacaine is more toxic, and some consider that it should not be used rou-

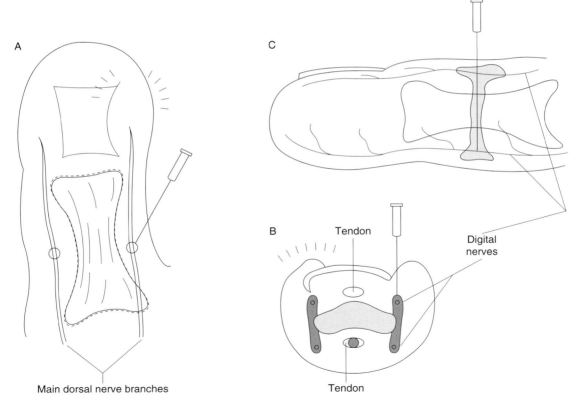

Figure 6.11 Digital blocks. Full-ring blocks should be avoided if at all possible. The toes are infiltrated at the base of the proximal phalanx as shown. For a total block, the lateral side should be infiltrated first, as the skin is looser. Dorsal to plantar injections are common for single sides. A full-ring block would encompass the whole toe; the volume should be strictly monitored in respect to the toe size and can cause a tourniquet effect. A, Dorsoplantar view. B, Lateral view. C, Cross-section showing position of nerves and tendons. The shaded area shows the deposit of anaesthetic.

tinely for this type of procedure, although there is no evidence to support this view. Failure to achieve sufficient analgesia may require changing the anaesthetic agent. A useful test is to place a blunt seeker down the painful nail sulcus to establish the depth of analgesia. Pricking the skin with syringe needles for this purpose is not advised as it will cause reactive wheals following histamine release; a clean blunt paper clip suffices.

Sterile field

Once anaesthesia has been achieved, the skin is prepared and a local sterile field established. The practitioner should be wearing sterile gloves. Non-invasive procedures can be performed in a clean clinical area with just a local sterile field. In the case of invasive techniques, particularly those affecting bone, a dedicated operating room is required with observation of the correct surgical protocol.

Equipment

Instruments should be freshly autoclaved or prepacked by a sterile supply department. A basic set of instruments for nail surgery is illustrated in Figure 6.12.

Tourniquet It is essential that exsanguination is achieved. A sterile ring tourniquet (Tournicot) or Esmarch band provides adequate haemostasis. Exsanguination should take place from the distal to the proximal end of the toe. Tourniquets should be retained for a minimum period, ideally under 30 minutes to avoid congestion and swelling later.

Non-invasive surgery

Total nail removal Total nail ablation requires separation of the hyponychial edge. An elevator is pushed under the plate, thus breaking the bond between the villus-like connection known as the onychodermal band (Fig. 6.13); the elevator is then pushed proximally under the plate until all resistance ceases. The eponychial fold is freed to prevent tearing. A mosquito or Spencer–

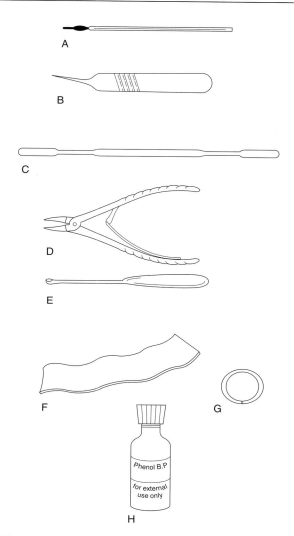

Figure 6.12 A basic set of instruments used for nail surgery. A, small probe (phenol application); B, nail splitter; C, nail elevator; D, straight forceps (Stamms shown); E, curette; F, Esmarch tourniquet; G, tournicot; H, correctly labelled phenol for external use only. The instrumentation also includes two Spencer-Wells forceps and a scalpel, as shown in Figure 6.1.

Wells forceps is clamped either side of the nail plate; a strong pair of forceps is recommended. The forceps are twisted to the centreline of the plate. The nail usually comes away in one piece. The nail bed is cleaned and dried. The practitioner must make sure that no small nail segments or loose pieces of skin remain.

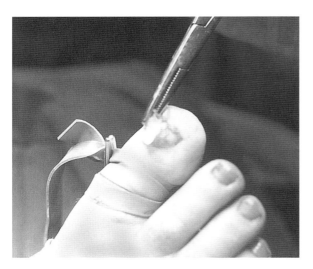

Figure 6.13 Nail ablation. Nail ablation is achieved by manual separation of the nail plate from the nail bed, working from the hyponychial (distal or free edge) border. The plate will separate easily once the onychodermal band has been freed.

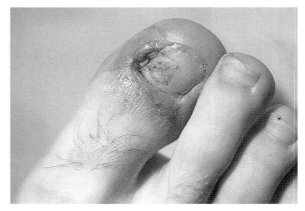

Figure 6.14 Partial nail ablation (PNA). The PNA is designed to remove up to 30% of the nail permanently when the matrix is destroyed. The illustration shows a PNA at first dressing. A small amount of inflammation is present around the base of the toe and on the medial side.

Partial nail removal Wedge or partial resection should ideally only remove 25–30% of the plate. The reason for this lies in the need to preserve some sensible cosmetic appearance (Fig. 6.14). If a greater proportion of nail is removed, the nail plate might just as well be removed in one piece. Once the tight adhesion of the most lateral side of the eponychial fold is released, by positioning an elevator to separate the two, a pair of fine, straight-sided nippers can be used to cut down the nail. The nippers are pushed firmly down the length of the nail plate until a point is reached when they either meet resistance or cannot progress further. If needed, a Beaver with a 61 blade (chisel-shaped) or nail splitter can be used to cut the remaining nail edge. The nail will give at the most proximal point. It must be appreciated that the most proximal limit of resistance is against the distal phalanx, which lies close to the interphalangeal joint. The risk of infection is greatest at this point. Forceps should grasp the spicule, rotating the piece towards the midline. It is incumbent upon the practitioner to check down the open sulcus and feel for deep fibrous attachments and broken nail; leaving a loose piece of nail in the sulcus will promote infection.

Destruction of the matrix Chemical and thermal treatments have been used to destroy the nail matrix. The following methods have been used:

- phenol (carbolic acid)
- sodium hydroxide
- trichloroacetic acid
- nitrous oxide
- carbon dioxide
- negative galvanism
- silver nitrate stick.

Phenol is by far the most popular method and is a powerful antibacterial agent, a point well established by Lister in 1865. Exsanguination (removal of blood) is essential, as blood will dilute the phenol as it coagulates protein on contact. Diluted phenol will effectively reduce the success of the operation. Phenol can be used at 80% strength or as a saturated solution. The former appears to be as effective as the saturated solution and may reduce the number of phenol burns.

There has been much speculation about the best way to apply phenol. Originally, three separate 1 minute applications were used. Phenol has a continuous action and is, therefore, probably not sensitive to time alone. Tissue uptake is likely to be more relevant. Fragile older tissue needs less time than young healthy tissue. The change from pink to dirty brown–white is a useful indication. Moist (hyperhidrotic) tissues may need longer.

The type of phenol is also important. Phenol should be fresh and have no pink tinge. This can best be achieved by disposing of small bottles of liquid or crystals after each use.

One of the problems associated with nail ablation techniques is regrowth. Andrew & Wallace (1979) found that, out of 107 patients, only 6% required further treatment after phenolic destruction of the matrix, compared with 18% following surgical excision. Ramsey & Caldwell (1985) provided evidence of only 3% of regrowth in 1013 cases. Chemical preparations, such as 10% sodium hydroxide and trichloroacetic acid, have also been used with success.

Freezing with gases such as nitrous oxide was reported by Tollafield (unpublished work, 1980). Healing appeared to be better than with phenol, but the apparatus to procure a freeze was expensive and it needed specialist probes. In a small research project of seven cases, patients experienced greater postoperative pain from nitrous oxide than phenol. Apfelberg (1987) described the use of carbon dioxide for nail ablation.

Polokoff described the use of negative galvanism in 1961 (see Polokoff 1987). This is an electrical technique that produces sodium hydroxide at the site of the active (cathode) electrode with a direct current, as opposed to an alternating current. Negative galvanism is performed without a tourniquet. Technically, this is not a popular technique in that it is time-consuming and produces a slight electrical hazard for patients with metal implants and pacemakers. Cautery loops have also been used. Thin metal wires heated with a small current offer another form of thermal destruction.

Invasive surgery

Zadik's matrix dissection   This procedure of surgical ablation by dissecting the matrix away (Zadik 1950) is difficult and should be reserved for experienced specialists, as partial regrowth is common. The process requires active debridement of the bone, peeling away the matrix carefully. The lines of incision must be carried on down the lateral sides of the nail apparatus to avoid spicular regrowth (Fig. 6.15A).

Winograd's partial matricectomy   Winograd described the partial matricectomy in 1929 (see Winograd 1987; Fig. 6.15B). The excised tissue is sutured afterwards. Any cells left behind commonly produce new nail growth. This tends to occur in partial removal at the proximal edge of the sulcus. The appearance is that of a little horn. If this occurs following healing, a small amount of liquid phenol can be placed on the site once the nail spicule has been ablated.

Other partial matricectomies (Frost and Steindler)   These two techniques differ from the Winograd procedure in that a flap of periungual

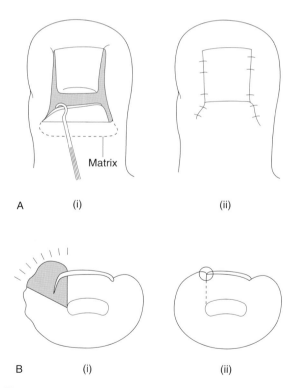

Figure 6.15   Various types of surgical nail ablation can be achieved by excising the matrices. A, Zadik's operation for total nail bed excision, showing incision lines (i) and sutured flaps (ii). B, Cross-sections through Winograd procedure for extensive paronychial tissue excision.

tissue is raised (Fig. 6.16). Sutures or sterile tapes can be used after deep dissection has been completed to secure the wound. Necrosis of flaps can occur if the skin is cut too thinly without regard for the blood supply. Postoperative healing is rapid (Fig. 6.17).

MANAGEMENT FOLLOWING NAIL SURGERY

The literature contains many regimens for management after nail surgery, ranging from packing the sulcus at the time of surgery to keeping the initial dressing on for 7 days before redressing. Some advocate bathing through the dressing by immersing toe and bandage in saline. Removal of the dressing after 24 hours is also practised. Daily bathing in a footbath is also common.

Packing the sulci after surgery, often with a paraffin tulle, results in the dressing becoming hard and may cause discomfort, especially when attempts are made to remove it. Some practitioners dislike the use of packing as they consider drainage may be prevented, particularly as phenol intentionally causes a discharge. There is no evidence to suggest that packing helps healing. Patients who keep their dressing on for 7 days may find that they develop a pungent odour, the dressing becomes discoloured and, in some cases, where there has been a discharge, strikethrough occurs. Immersion in a salt footbath with the dressing on does not appear to have any advantage over bathing with the dressing off, as long as a new dressing is reapplied. A suitable environment needs to be created for healing. The oedema and resultant exudate that may occur postsurgically may well reduce the rapidity of such a process. In most cases, postoperative resolution is achieved by simple cleansing and good hygiene. However, where the nail bed becomes

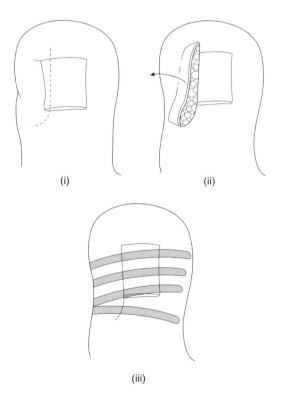

Figure 6.16 Steindler or Frost partial matricectomy. This approach is used for minimal exposure matrix excision (i, ii). Sterile tapes (Steristrips) have been used to close the wound (iii).

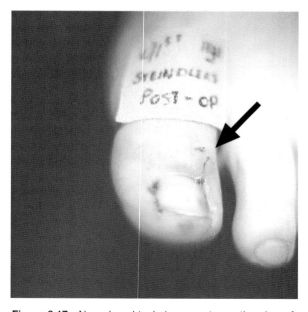

Figure 6.17 Non-phenol technique: postoperative view of Steindler procedure closed with Steristrip sutures.

macerated or a sulcus becomes particularly inflamed, an antiseptic should be used. Fucidin and cicatrin (topical antibiotic agents) are no more beneficial and may cause a risk of skin sensitivity. Creams such as Anaflex 10% cream have an anti-inflammatory effect, which is thought to be highly beneficial in drying the nail bed following surgery.

Altman et al (1990) considered other products applied topically after nail surgery. A control, silver sulfadiazine, and hydrocortisone 1% creams were used separately and in combination. Criteria used to judge success revolved around reduction of pain, discharge, inflammation and drainage. The combination product was slightly more effective in reducing the four associated criteria. The control did surprisingly well. Altman et al were able to show that using hydrocortisone did not impair healing and can be helpful in postoperative nail surgery care. Silver sulfadiazine is a topical medicament useful in the management of burns.

Complications arising from non-invasive nail ablation

Complications are not uncommon with nail surgery. Four weak links exist and give rise to problems in any surgical situation. These include the operator, the technique used, the environment and the patient.

Infection Phenol procedures have a slightly higher chance of becoming infected than do others. The reason for this lies in the resultant oedema in digital tissue, the open nature of the wound and the damaged tissue that is devitalized by the caustic. Infection should be treated with antiseptics in the early stages and by copious daily bathing, depending upon the patient's own capability and mobility. Antibiotics should be reserved for the occasion when the wound fails to respond to antiseptics, or where culture and sensitivity shows a positive infection. If poor healing (without proven infection) continues for several weeks, antibiotics appear to improve the situation. Tollafield & Parmar (1994) noted in a 5-year surgical audit that antibiotics often failed to give adequate relief unless the course was extended to 10–14 days for foot infections. *Staphylococcus aureus* is the most common infective agent and flucloxacillin is the drug of choice, at a dose of 250 mg (adult) four times a day. Allergies and sensitivities are not uncommon to this effective group of antibiotics, and erythromycin may be given as an alternative, at a dose of 250 mg every 6 hours.

Phenol burns Phenolization techniques may appear easy to apply, but they should not be employed by the inexperienced practitioner, who cannot appreciate the care required in applying an invisible caustic. The chemical often does not show its most potent effects for several hours, after the toe has lost its anaesthetic effect. Phenol spillage should be avoided as it provokes a pernicious response and may take many weeks to heal, even on healthy skin (Fig. 6.18). Burns from phenol spillage on the skin must be protected from infection and the patient must be warned about such a risk and told how to minimize the problem. Most toes heal in the end. Patience is more likely if the patient knows the risks from nail surgery in advance.

Delayed healing Healing is sometimes slow and can last from 1 week to 5 months. Drainage is common for 3–4 weeks but does not always sustain significant cultures. The larger the surface area phenolized, the more likely it is that a patient will heal slowly. However, it has been found that total ablations do not necessarily always follow this trend, because nails that have undergone this technique drain better than those that have undergone partial ablations. Likewise, age and tissue quality appear to have some bearing upon healing. The older skin tends to be weaker to the effects of phenol and may take longer to heal.

Periostitis Periostitis may occur following phenolization techniques, although it is rarely documented. Gilles et al (1986) reported the case of a 29-year-old woman who had a positive culture recorded with a pyrexic state of 37°C (98.6°F). Periosteal elevation, seen on X-ray film, is less evident in the absence of pus. X-ray views are important for ruling out osteomyelitis, which is indicated in the phalanges by radiolucency. Periosteal elevation is less likely unless there is

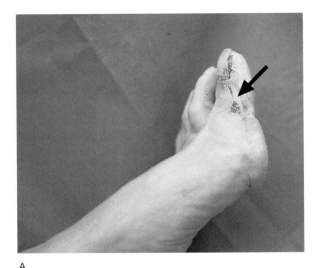

A

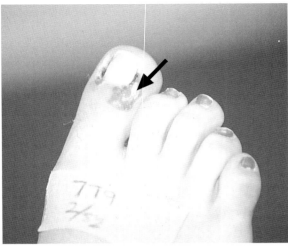

B

Figure 6.18 Phenolization. Phenol can leave considerable tissue damage if care is not taken. This burn took many weeks to recover despite the phenol only remaining on the skin briefly. A, Spillage down the side of the toe. B, Overzealous phenolization around the base of the hallux.

sufficient pus. If periostitis is suspected and the presence of infection has been ruled out, a Sher injection should be administered; this technique involves placing 0.1–0.2 ml corticosteroid into the epidermal edge under a ring block of anaesthesia. The injection should be performed at 90° to the surface, to avoid damaging the dermal blood supply.

Hypergranulation Hypergranulation (Fig. 6.10B) may be detrimental if left. The excessive vascular tissue can distort the toe and, if abundant, can recreate the problem, as seen in Figure 6.10A. Small amounts of pink tissue can be left without too much concern. The easiest technique for removing tissue is to cut it away with nippers (Stamm bone nippers) or to dissect it with an elliptical cut. The deeper and wider the cut, the more difficult it will be to close the wound. Larger sections of hypergranulation may need to be curetted when trimmed, in order to leave a clean granulating base. Phenol should not be allowed to seep into this part of the wound.

Postoperative pain. Pain that does not respond to basic analgesics such as paracetamol compounds should be carefully examined to rule out reflex sympathetic dystrophy. Radiographic features (Sudek's atrophy) may take several weeks to show. Vasomotor changes cause alarming colour patterns, such as hot flushed to a mottled cyanosed effect, either at the site or over the whole foot. The condition is poorly understood and pain is triggered by inconsequential trauma (Tollafield 1991). If pain cannot be alleviated within 4 weeks and there are no signs of infection, a pain clinic should be consulted.

Regrowth. Regrowth of nails following surgery is an accepted hazard. Practitioners will accept this inevitability at some time in their careers, but should take all steps to minimize its occurrence. Patients must be warned that not every case is successful and that rephenolization may be necessary; this can be achieved by dropping some phenol down the nail groove, once the spicule has been removed under local analgesia, if required.

Complications arising from invasive techniques

Sutures have been found to increase postoperative pain (Tollafield & Palmer 1994). The preferred method of closure is surgical taping for 2 weeks. Regrowth of nails following invasive surgery described above is higher than from phenolization by 30–40%. The infection rate seems no higher than that resulting from phenol techniques; it may even be a little lower. There are no risks from burns, but inclusion cysts do occur where nail cells become incorporated into the wound at the proximal edge.

INCISIONAL APPROACHES TO SURGERY

Indications

There are a number of reasons for incising the skin on the foot and these fall into four categories:

- to gain access to perform a surgical procedure to correct or ameliorate a problem that lies deep to the skin (Ch. 7)
- to release a deep-seated abscess from pressure of exudate and pus, to remove an old suture or to remove a foreign body, e.g. an inclusion cyst
- to remove a verruca that does not respond to conservative treatment
- to remove a section of a lesion for histological investigation when its precise nature is unclear.

Each of the above results in the need for a surgical operation that will require anaesthesia, haemostasis and appropriate postsurgical care. The instruments used will vary according to personal preference. Such instruments should ideally be prepacked and sterilized by a licensed department, together with drapes and dressings. The majority of techniques described in this chapter use instruments that can be packed in small presterilized bags. Surgery performed to a depth greater than that of the subcutaneous layers requires specialized instruments. The description and discussion of the various uses of such instruments is left to other texts.

Techniques

Principles of incision

The following discussion concerns the general principles behind skin incisions. All operative techniques should be planned to provide the best result possible. The site and direction of the incision are important considerations. An incision should be long enough to gain access to the anatomy. It may be easily lengthened but should not be stretched so that blood vessels near the surface are damaged. Linear (straight) incisions are easier to close (with suture repair) than tortuous or lacerated wounds. The blade that cuts through the epidermis must do so vertically to avoid stripping the delicate neurovascular supply between the dermis and epidermis. Careful tissue handling is imperative in order to avoid large contusions (bruises) below the surface and trauma that might create necrosis. Such problems will lead to sloughing and raise the risks of infection and hypertrophic scarring. The epidermal skin must not be squeezed tightly or pulled under tension needlessly with forcep-type instruments.

For many years, the plantar surface of the foot has been considered as a 'no go' area. However, some operations do require access through this surface. Where possible, the skin should be incised to one side of the metatarsal in order to prevent scarring over a load-bearing surface. Extrusion of plantar fat from a weight-bearing area is a sure way to invite a corn or intractable plantar keratoma.

Linear incisions are best curved around or over a joint. Cicatrization or scarring may limit movement and cause contraction. Examples of these areas include the dorsal metatarsophalangeal surface and the anterior surface of the ankle. The incision should curve so that potential contraction is spread in more than one direction. Known anatomical structures should be avoided.

There are parts of the foot where incision lines must be made in specific directions. If a round-bodied instrument, such as an awl, is inserted about 2.5 cm into the skin of these parts, the wound lengthens rather than showing up as a round hole. This phenomenon was identified by Dupuytren in 1834 and expounded by Langer in 1861: hence the term Langer lines. When sufficient holes were made in a cadaver, they formed the pattern of these lines. Langer found that the connective tissue attached to muscle underlying the skin was disturbed and affected the constant tension within the skin. Such lines run perpendicular to the action of muscles and may or may not coincide with wrinkle lines. Scars made along the Langer lines are considered to interfere less with body dynamics when placed transversely (perpendicular to the action) across muscles and joints. Testing for these lines can give rise to variance, as found by Cox in 1941 (McGlamry 1987). Pinching the skin deeply, to take in underlying tissues, shows resistance in one direction. By pinching in a direction perpendicular to this, the skin is picked up more easily. If the skin is squeezed too superficially, it will be difficult to differentiate the line of relaxed tension. The use of tension can assist in a simple skin biopsy.

Planning surgery in advance

Once an excisional wound has been created, the surgeon cannot always rely upon closure from double ellipse incision. Faced with a gap, two alternatives arise. The gap can be left – if it is closed, the blood supply will be compromised by tension of the skin – or the skin can be incised in such a way as to allow the defect (or gap) to be repaired as well. Naturally there are situations where skin autografts are required (e.g. where the defect is large). Surgery that may lead to possible unpredictable problems must be performed by trained surgeons in the correct theatre setting, where equipment and hospital can provide adequate support for any unexpected needs.

Curettage

Curettage means literally 'to clear out'. Verrucae with well-defined circumscribed outlines respond well to this technique; however, other, non-surgical treatments do exist and will be described in Chapter 15. Curettage is also a valuable technique for scraping the base of wounds such as ulcers and for hypergranulation, pyogenic granuloma and the base of excised verrucae. Curettage is often performed with electrocautery, which offers haemostasis. This technique should only be used for small lesions that will not produce extensive scarring on healing. Larger lesions are better dealt with by incision and suturing in order that healing can occur by primary intention.

The force required to curette a lesion within the epidermis is significant. In order to reduce the size of this force, the lesion should initially be incised in a circular manner, using a scalpel to the level of dermis. The sharp edge of the curette is then inserted into the incision. Curettage is not the method of choice for producing histology samples, as too much cellular damage may occur.

Biopsy techniques

Biopsy involves the removal of a part, or all, of a lesion for histopathological testing. Three techniques can be used: excisional, shave or puncture biopsy. Excisional biopsy has the advantage of providing a tissue sample and treatment at the same time. The excisional biopsy technique comprises a double ellipse incision around the skin lesion. The length needs to be four times the width, in order to achieve adequate closure of the wound. The shave biopsy is achieved by pinching up the skin and slicing the lesion across; this allows fat and dermis to remain. The main difficulty with this technique lies in the need to ensure that all cells are adequately biopsied, reducing the need for further tissue samples. This technique is rarely used on the foot.

A punch biopsy can be used to provide a sample from a large lesion but brings with it the disadvantage that a further operation may be needed later.

Wound closure

Having incised the skin, it is essential that the appropriate environment is created to ensure that healing takes place. The principles of repair are as follows:

- control haemorrhage
- provide good tissue apposition
- enhance repair
- minimize scarring
- restore function.

Suture materials The following materials can be used for sutures (*sutura* – Lat. 'seam'):

- adhesive surgical tape (various sizes)
- synthetic braided threads
- synthetic monofilament threads, e.g. nylon, polypropylene
- natural materials, e.g. silk, cotton.

Sutures are either absorbable or non-absorbable. Absorbable sutures are subject to degradation within human tissue. Suture strength is determined by the type of material and size and by the suture technique used. As a

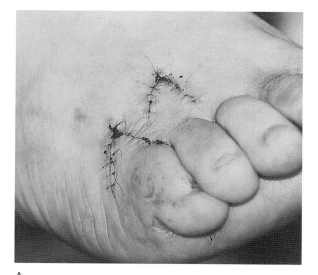

A

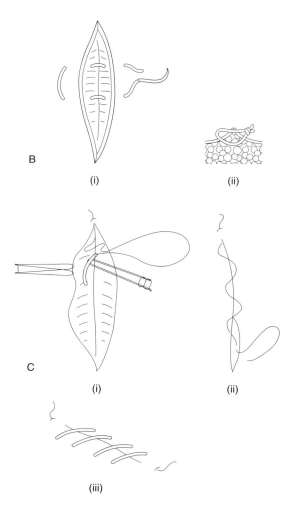

B

(i)   (ii)

C

(i)   (ii)

(iii)

Figure 6.19 Methods of suturing. A, Simple suture. This is formed from a single loop of thread, which is tied off as a reef knot. The advantage lies in the fact that it is easy to perform and the wound has an even spread of tension along its length, as long as the sutures are spaced evenly. If an infection arises, one or more sutures can be removed without compromising the wound. The wound in this figure has been incised with two V–Y flaps to reduce the fourth and fifth toes. 5/0 sutures of polypropylene have been used to minimize damage to the sensitive blood supply under the skin. B, Horizontal mattress. This type of suture offers two main advantages. First, the suture is made up of two loops and, therefore, closure is faster than with the simple suture (i). This suture is also harder to remove than the simple suture. Second, the wound haemostasis is improved because the skin is compressed (ii). C, Subcuticular suture. This is chosen for its cosmetic post-surgical results. It cannot be placed in a wound where tension is required. The suture is placed through the skin below the dermal-epidermal junction (i). By pulling on both ends, the wound pulls together (ii). Absorbable sutures do need to be bridged. Sterile tape is often used to support the wound after closure (iii). (Adapted from Mercado (1976).)

rule, this strength is measured in days. Catgut (collagen from the intestines of sheep) lasts about 1 week before it loses its strength. It is highly reactive and not used in the foot very often. Chroming the catgut (tanning) will increase the strength to 3 weeks. Common absorbable sutures used are polyglactin 910 or polyglycolic acid, and these can retain their strength for 40–60 days.

Non-absorbable sutures are derived from modern plastics, although cotton, silk and steel wire are still available. The two most commonly used sutures are polypropylene and polyethylene. Such materials are hypoallergenic and, therefore, relatively inert.

The size of a suture is determined by its gauge. '000' or '3/0' lies in the middle of the range of common surgical sutures: 1/0 is large and thick, while 6/0 is small and fine.

Needles Each suture is suaged to a needle. This means that the small attachment of suture to needle does not result in skin being stretched at the point of skin exit, as there is no 'eye' spreading out behind the needle. Needles come in all shapes. The curved shape allows the needle to be recovered easily from the opposing side of the wound. Larger sutures and their needles tend to have larger curvatures. Quarter circles of 19–20 mm are the commonest size for foot surgery. The length of needle represents its length before curvature. Half-circle needles are useful for deep wounds.

The cross-section of the needle is important for its function. A rounded cross-section might be fine for fat or mucous tissues, but epidermis is tough and will bend the needle quickly. A triangular cross-section with a trocar point offers strength and ease of application. Cutting and reverse-cutting needles are popular for use in the tough tissues of the foot.

Suture techniques The techniques used to close wounds must ensure that the skin edges are brought together and not buried, otherwise an epidermoid cyst could result. Three common techniques are shown in Figure 6.19, although there are many other variations that can be found in surgical texts.

General considerations when suturing include:

- wounds should never be closed in the presence of infection
- sutures should never be placed under tension
- sutures in the foot should be removed after 10 to 21 days; plantar repair requires 21 days
- stitch abscesses can occur as a result of intraepidermal irritation from buried suture ends.

SUMMARY

This chapter has covered the range of basic operative techniques that can be used to treat lesions affecting the epidermis and dermis, including the nail apparatus.

A number of examples have illustrated the breadth of clinical skills required. The general considerations and complications that may occur have been discussed, together with their management. The chapter has provided a broad overview but does not purport to provide sufficient depth for all types of foot surgery. It is essential that the reader consults more detailed texts.

REFERENCES

Altman M I, Sulensky C, de Lisle R, De Velasco M. 1990 Silver sulfadiazine and hydrocortisone cream in the management of phenol matricectomy. Journal of American Podiatric Medical Association 80: 545–547

Andrew T, Wallace W A 1979 Nail bed ablation: excise or cauterise? A controlled study. British Medical Journal 9: 1539

Apfelberg D B 1987 In: McGlamry E D, Banks A S, Downey M S (eds) Comprehensive textbook of foot surgery. Williams & Wilkins, Baltimore, vol 1, p 24

Gilles G A, Dennis K J, Harkless L B 1986 Periostitis associated with phenol matrictomies. Journal of the American Podiatric Medical Association 76: 469–471

McGlamry E D, Banks A S, Downey M S (eds) 1987 Comprehensive textbook of foot surgery. Williams & Wilkins, Baltimore, MD, vol 2, p 685–688

Mercado O A 1976 Podiatric surgical dissection. Fundamental skills. Corolando Education Materials for Podiatric Medicine, Illinois, p 20–23

Polokoff M 1987 Digital surgery. In: McGlamry E D, Banks A S, Downey M S (eds) Comprehensive textbook of foot surgery. Williams & Wilkins, Baltimore, MD, vol 1, p 23

Ramsey G, Caldwell 1985 Phenol cauterization for ingrown toenails: unreviewed reports. British Medical Journal 291: 110

Tollafield D R 1991 Reflex sympathetic dystrophy in day case foot surgery. British Journal of Podiatric Medicine and Surgery 3: 2–6

Tollafield D R, Parmar D G 1994 Setting standards for day care foot surgery. A quinquennial review. British Journal of Podiatric Medicine and Surgery 6: 7–20

Winograd A M 1987 Surgery of the nail. In: McGlamry E D, Banks A S, Downey M S (eds) Comprehensive textbook of foot surgery. Williams & Wilkins, Baltimore, MD, vol 1, p 19

Zadik F R 1950 Obliteration of the nail bed of the great toe without shortening the terminal phalanx. Journal of Bone and Joint Surgery 32B: 66–67

7

Surgery and the foot

David R. Tollafield

INTRODUCTION

No book written about the foot and its treatment would be complete without some reference to surgery. Much of the content of this chapter is intended for reference but the novice surgeon will find the contents valuable as an overview and introduction to a career in foot surgery.

The decision to initiate surgery lies with the patient's medical physician or health care practitioner. For this reason it is quite likely that patients likely to need surgery will seek preliminary advise from a non-surgeon. Surgery can be undertaken in a hospital or in a dedicated surgical day centre. Specific details on foot surgery and further details of anaesthetic management can be found in specialized texts for those wishing to study the art and science to a level suited to practice. Trauma, while being another important reason for surgery, would take this chapter outside its introductory remit. The unpretentious examples provided relate to patients seeking elective (voluntary) rather than emergency surgery.

Podiatry is the study of foot health and treatment of foot and ankle pathology by established medical, surgical and mechanical methods. While the most desirable form of treatment is conservative care, 20–40% of patients might end up with some type of surgery, particularly where deformity, trauma, pain or infection occur (Fig. 7.1). The surgical specialist is likely to receive patients for pain as the primary reason for referral, often after conservative care has been undertaken. Violation of tissue viability causes both morbidity as well as immobility, which may be affected by deformity or by functional instability. Priority for referral is judged often by intensity of pain and lack of improvement. Most patients will find management from podiatrists without the need for surgery but 5% of patients are unlikely to be treated with any type of success from management, which provides a sobering thought. Satisfaction and success is often viewed differently by patient and practitioner. The practitioner's role, in addition to considering the merits of surgical intervention, is to advise patients of the pitfalls of, and likely benefits from, such an intervention. Some knowledge of surgery is particularly helpful when providing patients with advice following previous episodes of foot surgery. Either way, the quality of advice offered by practitioners is closely allied to their understanding of surgical principles.

It is assumed in this chapter that a patient's medical health has already satisfied the requirements for safe admission, either as a day patient or as an inpatient. A patient's personal and social background forms a significant part of preselection for surgery and may prove to be more important than their medical welfare when taken alone.

Clinical governance impacting on surgery

The health care practitioner is responsible initially for generating a referral; in so doing, he or she must understand that, even in the hands of a meticulous surgeon, surgery is not without complication. The implications of failure must be included in any advice given to the patient, ideally before referral. In this chapter, discussion covers the likely complications, which are perhaps better termed as 'sequelae': events arising from surgery, which may be either foreseeable or less-obvious postoperative events.

During the 1990s, an explosion of health care political correctness fragmented many of the older philosophies. 'Safe care in our hands' is no longer accepted as the norm. Clinical governance has placed pressures on health care professionals to alter the perspective of treatment. Greater patient understanding must be included within the management process. The process of consent is very much part of selection and paramount in providing the best care. In this chapter, consent pertinent to surgery is considered more closely. When discussing patient selection in the next section, it is worth revisiting how consent and negligence become interwoven. Good planning and communication with the patient is principally to reassure the patient, but it is also necessary to protect against the soaring costs involved in defending a case where better planning might have avoided unnecessary litigation.

SELECTING PATIENTS FOR SURGERY

Referral urgency and appropriateness

Timely surgery allows the surgeon to prevent deterioration. Failure to make an appropriate referral to the surgeon (podiatric or orthopaedic) may alter the ideal prognosis. The converse of timely referral is to ensure that all appropriate measures have been carried out: orthotic management, local tissue management and, if appropriate, drug management. In reality, drug management should be brief and avoid medication side-effects. An example of a common problem

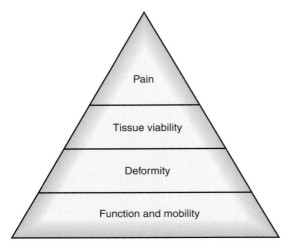

Figure 7.1 Four key aims in managing the foot by surgery.

Pain

Tissue viability

Deformity

Function and mobility

associated with inappropriate medication results from overuse and extended use of non-steroidal anti-inflammatory drugs (NSAIDs), where gastric irritation causes stomach pain and may lead to gastric bleeding. While analgesic medication may alleviate pain, such strategies should be limited to short periods – measured in weeks – or until a referral is made. Patient referrals should be as detailed as possible and if urgent should say so. As a guide, the health practitioner should consider the effect that the foot problem has on the patient (Table 7.1).

Tripartite nature of decision-making

Case study 7.1 illustrates the tripartite nature of the decision-making process: the practitioner, the patient and the surgeon will each have a different set of criteria, which will influence the acceptability of surgical intervention.

The practitioner will need to answer a number of questions before deciding to refer a patient for surgery:

- is surgery applicable?
- will surgery ameliorate the problem efficiently, with little disruption to the patient's lifestyle or occupation?
- can surgery be undertaken effectively at reasonable cost without
  - affecting the patient's income adversely, or
  - incurring unreasonable overheads if the outcome is unpredictable?
- will surgery place the patient's health at risk?
- can surgery prevent the problem from deteriorating?
- can the patient's quality of life be improved by surgery?
- will such intervention extend the patient's lifespan? (This question should also consider longer term success expected from surgery.)

Table 7.1 Criteria for referral[a]

Criteria	Routine	Urgent
Pain intensity	Varies but not all the time	Constant level increasing above scale 5 (0–10)
Pain duration	Comes and goes	Lasts especially at rest and seems to be increasing above scale 3 (0–10)
Need for analgesia	None	Becoming dependent and increasing doses and strength. Side effects present
Mobility	Some effect but can climb, walk and run to an extent	Any or all movements affected
Effect on daily function	Can do most things in the house/garden and can do shopping	Many simple activities are affected and routines have altered, including driving
Effect on work	Can go to work, affected by condition but not unduly	Patient has had time off work, or continues to have time off work
Effect on social habits and recreation	Can walk, play games undertake interests	Has had to stop games, and cannot undertake activities or even contemplate holidays
Presence of infection	Nil/well contained	Deeper tissue affected, or where tissue breakdown on a recurrent basis. Antibiotics needed frequently
Presence of ulceration or tissue breakdown	No presence of tissue damage or tissue is completely intact	Tissue is constantly breached, risk of infection and need to use antibiotics on more than three occasions

[a]Referrals are often delayed because of insufficient information. Practitioners should read their own correspondence where feasible and decide the urgency and need contained within the letter. Poor referrals are those without sufficient explanation while quality referrals contain key statements exemplified by the table. Scales refer to pain levels 0–10 where 10 is the most painful experience or response.

Case study 7.1   The tripartite nature of the decision-making process

A 54-year-old company manager was referred to a podiatrist by his family GP. The complaint was a fixed flexion deformity associated with the proximal IP joint of the second toe. The patient was suited to surgery because permanent relief of his symptoms could be achieved, but he declined surgical intervention.

The patient sought his GP's view regarding the complaint. Referral to the podiatrist was considered reasonable in light of the patient having no existing medical problems. Having assessed the patient's complaint, the podiatrist concluded that conservative treatment was less likely to result in a satisfactory outcome than surgical intervention. Taking account of patient motivation, medical welfare, home support and the ability to manage after surgery, the podiatrist was satisfied that surgery was in the patient's best interest.

The patient was fully informed and provided with a description of the surgical process. As part of the information, he was sent an informed consent by post, in advance of surgery. The patient read the consent and declined surgery because he felt that the stated risks were unreasonable and because a period of immobility was recommended. The risks highlighted on the consent form included possible infection, swelling and pain; it was also stated that there was a need to rest the foot for several weeks before returning to work.

Comment: Hospital consent forms rarely describe specific risks – such risks as are applicable are often left to a personal discussion before the operation. More often than not, consent forms are signed by the patient on the day of admission.

The GP, the podiatric surgeon and the patient each had their own criteria preset for the treatment involved. The referral was correct, the procedure selected carried the likelihood of a successful outcome; however, the patient believed that the risks stated on his consent sheet outweighed the benefits offered by surgery. Additionally, the patient felt that he could not take the recommended period of time off work.

Health status

A full medical assessment should be undertaken to avoid any known existing disorders that could place the patient at risk.

Many patients fail to see the risks that might arise from treatment. The desire to be cured may suppress the reality that a procedure can make some patients worse. Personal and social factors can have a greater impact on success from surgical management than health welfare alone. The decision to operate must take into consideration a variety of factors not related to health:

- support at home (social)
- occupation (financial)
- mobility (after surgery)
- accepted risk (complications)
- chances of success (rated outcome)
- patient motivation and attitude
- age.

Social circumstances

Patients should not be left alone following their discharge from the hospital or surgical centre. They should have a telephone in case of problems and should be able to reach the hospital or

surgical centre easily to attend follow-up appointments. The patient's lifestyle and home support can make a considerable difference, particularly where the patient has a dependant (children/parents). The patient's partner has to assume many of the patient's responsibilities, and tension can rise, particularly where recovery may be prolonged.

Occupation

Some employers provide few benefits for those in lower paid jobs. Examination of the patient's occupational circumstances is essential before agreeing to an operative solution, unless of course the operation is essential or is likely to have minimal effects on mobility. Prolonged periods off work are particularly hard for single-parent families, those without a partner's support and those in demanding positions at work.

Mobility

The effect of surgery on feet clearly has a marked impact on the ability to walk and carry out normal ambulatory functions, such as climbing stairs, driving, shopping, going to work and undertaking hobbies. While surgery performed on both feet at the same time may not be proportionally twice as painful, and the cost to the service may appear less, the resultant immobility can have a marked effect on ambulation. The postoperative requirements of bilateral surgery must be discussed to ensure that the patient fully understands the likely limitations. Prolonged bed rest poses a risk of deep vein thrombosis (DVT) and pulmonary thrombosis.

Risk

Infection, swelling and pain are commonplace in foot surgery. In some cases, it may not be possible to wear shoes for anything from 6 weeks to 6 months. Such conditions need to be discussed with the patient, in terms of how long each phase will last and what steps will be taken to ameliorate the problem.

Dysfunction, loss of sensation, poor tissue healing and hyperaesthesia form a second, albeit lower, set of risks. Nonetheless, if a patient should have any of these, resolution may take much longer. Sequelae arising from surgery are discussed later on in this chapter.

Success

Successful treatment can never be guaranteed. Careful audit of treatment provides an indication of the likely outcome. Patients will want to know how successful a particular procedure will be. Audit should be incorporated into the practitioner's routine, so that outcome can be expressed in terms of a percentage success rate. In each case, likely success and shortfall should be discussed with the patient in an unbiased manner. The final decision should be taken by the patient, based on the evidence presented. This activity, together with the risk element, forms the basis of obtaining consent.

Motivation

Expected patient compliance is an important part of planned management. A patient who fails to understand or even agree with the suggested

surgery may spell disaster. Well-informed patients recover more quickly and generally do better than those who remain ignorant.

Age

While age should be considered, age as a sole factor should not preclude a patient from surgery. On the contrary, many older people fair better than younger patients, despite the fact that youth suggests better health and quicker healing. The truth is that each age group presents the practitioner with different problems.

Consent

Once the patient has been referred and surgery is considered the best route for management, then the person who undertakes the surgical management must undertake the process of consent. Consent has three components and can only be carried out by someone qualified in the specific area of practice. While the quality of referral is essential for the reasons already given, inaccurate explanation by the uninitiated could cause greater miscommunication. Only the surgeon ultimately knows the best and preferred technique. Often there are several operative procedures that could be used so no one technique should be considered correct or incorrect.

Informed consent is a North American term although the same end result may take place. Informed consent implies that every little detail is imparted and this may not be appropriate in all cases. Unjustified detail can prevent some patients from benefiting from effective treatment as alarm may set in and a useful procedure is declined (see Case study 7.1).

The patient must be able to understand the nature of their condition and their treatment, the effects of treatment and any foreseeable risks that might arise. The patient should have sufficient mental capacity to make a decision. The consent should realistically be confirmed as near to treatment as possible or at least reconfirmed to ensure that no changes (in health or condition) have occurred since the patient was last seen. For instance, it would be inappropriate for any patient to provide written consent 12 months before an operation in a way that this was relied upon. A new consent would be better. On many occasions, the foot problem may alter and additional procedures might need to be added or even subtracted from the planned intervention. Children (under 16 years) may consent, often best with parental support although a child cannot refuse treatment where a parent has consented on their behalf in English law. It is important that practitioners know the legal position when treating all groups of patients. The examples in Case study 7.2 may be useful. The last point worth bearing in mind lies with the fact that written consent is not actually required. The patient may agree orally. It is an unwise practitioner, however, that relies on oral consent for an invasive procedure. Written consent confirms that consent has been undertaken. In law, and where negligence is alleged the complainant must prove that consent was not carried out. This is not easy unless proof of consent cannot be shown or where the clinical notes show that no process has taken place. There is no space in this chapter for greater detail associated with consent, law and negligence, but it is worthwhile bearing in mind that the foot does carry a high litigative risk, particularly for metatarsal osteotomies (Thomas 1991).

PRINCIPLES OF FOOT SURGERY

Surgery aims to reduce deformity, restore function, limit tissue damage and ameliorate pain; for some patients, all four aims will be achieved (see Fig. 7.1). Building evidence from blood tests, biopsy, imaging studies, neurological function tests and good clinical judgement will guide referral. In some cases, however, the surgeon involved should carry out these tests, unless the physician requires such data to direct clinical management. Early communication between practitioner and surgeon may help to ensure that tests are undertaken at the most appropriate time, thus avoiding repetition and unnecessary costs.

The methods available for surgical management of the foot can be summarized in terms of their individual principles and their perceived indications and limitations. The advent of new technology and ideas, supported by research studies, has allowed many fundamental techniques to be modified. Increasingly, simple carpentry tools such as chisels and hammers have been replaced by precision power tools, which

---

Case study 7.2 Consent and implications with surgery

Case 1

A patient suggests that the practitioner makes the decision. This is not an ideal situation, the patient must have all the facts explained. However, it is possible following full discussion to widen consent to cover each event so as to allow the practitioner to make the best judgement (i.e. if circumstances arise where a procedure would be less satisfactory then alteration would be permissible as it would have been agreed in advance).

Case 2

A patient attended clinic with her husband and was unable to understand the condition, potential treatment or the effects of such treatment. The husband suggested that he would make the decision for her. Again under English law this would be unacceptable as no one but the patient can make the decision except under mental incapacity, where the emphasis is placed on clinical intervention where, if it was not carried out, the patient's life might be affected.

Case 3

A patient underwent surgery with sedation. The surgeon realized that an additional procedure would have been ideal but had not taken consent where the possibility of additional intervention was discussed. Because the patient would not be able to make any reasoned decision owing to the altered effects brought about by sedation, any surgery performed without the usual system of presurgical consent might be invalid. The surgeon carries a risk of assault and battery should a foreseeable consequence arise. Presurgical assessment should consider all reasonable aspects of care prior to anaesthesia.

function with greater speed and accuracy. Biocompatible products, such as absorbable rods and screws, promise to minimize the need for later removal. Nine fundamental techniques associated with foot surgery are considered here:

- excision
- excisional arthroplasty
- replacement arthroplasty
- arthrodesis
- osteotomy
- soft tissue surgery
- tissue replacement
- amputation
- fixation.

Excision

The removal of tissue is the common method for dealing with swelling or prominences. Soft tissue is excised when it is thought to be malignant or where its presence causes infection or pain. Bone is excised when it is found to create pressure between bone and skin, and skin and footwear. Excision can be performed by minimal incisional exposure surgery or by full (open) surgical exposure.

Percutaneous excision of bone, for example, provides entry by a small incision in the skin. The additional term 'keyhole surgery', for percutaneous surgery, has been popularized in some circles. However, this has received poor press, particularly where a complicated procedure has been attempted without the benefit of a clear operative view – damage resulting from obscurity is hard to repair. *Osteotripsy* is synonymous with the percutaneous technique to reduce bony prominences. A manual rasp or power burr is introduced through the incisional aperture to reduce overlying bony projections (Fig. 7.2). The advantage of minimal incisional techniques is that they permit rapid recovery with minimal exposure of tissue; however, the risks associated with infection may still arise.

Arthroscopy is an ideal way of inspecting joint surfaces and offers the option to biopsy and excise tissue at the same time. The arthroscopic technique has been included in this section

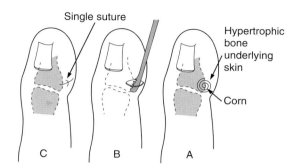

Figure 7.2 Osteotripsy. An example of minimal incisory surgery is associated with the fifth toe. An interdigital corn caused by a hypertrophic phalanx (A) is reduced using a percutaneous incisory technique (B). Before the wound is closed with a single suture (C), bone paste from the process of rasping is flushed out with saline.

because, unlike blind percutaneous surgery, it is a very accurate method of undertaking excision. The arthroscope provides an instant visual diagnosis using an optic camera through a small hole in the skin (Fig. 7.3). Investigative surgery associated with small foot joints and structures (e.g. metatarsophalangeal (MTP) joints, subtalar (ST) joints, fascia and nerve releases) has been developed as the heads of optic cameras and adjunctive equipment have become smaller and more refined.

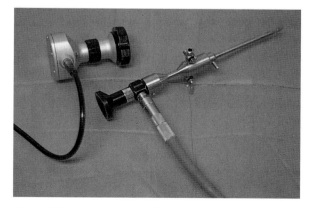

Figure 7.3 An arthroscope allows percutaneous diagnostic examination of a joint. The surgeon may have the option to perform either excisional or osteotripsy surgery. Defects in cartilage can be curetted and abnormal synovial debris removed. The camera attachment (shorter body) fits into the optical probe (longer body). The lenses are designed at different angles to provide the best visibility.

Two portals of entry are required to provide a clear picture. One portal conveys water to insufflate the joint space, while the other maximizes the optical position of the camera. The range of arthroscopy instrumentation is wide and includes grasping forceps, burrs, probes and suction systems. Laser has recently been introduced into arthroscopy and promises controlled, precise destruction of inflamed tissue and other defects, offering faster recovery than from manual/power equipment.

Older patients presenting with areas of ulceration and breakdown over common sites, such as the medial first metatarsal, may benefit from an exostectomy. This procedure is an example of the full, or open exposure technique, often requiring redundant skin to be trimmed after the bony eminence has been removed. No corrective benefit is achieved where a concomitant hallux valgus deformity coexists (Fig. 7.4). The tissue will heal quickly and provide relief of symptoms. This is particularly beneficial for the patient, reducing the risk of recurrent infections from intractable pressure.

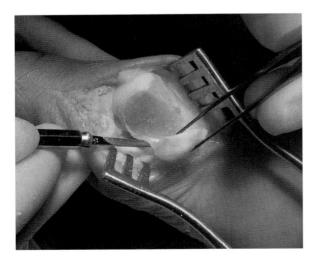

Figure 7.4 Exostectomy. Bony prominences can be removed to prevent underlying tissue and skin irritation. The procedure essentially offers 'salvage' in situations that may not be suited to extensive surgery, e.g. the elderly and infirm and those at higher risk of infection. A medial first metatarsal exostosis is illustrated; the exostosis fragment has been displaced medially, showing a smooth cancellous bone surface.

Cheilectomy is the excision by open surgery of small portions of bone formed by osteophytes (Fig. 7.5). Osteophytic degeneration associated with osteoarthritis distorts skin and reduces joint spaces. Cheilectomy is useful where joint replacement may not be appropriate. The metatarsal can be trimmed so that skin is not distorted and damaged, and any irritation of the synovial lining is minimized: active synovitis can cause greater discomfort than a stiff joint.

Excisional arthroplasty

An arthroplasty may involve the removal of either one or both sides of a joint surface. The extent of excision is dependent upon the type of operation. The term arthroplasty is misleading in that a new joint is not really formed. The gaps created by excising joints fill in with scar tissue. Lesser toes and interphalangeal (IP) joints usually remain stiff after such surgery but can become flexible, depending upon the extent of bone removed. Postoperative swelling can arise and will be discussed under sequelae. The patient needs to be advised about increased flexibility, loss of toe purchase power, stiffness and early discomfort caused by metatarsalgia.

Degenerative joints with synovitis can be relieved by excisional arthroplasty (Fig. 7.5). Deformity may be reduced but not always corrected. The procedure is destructive, and careful biomechanical consideration should be included in any assessment. Such techniques are often known as salvage procedures. In the case of *Keller's excisional arthroplasty* for hallux valgus, the toe position may be improved but the deformity can recur (Fig. 7.6). The foot may experience a transfer of pressure over lesser metatarsal heads as load shifts laterally. This arises because the hallux is shortened during surgery and has less purchase on the ground (Henry & Waugh 1975). While arthroplasties are often considered more appropriate in older patients, younger patients may well benefit from excisional arthroplasty; however, the surgeon should not wantonly destroy the biomechanics of the first ray. Other options should be considered to preserve the joint in the younger patient.

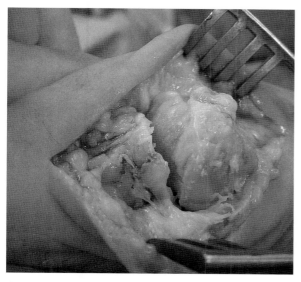

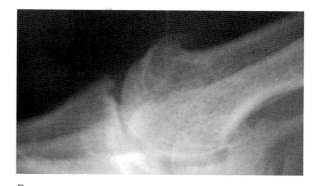

A   B

Figure 7.5 Osteoarthrosis (first MTP joint) may be treated with surgery by using joint salvage techniques. In both figures some of the joint pathology is shown between X-ray and in vivo clinical photographs. (A) The dorsal rim around the metatarsal head demonstrates a high spur, while the joint has lost the majority of the cartilage surface. The proximal phalanx fares no better. Such a joint may benefit significantly from a replacement implant. (B) This figure provides some idea of the height to which these spurs can project, often punching a hole or creating a rent in the capsule itself. Plain X-rays alone fail to qualify the extent of joint damage and act only as a guide. The surgeon has to be prepared to make a decision during the operation, ensuring that consent covers several options if at all possible.

Excisional arthroplasty is commonly used for problems associated with MTP and IP joints. The use of arthroplasty in the lesser MTP joints is less common than in the first MTP joint. The bases of proximal phalanges are trimmed in severe lesser toe deformities, but in most cases an arthroplasty technique will cause toe shortening: something the patient should be aware of beforehand.

The *pan metatarsal head* excision is an arthroplasty technique reserved for multiple toe deformity and pressure over the metatarsal heads. Pan metatarsal head excision has many names and tends to be reserved for rheumatoid and psoriatic arthritis, but it may be used in recalcitrant metatarsalgia and gross callus with deep small vessel infiltration. This procedure offers the patient a highly effective, although seemingly destructive, operation to manage pain associated with synovitis, deformity from deranged MTP joints and poor tissue viability. The result-

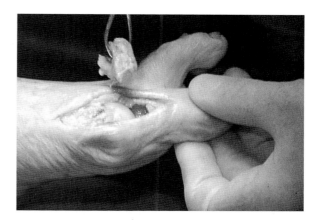

Figure 7.6 Keller's excisional arthroplasty consists of removing the base of the proximal phalanx and exostosis (see Fig. 7.4). The reason for the higher failure rate of this otherwise successful procedure is associated with too much bone being excised. The illustration shows removal prior to a first toe implant and, therefore, a slightly shorter length than usual is removed. One-third of the length of phalanx provides sufficient correction and moderate shortening without the toe becoming frail. The procedure can be combined with osteotomies.

ant effect leaves the foot remarkably more functional than if it were left untreated.

Replacement arthroplasty

A new joint is usually referred to as a replacement arthroplasty. In some cases, namely first MTP joints, lesser MTP joints and IP joints, silastic or dual metal–polypropylene implants can be used to replace the joint completely. Replacement of large joints in the foot, such as the ankle, appear to do less well than those of the hip and knee.

Replacement joints (prosthetic implants) can only be used where there is no infection and where the bone substance has adequate quality. Selection of implants is currently based upon the extent of joint damage and age. An older patient is likely to be less active than a younger patient, and, therefore, lower loads are experienced and wear and tear occurs more slowly. Conversely, younger patients have better 'bone stock' for receiving implants, compared with older bones with poor mineralization. Older patients have fewer expectations of postoperative joint motion and will demand less, physically, of their new

joint. Revision is necessary where patients expose the replaced joint to too much stress.

The silastic 'spacer' implant has a hinged concept (Swanson et al 1991). Figure 7.7 illustrates the silastic implant with metal grommets and in position after surgery, as seen by radiograph. Metal grommets (square washers), when used, may well improve the longevity of the implant. The grommet allows the metal, rather than the bone, to take the load from pistoning forces that build up. Silastic implants are soft and can tear and even pop out of the reamed square holes in which the two stems sit. Single-stem implants have fallen from favour at present, even though

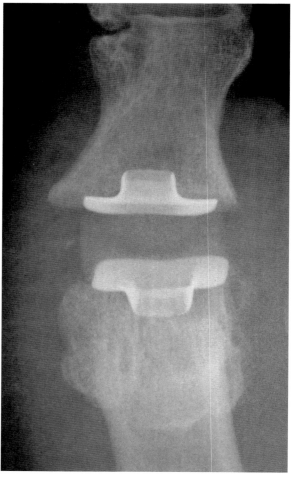

B

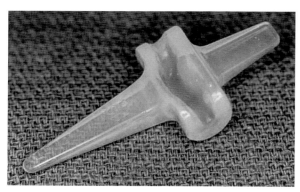

A

Figure 7.7 Osteoarthrosis and surgery using replacement arthroplasty. A, The implant made of silastic material (Swanson design) is sited between the proximal phalanx and metatarsal. Metal grommets can be seen providing a solid surface against the bone against which pistoning of the plastic joint is minimized. B, The implant is seen in a radiograph, highlighting the grommets. The two stems are outlined.

the hinged implant offers less freedom of movement and is restricted to sagittal plane motion.

Replacement joints made of two components, metal titanium and plastic, have been used in foot surgery. The latest design from Europe is a two-component prosthesis made from zirconium–ceramic material (Werner 2001). The earlier joint has been withdrawn for the newer press fit, which affords simpler technical application probably on par with the older silastic implants. Other two component systems perhaps require greater technical skills with special reaming guides. There have been insufficient longitudinal studies to predict the success of the two-component joint system to date. However, the ball and socket component replicates the mechanical function of the actual MTP joint more closely than does the hinge system.

A silastic joint replacement may allow the patient to bear weight actively within a short period although manufacturers may advise delay for a week after surgery in the author's experience (Vogiatzolglou et al 2000). Physiotherapy is advocated early to encourage movement and prevent the implant stiffening prematurely. Acute pain from the diseased joint should recede during this same postoperative period. Joint replacement requires extensive tissue handling and postoperative pain will be marked. UK surgical bodies such as the College of Podiatrists (Faculty of Surgery) and the British Orthopaedic Association have different attitudes toward prophylactic broad-spectrum antibiotics for implant surgery.

The most common joint replaced in the foot is the first MTP joint, as illustrated in Figure 7.7. The patient should be aware that movement expected from the joint after surgery can vary. Fibrotic infill along the hinge in the silastic implant can build up quickly from an initial haematoma; early mobility is preferred for this reason.

Complications from silastic implants have been noted and patients need to be advised of these. While problems are rare, bone abnormalities include fibrous hyperplasia, bone cysts and degenerative erosion. Potential problems associated with the implant material include foreign body granuloma and reactive synovitis from silicone. Fracture of the material may arise from fatigue; accidental damage from sharp instruments during surgery can sometimes contribute to this. Such complications have not been exclusive to silastic material. Loose implants, which have occurred with metal such as titanium, can cause pain, bone erosion, bone absorption and/or metallosis. The material found inside the joint is a dark loose soft breakdown product (Medical Devices Agency 2002).

Arthrodesis

In arthrodesis, all cartilage covering the bone ends must be completely removed and the denuded surfaces apposed and allowed to fuse together. The patient must understand that restriction of movement is permanent. Fixation can be achieved by autogenous materials (i.e. bone from the body itself) or exogenous materials from other species. Material from other species may be rejected depending upon the tissue used. Metal fixation materials come in the form of screws, wires, plates and pins.

Arthrodesis not only corrects the primary deformity but will also improve the function of weaker muscles and tendons that pass around the joint and adjacent bones. In the case of paralysis or congenital instability, a healthy muscle/tendon can be transferred. The arthrodesed joint will provide a stronger mechanical beam and thereby restore foot stability. Further description of tendon transfers is given below (see p. 137). The ends of bones can be reshaped to correct moderate deformity as well as to reduce joint pain.

Arthrodesis has become popular for flexed deformities of the lesser toes because each toe is turned into a rigid lever. Patients should be aware not only that IP joint movement will be lost as a result of surgery, but also that, because failure of fusion can arise, toes can swell. Lack of fusion results from too much fibrous replacement, with poor phalangeal compression in the presence of movement in the toe.

Midtarsal joints including the first medial cuneiform joint benefit from surgical fusion for midfoot pain. While the entity is poorly recognized and documented, continuous pain affecting patient lifestyles can benefit from fusion. The base of the first metatarsal (articulating with the medial cuneiform bone) is probably the most common form of midfoot fusion and is known as a *Lapidus operation*.

Where an arthrodesis is used in the foot, compensation may develop in distal or proximal joints to account for deficient movement; for example, an ankle arthrodesis can lead to greater ST and midtarsal joint movement. As a consequence, pain can arise in these otherwise normal joints where function has had to change. Recalcitrant painful flat foot problems may require surgery to fuse the medial border of the foot, raising the arch and improving tibialis anterior and posterior muscle function. The foot may adopt severe ST joint pronation, causing disability with gait problems. The ST joint arthrodesis is effective for recalcitrant pain in the hindfoot with severe deformity. The calcaneus is fused to the talus to limit pain, prevent further deformity and stabilize the hindfoot. The calcaneus may be fused to the talus, the talus fused to the navicular and the calcaneus fused to the cuboid bones collectively (Fig. 7.8). Where all three articulations are fused, the procedure is known as a *triple ST joint arthrodesis*. This procedure is usually regarded as the most extensive

form of arthrodesis in the foot. In many cases, single or double arthrodeses affecting one or two of the aforementioned joints will suffice.

Supinated foot deformity, as in the case of pes cavus, presenting with a marked forefoot equinus, may also benefit from arthrodesis. The navicular can be morticed or cut back into the talus, thus lifting the forefoot up. The articular surfaces can be fashioned to alter the position of the deformity. Many modifications of hindfoot arthrodesis have been developed; bone is trimmed to produce the correction desired: each modification might be named after the author and the abundance of named procedures today can easily cause confusion.

Cutting bone with recesses, holes and pegs provides a superior form of fixation. The surgeon will make use of shortening bone to correct deformity by also relaxing contracted tissue around joints. The most effective arthrodesis ensures that bone-to-bone contact is well apposed, using screws, staples and plates to achieve adequate compression. When a patient is advised that surgery can assist with the foot condition, the practitioner must discuss the use of 'hardware', a colloquial term for any internal fixation. It usually makes sense to suggest to the patient that all hardware will require removing eventually.

Osteotomy

Bone deformity can be corrected by arthrodesis, but the resulting stiffness across joints causes compensation, as movement must develop from other joints. When an arthrodesis associated with the first MTP joint is used, the type of footwear and heel height may be restricted. An osteotomy is carried out by surgically dividing the bone away from the joint. Not only will deformity be corrected, but also the joints can be spared surgical fusion.

Osteotomies in the foot are reserved for pain and deformity, but the end result will hopefully increase the life of a joint before degeneration becomes irreversible. Where cartilage is thinned out, shear stress increases (Radin et al 1992). The bone should have adequate mineral density

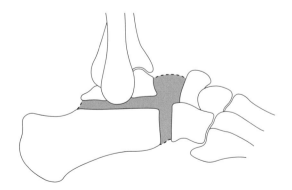

Figure 7.8 Arthrodesis. The triple arthrodesis shown is for stabilizing the hindfoot at the talocalcaneal joint, the calcaneocuboid joint and the talonavicular joint. The technique allows for the surfaces (shaded) to be refashioned, changing the relationship of any deformity present.

(bone stock) to accept surgical fixation across the surgical division.

After division, the abnormal bone position can be realigned to improve the biomechanics of the joint. Once decompression has been achieved, any inflammatory changes associated with synovitis may settle. Propagating cracks known as fibrillation will be prevented if abnormal stresses across the surface can be dissipated by improving the cartilage–surface relationship. Carrying out an osteotomy in someone with an arthritic condition is based on the hope that such surgery will create a remission of symptoms and pathology. If adverse joint changes can be resolved, the use of other destructive surgical techniques may be averted.

There are many osteotomy techniques in existence. With better clinical evidence – mainly through American literature – techniques are more restricted to well-tried and tested methods. Unfortunately, to confuse most newcomers to surgery, procedures carry the originating surgeon's name. European and American techniques may be similar but are obfuscated by names, where descriptions are probably better. Take Weil and Helal osteotomies as an example. The Weil is an excellent lesser metatarsal osteotomy but may be more appropriately described as a proximal capital displacement osteotomy; the Helal is an unfixed dorsal elevatory free-floating osteotomy. Osteotomies are applied to most foot bones alike, although the appropriateness of fixation is dependent on the quality of mineralization and joint quality.

Sliding, rotational, closing and opening wedge osteotomies are the principal types of osteotomy performed. While the principle of this surgical technique is directed at changing bone alignment, bone can also be lengthened or shortened; this is explained below. Careful preservation of neurovascular tissues is required in lengthening procedures.

A base (closing) wedge osteotomy is shown in Figure 7.9, which illustrates how hallux valgus can be corrected with lateral capital displacement. The MTP joint is aligned, and the intermetatarsal angle reduced by surgery. Release of the adductor hallucis and lateral capsule may be

necessary. Shortening of the metatarsal often relaxes tissues, saving unnecessary dissection.

A closing wedge osteotomy is performed by removing a triangular section of bone; one or two planes of deformity can be corrected simultaneously. Rotational osteotomies correct torsion in bone and are more commonly performed in the tibia and femur than in the foot. In the case of a hallux valgus deformity with an abnormal proximal articular set angle, both the cartilage surface and the distal metatarsal position can be influenced (Fig. 7.10). The metatarsal is shortened but the cartilage surface is preserved after the joint space has been increased. The hallux valgus is improved as the distal head of the metatarsal is displaced laterally (not shown in the illustrations). By combining different types of osteotomy, correction can be influenced in more than one plane. While a fuller description would not be appropriate in a general text such as this, most osteotomies, except for the open wedge type, can affect the length of a metatarsal. The surgeon must guard against removing too much bone in the first metatarsal, to avoid increasing mechanical stress over the second or third metatarsals. Usually the effects of such shortening are to cause callus or increased shaft thickness of the metatarsal, which can be seen on X-ray film. Presurgical judgement should take account of the corresponding second and first metatarsal lengths. The opening wedge osteotomy uses autogenous bone or bone from other sources, such as attenuated bovine bone, to lengthen one side. The wedge osteotomy avoids problems associated with shortening, but technically the procedure is more difficult and problems can arise with normal bony union. Wherever possible, autogenous (homogeneous) bone from the patient should be used as this is less likely to be rejected.

The osteotomy principle can be used anywhere in the foot. Flexible flat foot with a pronated shorter lateral border (without metatarsus adductus) can be treated by an open wedge osteotomy to lengthen the lateral border (Fig. 7.11). The medial border is stabilized simultaneously by fusing the navicular and cuneiform bones together. Pes cavus associated with a high

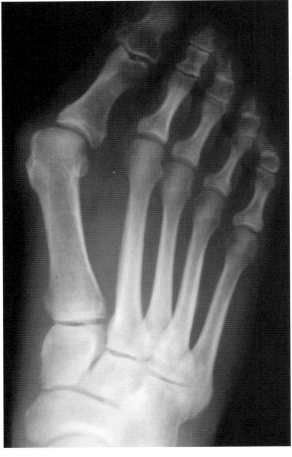

A

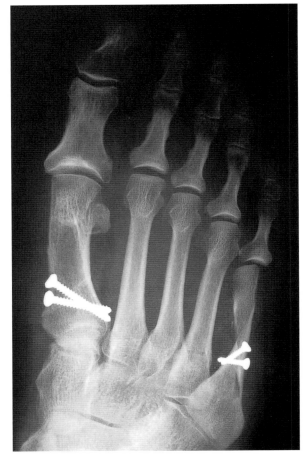

B

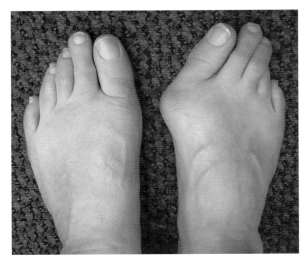

C

Figure 7.9 Closing wedge osteotomy: the cortex is breached with two-screw fixation to prevent rotation of the first metatarsal; the cortex is preserved in the fifth metatarsal. A, Preoperative view (X-ray). B, Postoperative view: the forefoot is narrowed, the metatarsal length preserved and the sesamoids are aligned. C, The clinical picture: the corrected hallux valgus is on the left side. Prior to osteotomy, the left foot was identical to the untreated right foot.

inclination angle of the calcaneus can be improved by rotational osteotomies or wedge osteotomies. Figure 7.12 illustrates combining hindfoot and forefoot osteotomies to change frontal and sagittal plane deformity.

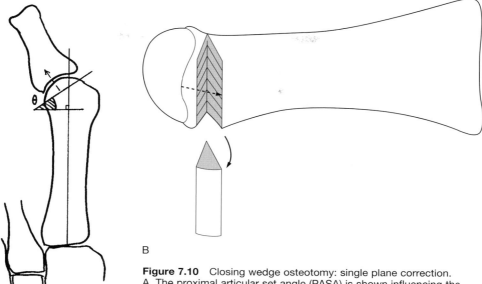

B

Figure 7.10 Closing wedge osteotomy: single plane correction. A, The proximal articular set angle (PASA) is shown influencing the direction of hallux deformity. B, A wedge is removed to correct the articular alignment and decompress the joint.

A

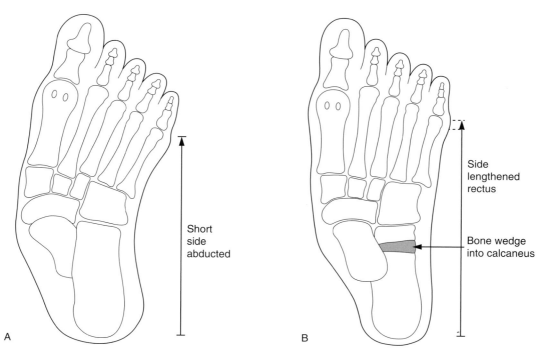

Short side abducted

Side lengthened rectus

Bone wedge into calcaneus

A

B

Figure 7.11 Opening wedge osteotomy. A, The lateral side is shortened by the abduction associated with foot pronation. B, Bone graft inserted into the calcaneus will lengthen the lateral side of the foot. This simplified illustration does not indicate the potential surgery required on the medial side.

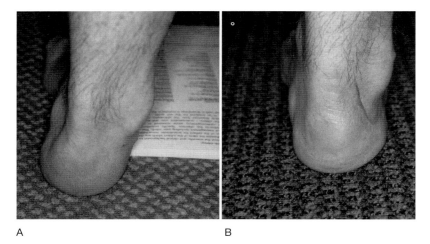

A   B

Figure 7.12 This 17-year-old man had marked pes cavus predominantly affecting his right foot. Surgery comprised a calcaneal (Dwyer) closing wedge osteotomy of the hindfoot, together with correction of his first metatarsal with a dorsiflexory closing wedge osteotomy; interphalangeal joint toe fusion and tendon (Jones) transfer of extensor hallucis to the first metatarsal. A, His foot is shown as markedly inverted by the Coleman test. In this test, a book is placed under the lateral border. If the hindfoot straightens in the frontal plane, the foot is correctable by orthoses; if not then surgery may be required. B, Foot correction is shown at 12 months, after much of the swelling has reduced. The wedge was taken with the widest side being on the medial portion. Appropriate alignment is essential and any surgeon using this technique is directed to a dedicated text for accurate placement of the wedge.

Soft tissue surgery

Some deformities are caused by soft tissue rather than by bone alone. Tendons and capsules contract, maintaining deformity. Simple surgery may release these tissues but, unfortunately, often fails unless the patient is young. A large number of terms exist for operating on soft tissue: the use of a prefix (associated with the anatomical structure) is followed by *-otomy* or *-desis*. The suffix will mean to incise, to divide or to limit movement. To add confusion to surgical terminology, some surgical techniques may have more than one form of nomenclature. *Capsulotomy* and *arthrotomy* involve an incision into a joint. As most joint surgery involves incising all the structures affecting a joint, the descriptors tend to refer to the general method employed, for example arthroscopy of the ankle, arthrodesis with capsulotomy of the MTP joint.

Where bones remain relatively soft (compared with tendons and capsule) and have not as yet been irreversibly affected by ankylosis (fibrous fusion) and torsion (permanent twisting of bone), surgery is indicated. If a deformity is left, the potential for successful restoration by division or incision reduces proportionally with age. As the patient ages, the adaptation by bone and soft tissue requires attention together, because the latter tissue will atrophy and contract. The child with club foot (congenital talipes equinovarus), therefore, responds better to early surgical intervention because most of the deformity is associated with tendons contracting abnormally during foot development.

Tenotomy is a technique involving transection of a tendon. A digital deformity in an 8-year-old child will benefit from this quick, minimal exposure procedure. The flexor tendons can be transected through a small percutaneous incision; the toes can be splinted with soft betadine soaks without sutures and the child can return to walking immediately. The toes can then be splinted for 6 months with silicone orthodigita to ensure that constant tension allows the flexor tendons to retain their length as they heal. If surgery is delayed beyond adolescence, then the deformity associated with flexion of the IP joints leads to ankylosis, necessitating an arthrodesis. Early intervention is successful and causes little stress to children, although a short general anaesthetic (GA) may be preferred.

Tendon transfers are indicated where muscle function needs to be reestablished. Miller (1992) identified the goals of tendon transfer:

- to improve motor function
- to eliminate deforming forces
- to restore loss of power
- to improve muscle balance
- to eliminate the need for bracing
- to improve foot appearance.

When a transfer is considered, joints should have minimal disease and have free mobility on clinical examination. Surgery should ensure that the biomechanics associated with transfer maintains the joint axis as close to perpendicular as possible with the new insertion. Faulty muscles attached to bone through their tendons may require detaching and moving proximally. The case of the triggered hallux associated with pes cavus in Charcot–Marie–Tooth is well documented (McGlamry et al 1992, Mann & Coughlin 1993). The flexible hallux at the MTP joint is stabilized once the long extensor tendon is moved from its insertion to a new point through the metatarsal neck. The IP joint must be turned into a rigid beam by an arthrodesis, otherwise propulsion would be affected. The newly positioned tendon lifts the first metatarsal, reducing the effect of plantarflexion, which maintains the hallux in retraction.

Split tendon transfers may be used to divide the power of tendons where spasticity causes an overpull. The tibialis anterior provides a good example in cerebral palsy. The forefoot inverts with spasticity. The split anterior tibial tendon transfer reduces the inversion power by transferring the moment of force to the lateral side of the foot. The site of insertion may involve either the peroneus tertius tendon or the cuboid bone.

A tendon may be transferred or split in order to route it to another site to enhance foot function. Abnormally tight tendons such as the tendo Achilles must be lengthened to avoid problems with inefficient heel contact. The foot adapts to ankle equinus through the midtarsal or ST joints. The efficiency of midfoot tendon transfers will be severely affected if the tendo Achilles is not attended to at the same time.

There are many examples of tendon transfer techniques. Research using electromyographic studies should ideally be used before surgery is attempted, to analyse the effect of such surgery. Foot pressure analysis with Harris ink mats and pedobarographs, for example, will allow the surgeon to evaluate successful weight-bearing changes after surgery. Many more examples of measuring foot pressure are available, but the two methods mentioned have been in practice the longest.

Soft tissue surgery may involve dividing ligaments, tendons and capsular structures. An adductovarus fifth toe position may improve after a simple capsulotomy with tenotomy, or adjunctive skin lengthening may also be required. One of the problems affecting toes following minimal surgery relates to scar tissue forming around MTP joints. The toe becomes dorsiflexed after a short period of success. The toe gradually lifts with contracture, particularly where the short and long extensor tendons fuse together forming a thick knot. Transfer of small tendons, such as the toe extensors, can be routed into metatarsal heads. Alternatively, a portion of tendon can be removed; this procedure, known as a *tenectomy*, may prevent some recurrence of the contracture. Established contracture around the MTP joint will require removal of bone, such as the base of the phalanx, and an osteotomy if the deformity cannot be corrected or improved.

Skin incisions used to correct deformity should be planned carefully to take advantage of potential lengthening. The use of a Z-plasty will allow scar tissue to be sited to a different position, minimizing recurrence of the contracture (Fig. 7.13). Care in relation to skin incisions is described in Chapter 6 (see p. 115).

Tendons and ligaments may be shortened or lengthened. Shortening, or *plication*, is not very common although it may be beneficial in conditions such as congenital convex pes planus. In this condition, the head of the talus sits in a vertical position and stretches the tibialis posterior and short/long flexor tendons, together with the medial deltoid ligament. As the calcaneus everts, the ligaments of the lateral side of the ankle shorten. The medial side is plicated and the lateral side is divided prior to holding the foot in a leg cast. As with congenital talipes equinovarus, congenital convex pes planus must be corrected shortly after birth to offer the best prognosis.

Tendons are lengthened not only to reduce deformity but also to improve the biomechanics of the foot. The tendo Achilles is perhaps the most common musculotendon group to be operated on. Ankle equinus is responsible for maintaining a flexible flat foot deformity in both normal and spastic patients. Too much lengthening will weaken the tendo Achilles. A Z-plasty is applied to the tendon in a different manner to that described for skin (Fig. 7.14). Downey (1992)

described lengthening of the tendo Achilles by distal recession. It is reasoned that recovery from surgery is improved if only the gastrocnemius component is lengthened. Full-thickness lengthening is commonly described in surgical texts. Smaller tendons can be lengthened by exactly the same technique, although repairing the paratenon is much more difficult. The paratenon is the very thin diaphanous membrane that surrounds the tendon and carries the fine vascular supply (Fig. 7.15).

Tissue replacement

Tissue from sources other than humans can be implanted into the foot. Specialized bone from bovine sources (xenograft) or from other humans (allograft) can be used as a matrix into which new bone cells will migrate (Fig. 7.16). Bone grafts may come from the iliac crest, tibia, fibula or calcaneus. Homogenous (autograft) bone is preferred; the donor site is usually from the iliac crest where the graft yields three sides of strong cortex (Fig. 7.17). Grafts include small cancellous

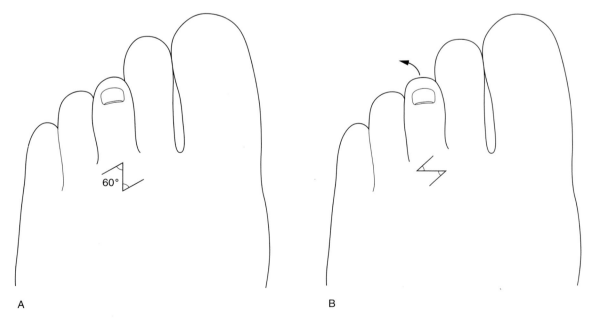

A   B

Figure 7.13 A Z-skin plasty is a popular method of rotating skin to a new position with the effect of increasing length. The central line represents the direction in which the scar has been moved so that less contracture is placed proximal to the digit.

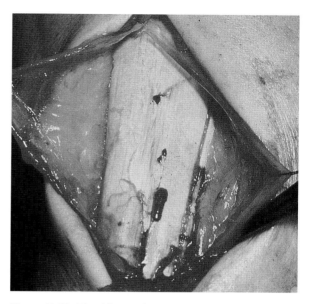

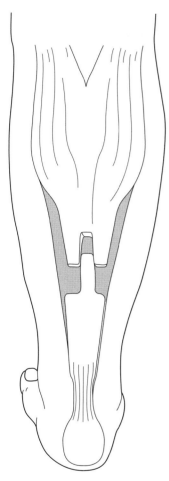

Figure 7.14   Soft tissue surgery: gastrocnemius recession for ankle equinus position. (Adapted from Downey (1992).)

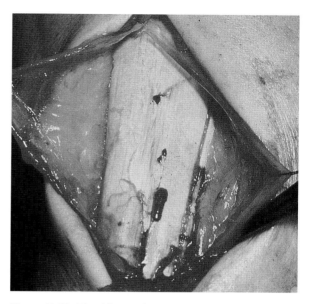

Figure 7.15   The thin membrane surrounding the tendo Achilles should be carefully preserved because of the vascular network. (Reproduced with permission from the Courtesy Fifth Avenue Hospital, Seattle.)

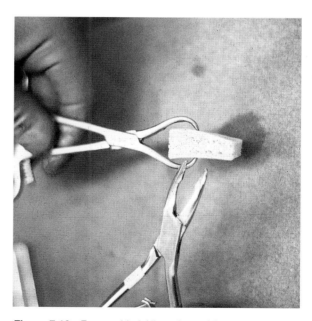

Figure 7.16   Freeze-dried Allograft used for open wedge osteotomy. Human donated bone is specially prepared and treated according to standards laid down by statutory bodies such as the US Centers for Disease Control and Prevention.

chips, slivers of cancellous bone and slab grafts. Bone grafts can be used to assist heal-delayed fractures and bone defects, can act as a fixation component for arthrodesis and can repair congenital defects.

Skin from sources such as a porcine graft is less readily accepted than skin from human sources and it may only act as a temporary cover to be replaced later by homogenous skin from the thigh. The thigh provides a wide expanse of skin from which a graft large enough for the foot is available (Fig. 7.18). The donor site may be

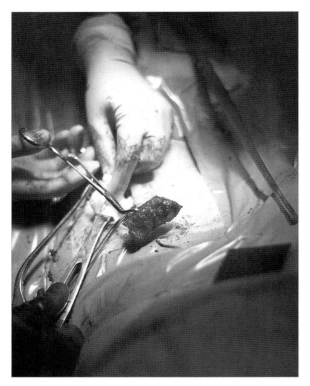

Figure 7.17 Bone taken from the iliac crest for implantation into the foot of the same patient. This is known as homogenous or autografted bone.

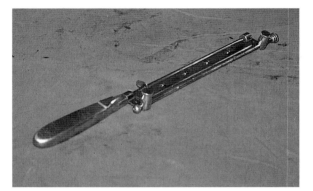

A

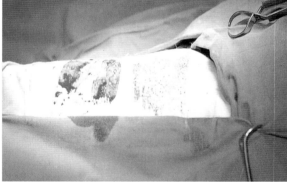

B

more painful than the recipient site, since the thickness of the graft usually exposes fine nerve endings, as shown in Figure 7.18C. Thinner grafts heal more quickly than thicker ones and can be perforated to stretch further and prevent build-up of exudate and haematoma. In the latter case, the graft might perish causing an infection to set in.

Where tissues are devitalized, as in the case of diabetics, specialist centres can offer myocutaneous flaps to cover larger avascular defects. The concept behind these flaps is to allow a large blood supply to be transposed with muscle. The muscle, with its rich supply, will provide nutrient and bulky covering to the skin (Fig. 7.19).

Skin grafting can be used after trauma from chemical and physical burns or after surgery

C

Figure 7.18 Skin for grafting. A, A Humby knife is used to remove a fine layer of skin. A number of systems, including electric roller/cutters, are available. B, The skin is kept taught using 'two slabs' of wood as shown. The skin is rolled up and kept moist before being carefully unravelled over the recipient site. C, Three areas of skin have been removed from the thigh (donor site). (Reproduced with permission from Mr J D Bromage, Kettering General Hospital.)

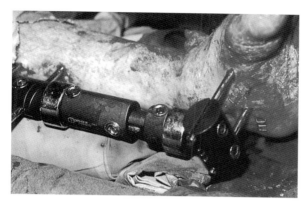

Figure 7.19 Myocutaneous graft used to cover bone and defects where little blood supply would allow a skin graft to take. A fixator is valuable when the wound is infected and the tissue cannot be closed. Bone can still be immobilized and grafting can be undertaken later on. (Reproduced with permission from Dr Ira Fox, Atlantic City, USA.)

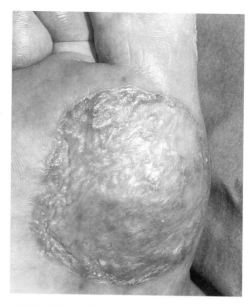

Figure 7.20 Skin graft used to cover a defect following surgical excision of a positive biopsy for malignant melanoma. (Reproduced with permission from Manor Hospital, Medical Photography Department, Walsall, UK.)

where tissue has been sacrificed. This last indication might include neoplasia (Case study 7.3; Fig. 7.20).

Tissue replacement with internal prostheses has been successful elsewhere in the human body: Dacron for blood vessels, heart valve replacement, and metal prostheses following removal of bone tumours. The foot has to withstand remarkable loads and the types of prosthesis used most frequently are associated with smaller joints. The most common joints include the ankle and the IP and MTP joints. The ST arthroeresis peg is unique to the foot. Made of silicone, the peg fits under the lateral side of the talus body and reduces the influence of pronation during development. The ST arthroeresis peg is later removed and orthoses may still be required to maintain the corrected position. This peg is not widely used in the UK.

Case study 7.3   Skin graft after malignant melanoma excision

A 74-year-old male was referred by his GP with a wart under the right first metatarsal head. The patient's history was complicated by respiratory disease and psoriasis. The GP had used the usual preparations on the lesion, which covered the metatarsal head. Upon admission to the day surgery unit, a dark pigmented nodular lesion was identified. The borders were irregular and the lesion was bleeding. The appearance was complicated by the use of keratolytics. A large excisional biopsy was taken under regional ankle block and the lesion was found to penetrate to, and include, the capsule of the first MTP joint. An underlying sesamoid was trimmed and the skin sample sent to histopathology. Two days later, preliminary stains strongly suggested a malignant melanoma, which was subsequently diagnosed as an acral lentiginous melanoma. Good closure was affected, but the lesion required further excision, necessitating a split skin graft (Fig. 7.20) rather than a full ray excision.

Comment: Despite some doubts about the skin graft failing, the lesion covered the defect without any Koebner phenomenon from psoriasis. The use of skin grafting provided an alternative form of management to loss of part of the first ray in a patient already ill with respiratory disease. The poor long-term prognosis expected with the malignancy of the acral lentiginous melanoma was accompanied by an adjunctive medical condition. Skin grafts can be successfully used on the plantar surface of the foot.

Amputation

While the practitioner strives to maintain tissue viability and function wherever possible, amputation has a place in surgical management. The indications for amputation are:

- recalcitrant pain
- gross deformity
- necrotic change
  - thermal damage
  - vascular impairment
- expansile neoplastic change
- severe disabling injury
- failed surgery.

When planning an amputation, the practitioner should be sensitive in the care taken with the patient. In most cases, patients understand the need for surgery but are less able to comprehend the effects that an amputation can have on their lives, for example psychological effects, dysfunction and, later, the need for a prosthesis.

Following amputation, symptoms would be expected to resolve. The loss of part of the anatomy of the foot inevitably may leave some reduced function. Most patients accept the loss of a lesser toe well (Fig. 7.21). The practitioner must point out that the gap may fill in with a drifting toe, as in the case of hallux valgus, but otherwise no functional disruption should arise. In fact, of all the toes, only the first toe will cause problems with balance. Any deficit of first ray or hallux function can be successfully compensated by a prosthesis (see Ch. 12). The patient should be aware that hammer toes may arise following first toe amputation. Toes are occasionally removed to replace lost thumbs in order to retain the pincer effect with the index finger.

Multiple toe amputations will cause a rise in vertical contact forces and pressure under the metatarsals. Ideally, the patient will be fitted with an insole or forefoot extension prosthesis to assist the shortened foot fit in a regular shoe.

Midfoot or transmetatarsal amputations (Fig. 7.22), ray excisions and those through the midtarsal joint will seriously affect biomechanical function. Tendons from the leg should ideally be inserted into remaining bone to maintain some function. The fascia should be retained wherever possible to support weight-bearing heel stumps. Skin flaps that bear weight should have as much deep soft tissue transposed at the time of surgery as possible, otherwise nerve entrapment and scar line corns will form, increasing pain and patient distress. While the retention of the talus and calcaneus together is better if a full foot prosthesis is required (Choparts's amputation), the calcaneus and talus can be removed if the underlying fat pad is large enough and viable to sustain weight bearing. The traditional Syme's amputation, named after the Edinburgh surgeon Sir James Syme in 1843, not only successfully removes the talus but also trims the malleoli (Fig. 7.23).

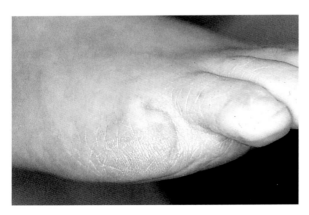

Figure 7.21 Amputation of the fifth toe, with a skin flap fashioned to retain underlying fat and a healthy blood supply.

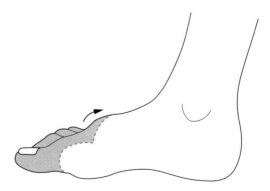

Figure 7.22 Lateral view of transmetatarsal amputation for the forefoot. A plantar flap is created and brought onto the dorsum.

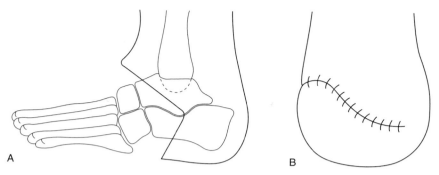

Figure 7.23 Amputation. A, Syme's whole foot amputation. B, A moccasin prosthesis would be required.

The use of amputation for the dysvascular foot, particularly in diabetic patients, is somewhat controversial. The common difficulty lies with wound healing and closure: if the wound were to become infected, it could lead to a below-knee amputation. Earlier intervention with a below-knee amputation may forestall many of the problems encountered by failed local amputations, metatarsal ray or trans-metatarsal surgery. While the surgeon ideally wishes to maintain as much of the original structure as possible, unless the timing of surgical intervention is appropriate, the foot may have deteriorated too far. Below-knee amputations are, therefore, often performed at the outset of deterioration. In the case of the diabetic patient or the patient with vascular patient, the main aim is to keep the patient alive – the fewer operations required, the more likely it is that this objective will be achieved.

Fixation

In much the same way that skin can be held together by sutures, bone can be sutured with fine gauge wire. Malleable surgical stainless steel wire can be placed through drill holes and twisted to bring the ends together. This technique, known as *cerclage wire*, is still in common practice, but is probably used less frequently now with the advent of AO (*Arbeitgemeinschaft für osteosythesisfragen*) fixation. The Association of the Study of Internal Fixation (ASIF), developed in Switzerland in 1958, led to the formation of

the study group that heralded AO fixation methods.

Internal fixation

Osteotomies or fractures heal best when well apposed and compressed at the ends. In the UK, as in the USA, the podiatric view that bone should be fixed by some mechanism is based on the premise that bone ends can move and thus delay union. As bones in the foot take, on average, 12 weeks to unite adequately, weight bearing is limited following surgery. The use of casting is helpful but very restrictive, and it can create an element of demineralization within the bone. Early ambulation following surgery is ideal, as the constant weight bearing will increase new bone formation and not only reduce potential cast disease (pain with demineralized bone and tissue swelling), but also limit the risk of DVT and complex regional pain syndrome through postoperative disuse.

There is a wide variety of fixation hardware: pins, screws, staples and plates. New designs of screws have flooded the surgical market, many bearing similarities to the AO system. Designs include self-tapping and cannulated screws, which reduce the need systematically to tap the drill hole each time. The cannulated screw system makes use of a hollow shaft. The screw fits over a pin called a Kirschner wire (K-wire). The K-wire keeps the screw in correct line and reduces the need for some of the usual AO over-drilling as well as tapping. A clamp is used to ensure that the bone ends do not move as the screw is inserted into the predrilled hole. The lag effect is used by ensuring that the furthermost hole is tighter. In this way, the pitch of the screw can bite into the bone substance drawing the ends closely together.

Plates are used when screws alone will not provide the stability required (Fig. 7.24). Access to some fracture sites is considerably limited. The plate is usually prestressed and has screw holes drilled eccentrically away from the fracture line. As the tapered screw heads make contact with the plate holes, the fragments are compressed together (Corey & Ruch 1992).

Pins are commonly used to achieve the same result as screws, but their compression ability is poor. Pin thickness varies from 1.25 to 1.6 mm, although smaller and thicker wires are available. These wires are used for stabilizing small bones as in the case of toes (arthrodesis) and metatarsal osteotomies. Pins may be smooth or threaded. Threaded pins tend to act like small screws because the thread turns in one direction, biting bone as it pierces the cortex. The advantage of such a product lies in its purchase and in the fact that it moves less frequently than the smooth version. No special equipment is necessary and the introduction is quick and efficient. Premature removal is most difficult because, unlike screws, no head exists into which a screwdriver will fit. Pins have to be overdrilled out. Percutaneous

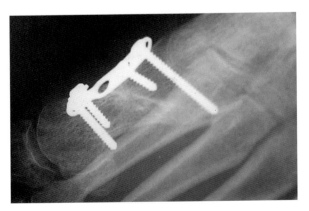

Figure 7.24 A plate with four AO screws is illustrated after an osteotomy of the first metatarsal, which failed to heal adequately at 6 weeks.

positioning works less well, as the thread wraps around soft tissue causing damage.

In the hindfoot, particularly the calcaneus, thicker *Steinman* pins are used because they can carry greater loads than Kirschner wires. Pins are generally designed to stabilize bones rather than take the load of weight bearing.

Staples have always been used, but from time to time they become unpopular. With the advent of power-driven staples, a quick system is now available to secure clean bone division. New technology has recently produced a metal staple sensitive to heat. Once the staple has been inserted, the body heat causes the metal to contract, forcing the two fracture ends closer together.

Absorbable fixation The technology used in biodegradable sutures is now being applied to rods and screws. One of the first designs, Orthosorb (Johnson & Johnson), has been used by orthopaedic and podiatric surgeons in the UK. The rod works on the basis that it locates the bone in its ideal position. Based on polyglycolic acid, the rod swells, making the alignment firmer. Osteotomies are not compressed, but nor would they be with smooth K-wires. Current research looks encouraging and side-effects are minimal, although additional swelling in toes has been noted.

Polymers of lactide and glycolide have been used to develop a range of screws. Development of this new product has been undertaken in the USA, but it awaits approval by the Medical Devices Agency in the UK. The screw, made of poly-L-lactide, promises to carry the load for fracture fixation but then disappear after the bone has regained its strength. The makers of SmartScrew (Bionix) offer a wide range of screw diameters. Lengths can be cut to suit the depth required. This means that less equipment (and a smaller range of stock) is required, and surgical removal is obviated, both providing resource savings that would look attractive to any surgical department.

External fixation

Although internal fixation provides the patient with an invisible reduction device, a place does exist for external fixation, mainly in trauma. Pins can be introduced through undisplaced bone using an image intensifier. The main advantage in having a wire externally sited lies in the minimal surgical exposure required and the ease of removal. Pins can be easily removed from bone, providing that insertion is not too deep. In this case, local anaesthetic (LA) is advised to remove firmer pins. Sharp ends of pins should be protected by some cover, such as a 'Jurgan ball' (Fig. 7.25) (Tollafield 1995). The risk of infection and loosening should be discussed with the patient.

External fixation can be achieved using a fixator (Figs 7.19 and 7.26). The external applicator is beneficial where an open wound needs constant care or is awaiting skin grafting, because this can be done without affecting bone repair. Smaller fixators are not that common because walking is impeded; traction is one advantage the internal fixation does not offer.

SEQUELAE ASSOCIATED WITH FOOT SURGERY

Earlier in this chapter, the risks associated with surgery were highlighted. The referring health practitioner will ideally select the surgeon best capable of dealing with a specific foot problem. However, no matter how experienced the surgeon, problems will arise. While it may have taken the aftermath of the 'Bristol heart cases' to change perception about information responsibility and audit, in reality many professions had already acknowledged the need for better clinical governance, protocol and pathways. For the most

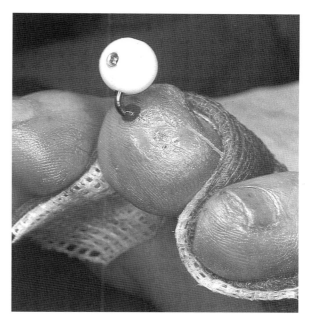

Figure 7.25 Jurgan ball (RFO Medical) placed on the end of the Kirschner wire to protect the point. The balls can be adjusted by a small grub screw and tightened against the wire. While corks and other methods are not recyclable, Jurgan balls withstand sterilizing through an approved HSDU/CSSD. The procedure shown is an arthrodesis of a third clawed toe.

part, problems will relate to minor inconveniences; however, the practitioner must always bear in mind that a minor inconvenience may be perceived by the patient as a major difficulty.

Many problems that beset patients following surgical intervention arise because they become impatient and attempt to undertake more than is wise during the postoperative period of recov-

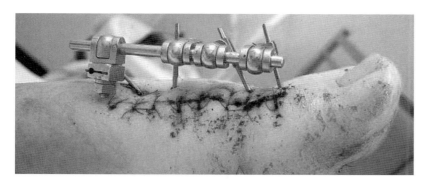

Figure 7.26 External fixator to provide traction at the first metatarsophalangeal joint, preventing contracture.

ery. The referring practitioner expects the dutiful surgeon to provide sufficient information to limit misunderstanding and prepare the patient for aftercare (Table 7.2). Both podiatric and orthopaedics surgeons specializing in foot surgery will discuss common postoperative events. Information sheets and publications are more accessible to the public and may play a part in clinical discussion when referral is considered. The referring practitioner may need to offer the patient advice about surgery but should only consider sequelae in general terms. The role that practitioners play in surgery will vary from advice to acting upon a problem to seeking best referral agent as second opinion. Surgeons, however, are best involved with problems that arise, as their network of cospecialists may offer a quicker solution. Caution must be taken over reacting to some common sequelae. An alarmed patient may not be helpful when considering other options.

Swelling

The extent of the inflammatory process varies between patients and surgical procedures. Certain parts of the foot, such as the toes, have a greater tendency to swell than others. Toes probably suffer most, as the return of fluid is least efficient here as swelling blocks natural drainage.

Heat, particularly during the hotter times of the year, too much standing and insufficient daily rest can lead to localized swelling. Healing of skin in healthy patients will only take 2–3 weeks, at which time sutures are normally removed. The non-compliant patient can burst stitches and any residual swelling that develops may place abnormal pressure on the wound. In this case, the sutures will need to be released immediately to safeguard the local tissue. Feet rarely stay swollen for long; if they do, the practitioner must suspect infection, DVT, non-union of bone or overuse (by the patient).

Management of swelling can be achieved with physical therapy such as the cryogenic boot (Aircast; Fig. 7.27). Simple home remedies can also be used and should include raising the leg

Table 7.2 Quick reference for postoperative sequelae[a]

Sequela	Brief comment
Poor pain control	7–20% risk
Medication side-effect	Older patients and known gastrointestinal problems
Swelling abnormal	Not uncommon with larger surgery at 3 months
Postoperative nausea and vomiting (PONV)	Associated with general anaesthetic
Pain at surgical site	Not expected beyond healing; may continue as twinges and be abating
Patient poor compliance	Consequences of not following instructions
Recurrence	Pain not improved, deformity not corrected
Incision line healing	Edges fail to come together
Scar line changes	Raised, thickened, discoloured and very tender
Fixation movement	Wires, screws – expected incidence 10–20%; plates may need to be removed more frequently than screws alone
Infection suspected	Appears infected: clinical best guess 4–8% chance
Infection proven	Sufficient material to culture organism required 2% chance
Joint pain stiffness	Surgery produces stiffness, which is uncomfortable
Sensory loss (small)	Can be expected with most surgeries. Skin level within small surgical area
Stump neuroma	Neuroma surgery (e.g. Morton's metatarsalgia)
Stitch problem	Suture reaction does arise, causing thick scars and inflamed skin
Digital periostis	More common in lesser toes where an arthroplasty has been performed
Haematoma	Bleeding into tissues swells. High risk of infection
Transfer metatarsalgia	Often because of first metatarsal shortening or inefficiency
Callus development	Following any forefoot surgery affecting metatarsals

Continued

Table 7.2   *Continued*

Sequela	Brief comment
Skin necrosis	Local skin embarrassment restricted to incision line, good recovery expected
Fracture of fixation hardware	Across joints more common, e.g. in arthrodesis
Inability to wear shoes	Return to all shoes is not expected, especially female designs. Limited footwear may be a problem
Joint prosthesis problem	All designs can give rise to revision and rejection
Avascular necrosis	Bone collapse. First metatarsals more common although a rare complication following osteotomy
Bone union delay	More often associated with non-fixation or reliance on casting of the foot
Metatarsal fracture (transfer load)	Can arise after first metatarsal osteotomies, e.g. second metatarsal stress fracture
Osteomyelitis	Unacceptable complication after elective surgery. Haematogeneous forms might prove difficult to avoid. Risk very rare
Deep vein thrombosis	Risk 2% of suspicion but proven DVT is rare and pulmonary form may arise outside surgery period
Sensory loss large	More common to anaesthetic needle damage affecting regional nerve branch, e.g. common peroneal nerve
Motor power loss	Associated with regional branch damage to muscles (as above)
Mortality	Greater risks from patients on polypharmacy, with unknown allergies, undergoing general anaesthetic when unfit, sudden cardiac disturbance in conduction: very rare in foot surgery (no cases cited since 1970s)
Complex regional pain syndrome	Unresponsive pain syndrome with varying level of disability. Can be severe. Serious manifestation probably 0.05%. Minor forms 0.2%, more often associated with repeated forefoot surgery
Ischaemia (greater part)	Caused by infection, thrombosis, anaesthetic technique, sickle cell,

Continued

Table 7.2   *Continued*

Sequela	Brief comment
	peripheral vascular disease. Serious complication
Poor healing	Caused by infection, blood supply, compliance, drug interactions and chemicals causing toxicity, e.g. phenol

[a]Covers the most common conditions; many of these may be discussed with the patient prior to surgery taking place. Comments in the table will illustrate the wide range of problems encountered with foot surgery. Data given are based on experience using the surgical audit system PASCOM (Rudge and Tollafield 2002). The advisory working party to the Society of Chiropodists and Podiatrists, Faculty of Surgery submitted their first pilot study of work undertaken by podiatric surgeons over a period from 1992 to 2001. One of the principles of surgery was the recognition of common problems known as sequelae: this has been widely defined and continues to expand.

above the heart. The knee should be slightly flexed to prevent tension on the sciatic nerve. Ice, crushed in plastic bags or frozen peas, can be wrapped around the ankle for 20–30 minutes every few hours, provided that the patient does not fall asleep: ice can cause ischaemia.

Walking aids such as crutches should limit the weight taken by the foot for the advised period of non-weight bearing. Dressings should be firm and should compress the wound evenly. They should be carefully placed to avoid nerve pressure.

Recalcitrant swelling in toes after surgery may be treated, provided that infection is not present, with a single injection of corticosteroid with LA. The patient should be told that toes can remain swollen for many months as a matter of course. Swelling associated with congenital lymphatic disorders, inguinal tumours, dependent oedema from heart failure and varicose veins will inevitably add to the problem. Diuretics to reduce retained interstitial oedema must be used with some caution, because the patient will need to go to the toilet more frequently. Previous trauma around the ankle will also encourage swelling. Both feet should always be compared and more serious problems excluded.

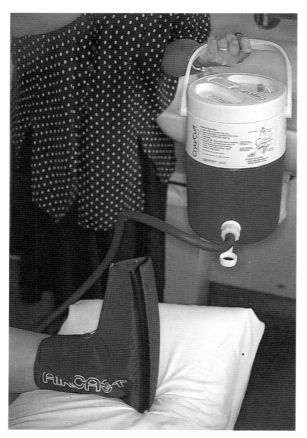

Figure 7.27 An Aircast cryogenic boot will allow iced water to recirculate in a closed system. The effects of the coldness and compression can last for many hours before a change of water is necessary. Patients should not attempt to fall asleep with the device attached, in order to avoid adverse effects of cold on the tissues. Recyling of the iced water is achieved by elevating the reservoir above the body.

Deep vein thrombosis

DVT can arise following foot surgery, although this should only account for a small percentage of patients with this condition. DVT has already been discussed in Chapter 4.

Prevention

Those at risk from DVT should be given prophylactic heparin before surgery. The risk of venous stasis increases with bed rest. DVT is inevitably reduced if patients can walk early and exercise their calf muscles. While the patient has to rest, hourly exercise should be undertaken using knee movement. Younger females taking the pill are at risk, as much as older females, from the effects of DVT. Any decision to stop contraception should be discussed with the patient's physician as a matter of course. The view upheld by the medical profession to cease contraceptive therapy before surgery is less than clear for elective minor surgery. Major surgery tends to be viewed differently, especially if a period of stasis arises.

DVT presents with alarming calf pain. The foot and leg may be very swollen and colour changes may be noted. The sudden hardness to palpation provides a strong clue. On examination, pressure should not be applied to the deep tibial vein in case an embolus arises. The circumference should be noted as soon as possible to monitor deterioration or improvement. The next stage of treatment may require a venogram if the condition is thought to be progressive, although colour Dopplex is popular to rule out upper leg clots. Admission to hospital allows the patient to be monitored. The silent DVT occurs without warning. Chest pain with shortness of breath indicates a pulmonary embolus. The patient will be in extreme distress, requiring pain control and thrombolysing with the hospital's standard protocol, e.g. streptokinase, alteplase and anistreplase.

In both DVT and pulmonary thrombosis, a team approach is essential. Both problems are uncommon in practice and are not necessarily associated with major surgery. If patients have not had a DVT before, then postoperative risk can only be suspected. Blood-clotting screens may help raise a concern but cannot be used to provide a definitive confirmation of the risk. The best standard blood assay in patients unknown to have a DVT propensity is still the platelet count as it is sensible and cost-effective. The problem of DVT is more likely to arise in females, long surgeries and where periods of immobility are prolonged. DVT symptoms can arise within a few days to several weeks. The practitioner should explain such risks with a view to educating the patient to call for assistance as a matter of urgency.

Infection

The foot is more commonly infected following surgery than many other sites on the body. Audited data seem to suggest that some 2% of podiatry operations may lead to infection (Tollafield & Parmar 1994). Infection is associated with swelling and the patient is in discomfort more often than not. Signs of cellulitis are identified as a demarcation of colour, the skin is tense and may be shiny. Lymphangitis and lymphadenitis may be present. Pyrexic change suggests serious levels of toxicity. Blood assay should include full blood count and erythrocyte sedimentation rate, as well as a white cell count to establish the severity of any infection and monitor improvement.

Infection is likely to arise after 24–72 hours. Infection should be suspected if pain is difficult to control after the immediate postoperative period. Early antibiosis is likely to provide a favourable reduction in symptoms within 48 hours. Most infections affecting the foot following surgery are associated with *Staphylococcus aureus* unless contracted from within a hospital (nosocomial infection).

Oral antibiosis is usually satisfactory although an initial double dose as a bolus may help to increase the blood level of antibiotic. All the principles of ice, rest and elevation should be applied and the patient should refrain from walking; full rest with elevation is the key to the best resolution.

Where infection does not resolve, pus may be in evidence, causing a rise in pressure at the site of the wound. The wound dehisces, exposing the area to further infection. Necrotic tissue should be debrided until healthy bleeding is visible. The wound is laid open to drain and then packed. The course of management in complicated infections is described in Case study 7.4 and illustrated in Figure 7.28.

Osteomyelitis imposes a protracted period of care. Antibiotics used for osteomyelitis may involve dual drug regimens and extended use of antibiotics. In severe cases, admission to hospital for intravenous drug administration may be necessary. Surgical debridement of bone is advocated where sequestrae are identified, and where blood tests suggest high antibody activity and raised erythrocyte sedimentary rates. In all cases of infection, the patient can expect to remain off work for longer than normal.

Pain

Patients respond to pain in different ways. The elderly are often stoic and may need encouraging to take pain medication. Patients who are sensitive to pain can often be identified by asking about their analgesic medications used at home. Those patients who have no drugs in their house

---

Case study 7.4 Infection after surgery

A 48-year-old female had a base wedge osteotomy performed to correct her hallux valgus. Surgery was unremarkable but 1 week later the foot swelled and an infection was noted. The wound burst and oral antibiotics failed to contain the bacteria (*Staphylococcus aureus*). The internally placed screw loosened and backed out of the bone, revealing the head of the screw in the wound. The patient was readmitted to theatre and the hardware removed and deep infection thoroughly lavaged. Infection had produced a papery separation between the skin and the superficial fascia. Exudate had pushed under the skin causing it to separate. The wound was extensively debrided and the antibiotic strength was doubled and extended for 3 weeks. The wound was left open to drain and packed; dressings were changed three times a week. The wound took 3 months to settle and the bone required the use of an 'Aircast' to maintain fracture site stability.

Comment: This case was unusual in that the patient had complied with her postoperative instructions. The summer temperature had reached 32°C (90°F) and the patient had been unable to cope with it. The inflammatory response and infection had loosened the well-positioned screw as the bone dimensions had expanded slightly. The main concern lay in retaining good bone alignment and preventing an osteomyelitis from developing. The whole episode delayed the patient's recovery by 5 months, when 1 month was the anticipated recovery period. The end result was greater scarring with some loss of underlying tissue, causing a dented appearance. This settled in time, giving a flat scar line. All future procedures had an additional screw for fixation (see Fig. 7.9B)

A

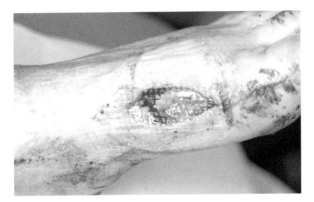

B

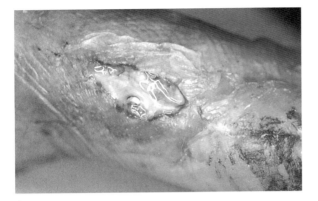

C

Figure 7.28 Complicated infections. A, A screw is seen in the wound in the presence of dehiscence and cellulitis. B, At 1 week after surgery, the screw has been removed and debridement has created a new bed of healing following drainage. C, At 12 weeks, the skin has healed by secondary intention.

probably cope better than those who constantly use analgesics and become tolerant to the lower-strength paracetamol/codeine compounds.

Unremitting pain through inadequate control is not acceptable: the cause must be identified. Suppression of pain should be achieved, after considering the patient's medical history, with appropriate drug therapy. In particular, the health of the gastrointestinal tract should be considered, as many drugs can irritate the lining. Hiatus hernia, ulcers and gastric reflux are common ailments that will be irritated by NSAIDs. Use of adjunctive agents (e.g. diclofenac sodium with misoprostol) or single-dose intravenous NSAIDs can be helpful. Cyclo-oxygenase 2 (COX-2) agents (e.g. refecoxib) are less favourable now in overcoming gastrointestinal problems because of associated heart effects. Unfortunately, the ideal analgesic preparation that does not cause gastrointestinal disturbance does not reliably exist at present for all patients.

The patient should be provided with preemptive pain control suited to the type of operation. The main objective of pain control is to prevent the patient from becoming anxious, crying or losing sleep. The operative site may throb and be generally sore, but this should be controlled at a level commensurate with the patient being able to hold a conversation and to eat and drink as part of coping psychologically. The pain regimen should last for the shortest period at the lowest dose able to bring relief. Nausea and vomiting complicate pain control, and analgesics can be injected intramuscularly or used per rectum if these are a cause of stomach irritation. Antiemetics may be required if marked nausea and vomiting arises.

Local anaesthetic blockades are invaluable and work as well as morphine without causing hallucinogenic side-effects. The source of pain should always be identified and managed before increasing the level of pain medication. Ice and elevation are essential components of good analgesic postoperative pain management. Patients should know that pain normally lasts for only a short period and should be expected. Preoperative discussion of pain levels should always be undertaken. Overstating the anticipated pain level is far better than understating the problem: such psychoanalysis works wonders! The two most common problems to arise following surgery relate to pain medication not given early enough (and then only on demand) and to too weak a dose being given when pain control is provided.

Transcutaneous nerve stimulators (TNS) have a role in pain management. They should be placed above the ankle along the nerve routes. New products for pain management reach the health market constantly, although many appeal to the psychologically sensitive by autosuggestion rather than providing direct scientific benefit. Rest, ice and elevation provide important supportive strategies to analgesia that should not be underestimated.

Scar lines

All operations have scars; some patients are lucky enough to have only faint lines. The scar line starts off as vascular for some months. The incision line swells and then regresses slowly, appearing soft and flat. The surgeon normally elects to keep scar lines away from the surfaces most exposed to pressure; these include plantar metatarsals primarily and skin over the heel, which may come into contact with the heel counter of the shoe. Incision lines over joints may thicken, especially those just over tendon routes.

Both white and black skins can suffer from hypertrophic (thickened) scarring. Careful questioning before surgery should include discussion about the effects of previous surgery. Examination of previous scars should be carried out and noted in the records under the plan of care. Corticosteroid medication should be infiltrated under the sutured incision line to prevent unwarranted hypertrophy at surgery. Hypertrophy is a minor complication, which may not cause any discomfort, but it can result in severe elevation around lesser toes. A Z-plasty may be required to deal with contracture, but only after a period of at least 2 years, as scars slowly regress with time. Keloid is a condition where the wound heals outside the normal boundary expected. The scar is raised and has an

irregular edge, which can spread widely. Surgical revision is fraught with recurrence and the opinion of a plastic surgeon is worthwhile before further surgery is anticipated. Using intradermal steroid injectable products or using inert suture material may offer some protection. The scar line may be compressed with silicone gel pads for as many months as appears beneficial. Both practitioner and patient must adopt patience. Scars may take 2 years before they show any noticeable improvement (Fig. 7.29).

Necrosis

During the healing process, some swelling and colour change are normal and should cause little concern. Dressings should ideally be changed early to assess deterioration. Patients who seem not to understand instructions well must be reviewed early. Colour changes are associated with oxygenation and perfusion, swelling and skin tension. Dark mauve colours indicate severe trauma; with rest, the tissue recovers. High red areas indicate pre-ulcerative change. Monitoring such changes is essential every few days. Skin with darkened edges usually means that the tissue edges have been traumatized or that the skin was handled roughly during surgery. Local sloughing is of little consequence but will result in healing by secondary intention. Distal darkening, red to black, is of greater concern, particularly if the area is extensive. The skin will slough, leaving a healthy pink underlayer. During the rather alarming postoperative period of change, the patient should have the wound dressed and kept clean. Antibiotic cover should be used if the wound weeps or appears fragile. The attraction of anaerobes is as unwelcome as aerobes at this point. Vascular studies (e.g. Doppler, thermography or digital subtractive angiography) may help to determine blood flow. Any tight sutures should be removed immediately; resuturing should never be attempted.

If the patient loses tissue or the tissue ulcerates, a split thickness skin graft can be used after the base has healed. If the circulation is compromised, the part will have to be debrided until healthy circulation can be established. The

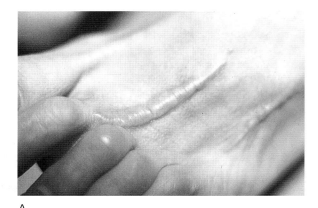

A

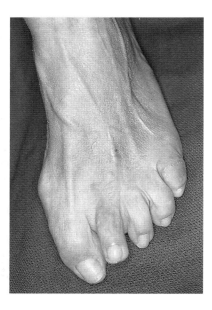

B

Figure 7.29 Hypertrophic scarring has arisen over the dorsum of the foot in a white 57-year-old female. A, After surgery. B, Two years later, the scar has settled over the second metatarsal. At no time was the scar painful, merely unsightly.

patient will need to be protected by intravenous/oral antibiotics.

Loss of sensation

Localized sensory loss is common after surgery. Small nerve fibres become damaged during surgical dissection. The permanency of this damage depends upon the site and the type of destruction imposed. Regeneration may take 9 months; after this period of time, any areas of sensory loss will most likely be permanent.

In hallux valgus surgery, the medial branch of the superficial peroneal nerve is commonly transected. The medial skin of the great toe may become insensate. Most patients tend to recover after 2 months. Ankle (arthroscopy) surgery and surgery using percutaneous techniques can inadvertently damage both nerve and blood vessels.

Repair of damaged nerves should be referred to a neurosurgeon only where the function of the foot and quality of life is affected. Damage to the plantar surface, for example, could lead to pressure ulcers as a result of an iatrogenic neuropathy. Nerve conduction studies may provide assistance in determining early damage, but the distal nerves in the foot are difficult to monitor accurately. Postsurgical compartment syndrome will require a fasciotomy to be performed as a matter of urgency. Increased interstitial fluid builds up under tension and can cause the circulation to become compromised.

Increased sensation and dysfunction

While surgery can damage nerves, reducing their ability to transmit signals, nerves can also be affected by increased sensitivity: hyperaesthesia. Entrapment neuromata arise within scar tissue between tissue layers or within the skin. A sensitive scar line may have to be reexcised if it does not settle within 3 months. Postneurectomy pain may trouble patients following Morton's neuroma resection. A stump forms in the intermetatarsal tissue and is actively excited as it becomes irritated. The surgeon may have correctly biopsied the nerve tissue, confirming the original diagnosis, but revision can still be required. Plantar surface exposure identifies amputated nerve endings, which can become surprisingly thickened. Patients with recurrent symptoms may require a magnetic resonance imaging or ultrasound scan to show the presence of the nerve. A high suspicion warrants surgery and this should be offered after

9–12 months if conservative injections fail to achieve improvement.

Hyperaesthesia is a highly sensitive response even to light touch. Two forms are described. The first, *causalgia*, may result in burning pain along a specific peripheral nerve route, but this usually follows a known injury. Nerves should be identified and the appropriate specialty consulted. The second, complex regional pain syndrome (CRPS; formerly know as reflex sympathetic dystrophy), provides the most alarming and serious side-effect seen after surgery, particularly associated with hands or feet. CRPS is not exclusive to surgical trauma. While minor injury can cause the problem, the reaction to such minimal injury is highly aggressive. Known patients with CRPS or even those suspected as presenting with CRPS should be evaluated by a pain specialist before surgery is attempted. The cardinal signs of CRPS include vasomotor colour changes, hyperalgesia, bone atrophy, known as Sudek's atrophy, and stiffness. A psychological diathesis may well be associated with the type of person likely to suffer; another theory behind the cause relates to a hypersympathetic reaction, similar to the Raynaud's sufferer.

Whether temperament or autonomic control forms the basis for CRPS, the normal inflammatory response fails to turn off the pain transmitters histamine, bradykinin and substance P. CRPS can vary in magnitude from mild symptoms to major symptoms. The latter causes gross disability and dependency on crutches or a wheelchair and can affect the contralateral side. Patients soon become labelled, and in children the condition can affect the stability of the family unit.

Treatment is poorly defined. If the signs and symptoms can be recognized early – within weeks – mobility can be improved with spinal blocks of guanethidine or LA. Sympathectomy is used and has some success, but no treatment offers a definitive outcome. The earlier that mobility can be restored, the faster the pain cycle is broken and vasomotor control settles. This condition is one where, after a while, the patient is often driven to seek legal resolve.

Bone union

While power instrumentation improves the surgeon's efficiency, the rapid oscillation of saw blades can burn the ends of bone, causing necrosis.

Most problems with a delayed union result in too much movement across the fracture site. Well-positioned fixation can limit this problem. Non-union arises after 9 months, when radiographic evidence suggests that the bone has atrophied (demineralized) and the ends have failed to develop callus. In cases of delayed union, there are no signs of new bone formation at around 6–8 weeks. Bone reduced with screws may show little activity and should not be confused with a delay in union; furthermore, the area around the screw may show signs of osteopenia.

If bone union problems occur, the first stage in treatment is immobilization in a cast for 6 weeks. A walker cast can be used for a further 6 weeks until radiographic evidence supports improvement. Where the bone shows no signs of healing, revision surgery in which a plate is used to reduce the fracture site may be required. The ends of the bone should be cleared of fibrous material to allow new bleeding and osteoblastic activity to develop. Electrical bone stimulators have been used to improve bone activity by piezoelectric effect of calcium hydroxyapatite crystals. Vitamin D/calciferol and calcium supplements can be given, and there is a role for hormonal replacement therapy in postmenopausal women; supplements of this nature, can support new bony mineralization if the patient is likely to have some immobility.

Pain may result from poor union, but once the correct diagnosis has been made, treatment is usually effective. The patient should know that postsurgical recovery can be delayed for up to 6–12 months.

TOURNIQUET USE AND EFFECTS

The use of a tourniquet has been described for nail surgery (Ch. 6). A tourniquet controls bleeding. This allows for surgery to be performed faster than if bleeding were allowed. Better discrimination between anatomical tissues ensures optimum care with dissection, minimal damage and easier definition. Whether a tourniquet is applied under GA or LA there is a finite time after which tissue, skin, muscle and fat, starts to show vascular impairment (Jones & Tollafield 1994). Surgery should be performed as quickly as possible for this reason; if the surgery is extended, the tourniquet should be released for 20 minutes before reinflating. Ankle tourniquets can be left on for 90–100 minutes, while thigh tourniquets may be elevated for longer periods 90–120 minutes. It is best if surgeons can work within an hour simply because this provides minimal adverse tissue effects and postoperative comfort. Even after a GA, pain from cuff pressure can be most unpleasant. In one study, Tollafield et al (1995) showed that 45 minutes was ideal for ankle tourniquets for foot surgery. When applied with sufficient protection, the ankle tourniquet is superior for unsedated patients as it is well tolerated after a short period of acclimatization (1–3 minutes). If tourniquets continue to cause discomfort or worse, distress, then immediate deflation is required. The ankle tourniquet is perfectly safe when placed above the ankle malleoli and well padded. When placed around the calf, the cuff is less well tolerated by patients. Cuffs at the ankle site, if painful after 5–10 minutes, will not be tolerated and should be deflated. Once pain arises in conscious patients the surgeon has to determine whether it is reasonable to continue; on balance it is kinder to deflate the cuff if the procedure requires more than 10 minutes delay in completion despite the unhelpful increase in bleeding. Negotiation with the conscious patient is the best course to take.

Patients under sedation do better but higher regional blocks such as high popliteal and common peroneal blockade can produce remarkable profound skin and muscle anaesthesia, making the tourniquet very tolerable and lasting for most surgical periods up to 100 minutes.

Thigh tourniquets can only be safely applied when patients are asleep (under GA). The pressure has to be higher above systolic pressure than required at the ankles and would be too painful otherwise. The ankle tourniquet functions well at 250–280 mmHg but should not be used on poor tissue ankle, in patients taking high levels of steroids or where bone pain exists.

Tourniquets tend to become unsafe when incorrectly applied and used. Training is essential and where deflation is carried out the appropriate respite periods should be observed.

ANAESTHETIC TECHNIQUES FOR FOOT SURGERY

The practitioner may be asked questions by the patient concerning the most suitable anaesthetic technique for surgery. A variety of anaesthetic methods are available for surgery on the foot (Fig. 7.30). All the techniques described should be performed in a hospital. The exception to this rule is LA infiltration for short day-case surgery, but all units should have provision for basic resuscitation, which ideally includes measuring oxygen saturation measurement. Oxygen should be available with separate masks, an ambou bag, Guedal airway and an approved defibrillator with heart monitor. The use of intravenous cannulae providing access to the vascular system is still debated where only LA is used. Higher-dose LA infiltrated near veins carries risks of cardiac arrhythmias and for this reason an indwelling plastic cannula (e.g. Veflon) might be preferred for easy access. Where intravenous drugs are used though cannulae, an indwelling cannula should be retained in the vein rather than using a syringe, which can easily be knocked and once removed is hard to keeping replacing back in a bruised vein.

General anaesthetics

The patient is unconscious during the operation, having been sedated initially (oral drug), anaesthetized and provided with an intraoperative analgesic. Full patient monitoring is essential throughout. Gas inhalation is commonly used to maintain the level of anaesthesia (Fig. 7.31). Modern anaesthetic techniques are safe and newer anaesthetic agents are easier to recover from than was previously the case. The ideal

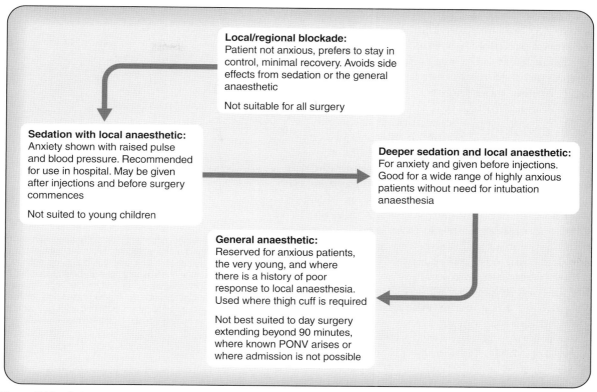

Local/regional blockade:
Patient not anxious, prefers to stay in control, minimal recovery. Avoids side effects from sedation or the general anaesthetic

Not suitable for all surgery

Sedation with local anaesthetic:
Anxiety shown with raised pulse and blood pressure. Recommended for use in hospital. May be given after injections and before surgery commences

Not suited to young children

Deeper sedation and local anaesthetic:
For anxiety and given before injections. Good for a wide range of highly anxious patients without need for intubation anaesthesia

General anaesthetic:
Reserved for anxious patients, the very young, and where there is a history of poor response to local anaesthesia. Used where thigh cuff is required

Not best suited to day surgery extending beyond 90 minutes, where known PONV arises or where admission is not possible

Figure 7.30 Quick anaesthetic reference. The preferred techniques for anaesthesia must be considered in parallel with the specific requirements for each patient. No one method applies to all. The arrows represent the next choice in order of preference. PONV, postoperative nausea and vomiting.

anaesthetic does not result in postoperative nausea and vomiting (PONV), and recovery is rapid.

The *advantages* of GA are rapid induction, elimination of anxiety and improved case load efficiency, as anaesthesia is predictable compared with use of an LA. Longer surgical operations may be easier under GA, as patients might find the duration difficult to tolerate under LA. Children and uncooperative patients may best be referred for GA for this reason.

The *disadvantages* of GA are associated with cost. An anaesthetist and recovery team is required. Patients may have to be admitted overnight if PONV is uncontrolled or any side-effects arise, such as low or high blood pressure. Procedures over 1 hour are more likely to require admission into hospital. Many drugs used in GA upset the hormone and biochemistry balance. The risks from cardiac arrest, anaphylaxis and

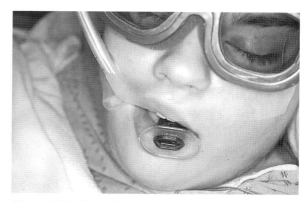

Figure 7.31 General anaesthetic with intubation and gas inhalation. A small Guedel oropharyngeal tube has been used to ensure that the teeth are protected.

malignant hyperthermia are rare but fatal. Aspiration of stomach contents poses another problem. Vomit and productive phlegm has to be managed by careful suction removal during recovery to prevent asphyxiation or postoperative respiratory problems. Prolonged operations may result in pressure sores where theatre staff are inattentive to tissue over prominences and correct turning procedure.

Local anaesthetics

Locally injected anaesthetic agents can be contrasted to GA for a range of surgical techniques. In minor biopsy surgery, for example, the anaesthetic can be infiltrated under the lesion, with or without epinephrine (adrenaline). Analgesia, rather than true anaesthesia, is achieved, while pain, temperature and sharp/deep pressure are removed; consciousness remains.

Ring blocks around toes allow access for nail ablations and IP joint arthrodesis. Regional ankle blocks using tibial nerve infiltration provides profound foot anaesthesia, allowing most distal ankle surgery to be performed safely and effectively (Fig. 7.32). Podiatrists favour regional blocks because a high volume of anaesthetic fluid is kept away from the surgical site and administration of these blocks is less painful to the patient. Blocks placed around the knee; popliteal and common peroneal nerve can create useful analgesia for hindfoot surgery. The patient must be warned, preferably with a written information sheet, about loss of motor function. The patient who inadvertently attempts to walk will fall over, with other unfortunate consequences.

The *advantages* of LA may reflect the reduced cost of the procedure. An anaesthetist is not required and the postoperative care team is replaced by intensive in-theatre care, which consists of a person caring for the patient, who remains awake throughout. The patient requires minimal recovery, does not suffer from PONV and rarely requires admission. Patient management is more predictable than under GA. LA can be used in selected patients with high blood pressure, kidney and liver disease, and it disturbs diabetic metabolism less than a GA. Patients do not have to fast and must be reminded to eat before surgery to avoid low blood

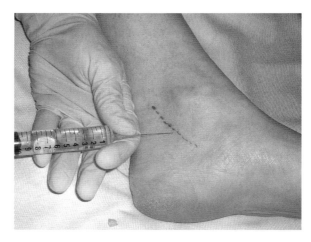

Figure 7.32 The tibial block is quick and easy to perform. The needle is placed along a line 45° from the medial malleolus to the calcaneus. The artery is palpated and the needle runs under the vascular bundle. Paraesthesia should be avoided but does occur. When this sign arises, the needle should be backed off. A good blockade for foot surgery needs 6–10 ml of local anaesthetic with or without vasoconstrictor. In skilled hands, this technique is very comfortable.

sugar, which can lead to unexpected syncope. However, patients undergoing longer interventions under planned LA may need to fast, if the option to convert to GA is available. Such conversion is prevented if food has been recently ingested (i.e. 6–8 hours).

The *disadvantages* of LA lie in the delay associated with regional blocks. Some blocks can take 60 minutes to perform satisfactorily. Anxious patients are difficult to manage in this situation; in rare cases, practitioners may find that anaesthesia is impossible to achieve, despite flooding the area locally. It has been estimated that 2–4% require a GA in podiatric practice: 0.5–2% of regional blocks fail, and this figure has been recorded at higher levels by some surgeons. Sedation in young patients is often unsatisfactory and unreliable. Paediatric clients are less reliable for LA and 60–75% of 12–16 year olds will require GA, while the numbers are even higher among those under 12 years of age.

While problems associated with LA are rare, all such drugs should be used in volumes that are within the optimum dose recommended by the manufacturer. Too great a volume of anaesthetic can cause ischaemia, even without the use of vasoconstrictors. Side-effects can arise, causing serious central nervous system and cardiovascular depression, e.g. fitting and cardiovascular hypotension and cardiac arrest.

Sedation anaesthesia

Sedation anaesthesia is another form of GA. Drugs used to provide sedation include the benzodiazepines, such as diazepam and midazolam. If these are given in small doses, the patient may remain awake, while larger doses will produce sleep although arousal is possible. Many intravenous and intramuscular drugs produce a range of effects that can give rise to different levels of anaesthesia. Intravenous midazolam sedation is preferred because the dose can be titred providing the desired effect: drowsy sleepiness or reduced anxiety with wakefulness. This drug is unsuitable for young children as it is unpredictable, as stated above. The elderly are sensitive to the drug and much smaller doses are needed. Sensibly used, this medication is excellent for day-case surgery patients. Anxiety elevates blood pressure, exacerbating cardiac output. Sedation will effectively lower blood pressure where hypertension itself is not the cause. All patients should have their blood pressure monitored and if necessary treated before surgery. Unfortunately, midazolam and also diazepam will not be helpful in extremely anxious patients and conversion to GA can be expected in a small number of patients. Propofol (Diprivan; Zeneca) is another useful drug, which, when combined with midazolam, allows the anaesthetist to control the patient's level of consciousness. LA must be given for pain control. This technique is often used with fentanyl, an opioid analgesic, which also contributes to sedation as well as controlling pain. Once several drugs have been combined an antiemetic is often required, highlighting some of the disadvantages to multiple sedation drugs. This is rarely a problem and has become very popular in both British and American podiatric surgery where the system is available.

Sedation anaesthesia has the *advantage* of providing the patient with the benefits of both LA and GA. PONV is very much less common and the patient's recovery is very quick, although drowsiness can last for an hour afterwards. The *disadvantages* are minimal in experienced hands, but too much sedation can require a longer recovery time than for a conventional short GA. The balance between each procedure requires careful planning before surgery, including advising patients about starving prior to admission. It is not always easy to predict who will benefit from which method, although a sensible guess is worthwhile with patient discussion.

Intravascular block

The Bier block uses low-strength LA, such as 0.5% plain lidocaine or prilocaine, infused into a vein below an ankle cuff. The tourniquet cuff is double chambered and monitored by the anaesthetist (Fig. 7.33). Intravascular leakage above the cuff can affect the brain and heart, given the high volumes (20–40 ml) required, and poses a greater risk than that from LA infiltrated around specific nerves. Intraosseous absorption can still arise despite the use of a tourniquet.

The *advantages* lie in a quick perfusion technique, which seeps into bone and soft tissue. *Disadvantages* lie in the high risk of convulsions from early release of the tourniquet or leaky cuffs. A full system of monitoring should be instituted and an intravenous cannula should be in place before any drug is administered. Surgery must last at least 30 minutes to allow absorption into the tissues before safely deflating the cuff. Bier block cannot be used for short cases.

Transcutaneous nerve stimulator – regional blocks

Recent advances with TNS have allowed accurate placement of regional blocks at the level of the sciatic nerve, but it can also be used at the level of common peroneal or tibial nerves (Fig. 7.34).

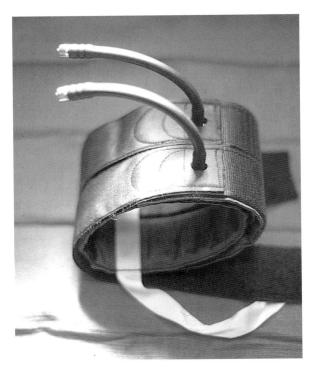

Figure 7.33 A double-cuffed chamber placed around the ankle in a Bier block. This provides an essential safety requirement to prevent premature vascular leakage affecting the heart or the central nervous system.

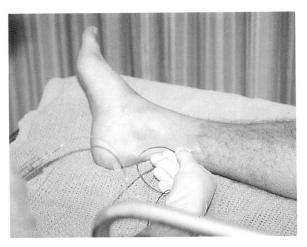

Figure 7.34 A nerve stimulator needle (stimulator not shown) is used with a tibial regional nerve block to effect plantar analgesia. (Reproduced with permission from Braun Medical, Aylesbury, UK.)

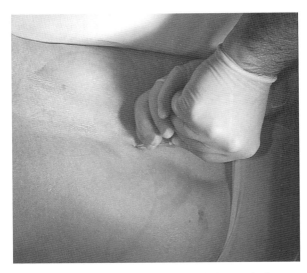

Figure 7.35 Spinal/epidural anaesthesia is popular in many centres, particularly where patients are at risk. One of the main complications is associated with a dramatic fall in blood pressure (see text).

The main *advantage* lies in a long-acting block used proximally, keeping anaesthesia away from the surgical site. The only nerve in the foot that must be separately infiltrated is the saphenous nerve. *Disadvantages* include failure; Dryden et al (1993) reported the need for GA in 10% of cases where the sciatic block failed. The patient cannot ambulate easily for 24 hours following surgery. This information is best given in writing and before surgery, as mobility is seriously hampered.

Spinal/epidural anaesthesia

Spinal/epidural anaesthesia provides an additional method for anaesthetizing the foot. Both forms have similar points of insertion but contrasting effects. In spinal analgesia, a fine needle is advanced until the subarachnoid space can be infiltrated (Fig. 7.35). In epidural analgesia, a thicker needle is used and the subarachnoid space is not breached. The main *advantage* lies in managing patients who might not be suited to GA.

There are several *disadvantages*. Both lower limbs are affected. Obese patients are difficult to inject, although it is the case that the obese patient will make anaesthetic more difficult in most operative procedures. As with most regional blocks, this technique is slower than GA and affects a great deal more than just the foot. Postoperative problems include induced hypotension following sympathetic paralysis and dilatation, anaphylaxis, local infection, backache, headaches and urinary retention. A skilled anaesthetist is also required.

SUMMARY

The principles of surgical management, their complications and methods of anaesthesia have been briefly outlined in this chapter.

In all cases of referral, the practitioner should ask four important questions:

- does the patient require surgery?
- will the patient be made better by surgery instead of other methods of management?
- is the surgery cost effective?
- will surgery create unwanted side-effects that can be avoided by using conservative care instead?

Referral of patients who are unsuitable for surgery creates unnecessary anxiety for those who might already fear such intervention. On the positive side, the changes in day surgery have offered a highly efficient service bringing many more benefits to patients. Earlier management, avoidance of bed blocking, reduced nosocomial infection and patient-friendly benefits are just a few of the advantages where the risks associated with such surgery are acceptable.

Much of the preparation for surgical referral can be achieved by good initial patient advice. As with all types of management, the practitioner must bear in mind that successful surgery relates to a partnership between the patient, the person undertaking the referral and the person undertaking treatment.

REFERENCES

Corey S V, Ruch J A 1992 Principles of internal fixation. In: McGlamry E D, Banks A S, Downey M S (eds) Comprehensive textbook of foot surgery, 2nd edn. Williams & Wilkins, Baltimore, MD, p 141

Downey M S 1992 Ankle equinus. In: McGlamry E D, Banks A S, Downey M S (eds) Comprehensive textbook of foot surgery, 2nd edn. Williams & Wilkins, Baltimore, MD, p 710–711

Dryden C M, Lloyd S M, Todd J G 1993 Sciatic nerve block as anaesthesia for foot surgery and the effect of preservatives in local anaesthetic solutions on the characteristic nerve block. The Foot 3: 184–186

Henry A P J, Waugh W 1975 The use of footprints in assessing the results of operations for hallux valgus. A comparison of Keller's operation with arthrodesis. Journal of Bone and Joint Surgery 57B: 478–481

Jones L A, Tollafield D R 1994 The use of the pneumatic ankle tourniquet with regional anaesthetic blockade. British Journal of Podiatric Medicine and Surgery 6,3: 57–59

Mann R A, Coughlin M J 1993 Surgery of the foot and ankle. Mosby, St Louis, MO, vol 1 and 2

McGlamry E D, Banks A S, Downey M S 1992 Comprehensive textbook of foot surgery, 2nd edn. Williams & Wilkins, Baltimore, MD, vol 1 and 2

Medical Devices Agency 2002 Screw-fit ceramic toe joint (metatarsophalangeal) replacement prosthesis: device alert. Medical Devices Agency, London, Crown Copyright DA2002(3), 9 May 2002

Miller S 1992 Principles of muscle tendon surgery and tendon transfers. In: McGlamry E D, Banks A S, Downey M S (eds) Comprehensive textbook of foot surgery, 2nd edn. Williams & Wilkins, Baltimore, MD, p 1306

Radin E L, Rose R M, Blaha J D, Litsky A S 1992 Practical biomechanics for the orthopaedic surgeon. Churchill Livingstone, New York, p 139–140

Rudge G, Tollafield D R 2003 A critical assessment of a new evaluation tool for podiatric surgical outcome analysis. British Journal of Podiatry 6(4): 115

Swanson A B, de Groot Swanson G, Maupin B K, Shi S 1991 The use of a grommet bone liner for flexible hinge implant arthroplasty of the great toe. Foot and Ankle 12: 149–155

Thomas T G 1991 Medical litigation and the foot. The Foot 1: 3–5

Tollafield D R 1995 Protecting Kirschner wires postoperatively. British Journal of Podiatric Medicine 7: 71

Tollafield D R, Parmar D G 1994 Setting standards for day care foot surgery. A quinquennial review. British Journal of Podiatric Medicine 6: 7–20

Tollafield D R, Kilmartin T K, Holdcroft D J, Quinn G 1995 Measurement of ankle cuff discomfort in unsedated patients undergoing day case foot surgery. Ambulatory Surgery 3: 91–96

Vogiatzolglou F, Ashford RL, Tollafield DR, Cassella JP 2000 A retrospective analysis of Swanson double-stemmed great toe implants following surgery for arthritic joint diseases. The Foot 10: 69–74

Werner D 2001 A ceramic prosthesis for hallux valgus. The Foot 11: 24–27

FURTHER READING

Cracchiolo A, III 1993 The rheumatoid foot and ankle: pathology and treatment. The Foot 3: 126–134

Lunn J N 1991 Lecture notes on anaesthetics. Blackwell Scientific, London

Paton R W, Galsko C S B 1991 Accurate structural assessment of idiopathic CTEV. The Foot 2: 71–73

Rosen J S, Grady J F 1986 Neuritic bunion syndrome. Journal of American Podiatric Medical Association 76: 641–644

Saxby T, Myerson M, Schon L 1993 Compartment syndrome of the foot following calcaneus fracture. The Foot 2: 157–161

Swanson A B, de Groot Swanson G, Mayhew D E, Khan AN 1987 Flexible hinged results in implant arthroplasty of the great toe. Rheumatology 11: 136–152

8

Pharmacology

David Gerrett

INTRODUCTION

There is a range of prescription-only and over-the-counter drugs that are involved in the management of foot problems. With the exception of antibiotics, the majority of these pharmacological preparations reduce and control the symptoms of the condition rather than address the underlying cause. In the management of foot problems, pharmacological treatments are often combined with non-pharmacological strategies in order to bring about the best therapeutic effect.

Drugs used in the management of foot problems are usually administered topically. Other routes, such as oral, subcutaneous and intravenous, are also used, but to a lesser extent. It is important that practitioners have a good working knowledge of the pharmaceutical properties, actions and contraindications associated with drugs they may use in the treatment of foot problems. For specific conditions, such as diabetes, it is also necessary to appreciate the drug implications in treatment. Practitioners must undertake a thorough assessment of the patient's medical history and be aware of past and current drug therapy for other health-related problems prior to prescribing pharmacological preparations. There are a whole range of contraindications associated with the use of drugs and these must be taken into account for each patient before a clinical decision is reached about whether pharmacological preparations should be used.

This chapter describes ways in which drugs can be administered and goes on to explore drugs used in diabetes plus the following thera-peutic drug groups used in the management of foot problems:

- analgesics
- anhidrotics
- anti-inflammatory drugs
- antimicrobial drugs
  - antibacterial drugs
  - antifungal drugs
  - antiviral drugs
- antipuritics
- caustics
- counter-irritants
- emollients.

Dressings and desloughing agents, as they are applicable to ulcer management, are addressed in Chapter 17.

TERMINOLOGY

In its widest sense, a *drug* is any substance that modifies normal physiological function. Normal hormones and neurotransmitters, such as hydrocortisone and epinephrine (adrenaline), must, therefore, be considered to be drugs, especially if they are used medicinally. A *medicine* is a preparation that contains one or more drugs made up in such a way that it is convenient to administer and from which the drugs can be absorbed efficiently and have the desired pharmacological effect.

All proprietary drugs have at least three names. The first of these is its *full chemical name*, for example (6R)-6-[(α-D-(4-hydroxyphenyl)gly-cylamino]penicillanic acid. Although this specifies the chemical in a way that would enable it to be 'built', for obvious reasons this name is seldom used, and never in clinical practice. The second name is the drug's *non-proprietary (official, approved,* or *generic) name.* For the chemical described above, this is amoxicillin. Note that the non-proprietary name is not spelled with a capital letter. Any company with rights to manufacture and sell a drug can use this non-proprietary name, and since each drug has only one of these, drugs mentioned in this chapter

are always referred to by their non-proprietary names. Drugs listed in the British National Formulary are arranged in therapeutic groups in the alphabetical order of their non-proprietary names (except for important drugs typical of their type, which are sometimes listed first, and out of alphabetical order). The third name is the *proprietary (trade) name.* In fact, one drug can have many proprietary names. The drug amoxicillin is sold under the name Amoxil, but it is also produced and sold under the name amoxicillin by many manufacturers of 'generics'. Note that proprietary names are proper nouns and always spelled with a capital letter. Proprietary names are the properties of individual companies and cannot be used by other companies without a contractual agreement between them. Companies initially patent chemical names and proprietary or 'brand' names. Once they have been granted a product licence or Product Authorization they have the right to manufacture and distribute that drug for a set period. Once the period is over, other companies can manufacture and distribute the drug but under its non-proprietary name. That is why you often see many labels for essentially the same drug. As a rule, non-proprietary drugs are made available at a lower cost than the branded proprietary equivalent.

The term 'generic' is often used instead of 'non-proprietary name', which is unfortunate because it means that there is no useful word to describe drugs belonging to a particular group or class. For example, 'barbiturate' and 'sulphonamide' are true generic names, embracing classes of drug, whereas the non-proprietary names of the individual barbiturates or sulphonamides are not truly generic – they are specific.

Most multiple-ingredient, fixed-dose formulations have only a proprietary name, although a few such medicines are recognized as being particularly worthy of recognition and are given non-proprietary names: for example, co-trimoxazole (a mixture of trimethoprim and sulfamethoxazole in the proportions of 1:5), co-amoxiclav (amoxicillin 250 mg plus clavulanic acid 125 mg per tablet) and co-proxamol tablets (dextropropoxy-phene hydrochloride 32.5 mg plus paracetamol 325 mg per tablet).

Non-proprietary names are generally designed to indicate the class to which the drug belongs. For example, all cephalosporin and cephalomycin antibiotics have 'cef' or 'ceph' in their non-proprietary names: cefaclor, cefadroxil, cefixime, cefodizime. Unfortunately, this standardization is only quite recent and older drugs may have non-proprietary names quite unrelated to other drugs with the same mechanism of action in the same therapeutic class, e.g. buprenorphine, dextromoramide, dipipanone, meptazinol, pentazocine, and pethidine are all opiates or endogenous neurochemicals that activate opiate receptors. Opioids are psychoactive drugs that originate from the opium poppy or that have a chemical structure like the drugs derived from opium. Such drugs include opium, codeine and morphine (derived from the plant).

MODE OF ADMINISTRATION

Before a drug can produce its effects, it must reach its site of action. The majority of drugs are not administered directly to the site of drug action, so that molecules of the drug must move from the site of administration to the site of action (Fig. 8.1). Exceptions to this are the topical application of drugs directly to a site and the injection of a drug into a joint.

In order to cross 'barriers' in the body, a drug must be able to cross cell membranes, which are largely composed of lipid or fat. To cross such membranes, drug molecules must be *lipid soluble, hydrophobic* (water hating) or *lipophilic* (fat loving). These are confusing terms because many lipid-soluble drugs also dissolve readily in water. When a drug is described as lipid soluble, it means that, when exposed to both a lipid or oil and water, the drug will dissolve preferentially in the oily fatty layer. Alternatively, if the drug is already dissolved in water then it will tend to move out of water (aqueous phase) into surrounding cell membranes (lipid phase). Lipid soluble is, therefore, a jargon short-hand term meaning 'high oil:water partition coefficient'.

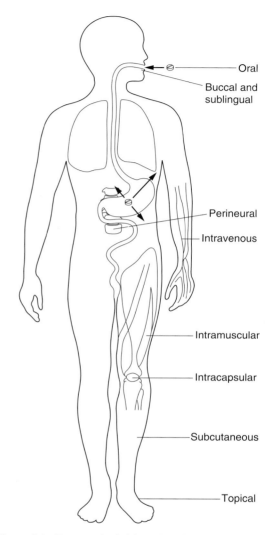

Figure 8.1 Routes of administration of drugs.

Sites of administration

Oral This is the most convenient form of drug administration. It is only effective for drugs that are lipid soluble, resistant to the acid environment of the stomach, which has a pH of 1.0 on the stomach wall, and not rapidly broken down by hepatic enzymes. The blood flow from all but the last 4 cm of the gastrointestinal tract passes first through the hepatic portal system, where drugs may be broken down by hepatic (liver) enzymes. This 'first-pass' effect results in, for example, only 30% of oral diamorphine entering the systemic circulation. The time to maximal plasma concentration after oral administration is considerably greater than after parenteral administration (by injection). Formulations for oral administration include liquids (often syrups or suspensions), capsules and tablets. Tablets are sometimes specially coated to protect the drug they contain from the activity of gastric acid and enzymes. Such tablets are known as *enteric-coated* tablets. Capsules are usually made of gelatin, which dissolves in the stomach releasing the active drug. There are also several other formulations designed to release the drug slowly over prolonged periods in order to extend the duration of action of the drug. These are known as *sustained-release* (or *controlled-release*) formulations.

Buccal and sublingual The mucous membrane of the mouth is very thin and richly supplied with blood vessels. Consequently, lipid-soluble drugs are readily absorbed from the lining of the mouth. This is the preferred route for drugs that are *lipophilic* but susceptible to hepatic first-pass metabolism, such as glyceryl trinitrate used to treat angina. This is because the venous drainage of the mucous lining of the mouth is not part of the hepatic portal system and, therefore, the drug enters the systemic circulation without passing through the liver.

Intravenous Drugs administered directly into a vein reach their peak plasma concentration virtually instantaneously. Plasma concentrations then fall continuously (Fig. 8.2). Intravenous injection is the preferred route when therapeutic concentrations must be achieved rapidly; for example, in life-threatening infections, or if the drug is too highly water soluble (hydrophilic, lipophobic) to be absorbed from the gastro-intestinal tract or too irritant to the body tissues to be given by any other route. The fast flowing bloodstream quickly dilutes injected chemicals, even so the rate of administration must be such as not to allow too great a concentration for tissue damage.

Intramuscular Skeletal muscle (gluteus, deltoid) is richly supplied with blood vessels; consequently, a drug injected into muscle will readily

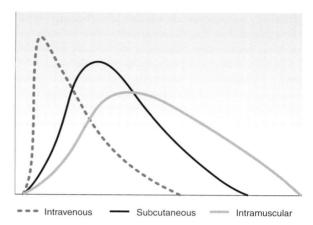

--- Intravenous   —— Subcutaneous   —— Intramuscular

Figure 8.2 Plasma drug concentration levels for intravenous, intramuscular and subcutaneous injections.

enter the systemic blood supply. Peak plasma concentrations are reached more slowly than they are after intravenous injection, but more quickly than after subcutaneous injection (see Fig. 8.2). This is the preferred route of injection as it does not involve the same level of administration skill as for intravenous injection and is suitable for most water-soluble drugs that are not irritant.

Subcutaneous There is a thin layer of fatty tissue immediately under the skin, supported with a poor blood supply. Drugs injected into this layer will, therefore, be absorbed quite slowly. After subcutaneous injection, the peak plasma concentration is reached more slowly than after either intramuscular or intravenous injection (see Fig. 8.2). Subcutaneous injection into the thigh or abdomen is the preferred route of injection for non-irritant, water-soluble drugs when a more sustained action is required than can be achieved by other routes (e.g. insulin).

Intracapsular Injection of a drug directly into a synovial cavity or capsule bypasses the diffusion barrier presented by the thick synovial membrane and allows therapeutic concentrations to be reached rapidly, for example corticosteroids used to treat inflammation in bone joints. Moreover, the membrane also slows diffusion of drug out of the capsule; as a result, the systemic concentration of the drug will be much lower than that inside the capsule. This is important for drugs that have a marked systemic effect, such as corticosteroids.

Perineural There are several ways in which drugs, for example local anaesthetics, can be injected so that they remain at high concentration around a nerve trunk. The principle is that because the blood supply to the area is so poor, the drug diffuses away slowly. When local anaesthetics are administered by infiltration, a vasoconstrictor drug is sometimes used to prolong the drug's action by reducing the local blood flow. In spinal and epidural anaesthesia, the local anaesthetic is injected either into the cerebrospinal fluid (CSF) of the spinal cord or into the epidural space surrounding a particular nerve root.

Topical Normally, the skin presents a more or less impermeable barrier to water-soluble drugs. Consequently, application of such drugs to the skin allows high concentrations to be achieved on the outer surface of the skin, with little if any absorption into the rest of the body. This enables systemically toxic drugs to be used against, for example, fungal infections of the skin. However, if the integrity of the skin is broken, for example by abrasions or burns, appreciable absorption can occur, leading to systemic toxicity. Similarly, if the skin becomes saturated with water, as under an occlusive dressing, water-soluble drugs can be absorbed. For lipid-soluble drugs, appreciable absorption will occur across the skin. This can be made use of in two ways. First, application to the skin is a convenient way of administering lipid-soluble drugs when prolonged action is required. Skin patches that deliver nicotine (for withdrawal from smoking), glyceryl trinitrate (for angina), oestrogen (for hormone replacement therapy and contraception) or hyoscine (for travel sickness) are now widely used. Second, by applying a high concentration of a lipid-soluble drug to a limited area of skin, relatively high concentrations will be achieved in the tissues underlying the area of application. If such administration is prolonged, the systemic concentration will eventually rise sufficiently for systemic rather than local effects to be produced. This will happen more readily if the area of application is large, if the drug is very lipid soluble, or if the skin integrity is reduced. It should be borne in mind that the surface/body mass ratio is much higher in children than in adults, so that topical administration to children is more likely to lead to significant systemic concentrations of drug.

Inhaled Drugs dissolved in vaporized microdroplets can be inhaled in the form of sprays. Absorption is aided by the 100 m² surface area of the 600 million alveoli sacks. A difficulty is to ensure correct inhalation technique so that drugs are not delivered to the back of the throat. This technique is useful to deliver drugs such as salbutamol used in asthma to the site of desired action in the lungs.

Examples of differing modes of administration

The options for insulin therapy in diabetes mellitus serve to demonstrate many of the principles described in this introduction. Diabetes is caused by varying degrees of insulin hyposecretion. Insulin is a peptide hormone secreted by the islets of Langerhans of the pancreas that enables circulating glucose in the bloodstream to enter cells. Drug treatment relies on artificially restoring insulin levels or making cells more sensitive to the actions of any circulating hormone.

Diabetes as a medical condition stands apart as the 'diabetic foot' causes more inpatient bed occupancy than all the other diabetic medical problems put together. Nerve damage (neuropathy) of the distal sensory type present as neuropathic foot ulcers on the soles of the foot, and peripheral vascular disease results in ischaemic ulcers in the distal ends of the toes.

The body's own physiological insulin peaks in 30 to 40 minutes after a meal then declines rapidly reaching 10 to 20% of the peak in 2 hours. Stomach acids break down insulin and, furthermore, it is water soluble and, therefore, not readily absorbed orally or topically from the skin. It could be given intravenously, but constant injections three or four times a day would result in venous damage, making this route of administration unavailable within 3 to 4 years. One option is subcutaneous injection.

Mimicking the 'normal' pattern is the goal of therapy, as failure to do so will result in long-term complications. For type one diabetes (fully insulin dependent), an option is to use Neutral Insulin, which is similarly water soluble (hydrophilic) and after subcutaneous injection appears in the circulation in 10 minutes, reaching peak concentrations after 2 hours then declines over 4–8 hours.

Diabetics could vary the amount and timing of soluble Neutral Insulin to fit with their meals but this would mean many injections and constant vigilance for signs of hyper- and hypoglycaemia. To make life more palatable, reduce injection frequency and increase concordance, further drug options are based on altering injected insulin's pharmacokinetics or absorption and distribution. In moving away from physiological human insulin, issues of reaction to the drug also become important.

By reversing two amino acids in insulin (insulin lispro), crystallizing insulin with zinc (lente insulin) or complexing insulin with protamine (isophane insulin) a multitude of options allow diabetics to tailor their treatment to individual lifestyles. The availability of beef, pork and human insulin variants allows for options should patients demonstrate any allergic reactions.

Diabetes demonstrates the principle of altering drug types to accommodate individual variation. It show how options for the route of administration are determined by the nature of the drug and that the goal of therapy is to find the right combination, form, presentation and type of drug that will optimally suit patients.

THERAPEUTIC DRUG GROUPS USED IN THE MANAGEMENT OF FOOT PROBLEMS

ANALGESICS

Analgesics are drugs that relieve pain. There are two main types. First, naturally occurring opioids or synthetic opiates, which stimulate the body's *opioid* (or *narcotic*) receptors and alter the perception of pain. Second, those that prevent prostaglandin synthesis. The second type refers to a group called non-steriodal anti-inflammatory drugs (NSAIDs), which have anti-inflammatory, analgesic and antipyretic activity. The latter activity is caused by the drug resetting the 'thermostat' in the hypothalamus to override the interleukin-induced increase in temperature.

Analgesics have a number of uses in the management of foot pain. They can be used:

- preoperatively to reduce postoperative pain
- to prevent pain during an operation (local anaesthetics)
- postoperatively to reduce pain
- to manage acute, non-surgically derived pain
- to manage chronic, non-surgically derived pain.

They can be administered orally, intravenously, intramuscularly and topically. The oral, intramuscular and topical routes are the most favoured.

The management of foot pain is complex. Every effort should be made to identify the cause of the pain and reduce or remove its effects. Where necessary, analgesics are a form of pharmacological treatment that has an important role to play in the management of pain alongside non-pharmacological strategies. If analgesics are to be used, it is essential that a thorough patient history is taken to determine the presence of allergies (especially those in whom attacks of asthma, angioedema, urticardia or rhinitis have been precipitated) and gastrointestinal ulcers or gastric reflux, all of which indicate caution in the use of NSAID analgesics. Specific NICE (http://www.nice.org.uk/National Institute of Clinical Excellence) guidance and Committee on Safety of Medicines (http://www.mca.gov.uk/aboutagency/regframework/csm/csmhome.htm) instructions are available in the British National Formulary to guide the use of these drugs. A wide range of analgesics is available over the counter. Patients require good advice as to which analgesics are appropriate for their pain, and they should be made well aware of the unwanted side-effects that may arise.

The following analgesics are discussed in the remainder of this section:

- opioid/opiate
- antipyretic
- local anaesthetics
- topical anaesthetics.

Opioid/opiate analgesics

Indications

The maximal degree of analgesia that is attainable with opioid or opiate analgesics varies. The naturally occurring opioid morphine and the synthetic opiate diamorphine ('heroin') have the highest ceiling effects, with the opiate pethidine considerably less. The opiate dihydrocodeine and the opioid codeine have intermediate and low ceiling effects, with the opiate dextropropoxyphene the least.

Although all the drugs described above are active after oral administration, diamorphine and morphine undergo considerable first-pass hepatic metabolism and, consequently, are usually administered by injection. Codeine, dihydrocodeine and dextropropoxyphene are well absorbed from the gastrointestinal tract and are less affected by first-pass metabolism. As a general rule, smaller doses of analgesics are needed to *prevent* pain than are necessary to abolish pain once it is present. Being very powerful analgesics, opioids and opiates are very helpful when repeated small doses are taken prior to elective surgery, as they prevent the onset of postoperative pain.

Mechanism of action

Opioids and opiates have the same mechanism of analgesic action. These analgesics produce their effects by interacting with receptors for enkephalins, endorphins and dynorphins, which are natural peptide transmitters involved in controlling our perception of pain and well-being.

Analgesia results from interference with both transmission of the pain signal up the spinal cord and its interpretation by the limbic system in the brain. Opioids and opiates are more effective against constant, general pain than against sharp pain, although they do help sharp pain. In addition to an analgesic action, the more powerful opioid and opiate analgesics cause some *euphoria* at therapeutic doses. This may contribute to the analgesic action by making the pain more bearable. The term *narcotic* is sometimes used because in high doses these drugs cause stupor and unconsciousness.

Unwanted effects

The most troubling unwanted effect for patients treated with these analgesics is constipation. The body does not accommodate to this effect, which is used therapeutically in diseases such as Crohn's disease and ulcerative colitis, where chronic diarrhoea is a problem. The most dangerous adverse effect is respiratory depression, and this is the usual cause of death from overdose. However, the respiratory depression is not accompanied by general cardiovascular depression, unlike most sedative/hypnotic/anxiolytics. Allied to respiratory depression is the ability these drugs have to suppress cough, an *antitussive* action. Codeine is a common ingredient of cough linctuses, as is pholcodeine. All the opioid/opiate analgesics suppress cough at subanalgesic doses.

Extended use of opioids and opiates results in *tolerance* and *physical dependence*; the patient needs progressively more of the drug to achieve the same degree of pain relief (tolerance), and withholding the drug causes the patient to suffer an entirely predictable *withdrawal* (or *abstinence*) *syndrome*. Withdrawal syndromes result when the body has adjusted to the presence of a drug so that normal function is disturbed when the drug is suddenly removed. As the body readjusts to the absence of the drug, the severity of the withdrawal syndrome declines. The signs and symptoms of withdrawal syndromes are generally the opposite of the actions of the drug. For the opioid/opiate analgesics, withdrawal of the drug from a physiologically or physically dependent patient results in a sense of extreme discomfort (*dysphoria*), pain from normally non-painful stimuli, such as the touch of clothing (*hyperalgesia*), profuse diarrhoea, dilated pupils (*mydriasis*), lack of sleep (*insomnia*) and hyperventilation. These are usually accompanied by a craving for the drug. The withdrawal syndrome can be abruptly terminated by giving an opioid or opiate. The drug of choice in this regard is naloxone because of its relatively shorter duration of action. All of the opioid and opiate analgesics, including the partial agonists such as buprenorphine, will substitute for one another in supporting a physical dependence although dosages vary according to potency.

The more rapidly the blood concentration of the drug falls, the more severe will be the syndrome. Hence the short-acting opioid morphine and opiate diamorphine produce more severe withdrawal syndromes than the more slowly eliminated drugs, such as dihydrocodeine or methadone (the opiate commonly used in treating those abusing drugs). It is most unlikely that a patient will become physically dependent on an opioid or opiate during treatment for acute pain. Furthermore, for pain of organic origin, appropriate use of these analgesics is not associated with the same levels of physical or psychological dependence as seen in abuse.

Antipyretic analgesics

Indications

The antipyretic analgesics are so named because they combine an analgesic action with the ability to lower body temperature in fever (*pyrexia*). In fact, most drugs in this group combine analgesic and antipyretic properties with anti-inflammatory properties. All of the NSAIDs are antipyretic analgesics (see p. 175). *Paracetamol* is atypical in that it is not a potent anti-inflammatory drug in peripheral tissue, which is why it is usually classed as an antipyretic analgesic as opposed to a NSAID. Paracetamol is a widely available pain-relieving drug. It may be combined with NSAIDs, such as aspirin, or opioids, such as codeine, thus complementing its action with either an anti-inflammatory effect in peripheral tissues or improving its pain-relieving capacity.

Mechanism of action

In fever and headache, antipyretic analgesics are effective because they inhibit cyclooxygenase (COX) (Fig. 8.3), which is an enzyme on the pathway for the production of prostaglandins in the brain. Fever has been shown to result from the central production of prostaglandins in response

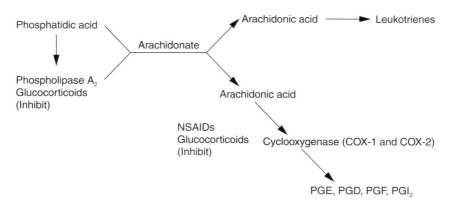

Figure 8.3 Synthetic pathway for the eicosanoids. Enzymes are shown in boxes; drugs are shown in italics. NSAIDs, non-steroidal anti-inflammatory drugs; PGE, prostaglandin E; prostacyclin is prostaglandin I_2.

to toxic substances (pyrogens) produced by foreign organisms, such as bacteria. Paracetamol selectively inhibits COX in the brain; it has a much lower activity against the form of the enzyme found in peripheral tissues.

Unwanted effects

In quite small overdose, for adults as little as two to three times the maximal therapeutic dose if combined with alcohol and three to four times in isolation, paracetamol can produce serious, potentially fatal, adverse effects. When the four possible pathways of liver enzymes responsible for the normal phase II metabolism of paracetamol become saturated, metabolism of paracetamol continues by phase I oxidation. However, this produces a toxic free-radical metabolite. At first, this toxic metabolite is inactivated by phase II conjugation with glutathione. Unfortunately, stores of glutathione in the liver are limited, and once these stores are used up, conjugation of the toxic metabolite ceases and the free-radical metabolite accumulates. The toxic metabolite binds to sulphydryl-containing proteins in the liver cell and causes lipid peroxidation, disrupting the cell membrane. These events eventually lead to cell death. Any organ that has P450 enzymes can suffer toxicity (e.g. liver, kidneys, heart and pancreas). Necrosis of liver and kidney cells typically begins 1 or 2 days after the overdose. Patients should be warned of the small margin of safety with paracetamol, especially when combined with alcohol.

Patients suspected of taking a paracetamol overdose should be urgently admitted to hospital, even if they show no signs of poisoning. Paracetamol levels in the blood indicate the potential risk and are interpreted according to the time of ingestion. Knowing this accurately is critical in determining treatment. The effective antidote to paracetamol overdose is *acetylcysteine* or *methionine*, used to increase the production of glutathione. To be effective, treatment must be started within a few hours of the overdose (6–8 hours), otherwise too much damage to the liver may have occurred. Treatments may be given up to 15 hours after ingestion depending on the local hospital accident and emergency or surgery policy.

Skin reactions are a common unwanted effect of NSAIDs, particularly with mefenamic acid (10–15% frequency). The condition varies from mild rashes, urticaria, and photosensitivity reactions to fatal diseases, which are fortunately very rare.

As stated, NSAIDs inhibit the action of the COX, the enzyme that converts arachidonic acid into prostaglandins such as PGE_2, prostacyclin and thromboxanes (Milner 2000) (see Fig. 8.3). A number of isoforms of COX exist. Of these, COX-1 is a constitutive enzyme responsible for cellular 'house keeping' functions. It is important for the physiological homeostasis of several systems, such as maintenance of renal blood flow, endothelial antithrombogenicity and gastric cytoprotection (Halliwell 1995). Notably, COX-2 is induced when tissues are exposed to traumatic or inflammatory stimuli and promotes the facilitation of inflammation and pain. Its inhibition is thought to be the method of analgesic action of NSAIDs, while many of the side-effects of these drugs are mediated by COX-1 inhibition. Prostaglandins have a protective effect on the gastrointestinal mucosa by direct inhibition of acid secretion, increased mucus secretion, increased bicarbonate output, increased mucosal blood flow and stimulation of cell growth and repair.

Consequently, NSAIDs that non-selectively inhibit prostaglandin synthesis can cause gastrointestinal mucosal damage. This is a systemic effect as NSAIDs are acidic and lipid soluble, which allows rapid diffusion and entrapment in the epithelial cells of the gastrointestinal tract. Topical application of NSAIDS may theoretically limit this systemic effect; however, they are not exempt from it. Research has led to the development of COX-2-selective inhibitors, which aim to reduce gastro-intestinal toxicity without reducing anti-inflammatory properties. A further potential advantage is that they may reduce the risk of gastrointestinal bleeding by not interfering with platelet aggregation, a COX-1 effect. Use of COX-2 drugs is currently advocated for patients at high risk of gastrointestinal problems.

Local anaesthesia

Indications

Local anaesthetics are primarily used to remove pain during a surgical procedure. They are increasingly being used for this purpose as they have a number of distinct advantages over general anaesthetics (Box 8.1). Local anaesthetics have non-surgical uses; they can be very effective, as a short-term measure, in reducing acute pain.

Most local anaesthetics are either *esters* (e.g. amethocaine, benzocaine) or *amides* (e.g. lidocaine, prilocaine, bupivacaine). Although some metabolism of the ester forms occurs in the tissue into which they are injected, termination of local anaesthesia depends mainly upon the drug being carried away from the tissue in the blood. Local anaesthesia prevents transmission in sympathetic vasoconstrictor fibres; consequently, blood flow in anaesthetized tissues usually increases. Prilocaine is unusual in that it does not cause vasodilatation. The most commonly used local anaesthetics are lidocaine, bupivacaine and prilocaine.

When using local anaesthetics, it is important that the optimum safe dosage is not exceeded.

Mechanism of action

Local anaesthetics (Greek: *an*, without; *aesthesia*, sensation) interfere with the development and transmission of nerve action potentials. They do not distinguish between sensory or motor nerves, somatic or autonomic nerves. As a result, local anaesthetics do not lead just to the loss of pain sensation but also to reduction or loss of other sensations and loss of function.

Box 8.1 Advantages of local anaesthetics

- Reduction in psychological stress
- Patient conscious
- Reduced costs
- Fewer fatalities
- Do not require anaesthetists to administer.

From McClure & Wildsmith (1991), with permission.

The small-diameter nerve fibres are anaesthetized faster than large diameter fibres. Type C nerve fibres are the most sensitive, whereas type A (motor) fibres are the least sensitive. This is simply because the former fibres have a greater surface area/volume ratio, so more of the drug enters the nerve fibre in unit time (Fick's law of diffusion). In addition, non-myelinated fibres become anaesthetized before myelinated fibres because the myelin sheath presents a diffusion barrier that the drug must penetrate before acting on the nerve itself.

It is only necessary for a short length of nerve to be anaesthetized for transmission to fail at that point. If a bundle of fibres are anaesthetized, the whole of the region of the body supplied by (or supplying) the nerves in the bundle will be paralysed

Normal activity in nerves depends upon transmission of action potentials. Action potentials are self-propagating waves of electrical activity that rely upon the electrical potential energy stored in the nerve fibre by virtue of its resting membrane potential. The membrane of excitable cells (mainly skeletal muscle and nerves fibres) is selectively permeable. It is moderately permeable to K^+, but highly impermeable to Na^+. Furthermore, there is a high concentration of K^+ and a low concentration of Na^+ inside cells. Extracellular fluid is conversely rich in Na^+ but poor in K^+. As a result, K^+ tends to leak out of the cell down the K^+ concentration gradient. As most of the negative charge inside cells is carried on proteins, which are too large to pass across the membrane, the leak of K^+ carries a net flux of positive charge out of the cell. The inside of the cell becomes progressively more negatively charged relative to the outside. As this negative charge builds up, it acts to oppose the leak of K^+, because these cations are attracted back into the cell by the intracellular negative charge. Consequently, there are two forces at work in opposition: a concentration gradient for K^+ directed out of the cell and an electrical gradient for K^+ directed into the cell. Eventually, these two forces are equal and the rate at which K^+ leave the cell under the concentration gradient exactly equals the rate at which other K^+ enter the cell under the electrical gradient. This electrical gradient is known as the *equilibrium potential* for potassium.

For this system to work, the cell has to be able to keep the intracellular concentration of K^+ high and the intracellular concentration of Na^+ low. This is achieved by a biochemical pump (*Na^+/K^+-ATPase*) that uses the energy provided by ATP (adenosine trisphosphate) to pump Na^+ out of the cell in exchange for K^+, which it pumps into the cell. The biochemical energy provided by the operation of the Na^+/K^+ pump running continuously is in the end responsible for the potential energy stored in the nerve fibre in the form of electrical potential: the *membrane potential*. In some ways, the nerve fibre can be viewed as an electrical accumulator that is constantly 'trickle charged' by the Na^+/K^+ pump.

During the transmission of an action potential, the electrical potential across the membrane falls (i.e. the inside becomes less negative). When this happens, the membrane changes its properties. Embedded in the nerve membrane, there are millions of specialized cylindrical protein structures that pass right through from the cytoplasmic side of the membrane to the extracellular surface. These have the ability to change their conformation and allow the passage of Na^+. These so-called 'Na^+ channels' have what amounts to two 'gates' that can open or close the central pore of the channel. These gates are known as the 'm' gate and the 'h' gate (Fig. 8.4A). At normal resting membrane potentials (typically $-120\,mV$), it is thought that the 'm' gates are closed and the 'h' gates open. When the membrane potential falls to a threshold level, the 'm' gates open quickly (*channel activation*), allowing Na^+ to enter the cell, carrying positive charge. This causes depolarization (i.e. the inside of the cell becomes less negative relative to the outside). This depolarization causes the 'h' gates to close, but they do this moderately slowly. Thus the Na^+ channels close (*inactivate*), stopping the fall in membrane potential. The depolarization also stimulates K^+ channels to open, and an efflux of K^+ through these channels helps the cell to repolarize quickly. Once the critical membrane potential is reached, the 'm' gates close rapidly and the 'h' gates slowly open again.

Until the 'h' gates are open, another action potential is impossible; the fibre is said to be *refractory*. As one part of the membrane depolarizes, it activates the Na^+ channels in the adjacent piece of membrane so that the action potential is propagated along the fibre rather like fire down a trail of gunpowder; the heat of burning grains of gunpowder sets fire to adjacent grains of gunpowder that set fire to adjacent grains, and so on.

Local anaesthetics block the movement of Na^+ through these channels, thereby preventing the depolarization that is necessary for an action potential to be transmitted along the fibre (Fig. 8.4B). Local anaesthetics do this in two ways. First, they are believed to dissolve in the nerve membrane, changing its physicochemical properties so that the protein of the Na^+ channels becomes distorted and less able to function. Second, some, if not all, of the local anaesthetics are believed to interact with a specific receptor site located inside the channel pore, near the intracellular end of the sodium channel. When a molecule of local anaesthetic is bound to this receptor, Na^+ cannot pass through the channel. Local anaesthetics do this by causing the 'h' gate to close. However, these receptor sites are not accessible to local anaesthetic molecules from the extracellular fluid. Local anaesthetic molecules can only bind to these receptor sites in the pore if they approach from the cytoplasm. This means that the drug must be able to enter the cytoplasm before it can exert this action.

To gain access to the cytoplasm, the drug must first pass through the cell membrane; only lipid-soluble forms of local anaesthetic molecules can do this. At pH 7.4 (tissue pH), local anaesthetics are partially ionized. Local anaesthetics are weak bases, and so the ionized form is a cation. Although only the non-ionized form diffuses across nerve cell membranes, it is the cationic form that combines with the receptor. Once the non-ionized form has crossed the membrane, it partially dissociates again (typically 80% exists in the ionized form at pH 7.4).

To prolong the duration of anaesthesia, some local anaesthetic preparations contain a vasoconstrictor to prevent vasodilatation. Two vasoconstrictors are available: *epinephrine* (adrenaline)

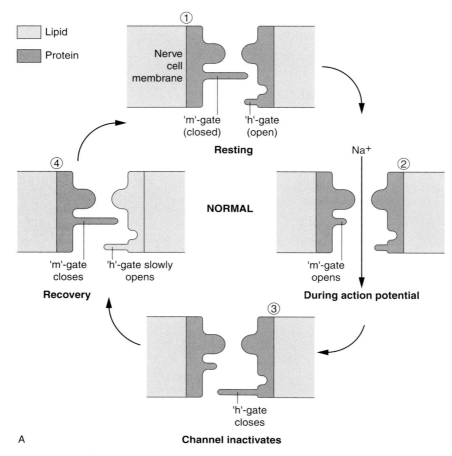

Figure 8.4 A, Mechanism of action of local anaesthetics. Normal mechanism for the generation of an action potential.

and *felypressin*. Epinephrine acts on adrenoceptors, much like norepinephrine (noradrenaline) released as a result of activity in sympathetic nerves. Felypressin is a peptide analogue of antidiuretic hormone (also known as vasopressin). Felypressin stimulates vasopressin receptors to cause vasoconstriction and is preferred if there is a risk that epinephrine may not be tolerated.

Unwanted effects

The main problems that may arise with the use of local anaesthetics are type 1 hypersensitivity reactions (anaphylaxis) and toxic reactions. Anaphylaxis is more common with the ester-type local anaesthetics. Toxic reactions occur in the presence of high plasma concentrations of the local anaesthetic. This initially leads to stimulation of the central nervous system (excitement, nausea, euphoria), followed by dizziness, shivering and drowsiness. In severe cases, the patient may have convulsions. These events are followed by depression of central nervous system activity, which may affect the cardiovascular system and can lead to circulatory collapse.

Irritation and inflammation are local effects that may occur as a result of injecting anaesthetics. If the local effects are severe, this may result in tissue damage and necrosis. The use of local anaesthetics combined with epinephrine or felypressin may lead to prolonged vasoconstriction.

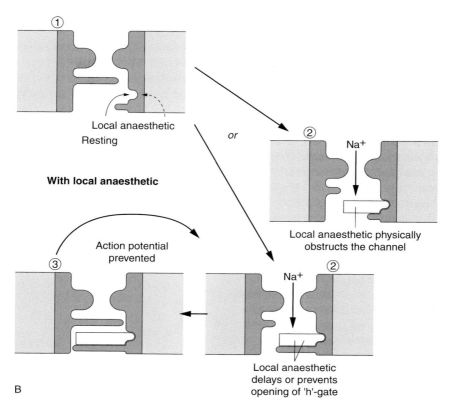

Figure 8.4 – *continued*   B, By physically obstructing the sodium channel or by interfering with the opening of the 'h' gate, local anaesthetics prevent sodium ion entry into the nerve. As a result, action potential generation is prevented.

This may have irreversible effects in digits, which have a large surface area to volume ratio. Ischaemic changes that lead to gangrene may ensue.

Tricyclic antidepressants act, at least in part, by reducing inactivation by uptake into nerve endings of epinephrine and norepinephrine. There is, therefore, a risk that patients taking tricyclic antidepressants may develop excessive vasoconstriction in response to epinephrine. Sometimes patients are given monoamine oxidase inhibitors to treat depression. These drugs inhibit the metabolism of epinephrine and there is a small risk of excessive vasoconstriction if epinephrine-containing local anaesthetic is used. Felypressin is not potentiated by either tricyclic antidepressants or monoamine oxidase inhibitors and, therefore, may be preferred.

Topical anaesthetics

Indications

Various preparations are used for topical anaesthesia: salicylates, benzocaine, amethocaine, lidocaine and prilocaine. These preparations may be combined, as in EMLA cream, which contains 2.5% lidocaine plus 2.5% prilocaine. The effectiveness of topical anaesthetics is questionable. Their use is often confined to analgesia of the skin prior to the administration of an injection. Additionally they may be incorporated into antipruritics.

Topical anaesthetics may be presented in lotions, creams, ointments, sprays or skin patches. Up to 10% of the free base in an oily vehicle has been found to be effective in achieving a small localized area of skin anaesthesia.

Mechanism of action

Local anaesthetics such as benzocaine and lidocaine produce analgesia when applied to mucous membranes and broken skin. Their action on intact skin is debatable. If applied to intact skin they must be applied for at least an hour, under occlusion, in order to penetrate the skin barrier and have any noticeable effects.

Salicylates, when administered orally, inhibit prostaglandin synthesis. It is known that salicylates are absorbed percutaneously; therefore, it is postulated that topical application of salicylates prevents the local synthesis of prostaglandins. As salicylates also have a known hyperaemic effect, it is also thought that their counter-irritant effect aids analgesia. It is believed that topical analgesics containing salicylates are best applied by massage; the action of massage is considered to aid rapid clearance of locally produced pain-inducing substances.

ANHIDROTICS

Indications

Anhidrotics are useful in the treatment of hyperhidrosis. The main anhidrotics are the aldehydes and aluminium salts. The aldehydes, for example glutaraldehyde and formaldehyde, can be very effective topically, especially in concentrations of 10%. Preparations based on the aluminium salts are the most popular and appear to be the most effective (e.g. 20% aluminium chloride hexa-hydrate and 19% aluminium hydroxychloride).

Mechanism of action

Most anhidrotics have a drying effect on the skin. This effect may be brought about by reversible damage to the eccrine glands, as anhidrotics reduce the size of the lumen, so that the production of sweat is reduced. Some astringents appear to act by producing a physical blockage of the sweat duct. Aluminium hydroxide is deposited within the distal intraepidermal portion of the eccrine duct and forms a plug.

Unwanted effects

There are no major unwanted effects. Care should be exercised with the use of aldehydes as sensitization can occur and the skin may also be stained brown when glutaraldehyde is used.

ANTI-INFLAMMATORY DRUGS

Inflammation is part of the body's defensive response to injury caused by trauma or invading organisms. Classical inflammation involves a local increase in blood flow (causing redness and heat), swelling, pain and impaired function. There are many chemical mediators of inflammation, but one particularly important group is the *prostaglandins*. Prostaglandins are 20-carbon fatty acids produced from the precursor arachidonic acid by a cascade of enzymes, the most important of which is COX (see Fig. 8.3). The prostaglandins are largely responsible for the swelling, vasodilation and pain that develops after the first 2 or 3 hours of an inflammatory response. The pain results not from direct activation of pain fibres by prostaglandins but from *sensitization* of pain receptors by prostaglandins, so that previously non-painful stimuli are felt as pain.

Anti-inflammatory drugs are widely used in the pharmacological management of inflammation in the foot. There is also a range of non-pharmacological strategies that can be very useful in the treatment of inflammation (see Ch. 9). Because of their effect on prostaglandin synthesis, some anti-inflammatory drugs are also effective analgesics and may be used because of this combined effect. Many factors can cause acute and chronic inflammation in the foot. The most likely causes are sudden or repeated trauma or invasion by pathogenic microorganisms. The other prime cause is the local or systemic effect of hypersensitivity and autoimmune reactions; examples are contact dermatitis (local) and rheumatoid arthritis (systemic). The majority of dermatological conditions also invoke an inflammatory reaction (e.g. psoriasis, eczema, lichen planus).

Anti-inflammatory drugs can be conveniently classified by their action, non-steroidal or steroidal. They are effective if administered orally, via intracapsular injections or topically. The two types of anti-inflammatory drugs are considered below, followed by a discussion of the administration of anti-inflammatory drugs parenterally and topically.

Non-steroidal anti-inflammatory drugs

Indications

The main NSAIDs are aspirin, ibuprofen, fenbufen, naproxen, ketoprofen, fenoprofen, diclofenac sodium, indometacin, piroxicam and mefenamic acid. The COX-2-selective NSAIDS are celecoxib, etodolac, meloxicam and rofecoxib. Although these drugs reduce pain, swelling and redness, and improve function, they have no effect on the underlying disease process.

Mechanism of action

NSAIDs act by inhibiting COX so that fewer prostaglandins are produced (see Fig. 8.3). This reduces local vasodilatation, swelling and pain. COX-2-selective inhibitors specifically inhibit an isoform of COX induced when tissues are exposed to traumatic or inflammatory stimuli. All the useful NSAIDs are quite well absorbed after oral administration.

Unwanted effects

Nearly all NSAIDs are weak acids that bind strongly to plasma proteins, which can lead to interactions with other drugs. By binding avidly to plasma proteins, NSAIDs can displace molecules of other drugs that were previously bound. This raises the free plasma concentration of the other, previously bound drug, so that the patient is effectively overdosed. Non-selective inhibitors of COX cause some degree of gastric bleeding by interfering with the production of the protective layer of mucus by the stomach lining, as production of this protective layer of mucus involves the local release of prostaglandins. This is a dose-dependent effect and is worse if the drug is chemically irritant (e.g. aspirin). Aspirin, being a weak acid, also tends to accumulate within cells lining the stomach, including the mucus-producing cells. This is because the acid environment causes the aspirin to be unionized and, therefore, more lipid soluble; as a result, it enters cells readily. Inside the cells, however, the pH is less acid (approximately 7.4), and a considerable proportion of the aspirin molecules dissociate, thereby becoming more water soluble and unable to diffuse out of the cells. This process is known as 'trapping'. Coating tablets so that they pass through the stomach without disintegrating can reduce the risk of gastric bleeding because the local concentration of drug in the stomach mucosa is reduced.

In patients with asthma, NSAIDs can precipitate asthmatic attacks, possibly by diverting the arachidonic acid pathway to produce bronchoconstrictor mediators such as leukotrienes (see Fig. 8.3).

Inhibition of prostaglandin synthesis in the kidney can lead to disturbed kidney function, and salt and water are retained. This can be particularly troublesome in patients with heart failure, as it can worsen the condition. Aspirin, but not other members of the group, also inhibits the renal excretion of uric acid. Aspirin is, therefore, contraindicated in gout.

Care must be taken with anticoagulants such as warfarin, as NSAIDs and possibly paracetamol will enhance their action.

Corticosteroids

Indications

The prime use of corticosteroids in the management of foot problems is to suppress inflammation. They may be administered orally for systemic problems; for example, the symptoms of rheumatoid arthritis are suppressed by glucocorticoids. They may be injected subcutaneously to suppress symptoms from a localized condition such as enthesopathy or plantar digital neuritis. Intracapsular injections may be used for acute arthritis. Topical anti-inflammatory drugs may be used to reduce inflammation of the skin associated with dermatological conditions such as psoriasis. It should be noted that if used topically when infection is present, they can mask the features of infection.

The corticosteroids (natural and artificial) are highly lipid soluble, which means that they are rapidly absorbed by all routes, even after topical administration. The most important synthetic corticosteroids can be classified as follows:

- *mainly glucocorticoid* but with appreciable mineralocorticoid activity, e.g. prednisolone
- *highly selective glucocorticoid activity,* e.g. betamethasone, beclometasone, dexamethasone, fluocinolone
- *highly selective mineralocorticoid activity,* e.g. fludrocortisone.

Mechanism of action

The adrenal cortex synthesizes and releases several closely related hormones, the corticosteroids. Most have very short half-lives once released from the adrenal cortex, whereas synthetic derivatives of the natural hormones have durations of action long enough to make them therapeutically useful.

The effects of the natural corticosteroids have been classified largely into two groups – glucocorticoid and mineralocorticoid actions. The major physiological mineralocorticoid is *aldosterone,* which has hardly any glucocorticoid activity. The major physiological corticosteroids are *hydrocortisone* (*cortisol*) and *cortisone,* both of which have some mineralocorticoid activity. Most useful synthetic corticosteroids are selective for either mineralocorticoid actions or glucocorticoid actions (Table 8.1).

The anti-inflammatory and immunosuppressant actions of the corticosteroids are mediated through the production of *lipocortins,* small messenger proteins. These lipocortins inhibit phopholipase A_2, the enzyme that begins the prostaglandin/leukotriene synthesis cascade (see Fig. 8.3).

Unwanted effects

Prolonged high doses produce a set of effects that resemble adrenal hyperactivity (Cushing's syndrome). These include salt and water retention, muscle wasting, osteoporosis, deposition of fat on the face ('moon face') and between the shoulder blades ('buffalo hump'), diabetes, susceptibility to infections and psychosis. Other effects include peptic ulceration, cataract and glaucoma. The immunosuppressive effect carries the hazard that the steroids are able to suppress the necessary protective responses to infection and can decrease essential healing processes. Suppression of the adrenal axis occurs with prolonged usage. The amount of steroid required for suppression varies according to the potency and route of administration.

After prolonged treatment, the adrenal cortex atrophies as a result of feedback inhibition of the release of adrenocorticotrophic hormone from the pituitary gland. When the exogenous corticosteroid is stopped, it takes time (months) for the atrophied adrenal cortex to start producing endogenous adrenocortical hormones, even though adrenocorticotrophic hormone levels rise almost immediately. During this time, the patient will show severe adrenocortical insufficiency. Corticosteroids should, therefore, be withdrawn slowly over a period of months to allow the hitherto involuted adrenal cortex to recover.

Injectable anti-inflammatory drugs

Indications

Corticosteroids, often combined with analgesics, may be used for injection into joints or subcutaneous tissues. Two main types of corticosteroid are used (all are more potent than hydrocortisone):

- methylprednisolone acetate
- fluorinated hydrocortisone, such as betamethasone, dexamethasone, triamcinolone.

Methylprednisolone acetate has approximately five times the glucocorticoid action of hydrocor-

Table 8.1 Effects of corticosteroids

Mineralocorticoid	Glucocorticoid
Na⁺ retention by kidney	Mobilization of peripheral amino acids
K⁺ loss by kidney	Decreased glucose uptake
	Increased gluconeogenesis
	Mobilization of fatty acids from fat stores
	Suppression of inflammation
	Suppression of the immune system

tisone and is 1.25–1.5 times stronger than prednisolone. Betamethasone is 8–10 times more potent than prednisolone. Methylprednisolone acetate can be used in all joints of the foot and plantar fascia. Table 8.2 provides a summary of the indications for methylprednisolone acetate and betamethasone (Tollafield & Williams 1996).

Injectable corticosteroids do not offer a panacea – as with all pharmacological preparations, they should be used with care. A thorough assessment to identify the underlying cause of the problem and the use of non-pharmacological strategies is necessary.

Greenfield et al (1984) found that patients with plantar digital neuritis preferred the use of injectable corticosteroids (with 1% lidocaine) to conservative treatment involving orthotic pre-

Table 8.2 Indications for the use of methylprednisolone and betamethasone

Methylprednisolone	Betamethasone
Rheumatoid arthritis	Capsulitis
Keloid	Heel pain
Granuloma annulare	Postoperative swelling
Synovitis	Neuroma
Tenosynovitis	Bursitis
Plantar fascitis	
Bursitis	

From Tollafield & Williams (1996), with permission.

scription and/or modification of footwear. In a retrospective study of 65 patients, a mean of three injections per patient was administered; 50% of the patients experienced temporary relief. Total relief was recorded in 14% of patients after one injection.

Corticosteroids should neither be injected into an infected joint nor used in immunocompromised patients.

Mechanism of action

The anti-inflammatory effect of injecting corticosteroids into joints is thought to involve:

- inhibition of chemotactic migration of white blood cells
- reduction in the permeability of the synovial membrane
- stabilization of leucocytic lysosomal membranes, which, in turn, prevents the release of cytotoxic enzymes
- inhibition of the formation of inflammatory prostaglandins through an inhibition of phospholipase A_2.

Unwanted reactions

Methylprednisolone acetate has been implicated as having a deleterious effect on cartilage. Hydroxyapatite crystal deposition following steroid injection has been found in experimental animals and this is thought to increase the effects of osteoarthritis (Ohira et al 1986). Loss of matrix glycosaminoglycans can lead to replacement with collagen, causing a reduction in the flexibility and resilience of cartilage. However, the overall effect on cartilage may not be completely detrimental, as decreased swelling protects synovial vessels and stabilizes chondroblasts and intimal cells of the synovium (Shoemaker et al 1992).

Corticosteroids can enter the circulation after injection into joints. Absorption from the joint cavity is affected by the lipid solubility of the drug, the dose and the surface area. Clinical problems with the use of injectable corticosteroids are rare. Greenfield et al (1984) and

Tollafield & Williams (1996) have reported 'steroid flares'.

Topical corticosteroids

Indications

Corticosteroids are the most potent and effective topical anti-inflammatory drugs. As they also have the ability to inhibit cell division, they are useful in the treatment of conditions such as psoriasis, which is characterized by a rapid epidermal cell transit time.

The effectiveness of topical corticosteroids is related to their potency and rate of absorption through the skin; the potency of topical steroids varies. Corticosteroids can be presented in a variety of vehicles: creams, ointments, sprays or gels. In general, ointments are better tolerated than creams or gels for dry skin as they form an occlusive layer and rehydrate the area..

Betamethasone sodium phosphate may be injected in small amounts into the lesion; this may be helpful in mucoid cysts, keloids or psoriatic plaques. Corticosteroids may also be incorporated with other topical preparations such as antifungal drugs (e.g. miconazole) or keratoplastics (commonly urea and lactic acid). It should be noted that the combined use of corticosteroids and antibacterial or antifungal preparations may mask the features of spreading infection.

Mechanism of action

There are marked regional variations in the percutaneous absorption of topical steroids; absorption through scrotal skin is much quicker than through the skin of the sole of the foot. Hydration of the skin markedly improves percutaneous absorption (increases four- to fivefold). If applied under an occlusive dressing, absorption may increase 100-fold. Topical steroids are far more easily absorbed through broken skin than through intact skin.

It is difficult to ascertain the optimal dose of topical steroids. Patients vary in the amount they apply and the frequency of application. On account of their side-effects, all topical steroids should be used sparingly. More potent topical steroids are contraindicated in infants under 1 year, and prolonged use of even low-potency steroids such as hydrocortisone should be avoided on the face.

Unwanted effects

Topical corticosteroids may lead to atrophy of the skin, telangiectasia, folliculitis and striae. If used over a prolonged period of time, systemic side-effects may occur as a result of topical absorption.

ANTIMICROBIAL DRUGS

There is no simple term that covers all the pathogenic organisms with which the body can be infected. The term 'microbe' probably comes closest to this and it is used here to refer to any foreign organism responsible for infection. Such organisms include bacteria, fungi, viruses, protozoa and metazoa. Drugs that are useful for dealing with invading organisms are different from most other drugs because they offer the prospect of a true cure for a disease, rather than modification of a disease process or a symptomatic treatment. These drugs achieve this by being toxic to the invading organism but not to the host.

Antibacterial drugs

Indications

At one time, the term 'antibiotic' was applied only to those antibacterial drugs extracted from biological sources, such as fungi or other bacteria. As many of these antibiotics can now be synthesized chemically, or are subjected to heavy chemical modification, this distinction is no longer sensible or workable. It is, therefore, unreasonable to deny the term to drugs such as the sulphonamides, which are totally synthetic. However, the term 'antibacterial' is used in this section to avoid this still somewhat contentious issue.

Bacterial infections occurring in the foot are usually caused by *Staphylococcus aureus*, although culture often reveals the presence of Gram-negative bacilli such as *Pseudomonas aeruginosa*. These Gram-negative bacilli are found as commensals of the gut. Their presence in the foot is usually a result of poor personal hygiene or contamination of antiseptics, in particular cetrimide, and medical equipment such as air hoses. Streptoccal infections are not common but, when present in the foot, can have major deleterious effects because of their rapid spread across and through tissues.

Most antibiotics are prescribed once infection has become established in the foot. Prophylactic antibiotics are increasingly being used preoperatively to prevent infection from becoming established. The use of preoperative antibiotics is indicated for patients who:

- are receiving implant surgery
- already have a surgical implant or prosthesis
- have a history of rheumatic fever or heart valve defect
- have previously been shown to be at risk of postoperative infection
- are about to undergo major surgery to the foot.

Mechanism of action

Antibacterial drugs are either *bacteriostatic* (i.e. they act by arresting the growth of the organism) or *bactericidal* (i.e. they kill the organism). Bacteriostatic drugs rely upon the body's immune system to destroy the organism once its multiplication has been stopped. Consequently, such drugs are ineffective in patients with impaired immune systems, whether this be because of disease, such as infection with the human immunodeficiency virus (HIV), or whether it be drug induced, for example by immunosuppressants used to prevent transplant rejection, or steroids for asthma or arthritis. Sometimes it is necessary to combine drugs to achieve effective treatment of infection. However, bacteriostatic and bactericidal drugs should not be combined, because each is likely markedly to

reduce the efficacy of the other. This is because bactericidal drugs are usually most effective on bacteria that are actively growing or dividing. Bacteriostatic drugs, therefore, protect bacteria from bactericidal drugs.

Unwanted reactions

One of the major problems with antibacterial drugs is the emergence of resistant bacterial strains. It is important, therefore, that the practitioner uses antibacterial drugs in the manner least likely to encourage the development of resistance. A further problem emerges with the use of antibiotics such as third-generation, orally active, cephalosporins that wipe out gastrointestinal tract normal flora and allow opportunistic overgrowth of, for example, *Clostridium difficile*, causing pseudomembranous colitis. Resistance to antibacterial drugs is acquired in several ways. In a population of bacteria of any one species, some will be naturally more resistant than others. These will be the last organisms to die when exposed to an antibacterial drug. Inadequate treatment will, therefore, leave the patient with an infection composed of the most drug-resistant strains of the organism.

In any population of bacteria, naturally more resistant strains are constantly evolving by spontaneous mutation. Only when non-resistant strains are killed by drugs are these resistant strains selected. The problem of resistance is further complicated by the ability of many bacteria to transmit genetic material to other bacteria, even to bacteria of different families. The genetic material comprises *plasmids*, strands of DNA-containing genes that encode enzymes that convey resistance. Another way in which genetic material can be transmitted is through viruses that infect bacteria (*bacteriophages*). A good example of transmission of resistance can be found in the enzyme beta-lactamase, which inactivates penicillins and cephalosporins. This has appeared in many strains of bacteria that did not originally possess the gene for the enzyme. The risk of encouraging resistance can be minimized if some basic rules are followed (Box 8.2).

Classes of antibacterial drugs

Beta-lactam drugs Beta-lactam drugs have a beta-lactam ring as the central feature of their structure (Fig. 8.5). The group includes the natural and semisynthetic penicillins, the cephalosporins, cephamycins, carbapenems and the monobactams. They are among the most highly selective and least toxic of all drugs, which means that very high plasma concentrations can be achieved, giving high kill-rates with a low incidence of adverse effects. These drugs interfere with the synthesis of the peptidoglycan layer of the bacterial cell wall. As a result, the cell swells as water enters by osmosis and eventually bursts. Beta-lactams are, therefore, bactericidal. They owe their high selectivity first to the fact that mammalian cells do not have susceptible cell walls and, second, to their being structural analogues of D-alanyl-D-alanine, a precursor of the peptidoglycan; mammalian cells do not have the capacity to use D-isomers of amino acids.

The spectrum of activity is similar for all the beta-lactams: all Gram-positive bacteria and Gram-negative cocci. Some of the newer drugs have a wider spectrum of activity than this. The chief reason for bacterial resistance to beta-lactams, among normally sensitive species, is the

Box 8.2 Factors to be addressed in order to prevent the development of resistant bacterial strains

- Do not use an antibacterial drug unless it is really necessary. Chronic infections may not need chemotherapy, whereas most acute infections do.
- Make the most precise diagnosis that the signs and symptoms allow. This will narrow the choice of drug by identifying the most likely organism. Samples for laboratory testing should be taken before treatment is started, but treatment should not be delayed until a bacteriology laboratory report is received, as this may take a day or more.
- Avoid the indiscriminate use of broad-spectrum drugs. Before the infecting organism has been identified by culture, there is a great temptation to use the broadest spectrum drug available to cover all eventualities. Only if precise identification of the organism is impossible should broad-spectrum drugs be used, and then it is best to avoid using the drugs with the broadest spectrum; these should be reserved for the most problematic infections.
- Give the drug for long enough to enable all organisms to be eliminated. This usually means at least 5 days, although disappearance of symptoms does not mean that all organisms have been eliminated.
- Use combination therapy when resistant strains are known to be responsible for the infection. The probability of an organism being resistant to two drugs is four times less than the probability of its being resistant to either one of the two drugs alone.
- Ensure that you have up-to-date knowledge of local resistance patterns. By being aware of local resistance patterns, the practitioner is less likely to use a drug that will encourage resistance to develop.
- Abide by agreements about reserving drugs for particular conditions. Most microbiologists and practitioners agree that new antibacterial drugs should not be used widely as long as older drugs still work. Some drugs are 'reserved' for treating infections with organisms that cause serious, life-threatening infections. If these drugs are used to treat trivial infections, resistance may develop and this resistance could be acquired by an organism responsible for a serious infection, thereby rendering the drug ineffective.

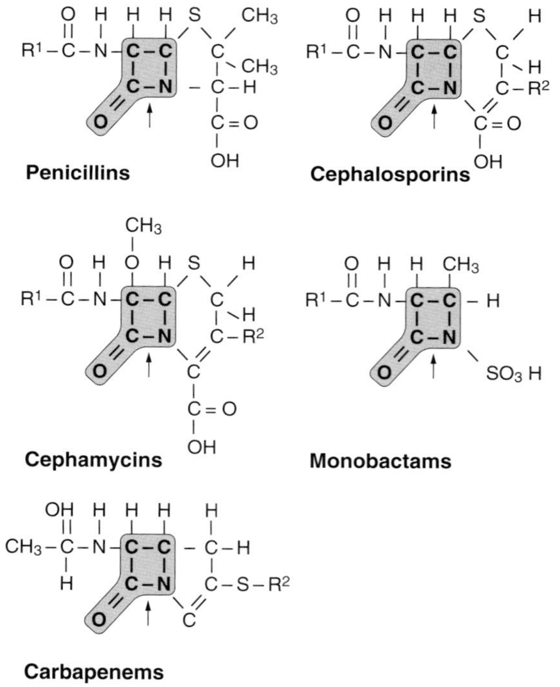

Figure 8.5 Beta-lactam antibacterial drugs. The lactam ring is shown bold. The arrow indicates the site of the action of inactivating beta-lactamases.

possession by the organism of an enzyme (beta-lactamase, penicillinase) capable of hydrolysing the lactam ring, thereby inactivating the drug. Most staphylococci are now resistant to beta-lactamase-sensitive antibacterial agents.

Although rare, some patients become hypersensitive to penicillin and an anaphylactic reaction develops on subsequent exposure. About 10% of such patients will also be allergic to cephalosporins.

Penicillins Penicillins are highly water-soluble and so penetrate the blood–brain barrier poorly. Some penicillins have enough lipid solubility to be absorbed after oral administration, but the original penicillin (benzylpenicillin) must be injected, partly because it is water soluble and partly because it is broken down by the acid in the stomach. The penicillins are weak acids and are actively secreted by the kidney tubule; consequently, the clearance of penicillin is very high (most of the penicillin entering the kidney is excreted in the urine). Probenecid interferes with the pump responsible for secreting penicillins from the kidney tubules and consequently extends the duration of action of the penicillin.

Benzylpenicillin (penicillin G) This early penicillin is susceptible to beta-lactamases but remains a drug of choice for streptococcal, pneumococcal, gonococcal and meningococcal infections. It is also recommended for anthrax, diphtheria, gas gangrene, leptospirosis, syphilis, tetanus, yaws and for Lyme disease in children.

Procaine penicillin This is an almost insoluble salt of benzylpenicillin and is suitable for intramuscular injection as a 'depot'. Penicillin is released slowly from the depot over a long period so that bactericidal tissue concentrations are maintained for at least 24 hours after a single injection.

Phenoxymethylpenicillin (penicillin V) This is less potent than benzylpenicillin but has essentially the same spectrum. Unlike benzylpenicillin, it is resistant to gastric acid and is, therefore, suitable for oral administration, although absorption is erratic because the drug is so water-soluble.

Cloxacillin and flucloxacillin These drugs are resistant to beta-lactamase and so are active against staphylococci that are resistant to the older penicillins. Flucloxacillin is more lipid-soluble than cloxacillin and so is better absorbed after oral administration.

Ampicillin This has a broader spectrum of action than the penicillins listed above, as it is active against some Gram-positive species as well as Gram-negative organisms, although it is sensitive to beta-lactamase. Most staphylococci, 50% of *Escherichia coli* strains and 15% of *Haemophilus influenzae* strains are now resistant to ampicillin. Absorption of ampicillin from the gut is poor and is further hampered by food. A combination of ampicillin and flucloxacillin is available as co-fulampicil.

Amoxycillin This has almost the same spectrum of activity as ampicillin but it is much better absorbed, so adequate bactericidal concentrations can be easily achieved with oral dosing. Other orally active wide-spectrum penicillins include *bacampicillin* and *pivampicillin*.

Clavulanic acid A fungal product that is structurally related to penicillin. Its value is that it inhibits bacterial beta-lactamase. Consequently, a mixture of clavulanic acid and an otherwise beta-lactamase-susceptible penicillin will be active against beta-lactamase-producing organisms. Clavulanic acid is available in a fixed-dose combination with amoxicillin, called co-amoxyclav.

Carbenicillin and ticarcillin (carboxypenicillins) These broad-spectrum penicillins are active against *Pseudomonas aeruginosa*. Ticarcillin is also active against *Proteus* species and *Bacteroides fragilis*. Azlocillin and piperacillin have a spectrum of activity similar to ticarcillin. Tazobactam, like clavulanic acid, is a beta-lactamase inhibitor and is available in combination with piperacillin.

Cephalosporins, cephamycins and other beta-lactams Cephalosporins have very similar properties to the broad-spectrum penicillins and share their dispositional characteristics. Cefradine and cefazolin are 'first-generation' cephalosporins, which have been superseded by second- and third-generation agents. Second-generation cephalosporins, such as cefuroxime and cefamandole, have more resistance to beta-lactamase than the older drugs. This gives them activity against *H. influenzae* and *Neisseria gonorrhoeae*. Cefalexin, cefradine and cefadroxil are orally active first-generation drugs. Cefaclor is an orally active second-generation cephalosporin.

Third generation cephalosporins tend to be more active than second-generation drugs against Gram-negative organisms, but less active against Gram-positive organisms. The third-generation cephalosporins are cefotaxime, ceftazidime, ceftoxime and cefodizime. Ceftriaxone has a very long half-life and is suitable for once-daily administration. *Pseudomonas* spp. are susceptible to cefsulodin and ceftazidime, for which they should be reserved. Cefixime is the longest-acting orally active cephalosporin, and has a Product Authorization or Product Licence (PL) for use in acute infections.

Cefoxitin is a cephamycin that has been found to be particularly useful in treating peritonitis because it is active against organisms found in the bowel. Aztreonam (a 'monobactam') is active only against Gram-negative aerobes and should, therefore, only be used when the infecting organism has been positively identified. Imipenem is a carbapenem that has a broad spectrum of activity, including aerobic and anaerobic Gram-positive and Gram-negative organisms. It is available in combination with cilastatin, an enzyme inhibitor that prevents the enzymic breakdown of imipenem in the kidney. Meropenem is similar to imipenam but is stable to the renal enzyme that inactivates it and, therefore, can be given without cilastatin. Meropenem has less seizure-inducing potential and is used to treat central nervous system infections.

Macrolides The macrolides, like the beta-lactams, inhibit bacterial cell wall synthesis, but they have a slightly different site of action. Consequently, their spectrum of activity is similar to the beta-lactams and they are often suitable alternatives for use in patients with penicillin (or cephalosporin) allergy. Erythromycin is indicated for respiratory infections in children, whooping cough, legionnaires' disease and enteritis caused by *Campylobacter* spp. Some of the macrolides are usually active against *Chlamydia* and *Mycoplasma* spp. Azithromycin and clarithromycin are concentrated in tissues and so achieve higher antibacterial concentrations with long tissue half-lives. Telithromycin

is a derivative of erythromycin often used for erythromycin resistant *Streptococcus pneumoniae* in community-acquired pneumonia.

Tetracyclines The tetracyclines are broad-spectrum antibacterial drugs that block protein synthesis by binding to aminoacyl-tRNA, preventing the ribosome from translocating along the mRNA template. The selectivity of tetracyclines for microorganisms results from their selective accumulation by the organisms through an ATP-driven active transport system. The tetracyclines bind avidly to metal ions such as calcium, aluminium, magnesium and iron (*chelation*) and consequently are poorly absorbed from the gastrointestinal tract if they are taken with, shortly before or after milk, antacids, iron-containing 'tonics' and haematinics, and calcium supplements. Tetracyclines also chelate with calcium in developing teeth and growing bones, causing unsightly staining of the teeth; consequently, they should not be given to children with developing teeth (under 12 years) or to pregnant women.

Although resistance to tetracyclines has been developing (largely by selection of strains that lack the accumulation system), tetracyclines are of vital importance in the treatment of infections with *Chlamydia*, *Rickettsia*, *Mycoplasma*, *Brucella* spp. and for Lyme disease. The spectrum of activity of all tetracyclines is similar, except that minocycline has activity against *Neisseria meningitidis*. The principal tetracyclines are tetracycline itself, doxycycline, demeclocycline, lymecycline and oxytetracycline.

Aminoglycosides The aminoglycoside antibacterials, for example vancomycin and gentamicin, inhibit protein synthesis in bacteria by binding irreversibly to part of the ribosome (the 30S subunit). This prevents aminoacyl-tRNA from binding to the acceptor site, and elaboration of the peptide chain ceases. Aminoglycosides selectively inhibit bacterial protein synthesis. Nevertheless, aminoglycoside antibiotics have only a narrow therapeutic window. They all cause permanent damage to the hair cells of the inner ear, causing deafness (ototoxicity) if the plasma concentration rises only a little above the effective bactericidal concentration.

Aminoglycosides are active against some Gram-positive and many Gram-negative organisms. Some (amikacin, gentamicin, tobramycin) are also active against *P. aeruginosa*. Streptomycin is active against *Mycobacterium tuberculosis* and should be reserved for treating tuberculosis.

All the aminoglycosides are highly water soluble and are, therefore, not absorbed after oral dosing. Their high water solubility also means that they are eliminated by filtration at the kidney, with a clearance that approximates to the glomerular filtration rate (approximately 100–120 ml/min). Injections are, therefore, usually given every 4–6 hours to maintain the narrow therapeutic range of plasma concentration needed to kill bacteria without causing ototoxicity. In patients with impaired kidney function, dosage adjustment is essential. An indication of impaired kidney function is provided by measurement of the plasma creatinine concentration. A raised concentration suggests that kidney function is impaired and that a careful evaluation of the dosage regimen is needed. This may include a full creatinine clearance assessment. Neomycin is too toxic for systemic use and can, therefore, only be used to treat skin and mucous membrane infections.

Sulphonamides and dapsone The sulphonamides were the first safe and effective antibacterial drugs to be developed. They came about because of Paul Ehrlich's observation that many bacteria could be selectively stained by certain synthetic dyes. He argued that it ought to be possible to attach a toxic group to the molecule and thus deliver a lethal message selectively to bacteria that took up the dye. Eventually a red dye (prontosil) was found that inhibited the growth of bacteria in culture and cured mice of otherwise lethal infection. It was first given to humans in the late 1920s and early 1930s. It was soon realized, however, that the effect of prontosil was from a metabolite, which was a sulphonamide. In the 1930s, the mechanism of action was elucidated and a number of potent and effective sulphonamides were in production by the 1940s.

Sulphonamides are structural analogues of *para*-aminobenzoate, which is used by bacteria to synthesize dihydrofolate (folic acid), an intermediate in the synthesis of the purine and pyrimidine bases needed during the manufacture of nucleic acids (Fig. 8.6). Mammals do not need to synthesize folic acid because it can pass through mammalian cell membranes; however, bacterial cell membranes/cell walls are impervious to folic acid, and thus need to manufacture it internally. Bacterial cell membranes/cell walls are impermeant to folic acid. Mammals do not need to synthesize it because it can pass through mammalian cell membranes. Sulphonamides are so similar in structure to *para*-aminobenzoate that they can react with the enzyme dihydropteroate synthetase in its place, but the complex does not dissociate readily and so the enzyme essential in the production of folic acid is inhibited. Sulphonamides are, therefore, bacteriostatic as they prevent cell division by limiting the availability of nucleic acids. However, most bacterial cells have reserves of dihydrofolate and tetrahydrofolate, so there is usually a time lag between inhibition of dihydropteroate synthetase and the stopping of bacterial cell division.

Sulphonamides are limited in value because many sulphonamide-resistant strains have appeared. The main value of sulphonamides (e.g. sulfadimidine) is in the treatment of urinary tract infections and meningococcal meningitis. *Dapsone* is a close chemical relative of the sulphonamides and is invaluable in the treatment of leprosy.

Trimethoprim Trimethoprim is not a sulphonamide but, like the sulphonamides, it inhibits nucleic acid synthesis. It does this by interfering with the enzyme dihydrofolate reductase. This enzyme takes as its substrate the dihydrofolate made by dihydropteroate synthetase and turns it into tetrahydrofolate. Although trimethoprim is used on its own, it is also available in combination with the sulphonamide sulfamethoxazole (the mixture is called co-trimoxazole). By interfering with nucleic acid synthesis by stopping two adjacent steps in the synthesis pathway, co-trimoxazole is less likely to produce resistant strains than either constituent drug given alone.

The 4-quinolones The 4-quinolones, for example ciproflaxin and nalidixic acid, inhibit the enzyme DNA gyrase (also known as topoisomerase II). This enzyme is normally responsible for winding the DNA helix into a so-called 'supercoiled' form. The drugs are selective for bacteria because the enzyme in bacteria is structurally different from that in mammals.

Ciproflaxin is effective against Gram-negative bacteria such as *Salmonella*, *Shigella*, *Campylobacter*, *Neisseria* and *Pseudomonas* spp. It has some activity against Gram-positive bacteria such as *S. pneumoniae* and *Streptococcus faecalis*. Ciproflaxin is also active against *Chlamydia* spp. and some mycobacteria, but it is inactive against most anaerobes. The main use for ciproflaxin is the treatment of respiratory and urinary tract infections, although it is not effective against pneumococcal pneumonia. Nalidixic acid is used almost exclusively for uncomplicated urinary tract infections.

The 4-quinolones are secreted into the urine, where they reach high concentrations and can crystallize unless adequate water intake is maintained. A potentially serious adverse effect of this group of antibacterial drugs is that they can precipitate convulsions in susceptible patients, particularly in patients with a history of epilepsy.

Nitroimidazoles The mechanism of action of the nitroimidazoles (metronidazole and tinidazole) is uncertain, but it may be that the drugs, or more likely their metabolites, cause breaks in the DNA of parasites. The selectivity is thought to result from selective appearance of these metabolites within parasites. Metronidazole was developed as an amoebicide, but in addition to activity against *Entamoeba histolytica* and *Giardia lamblia*, it is very effective against many anaerobes. It is, therefore, useful for surgical and gynaecological sepsis, especially infections with colonic anaerobes such as *Bacteroides fragilis* and *Clostridium difficile*. Both metronidazole and tinidazole are well absorbed after oral administration, but tinidazole has a longer duration of

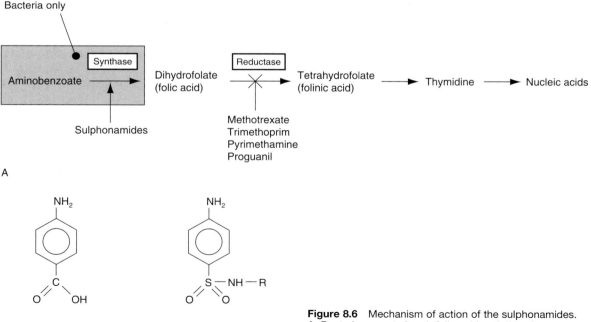

Figure 8.6 Mechanism of action of the sulphonamides. A, Bacteria cannot absorb folic acid and, therefore, must synthesize it from *p*-aminobenzoate and pteridine. B, Sulphonamides are close structural analogues of *p*-aminobenzoate.

action. Although most of a dose of metronidazole is excreted unchanged in the urine, some metabolism may occur; as the metabolites are strongly coloured, this gives the urine a dark brown colour.

The nitroimidazoles interfere with the enzyme aldehyde dehydrogenase, responsible for the second step in the metabolism of ethanol. This leads to an accumulation of acetaldehyde (ethanal) after the consumption of ethanol, which causes marked vasodilatation, headache, nausea, vomiting and a general feeling of malaise. Patients taking these drugs should not drink alcohol during treatment and for several days after stopping the drug.

Miscellaneous antibacterial agents Fusidic acid salts are extremely narrow-spectrum antibacterial drugs. They inhibit protein synthesis by preventing translocation of the ribosome along the mRNA chain of codons. Sodium fusidate is well absorbed after oral administration and is particularly useful because it penetrates and accumulates in bone. However, its narrow spectrum of action requires that it be used with another antistaphylococcal antibiotic, usually flucloxacillin or erythromycin, to limit the emergence of resistant strains.

Chloramphenicol is an extremely potent and valuable broad-spectrum antibacterial agent, the usefulness of which is limited by its propensity to cause fatal aplastic anaemia. The incidence of this adverse effect is about 1 in 50 000–100 000. Consequently, chloramphenicol is reserved for dealing with life-threatening infections, such as typhoid fever and *H. influenzae* septicaemia. Chloramphenicol inhibits protein synthesis by preventing the growth of the chain of amino acids as the ribosome moves along the mRNA molecule.

The *polymyxins* (colistin and polymyxin-B) are cationic detergents composed of peptide chains with hydrophilic and lipophilic amino acids. They have some selectivity for bacterial cell membranes, which are more susceptible to damage than mammalian cell membranes. They are bactericidal by disrupting the phospholipids of the membrane. These antibiotics are not absorbed after oral administration and so col-

istin can be used to 'sterilize' the gut (usually in conjunction with an antifungal agent such as nystatin). Both colistin and polymyxin-B are generally considered to be too toxic for systemic use, although colistin is available in a form suitable for injection. They are both active against Gram-negative organisms, including *P. aeruginosa*.

Antituberculous drugs Combination regimens have proved successful against *M. tuberculosis* with isoniazid, rifampicin, rifabutin, ethambutol and pyrazinamide as first-line drugs. Some second-line drugs include capreomycin, cycloserine and, rarely in the UK, streptomycin. A feature of many of these chemicals is enzyme induction, making them commonly implicated in drug–drug interactions. The mechanism of actions for the bacteriostatic isoniazid is unclear, although it may inhibit the synthesis of mycolic acids, important constituents of the cell wall and peculiar to mycobacteria. Rifampicin acts by binding to an inhibiting DNA-dependent RNA polymerase in prokaryotic but not eukaryotic cells. Ethambutol's mechanism of action is not yet known. Cycloserine prevents completion of the major building blocks of peptidoglycan.

Topical antibacterial drugs Topical antibacterials are traditionally termed antiseptics. Antiseptics are defined as substances applied to living tissues to destroy or inhibit the reproduction or metabolic activity of microorganisms. The term 'disinfectant' is reserved for the use of such substances on non-living material. In general, antiseptics are sensitive to their local environment, and hence their action may be impeded by the presence of tissue debris, blood or pus. Antiseptics are not usually effective against spores.

Some of the antibiotics discussed in the previous section can be used topically (e.g. neomycin). However, their popularity has reduced over the years, because of problems associated with resistance. It is difficult to control how much is used and where it is used, especially if the patient is self-applying the antibiotic. Unlike oral preparations, which are dispensed in carefully metered doses, topical antibiotics come in powder or cream form, the amount of which used can vary with each application.

Antifungal drugs

Indications

Antifungal drugs are usually administered either orally or topically. There have, in the past, been a number of unwanted effects associated with the oral antifungal drugs, which have restricted their use to severe infections. This situation is now being reversed with the arrival on the market of oral antifungal drugs with fewer unwanted effects. However, it is still primarily the topical antifungal preparations that are used.

There are a wide variety of over-the-counter preparations that come in a range of formulations: creams, ointments, sprays, paints and lotions. These preparations may be combined with 1% hydrocortisone, as fungal infection of the skin is often accompanied by an inflammatory response and pruritus. Penetration of topical agents to the site of infection in the treatment of onychomycosis may be problematic, which is why systemic therapy is considered to have a more beneficial effect.

When using topical antifungal preparations, it is important that their use is continued for up to 3 months after the signs and symptoms have resolved. This is because of spore formation; most topical antifungal drugs are not particularly effective against spores. With infected nails, treatment must continue until a new nail has grown (6 months for fingernails, 12 months for toenails). The treatment of fungal infection of the nails can be speeded up by the surgical or chemical (urea cream) removal of the nail prior to the application of the antifungal preparation. If this is not feasible, reduction of the nail with a nail drill will facilitate penetration of the antifungal agent into the nail.

Mechanism of action

As with antibacterial drugs, antifungal drugs may either be fungistatic (prevent growth) or fungicidal (kill). The classes of antifungal drug, their specific mechanism of action, adverse effects and mode of administration are considered below.

Polyenes Nystatin and amphotericin bind to ergosterol in the membrane of fungal cells and form channels through which the important intracellular components can diffuse, causing the cells effectively to starve to death. The polyenes are selective for fungal and yeast cells because mammalian cell membranes do not contain ergosterol. Nystatin is too toxic for systemic use but is so water soluble that it is not absorbed from the gut after oral administration and so can be effectively used to rid the gastrointestinal tract of candidal infection (thrush). It is commonly used in topical preparations.

Amphotericin is less toxic than nystatin but is also highly water soluble; hence for systemic treatment, it must be injected. However, it is still quite toxic, causing primarily renal damage, which may be permanent, and loss of potassium, which may be severe enough for the patient to require potassium supplements.

Imidazoles The imidazoles kill a wide range of fungi and yeasts. They act by preventing the synthesis of ergosterol, the main sterol in the fungal cell membrane. Miconazole is highly effective as a topical agent for some forms of ringworm. Other imidazole antifungal drugs available in creams for topical use include econazole, sulconazole, tioconazole and clotrimazole. Miconazole can be used orally to eliminate gastrointestinal fungal or yeast infection as it is highly water soluble and, therefore, poorly absorbed. It can also be injected for systemic infection (e.g. aspergillosis, candidiasis and cryptococcosis). Ketoconazole is absorbed moderately well after oral administration but has been reported to cause liver damage, which can be fatal. Fluconazole and itraconazole are safer alternatives, although the use of itraconazole in patients with significant liver disease is undesirable. Fluconazole, although water soluble, reaches antifungal drug concentrations in cerebrospinal fluid, whereas itraconazole does not penetrate the blood–brain barrier as effectively. Several 'new generation' azoles are undergoing phase III trials and voriconazol is now licensed for invasive aspergillosis or fluconazole-resistant candidiasis.

Allylamines The allylamines act by inhibiting squalene epoxidase, an enzyme that is required for fungal cell biosynthesis. The resulting build-up of squalene in the fungal cells kills the organism. Terbinafine and amorolfine are new antifungal drug agents available for systemic and topical application for use against tinea and candidiasis of the skin. Amorolfine is also available as a lacquer for use against onychomycosis.

Undecanoates Undecanoates (e.g. zinc undecanoate) were at one time the mainstay of topical treatments for fungal infection of the foot. They have been largely replaced by the imidazoles (e.g. clotrimazole, econazole, tioconazole, sulconazole and miconazole) for topical application. These substances also tend to be effective against yeasts. Tolnaftate is only available for topical application for dermatophytes such as tinea pedis but it is not effective against *Candida* spp.

Miscellaneous antifungal agents Griseofulvin is a narrow-spectrum antifungal agent isolated from the mould *Penicillium griseofulvum* in 1939. It acts by interfering with microtubule function and is fungistatic rather than fungicidal. Consequently, it must be given for long periods of time, otherwise regrowth and reinfection from the remaining inhibited, but not killed, fungal hyphae will occur. It is not particularly well absorbed after oral administration, but it is particularly useful against tinea infection of the skin and nails because it is selectively accumulated in these tissues as it binds to newly formed keratin. Treatment should continue until the infected keratin has been shed: perhaps a year or more for tinea infection of the toenails.

Flucytosine is active orally. It is converted in tissues into 5-fluorouracil, which blocks DNA synthesis by inhibiting thymidylate synthetase. Fungal cells convert flucytosine to 5-fluorouracil much more rapidly than do mammalian cells. The drug is well tolerated, with mild toxic effects such as gastrointestinal disturbances, although alopecia and neutropenia have been reported.

Antiviral agents

Considerable recent research has increased the breadth of antiviral drugs available. For herpes simplex and varicella–zoster, aciclovir, framciclovir (a prodrug of penciclovir), valaciclovir (an ester of aciclovir) and idoxuridine are effective. Zidovudine, a retroviral nucleoside reverse transcriptase inhibitor, delays the onset of full-blown acquired immunodeficiency syndrome AIDS in patients infected with HIV, but it does not cure the disease. Abacavir, didanosine, lamivudine, stavudine, tenofovir and zalcitabine are similar 'nucleoside analogues' that have become recently available. In the battle against HIV–AIDS, these have been augmented by amprenavir, indinavir, lopinavir, nelfinavir, titonavir and saquinavir. These are retroviral protease inhibitors; they are metabolized by cytochrome P450 and, therefore, have significant potential for drug–drug interaction. Efavirenz and nevirapine are two non-nucleoside reverse transcriptase inhibitors used in combination therapies against HIV–AIDS. Amantadine has some prophylactic value against influenza virus. There are currently no antiviral drugs for the treatment of verrucae pedis.

ANTIPURITICS

Indication

Pruritus may have systemic or local causes. It is a symptom of an underlying condition, such as a fungal infection. In many instances, treatment of the underlying cause, where known, will reduce the symptom. This is fortunate as there is no really effective antipruritic drug. A variety of preparations have some antipruritic effect.

Calamine, in lotion, cream or oily form, has been traditionally associated with the relief of pruritus, although its mechanism of action is unclear. Antihistamines, oral and topical, are considered to be useful where the underlying cause is an allergic reaction. Counter-irritants may also be used for pruritus; vasodilation is thought to 'block' the pruritic effect. As dry skin is associated with pruritus, emollients may also reduce the effects.

CAUSTICS

A caustic is defined as any substance that is destructive to living tissue. The following caustics are primarily used to treat corns and verrucae.

Salicylic acid This is caustic in concentrations greater than 6%. It acts by solubilizing the intercellular cement in the stratum corneum. Once this impermeable barrier has been damaged, water accumulates in the lower layers of the epidermis leading to maceration. Because of this maceration, salicylic acid is able to permeate into the lower layers of the epidermis, where it has a necrotic effect on cells undergoing keratinization. Salicylic acid is said to have a cumulative action and this, consequently, is why return periods should be relatively short (2–7 days) and why all affected skin should be debrided at subsequent visits. Salicylic acid is a common component of many proprietary preparations for corns and callus. Unfortunately, if the manufacturer's instructions are not followed carefully, unwanted side-effects, such as ulceration and infection, may occur.

Silver nitrate This is usually used in the form of a toughened stick produced by fusing silver salt with sodium chloride. Unlike salicylic acid, it has a superficial effect, forming a black eschar on the skin surface from the chemical reaction between silver nitrate and the constituents of sweat. On denuded skin such as hypergranulation tissue, it leads to shrinkage of the tissues. Silver nitrate should not be used on sensitive skin and should be avoided interdigitally unless used in lower strengths.

Mono-, di- and trichloroacetic acids These act by precipitating and coagulating skin proteins. They are effective local cauterizing agents most commonly used in the treatment of verrucae. Monochloroacetic acid is more destructive than trichloroacetic acid and is, therefore, a more useful preparation. Monochloroacetic acid combined with salicylic acid is a popular treatment for verrucae pedis.

COUNTER-IRRITANTS

Counter-irritants result in vasodilation, which aids the removal of metabolites and promotes resolution of lesions. Topical vasodilators are mainly the nicotinates (methyl, ethyl, phenethyl and thuryl) and essential oils such as turpentine, cajuput and capsicum. The massaging action used in applying these preparations is considered to play an adjunct role in promoting vasodilatation. There are many proprietary products on the market, all of which can be purchased without a prescription.

EMOLLIENTS

Indications

The normal water content of the skin is 10%. In patients with dry skin, the water content is much less. Dry skin may be a condition in itself or a complication of a local or systemic pathology (e.g. ischaemia). Patients with dry skin appear to be more prone to developing a range of dermatological conditions such as hyperkeratosis, seed corns or fissures. It is important that the water content of the skin is maintained in order to prevent these complications from occurring.

Mechanism of action

Water is the most important plasticizer of the epidermis. The application of an emollient increases the amount of water in the epidermis (Schwartz & Murray 1991, Loden 1992). In vitro, the stratum corneum can absorb as much as five times its own weight of water and can increase its volume up to three times when soaked in water.

Emollients achieve their effect by one or both of the following mechanisms:

- addition of water to the skin
- retention of water in the skin.

Addition of water is primarily achieved by the application of a water-based cream. Patients prefer this type of emollient as it is readily absorbed and does not leave a greasy film on the skin. Retention of water is achieved by the application of an oil-based preparation (e.g. ointment, water in oil preparation or silicone). These preparations leave an oily base and produce an occlusive barrier, preventing water from evaporating from the skin. Depending on the base, they may not be so user friendly. Some preparations achieve both of the above, adding water to the skin and keeping it there with a hydrophobic substance.

Urea-containing creams, especially those containing alpha-hydroxy acids such as lactic acid, produce prolonged hydration and help to remove scales and crusts. The active ingredients are hydrophilic and act by enhancing the ability of the stratum corneum to hold water and, thus, counteract the tendency of the skin to dry out. These preparations are referred to as *keratoplastics* because of their effect on the epidermis.

Salicylic acid at concentrations between 3 and 6% is keratoplastic as it causes softening of the horny layers and shedding of scales. It facilitates desquamation by solubilizing the intercellular cement and enhances the shedding of corneocytes by decreasing cell-to-cell adhesion.

Emollients have a very short lifespan as the epidermis is constantly desquamating. Therefore, they need to be applied on a regular basis, once or twice a day, to have any therapeutic effect.

PREMEDICATION PRIOR TO SURGERY

Some patients may be fearful or apprehensive of a surgical procedure undertaken under local anaesthesia. In such circumstances, it may be necessary to use drugs to assist the patient in coping with surgery.

Benzodiazepines

The benzodiazepines are useful because they allay the apprehension many patients have before surgery. The dose is chosen so as to produce light sedation. The shorter-acting benzodiazepines are more logical choices than the longer-acting drugs. In addition to sedation, benzodiazepines can induce a period of amnesia. If the dose is timed properly (perhaps 30–60 minutes before surgery), the patient may well have no memory of the stressful part of the procedure. For surgery carried out under local anaesthesia, this amnesic action of benzodiazepines can be very useful.

Benzodiazepines act mainly by increasing the effect of gamma-aminobutyric acid (GABA), the most abundant inhibitory neurotransmitter in the brain. Benzodiazepines also have a small, non-specific depressant effect on nerve cells in general by virtue of their lipid-soluble nature. None of the benzodiazepines has any antidepressant or antipsychotic properties. The anxiolytic action of the benzodiazepines is mediated through their action on GABAergic transmission in the limbic system. This is achieved at doses that are not sedative. All the benzodiazepines can cause dependence on prolonged use. The withdrawal syndrome is unlikely to be a problem if a patient has taken a long-acting benzodiazepine for less than 3 weeks, but it can develop within days for short-acting drugs. The withdrawal syndrome is characterized by effects that are the opposite of those of the drug. Consequently, if the drug has been prescribed to treat anxiety, stopping the drug may be associated with a return or worsening of the anxiety as a withdrawal effect. This can prompt a new prescription unless it is recognized as part of the withdrawal syndrome. The common benzodiazepines, their duration of action and common uses are given in Table 8.3.

The shorter-acting benzodiazepines (e.g. midazolam and temazepam) are useful as anaesthetic premedication agents as they allay fears and produce a period of amnesia. Diazepam is sometimes also used to produce sedation and amnesia for unpleasant procedures. The patient will be sedated or drowsy for some time and a second phase of sleep 4–6 hours after the dose is not uncommon. This is thought to be caused by the appearance of its active metabolite, nordiazepam.

Like all depressant drugs, benzodiazepines have an additive effect with other depressants, including alcohol and antihistamines. Consequently, patients must be warned that they should not take other depressant drugs. Those benzodiazepines with very long half-lives also accumulate when taken over a prolonged period of time. For a drug with a half-life of 80 hours (e.g. diazepam plus its active metabolites), the time taken to reach a steady-state blood level will be at least 3 weeks. Similarly, when the drug is stopped, it will take 3 or more weeks to be

Table 8.3   Properties of common benzodiazepines

Drug	Plasma half-life (h)	Half-life of active metabolites (h)	Uses
Chlordiazepoxide	20	30–200	Anxiety
Clobazam	35	40	Anxiety, epilepsy
Clonazepam	25	–	Epilepsy
Diazepam	30	30–200	Anxiety, epilepsy
Flurazepam	Inactive (prodrug)	30–200	Anxiety
Ketazolam	Inactive (prodrug)	30–200	Anxiety
Lorazepam	20	Inactive	Anxiety, insomnia
Medazepam	Inactive (prodrug)	30–200	Anxiety
Midazolam	3	Inactive	Insomnia, premedication
Nitrazepam	30	Inactive	Insomnia[a]
Oxazepam	7	Inactive	Anxiety
Temazepam	13	Inactive	Insomnia, premedication

[a]Although nitrazepam has a long half-life, it was promoted as a hypnotic. Its use in this role has been superseded by drugs with shorter half-lives.

eliminated. Benzodiazepines also interfere with the performance of tasks requiring vigilance and rapid reactions, such as driving or operating machinery. With long-acting benzodiazepines, a person may be unfit to drive the day after taking the drug.

Diazepam is active after oral administration and has a very long half-life (diazepam plus active metabolites is approximately 30–200 hours). This means that the drug can be given a considerable time before surgery. It also means that the patient is likely to suffer from a 'hangover' for some time after dosing. Temazepam has a much shorter duration of action than diazepam (half-life 8 hours) and is so lipid soluble that it is absorbed rapidly and completely from the gastrointestinal tract. Sedation and anxiolysis last for approximately 1–2 hours, after which the patient will be alert but drowsy. Lorazepam has a slightly longer duration of action (half-life 12 hours). Nitrazepam, which is promoted as an aid to sleep, nevertheless has a very long duration of action (half-life 28 hours). Patients are more likely to suffer from the after-effects of the drug the next day, with persistent sedation and drowsiness, than with short-acting drugs. Midazolam is similar in duration to the action of temazepam but is injected intramuscularly or intravenously rather than taken orally.

SUMMARY

Pharmacological preparations have a valuable role to play in the management of foot problems. As highlighted in the introduction, they are used, in many instances, to control and reduce symptoms rather than cure the underlying cause. Any pharmacological preparation should be used with care. It is essential that the practitioner, before deciding to use such a preparation, has undertaken a full assessment and is aware of the patient's current and previous medication, as well as the likelihood of any contraindications or adverse reactions. Specific Worldwide Web sites such as NICE and CSM contain up-to-date information to guide acceptable practice and the British National Formulary is a comprehensive, constantly updated resource for practitioners. When treating foot problems, the practitioner should be aware of concomitant drug therapy and the implication for practice such as drug interactions, synergistic combinations of drugs and recent advances in therapy. This chapter gives a brief overview as to the pharmacology that might be encountered; however, practition- ers are advised to have access to the publications in the Further reading as reference sources for greater detail in specific cases.

REFERENCES

Greenfield J, Rea J, Ilfield F 1984 Morton's interdigital neuroma: indications for treatment by local injections versus surgery. Clinical and Orthopedic Related Research 142–144

Halliwell R 1995 Adjuvant drugs for postoperative pain management. Current Anaesthesia and Critical Care 6: 81–86

Loden M 1992 The increase in skin hydration after application of emollients with different amounts of lipids. Acta DermatoVenereologica 72: 327–330

McClure J, Wildsmith J (eds) 1991 Mechanisms and management of conduction blockade for post operative analgesia. Edward Arnold, London

Milner Q 2000 Postoperative analgesia. Surgery 18: 198–201

Ohira T, Ishikawa K, Kumato S 1986 Hydroxyapatite deposition in articular cartilage by intra-articular injections of methylprednisolone. Journal of Bone and Joint Surgery 68A: 509–510

Schwartz S, Murray R 1991 Assessment of epithelial thickness by ultrasonic imaging. Decubitus 4: 29–30

Shoemaker R S, Bertone A L, Martin G S et al 1992 Effects of intra-articular administration of methylprednisolone acetate on normal articular cartilage and on healing of experimentally induced osteochondral defects in horses. American Journal of Veterinary Research 53: 1446–1453

Tollafield D R, Williams H A 1996 The use of two injectable corticosteroid preparations used in the management of foot problems: a clinic audit report. British Journal of Podiatric Medicine 51: 171–174

FURTHER READING

British National Formulary (BNF) 2003 British Medical Association and the Royal Pharmaceutical Society of Great Britain (Updated and published twice a year (March and September)), vol 46

Foster R W 1996 Basic pharmacology, 4th edn. Butterworths, London

Laurence D R, Bennett P N 1992 Clinical pharmacology, 7th edn. Churchill Livingstone, Edinburgh

Laurence D R, Carpenter J R 1994 A dictionary of pharmacology and clinical drug evaluation. UCL Press, London

Rang H P, Dale M M, Ritter J M, Moore P K 2003 Pharmcology, 5th edn. Churchill Livingstone, Edinburgh

Walker R, Edwards C 2003 Clinical pharmacy and thera- peutics, 3rd edn. Churchill Livingstone, Edinburgh

9

Physical therapy

*Warren A. Turner**

INTRODUCTION

Physical therapy can be used to treat feet therapeutically without the need for pharmacological preparations or invasive methods. The conjoint use of mechanical therapy will assist many foot problems after physical therapy has achieved the desirable effects of reversing, or at least stabilizing, any inflammatory process. Physical therapy will, therefore, generally employ heat and cold in the treatment of musculoskeletal conditions, injury or insult; indeed, heat and cold are the most common first-line treatments associated with this type of therapy. Electrical methods offer more sophisticated systems, producing similar results to thermal methods. The properties of enhancing the vascular system to local anatomy, as well as diminishing pain sensation, confer some of the essential benefits to the patient from a range of different physical modalities.

COLD AND HEAT

Cold and heat have been used in the management of trauma since as far back as 400 BC. The physiological effects of heat and cold help many of the local adverse pathological changes associated with tissue trauma. Pain may be reduced, healing aided and rehabilitation time improved.

*Warren Turner acknowledges the contributions of Steve Avil and Allen Hinde in the first edition of this chapter.

The effects of thermal treatment on tissue response are compared and contrasted in Table 9.1.

Physiology of cold and heat

Cold

The topical application of cold causes excitation of sympathetic adrenergic nerve fibres, which causes constriction of arterioles and venules and results in *vasoconstriction*. The direct effect of cold on the tissues is to reduce the metabolic rate, thus reducing the effect of chemical mediators associated with the inflammatory process. The demand for oxygen and nutrients will also be reduced and the inflammatory process can be minimized. A decrease in vascular permeability arises, with an increase in the viscosity of blood as the vessel walls constrict. Reduction of leakage of transudate from vessels will slow the acute inflammatory response and reduce the amount of swelling.

Heat

Conversely, the application of heat will cause a rise in the superficial skin temperature, resulting in *vasodilatation*. Temperature elevation increases the demand for oxygen and nutrients. This demand is met by increased blood flow from stimulated vasodilatation. *Vascular permeability* arises with the release of chemical mediators,

allowing leakage from the blood vessels. The resultant cellular activity will remove harmful substances, although inevitably this creates some of the problems that physical therapy is attempting to minimize. Therefore, the objective behind heat application is to encourage defence and repair. Heat should not be used where the circulation to the area is poor. Any increased metabolic effect will be deleterious to the local anatomy, causing the surrounding tissues to break down and ulcerate.

Heat will beneficially affect nerve conduction velocity, lowering pain perception; this, in turn, reduces muscle tone. Joint motion may be limited by spasm caused by tonic contraction. While spasm is protective, it nevertheless prevents the joint from functioning normally. In the foot, common joints affected by tonic spasm include the subtalar joint (peroneal muscle) and the first metatarsophalangeal joint (short flexor hallucis spasm). Heat will increase the extensibility of collagen and can be used to reduce scar tissue, particularly around joints. Initially, cold is used to minimize swelling and exudate, to reduce haematoma and to slow down the process producing scar tissue. Once the joint is stable, and adjacent soft tissues have been identified as not being torn and not requiring surgical repair, heat can be used to build up motion, muscle strength and flexibility. Joints kept immobilized for long periods become stiff and may have to be manipulated under anaesthetic. Early gentle movement and heat therapy will be used by the practitioner to ensure that immature scar tissue is stretched and mobilized. Intracapsular adhesions are, therefore, discouraged before they become a problem.

CRYOTHERAPY

Cryotherapy is the therapeutic application of cold. The methods employed range from the simple application of ice to more sophisticated and destructive systems, such as those used in the treatment of skin lesions. Cold is an ideal treatment for limiting the tissue response provoked by inflammation. Used in combination with non-steroidal anti-inflammatory drugs

Table 9.1 Effects of thermal treatment on tissue response

Cold	Heat
Vasoconstriction	Vasodilatation
Decreased pain	Decreased pain
Decreased muscle spasm	Decreased muscle spasm
Decreased vascular permeability	Increased vascular permeability
Decreased metabolism	Increased metabolism
Reduced swelling/oedema	

(NSAIDs), rest, compression and elevation, cryotherapy may be extremely effective for managing acute inflammation if used within 48 hours of initial injury.

The physiological effects of ice have been described above and in Table 9.1. All of these effects slow down the initial vascular response to trauma, assisting early rehabilitation by controlling some of the inflammatory mediators. Cold can be used in a number of forms:

- ice cube/frozen peas
- crushed ice in towels or cloths
- frozen gel packs
- cold or cooling sprays
- iced water or bowls of ice cubes
- cryogenic cuff.

Clinical indications

Ice Ice is readily available and cheap. Ice cubes wrapped in hand towels or water frozen in yoghurt pots supported by wooden spatulae may be massaged over injury sites. Massage may be continued for approximately 15 minutes at a time and may be repeated after an equal period of rest from the ice. Ice can be crushed in a strong plastic bag and wrapped in a soft towel or cloth. Frozen peas or sweet corn are as beneficial as crushed ice, conforming equally well to the uneven foot contours.

Ice packs These may be commercially purchased. The reagents, when crushed, create a temporary cooling effect from the chemical reaction evoked. Commercial products such as Koolpack (Williams Medical Supplies) have the advantage of easy storage over a system where ice has to be produced first. Practitioners treating sports persons in the field can carry the dry packs around safely, so that they are instantly ready for use on an acute foot injury.

Gel packs These have been available for many years. These products can be either frozen in a refrigerator or heated to deliver the appropriate temperature to the affected part. The problem with most ice delivery is that the beneficial coolant effect is eventually lost. A new cryogenic system is available (Aircast), however, comprising a zip-up boot that fits over the foot, with a tube containing a one-way valve delivering iced water from a reservoir held above foot/ankle level (see Fig. 7.27). This method of delivery offers a controllable dry cold application with an effective compression around the foot from the head of pressure. New iced water can be introduced by altering the pressure valve on the reservoir every 10–15 minutes.

Cold footbath immersion Cold therapy can also be achieved by immersing the foot into a bucket, or bowl of ice cubes, crushed ice, ice cubes in cold water or just cold water. Although cold water may not contain ice, the patient may not be able initially to tolerate the sensation. The short-term use of this system is to effect immediate analgesia. Immersion methods require the patient to submerge the foot below the level of liquid/crushed ice for approximately 3 minutes, or for as long as can be tolerated, up to 6 minutes. This may be repeated three or four times a day and is a useful home therapy.

Cold sprays The main use of cold sprays (Fig. 9.1) is in the acute phase of injury. The sprays are used in short blasts of 5–10 seconds, three or four times over a period of 2 minutes.

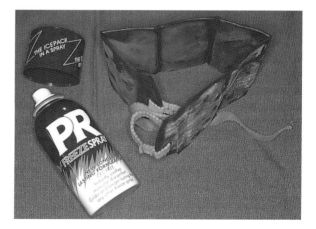

Figure 9.1 Cold can be applied as a spray from a pressurized canister. The cold spray acts momentarily, unlike gel pads, which can be prefrozen and applied as cold packs for 10–20 minutes. Gel pads can also be used as heated packs if required.

These are more commonly seen in use on a sports field. The value of such sprays prior to cutaneous injection of local anaesthetic is variable because the temperature at the nozzle end is dependent upon the chlorofluorocarbon (CFC) content. In the UK, CFCs are banned and, therefore, the environment takes precedence over the effectiveness of this type of coolant spray. The same problems of accessibility are not yet evident in the USA, where CFCs are still used in such sprays. The skin is cooled rapidly by the evaporation of the spray when it contacts the skin, producing the effects required to reduce pain, swelling and muscle spasm.

Contraindications

Cryotherapy should be avoided in patients with poor tissue viability. Impaired circulation will intensify the effect of the therapy, and ischaemia affecting the skin can arise, as well as ice burns and cold hypersensitivity. The practitioner should be aware of the sudden effect on the heart of immersion therapies, particularly on the elderly patient or those with a history of heart problems.

HEAT THERAPY

Infrared (IR) forms part of the electromagnetic spectrum. The wavelength is longer than visible light and so cannot be seen. All 'hot bodies' are sources of IR radiation. IR radiation is produced using a lamp that is either luminous or non-luminous. The terminology is self-explanatory, in that one form of IR can be seen while the other cannot.

Physical effects

The IR radiation emitted is absorbed into the body and converted into heat energy and can be applied to the chosen treatment site. *Non-luminous* forms penetrate to the epidermis, while *luminous* forms will penetrate to the dermis and the superficial fascia.

Method of application

All manufacturer's instructions should be carefully read when dealing with any equipment requiring or releasing energy. The lamp should be switched on and set up before the patient arrives. IR is directed (at a distance recommended by the manufacturer) at the uncovered site associated with the problem. Once the lamp has been heated up prior to treatment, it may be positioned at right angles to the surface of the skin. The skin should be monitored periodically to ensure that the response is normal and no blistering has arisen. The epidermis and dermis may be heated by gentle heat, which stimulates the free nerve endings producing some pain relief. A gentle hyperaemia should be apparent. The duration of each treatment should be no longer than 15–20 minutes. This may be repeated daily.

Clinical indications

IR can be used on chronic musculoskeletal and traumatic non-acute conditions; these may include sprains, strains, affections of joints, tendons, plantar fasciitis and conditions associated with non-infected arthritides.

Contraindications

The greatest danger lies in the possibility of thermal damage from burns where the lamp has been placed too close to the patient. Dressings and clothing over the site of treatment must be removed first to avoid blocking the IR radiation. The fibres found in these materials will retain heat, perpetuating the problem of skin burns. Any oil or embrocation must be removed first, as this may also enhance the heating effect. Large areas of skin should not be exposed to IR radiation in order to avoid the possibility of hypotension if the patient rises quickly following treatment. IR should not be used near flammable substances (e.g. alcoholic solutions).

ULTRASOUND

Ultrasound is a mechanical vibration (longitudinal wave) produced by the piezoelectric deformation of a crystal when subjected to a high frequency (0.75–3 MHz) of alternating electric current. The energy of the longitudinal wave will produce the mechanical effects of compression/rarefaction in the tissues through which it passes. The mechanical energy is dissipated by frictional losses at tissue interfaces. The dissipation is described in terms of the residual energy per unit distance from the site of application and is known as the 'half-value distance'. This distance is typically 5 cm for a 1 MHz output, the half-value reducing as the output frequency rises.

Physical properties

The physical effects on biological tissues are a result of the compression/rarefaction phases. Fluid is moved away from the treatment face of the equipment in a process called *acoustic streaming*. The mechanical energy frictional losses convert into thermal gains, increasing the temperature at the tissue interfaces. The beneficial physiological effects are associated with the result of acoustic streaming, which increases the tissue fluid flow rates at the site of application.

The compression/rarefaction wave action results in the following changes:

- increased capillary and cell permeability
- breakdown of complex biochemically active molecules
- decreased ground-substance viscosity.

The thermal gain results in all the normal changes brought about by heating tissues:

- rise in tissue temperature
- increased cell metabolic rate
- vasodilatation.

Methods of application

Ultrasound is applied either directly or indirectly (Fig. 9.2):

- directly: when the treatment face of the equipment is in contact with the skin via a coupling medium
- indirectly: when the part to be treated is immersed in water; the treatment face does not contact the skin directly because the water medium acts as the conductor.

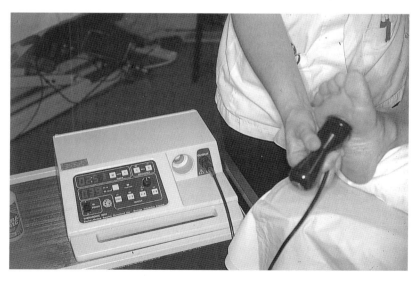

Figure 9.2 Ultrasound therapy uses high-frequency compression waves, offering a wide range of indications for foot problems: oedema, spasm of muscle, calcified tendinitis, synovitis and fasciitis.

In the direct method, it is essential to maintain continuous contact between the whole of the treatment face and the skin, if damage to the equipment or tissues is to be avoided. Some manufacturers of ultrasonic equipment supply a number of treatment heads to enable the practitioner to select the most appropriate diameter. Where the curvature of the part to be treated prevents complete contact being made, the immersion (indirect) technique is safer and more efficient. This applies to most of the foot and ankle region of the lower limb.

Prior to using ultrasound equipment with indirect application in a water bath, to prevent risk of electric shock, the practitioner should ensure that the ultrasound equipment is approved by its manufacturer for this method of application.

Once the absence of contraindications has been confirmed and the dangers noted, indirect treatment may commence. The following points should be noted:

- the part should be immersed in water
- air bubbles should be brushed from the skin and treatment face
- the dosage should be selected and applied
- the treatment face should be continually moved to direct the energy over the area
- the part should be dried and inspected.

As with all treatment, any values should be recorded in the patient's notes –dose, frequency, mode, time of application – plus follow-up instructions given to the patient.

When ultrasound is applied in the *continuous mode*, the thermal and mechanical effects are produced in the tissues through which the energy travels. When applied in the *pulsed mode*, the mechanical effects predominate. This is because the length of time during which the mechanical energy is produced is very short (typically 2 milliseconds) and the resting phase is relatively long (typically 8 milliseconds). The thermal gain is, therefore, limited and there is a period of heat dissipation before the next period of thermal gain. Manufacturers of ultrasound equipment sometimes offer the facility to adjust the pulsing ratios.

Clinical indications

The main indications for therapeutic ultrasound are listed in Table 9.2. Ultrasound waves will accelerate any active biological process at the time of application.

Dosage

For acute conditions, thermal effects should be avoided if further pain and tissue damage are to be avoided. The 'pulsed' mode should be chosen, with settings that give minimal energy input:

- low intensity output settings (< 0.75 W/cm^2)
- short time setting (< 3 minutes).

As the condition improves, either or both of these parameters may be increased so as to increase the energy input to the tissues.

Table 9.2 Indications for therapeutic ultrasound

Reduction of oedema	Reduction of pain	Mobilization of collagen
Acoustic streaming	Reducing the volume of any oedema	Depolymerization of the proteins, thus lowering the elastic modulus to allow stretching at lower forces
Increasing capillary permeability	Removal of the pain-stimulating chemicals released by trauma to the cells	
Increasing blood flow through the area	Reduction of relative ischaemia by increasing blood flow through the area	

As the acute inflammatory response reduces, the intensity and time settings may both be increased, gradually introducing thermal effects. Where chronic oedema is present, with adhesion formation, high-energy input is normally chosen:

- 'continuous' mode
- higher intensity output (> 0.75 W/cm^2)
- longer time settings (> 5 minutes).

The patient should always be warned that symptoms may increase 6–8 hours after treatment but should settle again 12 hours after treatment. This effect often results from the relatively arbitrary nature of deciding the dose to be applied and may be taken as an indication for the progression of the treatment:

- if post-treatment discomfort is great, reduce or repeat the settings at the next visit
- if no post-treatment discomfort has been felt, repeat or increase the settings at the next visit.

Contraindications

The use of ultrasound is contraindicated when:

- there is an infection in the area
- there is a bony prominence immediately below the surface of application
- there is a deep vein thrombosis or arterial disease
- tumours or tuberculosis are present
- the patient has haemophilia
- the patient is receiving radiation therapy.

Furthermore, caution must be exercised when:

- an area of skin is anaesthetized
- the underlying bone surface is concave
- there may be metal in the tissues
- there may be air-filled cavities in the area
- there is a suspected fracture.

Many of the dangers come from the possibility that energy reflected from the surface of bone, metal and air-filled cavities may create a point of high intensity in the tissues.

The waves of compression/rarefaction may cause cavitation in the tissues under treatment.

This effect can be prevented by ensuring that the treatment face is always moving over the skin and that light even pressure is applied. When the immersion technique is used, cavitation is less likely to occur, but movement should still be carried out. Air bubbles form on the treatment face and skin. These should be removed by brushing during the treatment, or the ultrasound will be attenuated before reaching the patient.

RADIOFREQUENCY HEATING

Radiofrequency heating is a general term covering those techniques that use shortwave (shortwave diathermy, SWD) or microwave (microwave diathermy, MWD) bands. Both forms of diathermy involve the generation of electrostatic or electromagnetic fields and are associated with the electromagnetic spectrum. SWD treatment is usually at the frequency of 27.12 MHz (wavelength 11 m), and MWD treatment is usually at the frequency of 2450 MHz (wavelength 122.5 mm). Technological advances in equipment generating radiofrequencies have resulted in a wider range of frequencies than those above being utilized. The output from the generator may be continuous or pulsed.

The physical consequence of the electrostatic or electromagnetic fields is to create heat in the tissues, as well as exerting a number of electrophysical field effects:

- the rotation of dipole molecules
- the distortion of non-polar molecules
- the vibration of ions
- the production of eddy current fields.

The fields created by the generators will tend to concentrate in those materials of low dielectric constant (e.g. blood and muscle) in preference to those of high dielectric constant (e.g. air and bone). Tissues with high fluid content will, therefore, be preferentially heated by using these techniques.

The physiological effects of applying radiofrequency heating result from the responses of tissues to heating, as listed in Table 9.1, and additionally include:

- reduction of muscle tone
- reduction in blood pressure
- rise in body temperature with time.

Method of application

The manufacturers of these heat sources supply a number of applicators to fit their machines. For SWD, there are a number of differently sized 'plates', either rigid and enclosed in plastic or glass holders or flexible and enclosed in rubber sheaths (Fig. 9.3). These produce their effects by creating electrostatic fields in the tissues. There may be a long cable enclosed in a rubber sheath. For MWD, there are usually a number of applicators, used singly, which are of different sizes to correspond with different body areas. The therapeutic effect is achieved by creating electromagnetic fields in the tissues.

The applicators are not placed in contact with the patient's skin but must always be separated by an air space or by dry padding. The size of the applicators must correspond to the size of the body part being treated (Fig. 9.3): too large an applicator will result in excess heating of the superficial tissues parallel with the field lines, while too small an applicator will result in field concentration in the tissues adjacent to the applicator and, consequently, excessive heating.

When selecting the applicator to be used for SWD, the choice of size or type will depend on the following points:

- for electrostatic fields, two plate electrodes are used, one for either side of the area to be treated; the plates should be slightly larger than the area and one may be flexible and one may be rigid, if necessary
- for electromagnetic fields, the cable enclosed in a rubber sheath is used.

The choice of applicator for MWD will be based on the size of the area to be treated and the range of applicators supplied with the generator. The sizes of the applicator and the area to be treated should be similar. For circular applicators, the maximum heating effect is around the outside of the field.

When using the cable, a choice of arrangement is available depending on the technique of heating required. If an electromagnetic field is desired, the centre of the cable is wound around the part to be treated, whereas an electrostatic field is produced by using the ends of the cable. The continuous modes of application are predominantly used for the thermal effects they produce, while in the pulsed mode there is a thermal effect during the 'on' phase, but the heat created will be dissipated during the 'off' phase. Manufacturers offer various pulsing ratios to allow the practitioner to select the appropriate thermal/non-thermal effects for the patient.

Many practitioners using SWD will select the cable technique and wind it around the calf and foot with approximately 2 cm of towelling between the patient and the cable as padding, or, alternatively, they will place two small applicators, separated with an air spacing, on either side of the area so that the field passes through the foot from the plantar to the dorsal aspects. If MWD is used, the smallest applicator is placed (with an air spacing) over the part to be treated.

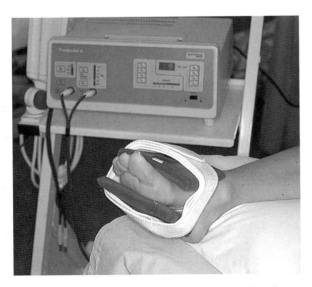

Figure 9.3 An electromagnetic current is applied to the right foot as short-wave diathermy. This type of physical therapy offers the deepest form of heat available to the practitioner/physiotherapist. Its uses for feet include degenerative joint disease, tenosynovitis/synovitis and haematoma.

The therapeutic benefits from radiofrequency heating are those that result from the thermal effects. In the pulsed mode, these thermal effects last for much shorter periods than in the continuous mode, typically 0.4 milliseconds and may be summarized as follows:

- an increase in the blood flow through the site
- stimulation of cell activity, e.g. skin growth in wounds
- a decrease in muscle tone
- a decrease in pain perception.

When the continuous mode is used, there will be a gradual increase in temperature of blood returning to the core. This will bring about a whole-body reflex vasodilatation in an attempt to control the body temperature, an effect which is called *reflex heating*. This vasodilatation results in a reduction in peripheral resistance and will, therefore, be accompanied by a reduction in blood pressure. Time must be allowed for the blood pressure to rise naturally before any exercise is commenced following treatment. A medical opinion may need to be sought before exposing patients with cardiac disorders to the demands imposed by radiofrequency treatment. Good communication and rapport with medical physicians will avoid placing patients at unnecessary risk.

Heating another site on the body, at a different location (with a healthy blood supply), will still cause a reflex vasodilatation at the impaired site. In this situation, the increased cellular metabolism created is less likely to create a deleterious problem than if applied directly to the impaired site.

When acute inflammatory conditions are being treated, low-energy levels should be applied. This may be achieved by using the pulsed mode at low intensity or, where the continuous mode is the only one available, by adjusting the output to a subthermal level, where no heat is perceived by the patient. As the acute response reduces, the thermal effects may gradually be introduced.

When there are chronic changes at the site to be treated, the generator is altered to produce different thermal effects best suited to deal with this level of pathology. Treatment may progress in the following way:

- if intolerable discomfort arises following treatment, reduce or repeat the settings
- if no discomfort arises after treatment, repeat or increase the settings.

Contraindications

The electromagnetic and electrostatic fields generated by the equipment may affect subjects other than the patients being treated. For this reason, departments using such generators must display signs at their entrances informing *all* people who intend to enter of the presence of the generators. Anyone who has a cardiac pacemaker must report the fact to the practitioner because its function may be affected by an external electrical field. Similar dangers exist for hearing aids. Any practitioner intending to switch on a radiofrequency generator must first check that no other patient in the room has a cardiac pacemaker.

The use of radiofrequency heating is contraindicated in the following situations:

- when *malignancies* are known or suspected to be in the treatment fields
- if *circulatory changes* are likely in the limb, such as those found in ischaemic conditions, thrombosis or phlebitis
- when *cardiovascular* pathologies are present, as they may be exacerbated by the increased circulation caused by treatment imposing an effect on blood pressure variation
- if there are metal or plastic *implants*, e.g. intrauterine contraceptive devices, in the treatment field, as they may be affected by radiofrequency heating
- if there is *infection* present, as it is exacerbated by the radiofrequency-generated treatment field
- excessive *fluid* in the treatment fields should be avoided; this could include non-inflammatory oedema, external wet dressings or even excessive perspiration on the skin
- if there is *haemorrhage* or if haemorrhage may be caused, as in the case of haemophilia

- where there is *impaired thermal sensation,* either hypo- or hypersensitivity, in which case the control settings should be reduced
- when patients are unable to understand the instructions concerning the treatment, in which case the practitioner may prefer to use a safer source of therapy.

Application of radiofrequencies to most parts of the calf and foot can be undertaken. The practitioner will choose the size and type of applicator to be used according to the patient's medical history and tissue sensitivity. In order to prevent an electric shock, the patient must not touch the generator or any other metal fittings. The part to be treated may, therefore, require supporting in order to mobilize the foot and limb safely. If toes are included in the treatment field, the spaces between the toes should be padded with small quantities of cotton wool to help prevent any build-up of perspiration and, therefore, the possibility of burns.

The practitioner needs to monitor the part being treated frequently. The level of heat applied should be no more than 'mild gentle heat' and should be applied for no longer than 20 minutes. On completion of the treatment, the patient's blood pressure should be given time to rise before the patient stands or begins to exercise.

HYDROTHERAPY

Hydrotherapy involves the use of a water medium in which the patient may perform movements against the water's resistance. Foot and leg hydrotherapy baths may include a spa effect, which can have additional benefits.

Therapeutic effects

By immersing either the body or the limb in water, the reduced effect of weight bearing and gravity will lower the stresses at the affected site while strengthening muscles and mobilizing joints. Rehabilitation is brought about by limiting pain while allowing active strengthening of damaged tissues. Mobility is increased and stiffness

discouraged by limiting adhesion formation. The water is usually heated and may have jets of air/water directed to provide massage at the same time. Pain-free movements can improve blood flow so as to stimulate tissue repair.

Method of application

The method of application will depend on the particular requirement but can range from directed exercises utilizing the non-weight-bearing state the patient can attain in the pool, with or without resistance to massage, to a simple application of heat. The body will need to be immersed in a pool to cover the injured site, with the patient either sitting or being supported while performing exercises.

Clinical indications

Hydrotherapy may be used as a method of upgrading fitness, strength, flexibility and cardiovascular fitness. Specific active or passive exercises with movements may help to relieve muscle spasm, produce relaxation and restoration of joint motions, increase muscle strengths, and enhance power and endurance. If used for patients with overuse injuries, hydrotherapy offers a medium in which training can be continued while limiting the effects of gravity yet maintaining muscle bulk and fitness.

It may be used for acute and chronic conditions associated with musculoskeletal or articular complaints.

Contraindications

Constant supervision should be arranged where whole-body immersion is used to avoid accidental drowning. Wounds should be protected to avoid excessive maceration, contamination of the water or further infection. Infected wounds should not be immersed.

Footbaths

Therapeutic heat or cold sources can be used in a variety of media, ranging from water to wax or mud. If required, medicaments may be added to the water baths for skin complaints or wounds. Warm saline baths may be used as a postoperative measure for phenolization treatments or following acid therapies as an attempt to neutralize too severe an action.

Methods of application

Hot footbaths The temperature of warm water should be 5–10°C above body temperature. The foot should be immersed in a bowl of the water for 15–20 minutes. This may be repeated two or three times per day. For cold footbaths, see cryotherapy (p. 194).

Contrast footbaths This type of therapy utilizes the physiological effects of cold and heat on the body (see Table 9.1). One hot footbath (40–50°C) and one cold (tap water) footbath are prepared. Colder mixtures may be made by adding ice cubes. The foot is placed into the cold footbath for 2 minutes and then into the hot footbath for the same length of time. This process is repeated, ending with a dip into the cold bath.

Wax footbaths Heated baths of paraffin wax are set at approximately 50°C. The patient's foot is immersed or dipped into the wax and then lifted out of it. A period of 15–20 seconds is allowed for this first coat to form on the skin before reimmersing. The process is repeated approximately six times so that a good coating of wax provides a strong envelope around the foot and retains heat. The foot is then wrapped in a plastic bag or plastic sheet and further wrapped in a blanket. The patient is then left to relax for 20–30 minutes. This process produces a comforting heat, ideal for arthritic complaints and chronic musculoskeletal injuries.

Contraindications

Footbaths should be avoided when skin wounds are open, except where antiseptic is added intentionally to assist with drainage for infections and ulcers. Hypersensitivity to hot and cold will adversely affect conditions such as reflex sympathetic dystrophy.

MISCELLANEOUS APPLICATIONS

MUSCLE STIMULATION

Interrupted direct current applied to nerve and muscle will produce a contraction of the muscle. Faradic-type currents are used on normally innervated muscle to produce a contraction (Fig. 9.4). The pulse duration is usually selected to be between 0.02 and 1 millisecond. A depolarized pulse is used to prevent electrolytic burns. The output must be surged to produce a tetanic-like response from the stimulated muscle. The contraction of the muscle itself will produce a number of physiological effects. Direct stimulation of motor neurons will produce a contraction in innervated muscle.

Therapeutic effects

Stimulation of muscle will invoke two effects. The stimulation of muscle tissue will raise its metabolic level, creating a reactive vasodilatation. Circulation must be adequate to cope with the required venous return. In addition, fibrous adhesions may be stretched, especially where the stimulation is preceded by a thermal treat-

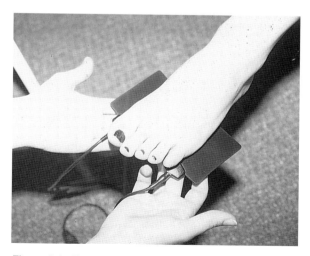

Figure 9.4 Two electrodes are placed under the left foot for muscle stimulation.

ment. The increased tone of muscle may well assist in reducing muscle discomfort and dynamic function.

Method of application

The output of the Faradic-type current is applied directly to the patient through metal (zinc) electrodes (Fig. 9.4). The electrodes can be covered with a wetted cloth and strapped onto the treatment site. Alternatively, the electrodes may be placed in a shallow water bath in which the foot is immersed so that the current may act over the treatment site. Both methods can be combined.

Muscles may be stimulated individually or in groups, depending on the specific aim of the treatment. The most efficient points for electrode location are on the peripheral nerve supplying the muscle and on the motor point of the muscle. The motor point of a skeletal muscle is that point where there is greater concentration of motor end plates. The position is typically at the junction of upper and middle thirds of the muscle belly.

In order to reduce the intensity of the sensory stimulus and at the same time produce an efficient contraction with the minimum current, it is advisable to wash the sites thoroughly for electrode placement. Soaking the calf and foot in hot water for approximately 10 minutes before treatment helps to reduce skin resistance and makes the treatment more comfortable for the patient. During this time, the equipment may be prepared.

One electrode is placed on the peripheral nerve supplying the muscles. If treating a single muscle (e.g. abductor hallucis), the other electrode is placed over the motor point of the muscle. The water bath method will usually be more efficient when treating an intrinsic muscle group. A shallow plastic tray is filled with water and the foot is placed into it. Electrodes are placed at each end of the tray in line with the muscles to be stimulated. When the current is flowing, the muscle will contract. The practitioner must regulate the frequency and intensity of the flow to bring about a painless contraction.

The patient can augment contraction by voluntarily activating the muscle (although this is difficult with intrinsic foot muscles).

During treatment, the intensity of the current is reduced. The muscle should be placed in its shortest position and the patient encouraged to maintain the strength of contraction. Once voluntary contraction can be maintained without the current being used, the electrodes can be removed. The skin should be dried and inspected for rashes brought about by chemical irritation at the electrode sites.

Clinical indications

Faradic-type stimulation is applied to muscle to improve contraction where the muscle is weak or has suffered some recent paralysis associated with deficient motor innervation. Once a popular method employed for all forms of flat-foot pathology, this technique is reserved for specific conditions and provides adjunctive rather than primary therapy, i.e.

- postsurgical-related pain inhibition preventing muscle function
- education of muscles after tendon transplantation (Ch. 7)
- to improve recent rather than long-standing muscle atrophy.

Secondary effects associated with stimulating muscle tissue improve tissue blood flow and venous/lymphatic drainage from the area.

Contraindications

Electrical stimulation should not be used in the following circumstances:

- on skin with loss of sensation
- over skin lesions, malignant or otherwise
- in the presence of infections
- where there is a presence of metal
- where there is ischaemia or abnormal local circulatory status
- where the patient may not be able to comprehend clinical instructions.

TRANSCUTANEOUS NERVE STIMULATORS

Transcutaneous electrical nerve stimulation (TNS) is another electrically modified method similar to Faradism, but rather than working to increase muscle tone, the small unit acts on nerve pathways to reduce pain via contact electrodes. A direct current is produced across the skin and deeper tissue. Non-thermal micro-massage and some motor stimulation are produced (with lower current (milliampere) levels and frequency).

Therapeutic effects

The precise mechanism associated with TNS therapy is still poorly understood. Much of the theory initially postulated was based upon Melzack & Wall's (1996) pain gate theory, which has now fallen out of favour. In this theory, an applied electrical current was thought to inter-fere with the transference of impulses along the nerve fibres, diminishing pain response. Large afferent nerves are particularly affected. The TNS system increases cell permeability and stim-ulates natural endogenous opiates associated with pain relief.

Method of application

Transducers are coated in a lubricating gel, which forms a contact medium. The transducer pads (Fig. 9.5) are fastened over the painful area or nerve route using hypoallergenic tape. The intensity of the current is increased to obtain a tingling effect. The current can then be adjusted after 2–3 minutes to maintain analgesia. The sen-sation should be pleasant. Too high a current will cause unpleasant muscle contractions. The treat-ment is designed to be used continuously and is powered by a portable battery unit. Therapy is set at the lowest level to confer analgesia. Many of these units are now economical enough for patients to purchase, although they are very basic. The unit shown in Figure 9.5 can utilize four electrode pads. The pulsing effect can be altered by altering the frequency and current, offering greater flexibility.

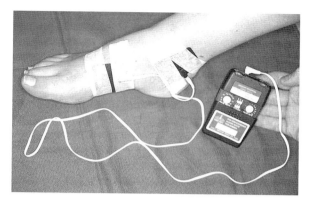

Figure 9.5 A portable transcutaneous nerve stimulator (TNS) provides an alternative form of analgesia. TNS has two (to four) electrodes applied along the medial plantar nerve branch as it passes through the ankle into the sole of the foot.

Clinical indications

Painful problems can be assisted with TNS, offering an alternative to analgesic drug therapy. The use of TNS units in feet has not been as well documented as their use with labour pain.

Another popular method of providing TNS therapy is via an acupuncture needle. The cur-rent is directed at the entry site rather than using a conducting pad.

Contraindications

TNS units may interfere with cardiac pace-makers. Where pain may be diminished follow-ing an application of TNS, the patient must not overuse the part to avoid further injury during desensitization.

MANUAL THERAPY

Massage, manipulation and mobilization to assist in the recovery from injury and disease were used by ancient civilizations over 5000 years ago. More recently, there has been a resur-gence in the use of hand massage and manipula-tion in the management of musculoskeletal dis-orders. While the foot and ankle offer a small area to work on, manual techniques used else-where on the body can still be used on the foot.

Massage

Soft tissue can be manipulated by effleurage (stroking), petrissage (deep friction) and kneading movements. The energy generated by the fingers creates the same beneficial effects as seen in methods using heat and electrical stimulation. Little clinical research has been offered to support the science of massage. However, the physical effects of touch produce relaxation and a feeling of well-being.

The therapeutic effects associated with stimulating local circulation with massage involve inflammatory mediators. Effleurage is used to push the circulatory volume towards the heart with the palms of the hand or pulpy tips of the fingers. Drainage is stimulated, especially with movements along the long arch and calf muscles. Effleurage is ideally performed prior to other manipulations.

Petrissage is applied by direct pressure to the area of chronic injury or damage with the tips of the fingers. Interfibril adhesions and scarring can be immobilized. This technique is useful on muscles, tendons and ligaments. Tissue compression and nerve excitation provide additional pain relief.

Kneading will enhance the analgesic effect and again can be used on the arch and calf areas. Soft tissue can be picked up and squeezed with a rolling manoeuvre against harder tissue. Collagen fibres that form abnormal cross-linkages can be mobilized by kneading. These areas of tissue may be palpated as 'masses' and 'knots'. The function of kneading will assist the reabsorption of these abnormal areas and create greater flexibility.

Contraindications

Massage should not be undertaken when infection is present. Apart from the additional pain created, infection could be forced further through the tissues. Phlebitis and thrombosis could be made worse by massage. Essentially, any undefined or unrecognizable inflammatory process or mass should be avoided.

Mobilization and manipulation

Method of application

Movements are performed with sudden thrusts at high speed. This technique should not be performed where joint motion is likely to be inhibited by a synostosis (bone bar). Mobilizations are passive movements aimed at restoring motion to stiff and painful joints. An oscillatory movement is performed on the patient within the joint's accepted anatomical range. Patients may perform some of these manoeuvres themselves.

Manipulation differs from mobilization in that it is a movement or thrust performed at high speed to a joint at the end of its range of motion. In these circumstances, the patient has little control of the movement and is not able to prevent it. Once again, the reason for the success of these techniques is poorly understood. The joint is taken through a range of motion and then stressed at the end of its range of excursion. Physiological function may be improved by actively stimulating the controlling mechanisms, such as the mechanoreceptors within the joint capsule. Manipulative stimulation can help to reduce pain. If the joint is too painful to move, traction may be applied for up to 20 seconds, or the joint may be compressed without movement.

Clinical indications

Mobilizations may be used for any joint where there is stiffness and reduction of normal range of motion with pain. Manipulations are used on stiff, pain-free joints, or on acute, locked joints following mobilization.

Contraindications

Contraindications to mobilization and manipulation are:

- bone disease/malignancy
- central nervous disease
- infection
- neoplasia
- acute nerve route compression

- spondylolisthesis
- gross joint instability
- inflammatory bone disorders
- fractures
- epiphyseal plate lesions.

LASERS

Lasers have become a popular addition to physical therapy. Laser is an acronym for 'light amplification by stimulated emission of radiation'. Initially, lasers used in medicine were high-powered devices, such as the carbon dioxide laser. These were used for tissue destruction by carbonization, vaporization and burn-off. These lasers are still commonly used in surgery, dermatology, gynaecology and ophthalmology, and are being used in arthroscopic surgery (Ch. 7).

Early research demonstrated that surgical wounds created by laser healed faster than wounds created by scalpel. This has led to much research into the effects of laser on tissue healing. Lasers operating at very low-power outputs were found to alter the rate of healing in experimentally induced wounds. Low-level (power) lasers have subsequently been developed to achieve this therapeutic objective and can significantly increase the rate of wound healing.

Physical properties

Lasers have several important characteristics: they are well collimated, wavelength specific, exhibit energy uniformity and are coherent.

Light emitted from a laser source will travel in a straight line, with relatively little divergence of the beam. The light is, therefore, said to be *collimated*. However, with most commercially available laser probes, some degree of divergence will be inevitable, making close contact between the probe and the skin essential.

Light emitted from a single laser probe will all be at the same wavelength. This has led some to low-level laser therapy (LLLT) being termed 'pure light' therapy. Wavelengths used in LLLT are usually in the range 660–950 nm and are found in the visible and IR parts of the electromagnetic spectrum.

Energy delivered by laser is consistent, because each photon of light 'carries' the same amount of energy. This *energy uniformity* is an important characteristic of laser.

Coherence of a laser is said to occur when all waves of light are in phase or 'in step' with one another. This property is not thought to be clinically important. Laser probes that produce coherent light are much more expensive than probes producing incoherent light; however, the value of coherence has not been established.

Laser energy is released on interaction with tissue, producing either a thermal effect or a photochemical effect, or both. It has been proposed that LLLT produces a photochemical effect, causing molecular changes to occur within cells, thus leading to metabolic changes. The effects of LLLT on tissue can be summarized as follows:

- increased ATP synthesis
- increased macrophage activity and phagocytosis
- increased fibroblast proliferation and collagen synthesis
- increased lymphocyte proliferation
- increased vasodilatation
- increased vascular permeability and mast cell degranulation.

Clinically, these effects are useful for treating a wide range of lower limb pathologies. The vascular and cellular effects augment cell-mediated immunity, making LLLT suitable as a therapy for verrucae. Increased collagen production and keratinocyte proliferation encourage wound granulation and reepithelialization. Sports and soft-tissue injuries respond well to LLLT, and relief from pain is achieved in conditions like rheumatoid arthritis and plantar heel pain.

Clinical indications

LLLT can result in improved local cell-mediated response and wound healing and can reduce pain.

Wavelength, pulse frequency and energy density are important factors to consider before starting a course of laser treatment. The most effective wavelengths for podiatric purposes are 660 and 820 nm; a 915 nm superpulse probe may be indicated for the treatment of bone lesions. A 660 nm probe will act fairly superficially and activate macrophages and fibroblasts and cause mast cell degranulation. The 660 nm probe is, therefore, appropriate for the treatment of verrucae and fungal infections, but it may also be used to encourage wound healing. An 820 nm probe has a deeper penetration and will also stimulate macrophage and fibroblast proliferation; it also appears to be more effective in the management of pain. The 820 nm probe is, therefore, appropriate for the treatment of chronic pain (as in rheumatoid arthritis) and deeper soft-tissue injuries.

Pulse frequency is also important. Most conditions will respond favourably to a frequency of 20 Hz, but frequencies between 10 and 20 kHz may be chosen. Stimulation of fibroblasts is most effective at 700 Hz, and infected conditions will respond best to frequencies between 1 and 20 kHz. If a condition fails to respond following a reasonable number of irradiations, changing the pulse frequency may be all that is necessary to bring about improvement.

Energy density is also an important consideration, since therapeutic effects are energy dependent. Too low or too high an energy density could result in negative effects. As a rule, energy densities of 8–12 J/cm^2 are the most widely used and effective, with 8 J/cm^2 appearing to be particularly beneficial. The energy density may be calculated from the following formula: energy density = [probe power (W) × irradiation time (s)]/area of irradiation (spot size, cm).

Close contact between the probe and the skin is important, and it is essential to keep the probe at 90° to the skin surface. For wounds and verrucae, irradiation around the perimeter of the lesion at 2 cm intervals is recommended, together with irradiation of the central lesion. For large wounds, irradiation of the central wound area may be better achieved with a multi-diode cluster probe. Some suggested treatment protocols are given in Table 9.3.

Contraindications

There are fewer contraindications associated with LLLT than with many other physical therapies. To avoid eye injury, laser operators, patients and any observers must wear goggles *appropriate to the wavelength of light* emitted by the device.

Lasers should not be used on pregnant mothers or patients with cancer. Lasers should not be used over an area that has recently (within the previous week) received a corticosteroid injection. Epileptic patients may receive laser therapy, providing the probe is shielded from the patient's view, using a towel or a sheet. Koebner's phenomenon at the site of laser irradiation in patients with psoriasis has been reported. Caution should be taken in photosensitive individuals and in patients with porphyria.

A notice warning that a laser is in use and restricting access to the room should be placed on the door of the clinic before the beam is switched on. The room should contain no highly

Table 9.3 Suggested irradiation protocols (Omega)

Condition	Wavelength (nm)	Energy density (J/cm^2)	Pulse frequency (Hz)	Frequency of treatment
Verrucae	660 or 820, followed by cluster	8–10	20	Twice weekly
Wound healing	660, followed by cluster	4–6	Range 20–10 000 (usually 700, but higher if infection present)	Weekly to twice weekly
Pain and injury	820	8–12	146	Weekly if chronic; as much as daily if acute

reflective surfaces, so as to reduce risk of laser reflection.

SUMMARY

Physical therapy uses heat and cold to modify inflammation and pain. There are many more methods to generate heat than there are to generate cold. Both approaches are used at specific points during the inflammatory phase: cold is applied during the early stages of trauma, while heat is usually applied later than cold and is predominantly used to promote early repair and to support analgesic care. Equipment has become more sophisticated, safer and more user friendly over the years. Contraindications exist and the method used should take account of the patient's health and conditions that can be directly affected by vasomotor and electrical changes. Physical therapy often produces beneficial responses without the need for other interventions described in this book; however, adjuvant therapy can often help to make physical therapy more effective.

REFERENCES

Melzack R, Wall P 1996 The challenge of pain, 2nd edn. Penguin Books, London

FURTHER READING

Low J, Reed A 1990 Electrotherapy explained: principles and practice

Wadsworth H, Chanmugam A P P 1988 Electrophysical agents in physiotherapy, 2nd edn. Science Press, Marrickville, Australia

10

An introduction to mechanical therapeutics

David Pratt
David R. Tollafield

INTRODUCTION

Mechanical therapy is a very broad subject. It is sometimes called biomechanics, but this is not particularly accurate since the term mechanical therapy is used to represent any treatment that influences foot function and includes relatively minor solutions, such as limiting pressure over the skin, as well as more major interventions, such as altering the load within joints. The type of therapy, therefore, varies widely, from simple dressings and taping to more complex made-to-measure devices. Biomechanics, by comparison, refers to the response by living tissue to physical forces. Mechanical therapy will, therefore, influence biomechanics.

There are a number of texts already in existence that deal in depth with the subject of biomechanics; consequently, only those fundamental elements of biomechanical principles and material science that are important to practitioners are presented here.

In this chapter and Chapters 11 and 12, the role played by mechanical therapy in alleviating foot pathology is discussed. Each chapter deals with different approaches to managing foot pathology, based on improving foot alignment. Chapter 11 concentrates on clinically based skills and products that can be dispensed without the use of expensive facilities. Chapter 12 focuses on orthoses that result from prescriptions and casts produced by a well-equipped orthotic laboratory.

In this chapter, the purpose of mechanical therapy is discussed and the concept of orthoses is introduced. A foot orthosis is an orthopaedic device that is used to support, to absorb shock, to correct a deformity, to relieve pressure or to improve the intrinsic function of the foot or of the whole body interfacing with the lower limb. Inlays, insoles, orthodigita and prostheses all have an orthotic function, and orthoses, therefore, act as conduits for mechanical therapy.

Also in this chapter, the types of material that are available in modern therapy, many of which are based on plastics technology, are described. Knowledge of these materials and mechanical principles (stresses and strains) forms the basis of an accurate laboratory prescription.

Mechanical therapy improves a patient's mobility by reducing the pain experienced during motion. It also offers an alternative to other treatments that may be less suitable for the patient. In particular, the patient may be averse to the idea of surgery or may not wish to depend on adhesive dressings and padding. A single treatment strategy will always appeal to patients; orthoses may often satisfy this need.

The ultimate objective of mechanical therapy is a complete discharge from the clinic; if this is not possible, one would aim at least to reduce the frequency of visits to the clinic. In this context a patient must be made aware that, while treatment is designed to alter the function of the foot, a complete cure is not always possible. It is in this latter case that the provision of orthoses is considered more beneficial than other techniques described in this book.

As there are many approaches to treating problems of the foot, a practitioner may find it desirable to combine mechanical therapy with other methods of management.

PRINCIPLES OF ORTHOTIC MANAGEMENT

Orthoses can be used to control the foot. Control involves stabilizing abnormal pronation, reducing shock against the foot and minimizing skin wear. In all cases, the aim of treatment is to reduce pain and inflammation in the anatomical structures. The presence of disease will offer

greater challenges to the practitioner and in many cases a compromise may be required. The objectives of orthotic therapy are summarized in Box 10.1.

There are three types of foot pathology:

- foot instability or deformity caused by muscle (or neuromuscular) weakness or imbalance
- foot instability or deformity caused by structural malalignment
- deformity arising from a loss of structural integrity within the foot.

In practice, two laws are used to describe the way in which tissues adapt to external stresses: Davis's law and Wolff's law. The former is used in relation to soft tissue, while the latter is used for bony tissue. Davis's law is more applicable to young feet prior to maturation, as developing collagenous structures are influenced more readily. Bone does not adapt as well to externally applied forces as it does to those internal forces applied through plates and pins, and yet the biological control mechanisms that produce the effects described in Wolff's law are still poorly understood (Burnstein & Wright 1994). Davis's

---

Box 10.1 Objectives of orthotic therapy

- Redistribution: relief of pressure from localized areas of stress, such as debrided keratoses or infected/ulcerated lesions, or from prominent structures subject to trauma from shoe pressure.
- Accommodation: rigid deformities cause pressure points which need containing. Better achieved by prescription orthoses or soft Plastazote inlays.
- Stabilization: realignment of bony structures (joints) in an attempt to improve function and improve soft tissue function.
- Compensation: use of cushioning or a shock-attenuation supplement to repeatedly traumatized areas, in some cases serving to augment areas of natural fibrofatty padding that have undergone atrophy or pathological displacement.
- Rest: reduction of the effects of excessive friction on the skin.
- Immobilization: inhibiting movement of a part by applying force to overcome motor power.
- Containment: a means of controlling the application of medicaments so that only the required site is subjected to the desired action.

law is described later in this book in direct relation to orthodigital function (Ch. 15).

In addition to managing soft tissue such as ligaments and bone around joints, the therapeutic objective must consider the protection of superficial (skin) lesions. In the following, some basic orthotic principles are discussed and are used to show that forces can improve foot function.

Stabilization

No matter what the underlying cause of the foot pathology, its orthotic management is always governed by the same principles (Pratt et al 1993). Many foot orthoses work by realigning the force between the foot and the ground (ground reaction force) in such a way as to reduce or counteract a deforming moment. However, this type of correction is usually temporary, lasting only for the duration that the orthosis is applied to the foot. However, the symptoms associated with the deformity or dysfunction can be ameliorated for much longer periods, since the aim is to reverse the effects of the pathology. In this case, a patient may well become dependent on an orthosis, once it has been found to be beneficial.

A simple example of this is the way in which a shoe can be modified to help to correct a pronated foot. With an unmodified shoe, the line of action of the ground reaction force will be lateral to the line of action of the weight (force) at heel strike, thus producing a valgus moment, which forces the subtalar joint into further pronation. This can be avoided by moving the point of initial contact medially so that the ground reaction force now produces a correcting varus moment. This can be achieved by flaring the heel of the shoe medially, as shown in Figure 10.1. Such a flare will not, however, have any effect upon the final position of the calcaneus relative to the ground, and this is required if pronation is to be controlled. The simplest way to adjust the position of the calcaneus would be to use a heel wedge, either placed in the heel of the shoe or, more effectively, built into an in-shoe orthosis (Fig. 10.2).

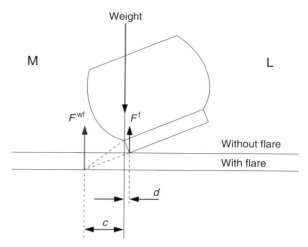

Figure 10.1 The effect of a flare on the heel designed to convert a deforming valgus ($F^f \times d$) moment to a correcting varus moment ($F^{wf} \times c$).

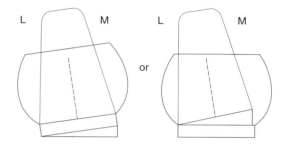

Figure 10.2 The principle of a rearfoot post on the resting calcaneal position.

Wedging, also known as posting, is one of the principles used in functional foot orthoses; the exact angle at which the rearfoot is canted forms part of the assessment of the patient. This approach can also be used for a supinated foot, with the wedges and flares applied in the opposite sense.

Three-point force systems are often used in the design of orthoses, for example in the management of hallux abductovalgus. This deformity comprises an abducted hallux at the metatarsophalangeal joint. The hallux may well deform the second toe and subsequent lateral toes. The metatarsal is adducted and, in severe cases, the medial side of the metatarsal becomes prominent with a bursal sac (bunion). Orthotic management of this deformity requires that the hallux be adducted and the first metatarsal shaft be abducted (Fig. 10.3). Two three-point force systems are used, with F^1, F^2 and F^3 correcting the hallux, and F^2, F^3 and F^4 correcting the first ray. Unfortunately, this can result in a very bulky device, although some orthoses, such as the Darco splint, are designed for daytime (Fig. 10.4). To keep the corrective forces small, they are applied as far from the joint centres as possible and the pressures are reduced by spreading the forces over large areas.

Redistribution

Often, pressures are increased to painful and damaging levels under fixed or depressed metatarsal heads. The therapeutic aim is either to move the metatarsal shaft back into alignment with the others or to redistribute the load under the fixed metatarsal head. In the former, a pad is used to push the shaft dorsally and thus realign it. If the deformity is only partially correctable or not correctable at all, then the area of increased pressure should be relieved (Fig. 10.5). To do this, the area under the plantarflexed head is excavated relative to the other heads, so that pressure is reduced and spread more evenly over each head (Whitney & Whitney 1990). This is a simplification, since in fact there are often multiple sites requiring relief, and the tissue viability of the skin and underlying structures may be poor, preventing the redistribution of pressure where it should ideally be placed.

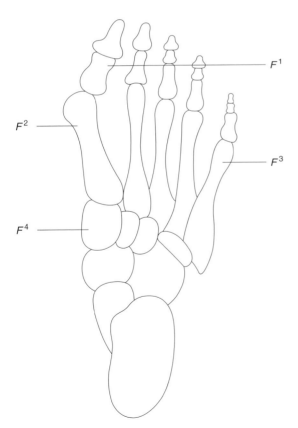

Figure 10.3 Two three-point force systems, (F^1, F^2, F^3) and (F^2, F^3, F^4), being used to correct a hallux abductovalgus deformity.

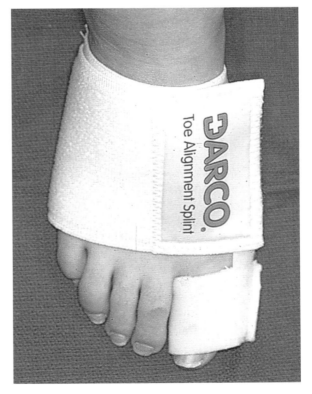

Figure 10.4 A Darco day splint for hallux valgus provides a simple example of the three-point force system.

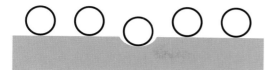

Figure 10.5 The principle of pressure reduction by spreading the forefoot load over as large an area as possible, instead of concentrating it on, in this case, the third metatarsal head.

Compensation

While redistribution forms the principal approach in managing symptoms, several other approaches may need to be dovetailed into orthotic management. In many cases, pain is caused by excessive shock transmission through the joints during walking or running, through loss of the natural shock-attenuating properties of the foot, particularly at the heel. Such excess shock can be harmful as well as painful and should be treated seriously (Collins & Whittle 1989). Simply replacing the lost shock attenuation property of the foot with a tissue-equivalent material is often sufficient to relieve the symptoms. This approach of increasing the attenuation of shock will compensate for loss of fibro-fatty (adipose) tissue, which is common with old age and certain disease processes. When selecting the material to be used, one must take account of factors such as the weight of the patient, the location of the pain, the conditions producing the discomfort, and the general health and activity of the patient. No one material can satisfy all of these constraints, but studies have been carried out on a range of materials and so there is much information available to help the practitioner to arrive at the most suitable selection (Campbell et al 1984, Oakley & Pratt 1988, Pratt 1990). Compensation is used where a limb has been shortened or where a part of the anatomy has been lost altogether. The loss is made up using additional material directly under the heel or on the outer sole. Where severe pain occurs, load has to be taken off the foot by using devices such as patella–tendon-bearing ankle foot orthoses (McIllmurray & Greenbaum 1958). Detailed discussion of this type of device is outside the scope of this text, although ankle foot orthoses are considered further in Chapter 12.

Accommodation

Accommodative orthoses primarily accommodate fixed deformities and are valuable in patients who are particularly 'at risk' from the effects of poor tissue viability (Janisse 1993). Casted orthoses are prescription orthoses prepared on positive moulds of the foot. They may conform to feet purely with the primary objective of moulding around lesions, offering compensation as well as redistribution from specific points affected by high load.

Summary

In conclusion, it should be noted that, sometimes, the therapeutic objectives outlined in Box 10.1 will overlap. For example, rest and immobilization might well be by-products of redistribution, stabilization or compensation.

The influence of the foot on the proximal skeletal structures, and vice versa, has been recognized as a significant component of gait. As such, this relationship must be assessed (Tollafield & Merriman 1995) and considered when taking the decision to use foot orthoses. No foot treatment should be considered without careful regard to proximal joint problems at the level of the knee, hip or back. The need to make adjustments must always be borne in mind, as the effect of torque forces will add to, rather than ameliorate, pathology.

MECHANICAL PRINCIPLES

In order for mechanical therapy to be effective, the practitioner will need to be able to select materials from a large range of products. In this next section, we will consider properties of the foundation materials (material science) of some common products described in this book, which are also widely advertised in journals.

Basic physics

The effects of forces on an object are often poorly understood, and the foot is no exception. Suffice it to say that forces generated by activities such as walking or standing cause stresses and strains in the foot that need to be taken into account when designing orthoses. It is equally important to be aware of the stresses and strains generated in the materials designed to assist the foot, as this will affect their choice.

In order to understand the effects of forces and levers on the skeletal structure when considering orthotic function, familiarity with a number of principles of physics and mechanics is required. Without this knowledge and an appreciation of the properties of materials used to produce an orthosis, mistakes are likely to be made when fitting and dispensing. Physical principles are used in the design of orthoses, and some practical examples are used here to illustrate some of the general points. A more detailed description can be found in Chapter 12.

Units

The SI system of units will be used throughout for all mechanical units. In everyday practice, the principles of biomechanics are increasingly encountered. Before specific quantities and principles are described, it is worth mentioning that there are two types of quantity: *scalars* and *vectors*. Scalar quantities are those that need only a magnitude to describe them fully, such as temperature, whereas vectors comprise both a magnitude and a direction. Examples of vectors include force and velocity, and these are discussed later in this section. This difference in the way quantities are specified also means that the methods by which they are added together (i.e. vector addition and scalar addition) are different. These two methods of addition are described below.

Displacement, velocity and acceleration

If an object is moved from one position to another then it has been displaced. Hence, the distance it has moved is its *displacement*. In order to specify its new position, however, it is not sufficient to say that the displacement is 5 metres (m), because the direction in which it has been moved is also required (therefore, this term is a vector). The direction is described using a set of three mutually orthogonal axes (x, y, z). This enables a complete description of the object's starting and finishing positions. The rate of change of displacement with time (t) is called velocity (v), and is measured in metres per second (m/s or m s^{-1}). It is sometimes written as ds/dt, which represents the change in position divided by the time taken for the change. Velocity is, therefore, also a vector, since both the magnitude and direction of motion are required to describe how it is moving. Speed, by comparison, is a scalar. When we say a car is moving at a speed of 30 mph, we do not need to specify the direction of motion; you *cannot* say that a car has a velocity of 30 mph unless you specify a direction: it is meaningless! The rate of change of velocity with time is called acceleration (a) and is measured in metres per second squared (m/s^2 or m s^{-2}). It is sometimes written as dv/dt. Again, this is a vector quantity.

Force

A force (F), measured in newtons (N), is defined as any action that produces, or tends to produce, acceleration of an object on which it acts. For example, if you push a wheelchair containing a patient, it will start to accelerate. Once moving, if there was no frictional force, it would continue to move at a uniform velocity until another force acted upon it. However, friction is present and, therefore, a small force input is required to keep the chair moving, although this is less than the initial force required to start the chair moving. If there was a heavier patient in the chair, the forces required to achieve the same velocity would be greater. The amount of matter that makes up an object, in this case the wheelchair and the patient, is called mass (m) with units of kilograms (kg). The force (in newtons) required to accelerate the wheelchair is given by

$$F = m \times a$$

This too is a vector quantity, requiring both magnitude and direction to describe it fully. At this point, we should note that weight is also a force and that it is the product of the mass of an object and the gravitational acceleration (g). In order to define the weight force fully, its point of application on the object has to be defined. This is called the centre of gravity and is, in effect, the same as centre of mass. It is the point at which the mass of the object may be considered as being concentrated.

Vector addition

As mentioned above, the addition of vectors is different from the addition of scalars. With scalars, the addition is simply the sum of the two numbers, but with vectors we need to use vector addition. This requires the use of vector diagrams.

Figure 10.6 shows two people pushing a bed, each with a different force (F^1 and F^2) and in a different direction. To find the total force acting on the bed and its direction of motion, we need to redraw the diagram as shown in Figure 10.7.

Here the two forces are represented by arrows. The length of each indicates the magnitude of the force, and the angle indicates the direction, or line, of action. The lines are drawn parallel to their actual positions: F^2 follows from the end of F^1. If there were more forces involved, they could be added to the end of the last arrow in any sequence. This results in a line of arrows with a start and a finish. The sum effect of all the forces is found by joining the two free ends with a new arrow to give a new force (R). The length denotes its magnitude and the angle gives its direction. This new force is called the resultant force.

This process is often used in reverse to produce two forces acting along specific axes from a single one. This may seem like a pointless activity, but it is helpful when adding the effects of forces. This is called 'resolution of forces' and Figure 10.8 shows how this is done. The force F has been resolved into two component forces, F^v vertically and F^h horizontally. These component forces (still in newtons) are given in terms of the original force by

$$F^h = F \cos \theta$$

$$F^v = F \sin \theta$$

Resolving forces is very useful; vertical and horizontal component forces can be simply added. These two final components can be added vectorially, as described above, to give the overall effect of all the forces; this simplifies the mathematics considerably.

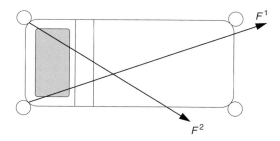

Figure 10.6 Diagram of two people pushing a bed with forces F_s^1 and F^2.

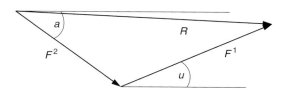

Figure 10.7 The principle of adding two forces, F^1 and F^2, vectorially to give a single resultant force.

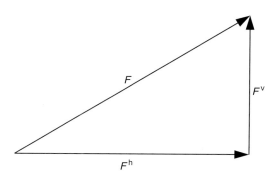

Figure 10.8 Resolution of the force F into two components, F^v vertically and F^h horizontally.

Moments of force

The moment of any force about a point is the product of the magnitude of the force and the perpendicular distance (d) between the point and the line of action of the force (the moment arm). Thus, in Figure 10.9, the moment of F, measured in newton metres (Nm), is given by

Moment = Fd

Moments can be used to find muscle and joint forces when used in conjunction with the concept of equilibrium. This concept states that when an object is at rest or moving with a uniform velocity, it is in equilibrium. Therefore, in this state, the net sum of all the forces and their moments about any point must be equal to zero.

Figure 10.10 shows a highly simplified schematic foot being held at 90° to the tibia by the action of the muscle force (P). In this simplified case, the muscle force is only required to resist the weight of the foot (W). Both of these forces are assumed to act vertically at distances a and b, respectively, from the point of rotation (the ankle joint centre). As this foot is at rest, it is in equilibrium, and hence all the forces and moments are equal. So we have a basic equation, $Pa = Wb$. If W can be measured, or calculated, and a and b are measured, then P can be found from $P = Wb/a$. In fact, in this case, as there are no other forces, one could simply say that $W = P$. In reality, however, the picture is more complicated than this, with many more forces acting at vary-

ing angles to each other in all three planes. In these circumstances, both force resolution and equilibration of moments are needed.

Pressure

Pressure and force should not be confused. They are different, although they are related by a single quantity: area. Pressure, measured in newtons per square metre (N/m^2) or pascals (Pa), is the force per unit area (F/A). So, if a force of, say, 100 N acts on two surfaces, one with an area of 10 m^2 and the other with an area of 20 m^2, the pressures will be 10 Pa (100/10) and 5 Pa (100/20), respectively. Thus, the pressure resulting from a force can be reduced by increasing the area over which it is applied. (Note: in many medical texts, millimetres of mercury (mmHg) are used as units for pressure; 1 mmHg = 133.322 Pa.)

While it may seem of little practical value to know about force, it does have some very practical applications. For example, orthoses function by applying forces to the body as a way of influencing the skeletal structure. The interface between the orthosis and the skin needs to be

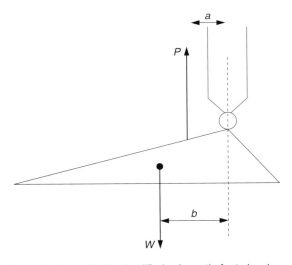

Figure 10.10 A highly simplified schematic foot showing the forces in the muscle (P) and that from the weight of the foot (W) in equilibrium. To balance the plantarflexion moment of $W \times b$, the muscle needs to apply a dorsiflexion moment of $P \times a$.

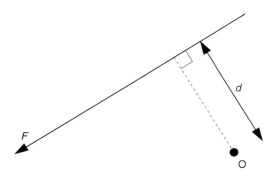

Figure 10.9 The moment of the force F about point O is related to the perpendicular distance between the line of action of F and O.

protected from forces that could damage the skin (Pratt 1994), and a few simple rules based on the above are invaluable.

The way in which the imposed force is distributed throughout the material is called stress. Stress (σ) is the force (F) divided by the cross-sectional area of the object at the point of interest (A). (Note that stress has the same units as pressure.) Therefore,

$$\sigma = F/A \text{ (Pa)}$$

There are three types of stress: tensile, compressive and shear. These usually act together at any point in an object (Fig. 10.11).

Strain arises when a force is applied to any structure, whether it be an organic or inorganic material. Strain is related to compression or tension and has no units as it is the ratio of the change in length to the original length. Pathology may well arise when there is no recovery in the length (e.g. of a ligament) after a force has been applied. Body tissues such as ligaments and tendons normally provide an element of recovery in length once the force (stress) applied has ceased. In the case of Davis's law, mentioned earlier, treatment may include the maintenance of exter-

nally applied stress to bring about a permanent change in length.

Compressive or tensile strain (ε) is given by change in length/original length:

$$\varepsilon = \delta l / l$$

Another quantity of interest is shear stress (τ). This type of stress is more complicated to define but Figure 10.12 shows its effect on an object of height L, where it causes the material to deform by a distance x on one surface, corresponding to an angular deformation ϕ. This angular deformation is know as the shear strain (measured in radians) and is given by x/L.

The ratio of the shear stress to shear strain is called the modulus of rigidity (G) and is measured in newtons per metre (N/m). Thus

$$G = \tau / \phi$$

If a piece of inorganic material such as metal is stressed, the strain increases linearly up to a point called the elastic limit (Fig. 10.13). If the stress is removed at any point up to this limit, the material will return to its original length. The slope of the line up to this limit is called the modulus of elasticity, or Young's modulus (E), and is a measure of the stiffness of a material. It is defined as

$$E = \sigma / \varepsilon$$

Young's modulus has the same units as stress (Pa). After the elastic limit has been reached, the

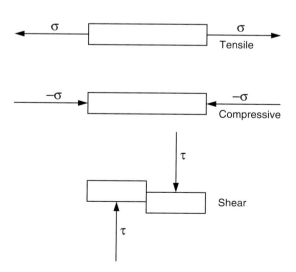

Figure 10.11 The three types of stress: tensile, compressive and shear.

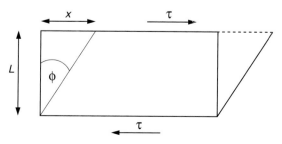

Figure 10.12 The effect of shear force on a rectangular object.

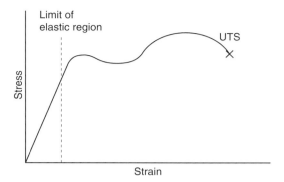

Figure 10.13 A typical stress–strain curve showing the limit of elasticity and the ultimate tensile strength (UTS).

relationship between stress and strain is no longer linear and the material enters a plastic region where permanent deformation takes place. At some point the material will fail, usually at a point lower than its maximum strength; this is known as its ultimate tensile strength (UTS).

Ductility and *brittleness* are terms that are often used to describe the performance of materials. A ductile material has the ability to demonstrate 'plasticity' over very large increases in stress before failing, whereas a brittle material undergoes little or no plastic deformation. In general, ductile materials are tougher (i.e. they are more able to withstand impact loads). Toughness is a measure of the energy needed to fracture a piece of material, and this is a function of ductility. Therefore, ductile materials are more suitable for use in orthotics or prosthetics, as their impending failure is signalled by the plastic deformation taking place.

A brittle failure gives no advance warning and as such can be dangerous for someone who is relying on the support that the device is providing. Furthermore, brittle materials that fracture (e.g. unmodified plastics) sometimes leave sharp fragments, which can lacerate the skin. Certain types of plastic (e.g. polythenes) are ductile and offer the ideal properties for many orthoses. The material will allow some structural change or 'give' without losing its shape. The resilience of plastic, while offering such ideal physical prop-erties, will inevitably vary between products because of the different polymeric structures used with chemical production techniques.

Let us now consider how these aspects of materials and mechanics can be used to establish principles that are useful for orthotic management and material selection. The subject of *orthopaedic biomechanics* is extensive and the detail is beyond the scope of this book. The interested reader is directed to the Further reading.

MATERIAL PROPERTIES

There is a constant influx of new materials onto the market, and the large number of materials to choose from can easily confuse the practitioner. While it is unnecessary for the practitioner to acquire the same knowledge as a chemist, a working knowledge of some of the newer technologies can help to differentiate those materials ideally suited to the situation at hand from those that are not. A keen practitioner who fails to be well informed will experience personal disappointment and patient dissatisfaction.

Foundation materials

Basic chemistry

Many of the materials used today are plastics, and these can be broadly divided into two categories: *thermoplastic* and *thermosetting*. The first of these, the thermoplastics, which include common plastics such as polystyrene, polyvinylchloride (PVC) and polyethylene, are materials that can be softened by heating, formed into a new shape and then allowed to harden by cooling. This process of softening and hardening can be repeated many times with no degradation to the plastic. Thermosetting materials, however, first soften on heating and then, with further heating, set hard and cannot be altered again by heating. An example of this is the old 'Bakelite' type of plastic used for door handles and old radio cabinets. These different behaviours are a result of chemical differences.

Plastics are materials with long chains of molecules called polymer chains. In thermoplastic materials, these long molecules are separate from each other. In thermosetting materials, heating or chemical reaction causes strong chemical links between chains to be formed (cross-links), thus linking them firmly together.

The term polymer has been used above and it is worthwhile describing the polymer molecule. Much of chemistry is concerned with molecules of between 2 and 50 atoms, which exist as solids, liquids and gases. However, there are many molecules that cannot be classified conveniently into these three types: fibres, such as wool or nylon; thermoplastics, which soften on heating to form thick viscous fluids instead of mobile liquids; and rubbers. All these substances consist of collections of large polymeric molecules joined together. The polyethylene (often called polythene) molecule, for example, has typically 1000 (CH_2CH_2) units linked end to end. The bulk thermoplastic has thousands of these chains packed together, sometimes regularly, sometimes tangled.

There is no precise point at which a line can be drawn between large and small molecules, but a molecule may be considered as large when it gives rise to substances that possess resinous, rubbery or fibre-like properties.

There are two basic chemical reactions by which long-chain molecules are formed: condensation and addition polymerization.

Condensation polymerization In condensation, a small molecule (usually water, ammonia or hydrochloric acid) is eliminated when an organic base (e.g. ethyl alcohol (ethanol)) condenses with an organic acid like acetic acid. Thus

$$C_2H_5OH + CH_3COOH =$$
$$C_2H_5OCOCH_3 + H_2O$$

If the base possesses two hydroxyl groups (OH) and the acid possesses two carboxyl groups (COOH), condensation produces an ester with a basic and an acidic group, which can condense further with another ester molecule. An example of this is polyethylene terephthalate (PET or terylene), made from the addition of terephthalicethylene acid and glycol:

$$HOOCC_6H_4COOH + HOCH_2CH_2OH =$$
$$HOOCC_6H_4COOCH_2CH_2OH + H_2O$$

A further condensation produces a diester:

$$HOOCC_6H_4COOH +$$
$$HOOCC_6H_4COOCH_2CH_2OH =$$
$$HOOCC_6H_4COOCH_2CH_2OCOC_6H_4COOC$$
$$H_2CH_2OH + H_2O$$

Further condensation produces the general form $H(OOCC_6H_4COOCH_2CH_2)_nOH$, which is a polyester (terylene). The nylons are another product of this type of reaction.

Addition polymerization Usually addition polymerization involves carbon–carbon double bonds. This process occurs in three steps.

1. *Initiation*

$$IN^* + C_2H_4 \rightarrow IN \cdot CH_2CH_2{}^*$$

The initiator (IN^*) may be an ion, resulting in ionic polymerization, or a free radical, resulting in a radical polymerization.

2. *Propagation*

$$IN \cdot CH_2CH_2{}^* + C_2H_4 \rightarrow IN \cdot CH_2CH_2CH_2CH_2{}^*$$

$$IN \cdot CH_2CH_2CH_2CH_2{}^* + C_2H_4 \rightarrow$$
$$IN \cdot CH_2CH_2CH_2CH_2CH_2CH_2{}^* \text{ etc.}$$

The chain grows rapidly with the evolution of heat until a termination stage is reached.

3. *Termination*

$$IN \cdot (CH_2)_nCH_2CH_2{}^+ \rightarrow$$
$$IN \cdot (CH_2)_nCH = CH_2 + H^+ \text{(solvated)}$$

Termination involves the loss of a proton from the chain end. In polyethylene, n is of the order of 1000. Examples of this type of plastic are PVC, polypropylene and polystyrene.

The repeating unit of a polymer (a monomer) can be either a straight chain molecule (aliphatic) or in the form of rings (aromatic). The aliphatic molecules have three divisions based upon the nature of the hydrocarbon bonds. Alkanes have a single bond, e.g.

$$H - \underset{\underset{H}{|}}{\overset{\overset{H}{|}}{C}} - \underset{\underset{H}{|}}{\overset{\overset{H}{|}}{C}} - H \qquad \text{(ethane)}$$

Alkenes have unsaturated hydrocarbon bonds in the form

$$\underset{\underset{H}{|}}{\overset{\overset{H}{|}}{C}} = \underset{\underset{H}{|}}{\overset{\overset{H}{|}}{C}} \qquad \text{(ethylene)}$$

Alkynes have even more unsaturated bonds, such as

$$H - C \equiv C - H \qquad \text{(ethyne)}$$

Monomers can be combined either as the same unit repeated (a homopolymer) or using different units (a copolymer), and the chains can be linear or branched and may be cross-linked.

Having outlined some of the structural and chemical principles of polymers, some of the many different types of polymer can now be described and their uses in mechanical therapy presented. It is not the intention here to list all possible polymers, as only those of value to mechanical therapy are relevant.

Polycarbonates

A polycarbonate is a thermoplastic polymer with linear polyesters of a carbonic acid with diphenylpropanol. Carbonic chloride is reacted with pyridine to form the polymer sheet. Polycarbonates are hygroscopic (i.e. they absorb water into the chemical structure). Before heat processing, they need to be thoroughly dried out, otherwise water bubbles form in the bulk of the material, causing a loss of mechanical strength. This drying takes about 24 hours at an elevated temperature, which is below the material's moulding temperature. Polycarbonates can be used for manufacturing orthotic plates (the basic shell vacuformed around a cast). During heat processing, care must be taken because overheating can result in the release of benzene gas, which is hazardous. Polycarbonates provide a high strength, but they are expensive and are, therefore, not often used in foot orthoses.

Polyvinylchloride

PVC is a thermoplastic polymer to which plasticizers may be added. These are materials that improve the elasticity of the polymer. They are used in sheet form to make rigid foot orthoses, although they are valuable as a cover material with or without a foam backing. PVC can be modified by adding cross-linkages and copolymerized to form an impact-modified PVC. If overheated, it also gives off benzene, phthalic anhydride and hydrogen chloride, all of which are hazardous.

The general structure of PVC is:

$$\left[CH_2 - \underset{\underset{Cl}{|}}{CH} \right]_n$$

Trade names are Pacton and Darvic (ICI Plastics).

Polyethylene (polythene)

This plastic is a thermoplastic polymer formed by addition polymerization. The properties that are most suitable for orthoses are found in the high-molecular-weight versions of polyethylene. These materials are ideal for use in semi-rigid orthoses, which have some flexibility while still possessing the controlling, non-deforming properties offered by acrylic, polycarbonate, polyester and high-impact PVC (trade name, ICI) materials used in rigid orthoses.

The general structure is:

$$\left[CH = CH \right]_n$$

The main advantage offered by this material is that there are few real dangers in the heat-processing stages, although acrid fumes are produced if it burns. Trade names are Ortholen and sub-Ortholen (Teufel).

This material can be foamed to produce closed cell foams. Foamed materials provide a matrix of individual bubbles or cells unconnected to their neighbours. In the foam form, it is used as a soft padding for insoles or, in the more rigid foam formulations, as a very light raise to compensate for leg length discrepancy. It does, however, suffer badly from compression set. This is when permanent collapse of the foam occurs under repeated loading (Pratt 1990).

The trade names of this foamed version are Plastazote (BXL) and Evazote (BP Plastics).

Polypropylene

Polypropylene is the most commonly used plastic for orthoses, being suitable for UCBL (University of California biomechanics laboratory) orthoses and ankle foot orthoses, as well as many other bespoke (made-to-measure) applications.

Polypropylene is a thermoplastic polymer made by addition and has many isomeric forms (an isomer is a different structural arrangement of the same monomeric units, often with very different physical and chemical properties). The general form of this polymer is

$$\left[CH_2 - \underset{\underset{CH_3}{|}}{CH} \right]_n$$

The three isomeric forms of significance are the isotactic, syndiotactic and atactic forms, which relate to the arrangement of the CH groups on the helical polymer chain. If all of these are on the same side of the chain, the isotactic isomer is formed, whereas if they alternate between sides then the isomer is in the syndiotactic form. The atactic form is more random, with areas where the groups are on the same side followed by alternating sections. This form is also non-crystalline and has a low softening temperature and poor mechanical properties.

Because of the excellent moulding properties of polypropylene and its resistance to mechanical failure, it is widely used in orthotics. It is found either as a homopolymer, which is comparatively brittle, or as a copolymer, the latter being the material of choice.

Dangers during processing include the release of toxic fumes if overheated, with a great deal of black smoke.

The trade name is Propylex (Courtalds).

Polymethylmethacrylate

Polymethylmethacrylate (PMMA) has both thermoplastic and thermosetting polymerplastic properties, depending upon the form in which it is used. PMMA has been modified by cross-linkages and copolymerization to give improved mechanical properties in the sheet form; it is very useful for rigid foot orthoses. It is available in a variety of thicknesses and colours.

The general form of this polymer is

$$\left[CH_2 - \underset{\underset{\underset{\underset{OCH_3}{|}}{C=O}}{\overset{\overset{CH_3}{|}}{C}}}{C} \right]_n$$

In powder form, when mixed with a polymerizing agent, PMMA is used to form rigid posts in functional foot orthoses. It is also sold as dental acrylic for the repair of dentures. In this form, the material has thermosetting properties.

The trade names are Perspex (ICI) as unmodified sheet, Novaplast (Kraemer) as modified sheet and Orthoresin (DeTrey) as a powder for posting orthoses.

The dangers of using this product depend upon the form being processed. If it is overheated during processing, small quantities of cyanide fumes can be released. In the two-part system, the liquid is very flammable, with a flash point of only 13°C. In recent years, the form known as Rohadur or Plexidur O has been withdrawn from production for environmental reasons.

Polyurethane

Polyurethanes have a complex structure and tend to be mixtures of crystalline and non-crystalline polymers that phase separately. There are two different types: polyether urethanes and polyester urethanes. They are all characterized by the urethane linkage (–NH–COO–) and exist in many forms too numerous to list here.

These polymers can be produced in sheets or as foam. The sheets are dense polymers that can be used to replace the loss of shock attenuation in the foot. However, many of these shock-attenuating properties can be found in polyurethane foam, which is produced by adding water during production. This produces carbon dioxide and hence foaming (Pratt 1988).

Trade names for the sheet form are Viscolas (Cabot) and Sorbothane (IEM Orthopaedics), while those for the foamed product are PPT (Langer Biomechanics), Poron (Rogers Corporation) and Cleron (Seaton and Price).

The dangers associated with use of this material depend upon how it is supplied. If supplied as a sheet, there are no specific dangers unless the product is burned. If supplied as two parts of the foam product to be mixed in situ, the liquid methylene diisocyanate can be a respiratory irritant.

Silicones (siloxanes)

The silicones are thermosetting inorganic polymers with rubber-like properties. They are formed by a condensation reaction to give a polymer of the general form

$$HO \left[\begin{array}{c} R \\ | \\ Si - O \\ | \\ R \end{array} \right]_n H$$

(where R is any of a range of organic groups).

Silicones can be produced in a gum form (e.g. bathroom sealants) and can then be used to make insoles (Pratt et al 1984). However, the preservative agent, acetic acid, makes this form rather noxious to use. In addition, silicones can be used in a two-part mix – gum with catalyst – to form protectors for the digits in situ. These can be used, for example, to protect toes from high pressures (Whitney & Whitney 1990). There are many silicone gums available and, combined with a catalyst as a paste or liquid, they will cure quickly (within 2 minutes), allowing the practitioner to dispense the plastic orthodigital device during the consultation. Otoform, a silicone introduced originally for hearing aid impressions, has remained popular for over a decade. Further applications of this substance are discussed in Chapter 11.

Trade names are Podiaform (Footman), Otoform (Dreve), Verone and KE20.

Table 10.1 outlines the comparative properties of most of the commonly used polymers in orthotic manufacture, together with some other potentially useful products. For full details of the dangers of processing plastics, the reader is referred to a publication by the Health and Safety Executive (1990). Practitioners directing or carrying out any form of manufacture with plastics must be aware of all the necessary safety precautions concerning respiration, and eye and ear protection, as well as ensuring that reasonable safety and guard protection are applied to moving parts.

Composite materials

The composites are a group of materials comprising both a plastic matrix and a reinforcing fibre. They are emerging as a useful addition to the field of orthotic application (Bader 1993). There are certain products on the market, based on carbon fibre, that are used primarily for selective strengthening of orthoses; these are moulded at the same time as the main plastic (Compcore, Becker Orthopaedic). Composite materials that offer a superior strength-to-weight ratio compared with conventional polymers (TL2100, Medical Materials Corp.) are also

Table 10.1 The comparative properties of most of the commonly used polymers in orthotic manufacture

Polymer	Density (kg/m^3)	Yield stress (MPa)	Modulus (GPa)	Impact strength (J/m)	Fatigue stress (MPa)	Maximum service temperature (°C)	Coefficient of friction	Relative flammability
Polycarbonate	1200	60	2.5	700	7	120	0.2	26
Polyvinyl chloride	1500	45	2.5	300	15	70	0.4	45
Polyethylene								
Low density	930	12	0.3	–	15	70	0.6	17
High density	960	27	0.7	800	15	80	0.25	17
Polypropylene	1120	85	5.0	100	20	110	–	16
Polymethylmethacrylate	–	150	12.0	–	–	200	–	16
Polyurethane								
Moulded	1100	22	0.3	–	–	120	–	–
Foamed	500	15	–	–	–	90	–	–

available for the production of rigid foot orthoses. The dangers of these materials are those associated with the matrix plastic, as outlined above, as well as those associated with the reinforcing fibre. The latter dangers are chiefly related to the production of small particles of fine fibres during the finishing process, which can act as respiratory irritants. As yet, carbonized orthoses are still in their infancy, although they are gaining in popularity.

Impression materials

Casting materials are important for taking impressions and replicating models from the foot and lower leg with varying degrees of accuracy. Further details of how these impressions are referred to professional laboratories, with a specific prescription format, will be provided in Chapter 12. The end product of this procedure is a bespoke orthosis. A number of these casting materials also play a role in limiting motion or acting to redistribute load from a central area of pathology, such as an ulcer. In this respect, casting has two main functions: impression taking and therapeutic function.

Traditionally, casts were made of plaster of Paris (calcium sulphate dihydrate). This material, while still useful, has been superseded for therapeutic use by mixtures of polymers, including composites, often used together with inorganic compounds. As this field is changing rapidly, it is only sensible to outline the general properties and leave specifics to the current journal publications.

Several studies have been carried out on these new materials, with a view to providing comparative data on their performance. Despite the number of newer materials, plaster of Paris is still used for many orthotic impressions because it rapidly sets to give a good pattern of the limb segment, is easily moulded around the limb, and is still cheap. Furthermore, although many of the newer products offer improved mechanical performance, they are much more expensive and less easily conformable. These latter problems are still being tackled by the producers. Rowley & Pratt (1986) examined most of the products available at that time and produced a comparative table (Table 10.2).

Alginates were originally used for taking dental impressions. This rubbery material is based upon alginic acid extracted from brown seaweed. Alginic acid comprises two stereoisomers, guluronic acid and mannuronic acid, and forms the basis of alginate. When combined, in powder form, with water, alginate creates cross-linking to produce insoluble calcium alginate from

Table 10.2 Comparison of casting materials available in 1986

Casting material	Density (kg/m³)	Yield strength (MPa)	Flexural modulus (GPa)	Fatigue life cycles	X-ray absorption coefficient (mm⁻¹)	Exotherm (°C)
Gypsona	740–810	1.53–2.62	0.642–0.828	13	0.18	27
Cellona	–	2.87	1.11	15	0.17	–
Zoroc	920	3.14	0.840	70	0.19	28
Crystona	950	1.36	0.227	60	0.13	29.3
Scotchcast	680	39.97	0.340	24 200	0.08	26.8
Scotchflex	380	13.70	0.133	18 500	0.05	25.3
Baycast +	410	7.86	0.660	3 200	0.01	25.6
Dynacast	–	36.30	0.690	30 000	0.07	–
Hexcelite	490	3.76	0.031–0.066	39 700	0.02	35–38

From: Rowley & Pratt (1986).

sodium alginate and calcium ions. The process of cross-linking is common to many thermosets, including polyurethane and polyester casts, which form by the same principle, whereby a soft material cures to a state in which it has greater strength.

Clinical materials

Many materials originally used for treating foot complaints have now been replaced by plastic products. There is little value in describing all the potential products, as new materials are introduced frequently and can be found in many journals that carry advertisements. Therapeutic selection will be better assisted with some fundamental knowledge of the types of material suited to foot management. Materials such as felt, foam rubber and strapping will be adhered to the foot or combined with ready-made products. Chiropody treatment was founded on such materials, but many have become obscured by the advent of easily dispensed, ready-made pads and insoles. The modern practitioner should make the appropriate selection of these useful adhesive products, particularly for short-term use.

Foot padding materials

Strapping and tapes are used in a variety of ways, either to limit motion or to allow adherence of dressings to the foot (Ch. 11).

Felt　Felt is made up by layering wool and then compressing and steaming it under rollers. Because felt is expensive, mixtures of synthetic material such as nylon reduce the wool content. Unfortunately, the market has been flooded with materials of low durability and high synthetic content that are not of the same quality as wool felts. In this respect, over-the-counter products, while expensive, have fewer resilient properties than felt purchased from main supply houses. It is common practice to describe felt as compressed or semi-compressed, although a durometer or hardness measurement, usually between 9 and 65 on a scale 0–100, is sometimes specified. Recent changes in the UK market have affected the quality of felt.

Rubber　Rubber has many applications in treating the foot. Rubber latex sheeting can be used for toe and tarsal loops as replaceable padding. An older but still occasionally practised technique uses liquid latex that cures as it dries. This is preserved in ammonia. Hallux and digital shields can be made by immersing plaster models of toes in dipping latex. Padding in foam latex is sandwiched between layers of dipping latex. Natural rubbers may be combined with synthetic rubbers to achieve the same physical properties as the original rubber, while offering greater shear strength; for example, isobutene and isoprene are combined to produce butyl rubber. A very common rubber is neoprene (2-chlorobutadiene; Du Pont), which is synthetic.

Spenco is still one of the most widely used synthetic rubbers (a neoprene). It is used for insoles and foam pads. Rubbers are also mixed with plastics, such as styrene butadiene rubber (SBR). These synthetic rubbers are less likely to perish with age but do not have the softness needed for clinical application. They can be used in compound manufacture, where a mixture of different products are selected for their combined physical properties. Ethylvinyl acetate (EVA), used in running shoes, is very popular as a wedging material or as a whole orthosis.

Foams Foams have been discussed above as being produced by a chemical process that causes plastics to expand. Rubber latex (natural isoprene rubber) is useful, although granular in nature, as a foam. When covered with a fabric, the material is less compressible and is remarkably long lasting.

PVC foams may be available as strips, very similar to tapes on a roll. They can be adhered over joints to prevent shear forces creating blisters. Fleece web and moleskin, not surprisingly, do not arise from either sheep or moles. Both are thin synthetic materials and are indicated for patients whose shoes cannot accommodate thicker materials. Fleece web has greater elasticity than moleskin, but only in one direction. Both are covering materials and are useful for binding foams together or for binding foams onto card in-socks as a temporary measure. Fleece web can tether the epidermis down, preventing deep shear stress or surface friction using the feature of one-directional stretch. Any form of tensionable strapping will offer varying degrees of therapeutic immobilization.

Adhesives

Felts and foams adhered to the foot tend to be affected by water and salts associated with sweat. Adhered materials were formerly made from a thin rubber backing on the desired material. Natural rubber made up the main base and was mixed with a resin known as colophony or one from a synthesized hydrocarbon. Plasticizers, such as lanolin or liquid paraffin, were added for flexibility. A filler, usually zinc oxide, was used to give the backing strength. This type of skin tactifier is no longer used because, whether it was used for strapping or for padding to the sole of the foot or toes, it would store poorly, become brittle and lose its stickiness, causing the padding to be less resilient. Clinically, many patients were recorded as having a zinc oxide allergy. In fact, the zinc oxide was rarely the allergen, the cause of the problem usually being the rubber or other preservatives. Many shoe components still create the same problems because of the wide use of rubber products and preservatives, dyes and allergenic linings.

Hypoallergenic taping

A wide range of hypoallergenic tapes is now available. The adhesives are made from methylmethacrylate as a polymerized monomer, or from other plastics such as polythene and PVC. The adhesives themselves are water or solvent based (Micropore, 3M).

Apart from the fact that patients have a greater tolerance for hypoallergenic tapes, the acrylic adhesives are light and can be applied very thinly, resulting in thinner tapes that are more easily accommodated in footwear than zinc oxide-based tapes. These tapes are primarily used for binding dressings and the range of padded dressings for the foot. However, hypoallergenic tapes are generally less suitable for strapping injuries and preventing motion around joints because they are light in composition and offer less strength. This problem has been addressed in newer products, which have elastic properties and offer an alternative to zinc oxide tapes. Zinc oxide tapes deteriorate much more quickly in storage and have less water resistance when applied to the skin surface. Modern tapes are dispensed on a roll or with a peelable backing and can be cut to the desired length. The wide availability of plastic polymers means that the practitioner has an everincreasing range of adhesives to choose from.

Cement is a broad term often used interchangeably with the term adhesive. Both are synthetic chemicals based on hydrocarbons. Glue, however, has its roots in animal by-products such as bone and hooves.

When manufacturing orthoses, the adhesive needs to run freely to prevent hard lumps forming. The appropriate viscosity should be selected. The drying rate will be influenced by the rate at which the solvent evaporates. 'Tack life' is a term used to describe the period of time after application during which there is still a possibility of making a good bond. The 'green strength' is the strength of the adhesive after making the bond. Again, given the range of materials now available, it is not good enough to rely on one adhesive for bonding all products.

The manufacturer's information must be followed to ensure that the material being used is bonded with the most appropriate adhesive. The effects of shear force upon materials, mentioned at the beginning of this chapter, can be observed in weak bonds, when the adhesive might behave in a brittle manner. Adhesives have to resist multidirectional forces, as well as the effects of varying pH within sweat.

Neoprenes (polychloroprene), polyurethane, epoxy resins and rubber solutions are four groups of adhesive that are used in different situations. *Primers* are often recommended for improving the bonding ability of adhesives. They have the effect of softening the surface, making the adhesive easier to attach, particularly to an asperitous surface. Some adhesives respond to reheating, allowing surfaces to rebond after being separated. This is known as reactivation.

Cohesive bonding

This is possible with materials such as PMMA and polyethylenes. This action occurs when similar molecules are bonded together. PMMA bonds as a resin, while polyethylene is heated so that the chains of molecules can recombine together, forming a very strong bond indeed. Plastic welding rods are available to enhance this process, as well as filling in any gaps between the parent material and the additional material being combined.

Safety

Adhesives are inflammable, and health and safety aspects are paramount in regard to their storage and fire prevention. Solvents can cause respiratory difficulties and depress the central nervous system, causing drowsiness. Good air circulation and venting is essential.

SUMMARY

This chapter has covered the general principles concerning the materials used in producing orthoses and highlighting the types of problem likely to influence their effectiveness.

Modern materials have the advantage of being lightweight while still offering strong mechanical properties, but even these have difficulty in overcoming the triplanar effects of movement of the body over the foot. Successful management with orthoses depends upon a healthy marriage between shoes, the type of orthosis prescribed and the patient's ultimate requirements.

REFERENCES

Bader D L 1993 The potential of advanced composites in orthotic applications. Journal of Orthotics and Prosthetics 1: 33–41

Burnstein A H, Wright T M 1994 Fundamentals of orthopaedic biomechanics. Williams & Wilkins, Baltimore, MD, p 200

Campbell G J, McLure A, Newell E N 1984 Compressive behaviour after simulated service conditions of some foamed materials intended as orthotic insoles. Journal of Rehabilitation Research and Development 21: 57–65

Collins J J, Whittle M W 1989 Impulsive forces during walking and their clinical implications. Clinical Biomechanics 4: 179–187

Health and Safety Executive 1990 The application of COSHH to plastics processing. HMSO, London

Janisse D J 1993 A scientific approach to insole design for the diabetic foot. The Foot 3: 105–108

McIllmurray W J, Greenbaum W 1958 A below-knee weight-bearing brace. Orthotics and Prosthetics Journal 12: 81–82

Oakley T, Pratt D J 1988 Skeletal transients during heel and toe strike running and the effectiveness of some materials in their attenuation. Clinical Biomechanics 3: 159–165

Pratt D J 1988 Polyurethanes in orthotics and orthopaedics. Cellular Polymers 7: 151–164

Pratt D J 1990 Long term comparison of some shock attenuating insoles. Prosthetics and Orthotics International 12: 59–62

Pratt D J 1994 Some aspects of modern orthotics. Physiological Measurement 15: 1–27

Pratt D J, Rees P H, Butterworth R H 1984 RTV silicone insoles. Prosthetics and Orthotics International 8: 54–55

Pratt D J, Tollafield D R, Johnson G R, Peacock C 1993 Foot orthosis. In: Bowker P M, Condie D N, Bader D L, Pratt D J (eds) Biomechanical basic for orthoses. Butterworths, London, p 72–98

Rowley D I, Pratt D J 1986 Orthopaedic bandage-form splinting materials. Clinical Materials 1: 1–8

Tollafield D R, Merriman L M 1995 Assessment of the locomotor system. In: Merriman L M, Tollafield D R (eds) Assessment of the lower limb. Churchill Livingstone, Edinburgh, p 146–147

Whitney A K, Whitney K A 1990 Padding and taping therapy. In: Levy L A, Hetherington V J (eds) Principles and practice of podiatric medicine. Churchill Livingstone, Edinburgh, ch 28

FURTHER READING

Bates B T, Osternig L R, Mason B et al 1979 Foot orthotic devices to modify selected aspects of lower extremity mechanics. American Journal of Sports Medicine 7: 338–342

Bowker P 1993 An update in essential mechanics. In: Bowker P, Bader D L, Pratt D J, Condie D N, Wallace W A (eds) The biomechanical basis of orthotic management. Butterworth-Heinemann, Oxford, ch 2

Radin E L, Rose R M, Blaha J D, Litsky A S 1992 Practical biomechanics for the orthopaedic surgeon, 2nd edn. Churchill Livingstone, New York

Robins R H C 1959 The ankle joint in relation to arthrodesis of the foot in poliomyelitis. Journal of Bone and Joint Surgery 41B: 337–341

Tollafield D R 1985 Mechanical therapeutic coursework. Nene College, UK

Wright D G, Desai S M, Henderson W H 1964 Action of the subtalar and ankle joint complex during the stance phase of gait. Journal of Bone and Joint Surgery 46A: 361–382

11

Mechanical therapeutics in the clinic

Michael Curran

INTRODUCTION

This chapter concerns foot problems that can be managed either wholly or in part by orthotic control at the time of consultation. Broadly, the philosophy of orthotic care provision is that a programme of temporary management is followed until a 'stock' or 'prescription' orthosis is considered more appropriate. The term 'stock' is used in this chapter to refer to ready-prepared orthoses. These are often prepackaged, such as Frelon, Formthotics and Vasyli. Patient versions of some of the aforementioned are now available over the pharmacy counter.

There are certain criteria that should be considered when deciding whether to use mechanical therapy, and these have been summarized in Box 11.1. Alongside the use of orthoses, there is also a role to be played by dressings and other more substantial materials, and this role is discussed below. These materials can provide considerable mechanical therapeutic benefit, even though traditionally they are not considered to be orthoses themselves.

Mechanical therapy can be provided without laboratory prescription in one of five ways:

- dressings and bandages
- clinical padded dressings
- limiting foot and ankle movement
- replaceable orthoses
- moulded thermosetting and thermoplastic orthoses.

Each of these five will be discussed in turn, and for each technique, the function and method of

---

Box 11.1 Criteria used in considering mechanical therapy

- Will the patient benefit from mechanical therapy?
- Is mechanical therapy likely to succeed for the condition being treated, e.g. skin lesions versus joint lesions?
- Will adjunctive therapy be required?
- Will more than one therapeutic modality be advantageous? Success may be improved by implementing more than one therapy; for example heel pain can be treated by heat, non-steroidal anti-inflammatory drugs, injectable steroid and a combination of mechanical modalities.
- What is the prognosis from applying such therapy? For example, will a fixed toe deformity be corrected or interdigital neuroma be relieved by orthoses rather than surgery?
- What is the patient's expectation?
- Does the patient understand what an orthosis is and what it can achieve? Does the patient realize the limitations imposed by orthoses used in more than one pair of shoes?
- Is the patient's footwear suitable?
- Can the patient fit the ideal orthosis into a shoe? If not, will successful treatment be thwarted and the patient become frustrated or even feel cheated?

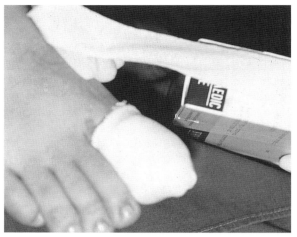

A

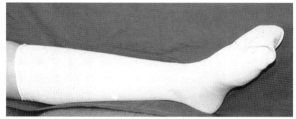

B

Figure 11.1 Examples of tubular dressings that offer the advantage of easy application during consultation (applicator not shown). A, Tubegauz 12. B, Tubigrip E.

application will be considered, highlighting its advantages and disadvantages.

The main objective of mechanical therapy is to resolve a problem as quickly as possible using physics and material science as the basis of treatment. Most orthotic management, whether it uses a simple dressing or a manufactured prescription (Ch. 12), is carried out with the aim of achieving one or more of the objectives described in Box 10.1.

DRESSINGS AND BANDAGES

Since the 1980s, there has been a considerable increase in the number of dressing materials available on the market, and to discuss all of them in detail would fill a chapter all by itself. Besides, all too frequently, information such as this rapidly becomes out of date. However, the practitioner should be aware of the main products on offer.

It is worth, however, mentioning the simple tubular bandage, which has revolutionized the speed at which dressings can be applied to digits, and which offers much greater security to the digit than previous methods (Fig. 11.1A). Gauze and adhesive dressings (formerly 'Bandaids' and 'sticky plasters') have also simplified the approach to dressing wounds.

In addition to the improvement in dressing materials, there have been a number of accompanying innovations (see Table 11.1). The application of tubular bandages, for example, has been greatly eased with the introduction of various applicator aids. Some of these applicators look like badminton shuttlecocks, while others resemble wire cages. The advantage of using an applicator is that there is minimal disturbance of the gauze dressing under the bandage, and also

Table 11.1 Bandage category of dressings

Type	Use
Non-tubular	
Open weave	Dressing lesions, e.g. K band, Kling
Crepe	BPC dressing for lesions and light support
Adherent	Rubberized elastic bandage, stretches, good antislip, highly compressive, e.g. Coban, 3M
Elastic material	Support ankles/knees
Wool 5–10 cm	Cast lining and thick dressing padding, e.g. Velband (Rayon, cotton wool bandage)
Polyurethane foam (PF)	Used for lining casts and bandages, partially water repellent, e.g. Deltatape
Animal wool	Lambswool used largely for insulation properties within tubular bandages
Polymer bandage	See below, compression and emollient properties, e.g. Silopad
Tubular non-elastic	Dressing lesions and supporting gauze against skin, e.g. Tubigauz (Scholl), Tubinette (Seton)
Sizes 01, 12	Digits, hallux
Size 34	Forefoot
Size 56	Whole foot
Size 78	Lower limb
Elasticated	Supporting joints, dressings, reducing oedema and haematoma, increasing shock absorption, lining casts. Water-repellent properties available, e.g. Tubiton (Seton)
Elastic net	A wide gauge net, offers good ventilation, good ability to stretch (Nylon)
Elastic interwoven	Bandage with coloured lines: whole foot and foot/leg for cast lining: red (small, 3.2 cm), green (5 cm) and blue (8 cm)
Stockinette	Sizes increase alphabetically in variable incremental size increases (e.g. Tubigrip (Seton): A (4.20 cm), C (6.75 cm), D (7.50 cm), E (8.75 cm), F (10 cm) and G (12 cm))
Open-cell foam bonded to bandage	Polyurethane (PU) padded on Tubigrip small (7 cm), medium (8 cm) and large (10 cm)
Foam-lined digital bandage	Single- or double-rolled (X) PU foam: A (15 mm) to D (25 mm), or AX to DX for digits
Non-foamed polymer	Digital, forefoot and heel bandages with pads incorporated within thin bandage, e.g. Silipos gel, Silopad
Heel anklet bandages	Heavy-duty bandages pre-formed to fit a variety of circumferences. Incorporation of silicone pads, e.g. Bauerfeind

the likelihood of compression causing a patient discomfort is reduced. Applicators are designed to slide dressings over toes, as well as over the whole limb (Fig. 11.1B).

Indications

Dressings fulfil a number of broad objectives. They protect a wound, allow the absorption of exudate, prevent infection from external sources and stimulate healing.

A dressing can assist with the restoration of limb function, even though its main objective is to reduce pain. An adhesive padded dressing prevents shear over the skin, as well as preventing the exposure of fine nerve endings to the outside environment. The ability to select dressings correctly comes both with the experience gained by 'doing it yourself' and from watching other practitioners.

Bandages are used to support feet and are available in a number of widths, usually between 5 and 10 cm, although 15 cm bandages can be obtained for use with larger feet. They are used to hold gauze dressings in place and are also valuable for strains and sprains, where movement needs to be restricted. Elastication provides compression and prevents slippage, as in the case of 'Tubigrip' bandages (Fig. 11.1B), and this means that oedema is likely to be reduced, thus limiting chronic inflammatory changes. The ankle joint benefits best from this type of wrap-around bandage. Generally, the heavier the material, the stronger the action. The lifespan of the material also tends to increase with weight; therefore, the heavier designs can usually be washed and reused.

A conforming or compression bandage can create skin abrasion and can even limit circulatory flow. Patients should be made aware of complications such as numbness, tingling and cyanotic or white colour changes around their digits, signifying impairment. Older patients, and those with weaker skin, can develop blisters between the toes if rubbing from dressings ensues.

Adhesive techniques are commonly used with all types of foot dressing, and the problem of skin damage must be considered before application. All forms of dressings, plasters or bandages can result in varying degrees of cutaneous moisture; an increase in the number of microbial flora under adhesive dressings can increase the mechanical damage resulting from long-term use.

Summary

Dressings offer a quick method to secure and support the area in question and usually allow a temporary programme of rest during which the lesion, open or otherwise, resolves. Some of the more heavy-duty products available as stock items are designed to last and may incorporate component padding, which in itself can offer emollient benefits.

Open lesions or lesions that have an inflammatory base are the most likely candidates for a dressing. Clinical padding may be incorporated within elasticated forms of bandages to enhance protection.

CLINICAL PADDED DRESSINGS

Padded dressings play a large part in conservative foot management. The many designs available have traditionally been taped to the foot with adhesive strapping. Used in this way, they provide a first-line method of treatment for both acute and chronic problems.

As a group, padded dressings include foamed pads, felt pads and thin coverings such as moleskin and fleece web (Table 11.2). Each material is characterized by different physical properties. Felt is used in conforming dressings, offering resilience sufficient to reduce pressure. Felt is frequently used with cut-outs and cavitations to limit pressure over the load-bearing parts of the foot with most symptoms. Foam has the elastic properties offered by synthetic plastic, acting as

Table 11.2 Clinical padding materials

Material	Description
Felt Semicompressed	Plain (no adhesive) 2, 5, 7 mm Hypoallergenic 5, 7 mm Membrane adhesives (thinner) 5, 7 mm *Properties:* hygroscopic (absorbs perspiration)
Compressed newer felts	Hypoallergenic 2, 5, 7 mm, 30% viscose added. Semicompressed only. Also available as 10 mm; otherwise as above
Foams	Polyurethane (PU open-cell foam) with cover or without. Thin cover provides greater strength, e.g. Fleece foam, Dalzofoam, Elite 5, 7 and 10 mm. Latex (rubber, closed-cell foamed) 4.5, 5 and 7 mm depending upon backing: Swanfoam, Molefoam have fabric covers to improve recovery upon foot loading as PU above. Adhesives vary as with felt
Fine coverings	Carded cotton, stretch two directions, e.g. Fleecy web. Thinnest single stretch covering is Moleskin or Stockinette

'rubber'. Foam lasts surprisingly long compared with felt, which has the disadvantage of absorbing moisture more readily. Cavities in foam are less effective than those in felt and are only necessary to improve foot skin contour. The thin covering pads limit surface shear and can anchor skin when it is placed under tension.

Indications

The main advantage offered by adhesive dressings lies in the fact that there is an element of some bulk positioned next to the lesion. Such dressings tend not to move once they are placed, although you should remember that patients do remove dressings and often replace them incorrectly. Nowadays, hypoallergenic adhesive backing is more common in clinical adhesive products than rubber-based zinc oxide, and so allergic reactions are few and far between. The movement of adhesive attachments, however, does sometimes cause sensitive skin to mimic allergy. Note that in this case there is usually an absence of blistering or of a red outline around the pad. True allergies can only be properly ascertained with a patch test, when a piece of the offensive material shows positive.

Adhesive padding offers selective immobilization by limiting tissue movement; herein lies the success of thin dressings that cover the skin and prevent frictional rub. Additionally, these thin materials take up little room in the shoe.

The practitioner is cautioned against allowing patients to become dependent upon the common padded dressing, because many of the benefits, while effective, are only temporary.

A list indicating some of the diverse uses of these dressings to ameliorate pain in the foot is provided in Box 11.2.

The mechanical basis of selection

When deciding which dressing to use in treatment and how to use that dressing, two questions need to be answered: what is the desired objective and what is the most appropriate material to use in achieving that? Below, we dis-

---

> **Box 11.2** Indications for the use of padded dressings
>
> - Corns: redistribution (plantar/dorsal/apical/inter-digital)
> - Ulcers: protection by redistribution (as for corns plus malleoli)
> - Bony alignment protection: prominences associated with hallux valgus, exostoses and Tailor's bunion
> - Increased alignment and loading of dysfunctioning metatarsals
> - Heel pad shock attenuation: posterior or plantar foam pad in 3–6 mm thicknesses
> - Digital deformity alignment: props under toes
> - Arch discomfort: infills (valgus pads for fascia strain)
> - Elevation of part of the foot: for Achilles tendon pain, limb length discrepancy
> - Inflammation and blistering: cutaneous or deeper trauma, skin movement limited
> - Tongue pads and heel protection: for shoes (see Ch. 13).

---

cuss this question of selection in terms of the objectives of orthotic management described in Box 10.1.

Redistribution

In order to reduce pressure, one must decrease the influencing force or increase the area over which that force acts. When an intermittent force is applied to a relatively small, localized area of the foot, adhesive padding can provide the increased surface area needed to dissipate that force.

The pad must be large enough to provide sufficient surface area to achieve the desired reduction in pressure; it must consist of a material that will resist compression; it must be positioned so as to achieve maximal protection without actually encroaching on the site; and its thickness must be such that it can be accommodated in the shoe. A successful result will not be achieved unless:

- the cause of the pressure is correctly diagnosed
- the direction of the pressure is correctly gauged

- an evaluation is made of the area to which pressure is to be redistributed.

Generally, the adhesive material used for the purposes of redistribution is semi-compressed felt. No scientific evidence supports such a selection and, as previously mentioned, foamed pads can offer equal benefit. Cavitations and cut-outs using felt probably work better than those in foam, but the reason for selecting felt is probably historical and based on the ease of handling such materials with scissors.

Compensation

The objective of compensation is shock attenuation, that is, to decrease the velocity of impact of the force causing the undesirable stress. A material placed over the area that is being stressed does this. The material needs to be sufficiently dense to be truly effective. Foams offer satisfactory resilience because of the cells created during the foaming process. The material acts as a pneumatic cushion; with foot-ground pressure, the foam deforms and air is expelled. When the pressure is released, air reenters the matrix, returning the pad to its original shape. Effective materials such as Sorbothane (Viscolas) and Silopad (Silipos) are reducing the popularity of adhesive cushioning.

Rest

Surface friction is often generated between the foot and the shoe. When this force becomes excessive, blisters form, which can lead to callosity. A thin material placed between the two surfaces will reduce tissue movement, as well as friction and shear stresses, the material itself absorbing the forces and the heat that is generated. The most widely used antifrictional material is a fleecy web comprising loosely knitted wool fibres on which an adhesive is spread. It is easily stretched and consequently conforms to the contours of the foot. Skin movement into the toe sulcus can be temporarily prevented by applying tension proximally with a fleece cover anchored just beneath the toes.

Stabilization

The temporary realignment of bony structures occurs when the force, and hence the weight, borne by an otherwise non-weight-bearing part is increased. This may occur, for instance, at the second metatarsal head, which becomes overloaded if the first metatarsal does not contact the ground efficiently; the manifestation of this extra load is usually seen as a callus. In this case, a pad is required to withstand compression. Compressed felt is preferred but is often too hard to adhere to the surface of the foot. It is used more frequently on insole bases.

Containment

Application of medication, such as emollients, keratolytics and caustics, within firm dressings is most effective when the medication is confined to a precisely defined area. This containment of medicaments is achieved by using a variety of shapes of dressing, e.g. crescents, cavities or complete apertures in the pad (Fig. 11.2).

Application of padded dressings

Individual dressing pads have evolved over time and there are now many variations in design. The discussion of various pads that follows does not purport to be a definitive one but merely aims to describe those that are most commonly used.

This group of firm dressings is almost always secured with strapping, and this means of holding pads in place will be considered first. (The term 'taping' is synonymous with 'strapping'; however, in the context of this book, taping has been used to describe a therapeutic technique (see later) and strapping is used to describe the securing of padded dressings.)

Strapping

Strapping can be used in many different ways. Whatever method is employed, the dressing should achieve the following: it should conform to the foot, provide the patient with comfort,

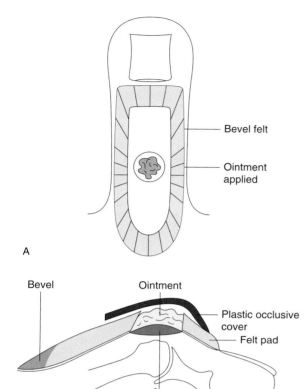

A

B

Figure 11.2 Containment of medications. A, The dorsal cover provides greater deflection of load over the interphalangeal joint of the digit, as well as providing a cavity or aperture through which medication can be introduced. B, A thin cover, cut from a plastic bag or sheet, will prevent any undue leakage of the medication.

have good adhesion, and maintain the correct position against the foot.

In order to achieve the above aims, one should ensure that the strapping does not create wrinkles in the skin, which can cause discomfort, that all edges of the padding are covered, and that the edges of the strapping are rounded so as to reduce the chances of it peeling away from the skin and taking the padding with it.

Particular care should be taken when strapping a digit; digital circulation must not be constricted. Modern elastic-type strapping is ideal for digits as it conforms neatly to contours and

will stretch if for any reason the digit should swell. Tubular toe bandages such as 'Tubegauz' are popular in securing digital pads.

Padding

The basic concept of a pad or firm dressing as described in this chapter should be modified to the requirements of the presenting problem. However, certain principles of construction should always be followed; these are described in Box 11.3.

Design of padded dressings

Digital padding

The digital pads described below are usually constructed from semi-compressed felt. Single, and in some cases multiple, pads are secured with 01/12 Tubegauz. Shaped adhesive strapping is used to ensure that there is no movement from the pad/dressing against the skin.

Dorsal digital cover The thickness of the dorsal digital cover lies on the dorsum of the toe and extends its complete length from the base of the nail. The distal border is slightly shaped to

---

Box 11.3 Summary of points to consider when applying padded dressings

- The shape of the pad should conform to the size and natural contours of the individual foot.
- The perimeter should be bevelled gradually to avoid bulky and uncomfortable ridges. The bulk of any pad should lie in the natural hollows of the anatomy and posterior to the structures to be protected.
- Bevels are angled cuts made on the top surface (top-bevelled) or undersurface-adhesive side (under-bevelled). The straight bevel can be cut along the edge or a pie crust bevel can be selected perpendicular to the edge, allowing the pad to curve. A double bevel is created by two parallel bevels made along the edge, thus widening the bevel.
- Cavities within the pad should be half the thickness of the material used and of sufficient depth to accommodate dressings and protuberances.
- Cavities and apertures may be optionally bevelled slightly on the adhesive side to aid conformity to tissue contours.

follow the base of the nail, the proximal border is slightly rounded, and both sides run longitudinally straight down the toe without extending down from the dorsum. The pad has a top bevel on all sides and a cavity on its adhesive aspect, or aperture, usually at the level of the proximal interphalangeal joint (IPJ). The indication for use is where redistribution of pressure from the proximal IPJ is required, and so the material of choice is felt (see Fig. 11.2).

The *dorsal digital crescent* is a modification of the dorsal cover and may be employed where less bulk is required within the shoe. The distal border lies proximal to the joint or lesion to be protected and is under-bevelled. A further modification involves the extension to a double or multiple crescent that serves adjoining toes (Fig. 11.3).

Horseshoe pad The horseshoe pad offers redistribution of pressure over a greater area than does the dorsal digital cover and offers a means of protecting a dorsal digital lesion that allows dressings to be changed without disturbing the pad. As the name suggests, the pad is roughly the shape of a horseshoe, with two longitudinal arms, which may lie, for instance, on the dorsum of toes 2 and 4, continuous with a central crescentic section, which sits immediately behind a lesion on toe 3 (Fig. 11.4). The pad is top-bevelled around its outer margin. Under-bevelling in the crescentic area proximal to the lesion is optional. A cavity or aperture in one of the longitudinal arms can be adapted to accommodate a second lesion on an adjacent toe.

Apical crescent The apical crescent is designed to redistribute pressure from a lesion at the apex of the toe. The pad sits around the pulp of the digit and is bevelled by small vertical cuts (pie crusting), allowing the pad to be shaped around the end of the digit (Fig. 11.5). The pad is commonly used where there is a degree of rigidity in the toe and straightening is not practical, and where lesions constantly develop on the tip or around the nail edge.

Digital prop and long prop The prop is designed to have an extension effect on the clawed toe, thus assisting with ground purchase. In the case of fixed toe deformities, it offers pro-

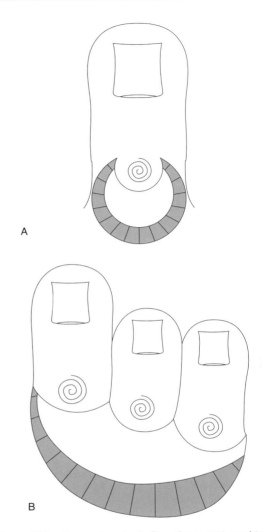

Figure 11.3 Crescent pads. A, Dorsal crescent used to create less bulk than dorsal cover; this is not as effective for holding medicaments. B, Multiple crescents for more than one toe, e.g. retracted toes with dorsal lesions. The bulk of this padded dressing can sit in the space created by the drawn back toes.

tection and redistribution of high loads. In this latter respect, there is some similarity to the apical crescent. The adhesive side is bevelled to fit into the toe crease and, where the toe is sufficiently flexible, to extend the distal IPJ forwards. The side bevels fit against the lateral toes, as shown in Figure 11.6. In its adhesive form, the pad is only suitable for short periods. It is usual to progress to silicone moulds or to a replaceable

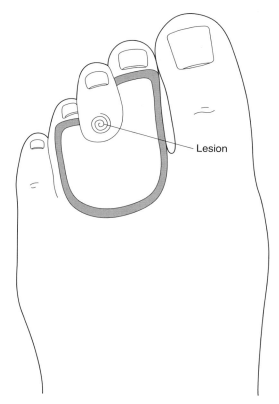

Figure 11.4 Adhesive horseshoe design: shaped to spread load across adjacent digits with bevel indicated and excellent for assisting healing ulceration over interphalangeal joints.

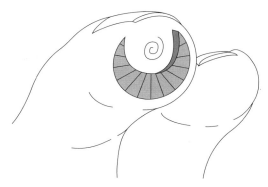

Figure 11.5 Apical crescent is best pie crust bevelled. This technique allows better conformation around the end of the toe and can then be secured with 01 or 12 Tubegauz.

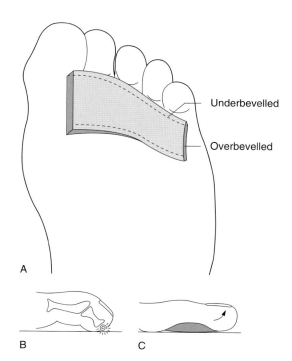

Figure 11.6 Props. A–C, The long prop shown is an extension of the single prop affecting the apex of toes: protective and partially corrective in function.

orthodigital device. The long prop is a modification of the single prop and is applied where additional toes need supporting; often, the three central toes need to be supported together. The prop can be secured with 1.25 cm wide tape.

Interdigital wedge/dumb-bell pad The interdigital wedge (IDW) is a protective dressing that separates adjoining toes, reducing the shear stresses. The IDW is shaped to fit the side of the toe; the under-bevelled base is shaped to fit the webbing, and the top-bevelled sides follow the shape of the toe distally and extend slightly in the dorsal and plantar directions. The distal border is either crescented to fit proximal to the lesion or extends almost the full length of the toe, in which case the pad will contain a cavity if redistribution of pressure is the aim. Some prac-

titioners prefer to strip the adhesive backing from the foam material, as the toes can hold the IDW with stockings adequately (Fig. 11.7A). This technique offers a non-adhesive removeable pad.

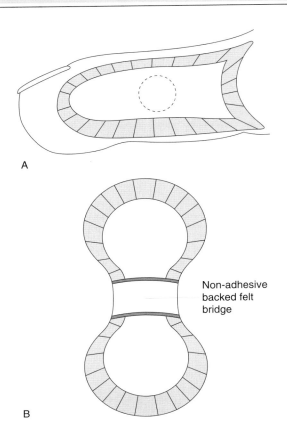

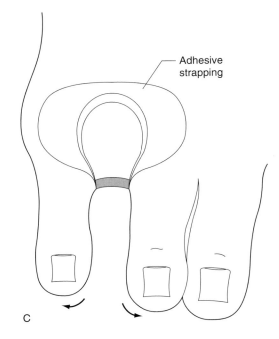

Figure 11.7 Interdigital dressings are a short-term alternative to silicones. A, This dressing provides a small degree of separation and uses a cavity. B, C, The dumb-bell pad. As show in (C), it spreads two toes where the lesion lies at the base of the cleft, commonly digits 4 and 5.

The dumb-bell pad is so-called because of its shape. The central stem of the dumb-bell is under-bevelled to strip away its adhesive and placed interdigitally at the base of the cleft. The two bulbous ends are top-bevelled and adhered to the foot on the dorsal and plantar aspects. The use of these pads has been largely superseded by silicone devices. The dumb-bell's main function is to spread two toes, particularly toes four and five, the cleft of which is a common site for soft corns. The pad is palliative and will rarely eradicate the problem and so is used for short periods to reduce symptoms (Fig. 11.7B,C). Adhesive tape is the preferred means of attaching the dorsal and plantar 'bulbous' ends to the skin.

Plantar phalangeal pad The plantar phalangeal pad is used almost exclusively for the hallux but is occasionally used for a lesser toe. It offers protection from a plantar lesion over the IPJ either by redistribution or by cushioning, depending upon the material used. Short-term alleviation from the symptoms of corns, cysts and bursae can be obtained. The dressing is shaped to resemble the plantar surface of the toe. The base is under-bevelled and follows the line of the toe as it joins the webbing. The top-bevelled sides follow the line of the toe distally and the distal border is rounded to the end of the toe. A cavity or aperture may be employed where necessary (Fig. 11.8).

Plantar padded dressings

In this section, four main plantar padded dressing techniques are described, each offering a different function. Unfortunately, few studies have been conducted into their effectiveness despite the use of pressure and force plate techniques to analyse load deflection. Plantar dressings of this nature often seem to work empirically in reducing foot pain. The practitioner is advised, as with many of these padding strategies, to prescribe

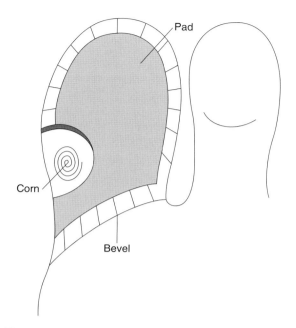

Figure 11.8 Plantar phalangeal pad used most commonly for the hallux.

the metatarsal pads on a short-term basis (i.e. 5–7 days) and then to consider conversion to an insole or alternative design should management appear successful. These padded dressings are strapped into place, overlapping the edges 50:50. The methods used to secure the pad vary: 'goal post' (boxing the pad in) and 'church door' (formation of an 'A' around the pad) strapping have in most cases been replaced by the overlapping horizontal method, which starts at the base of the pad and ends with the distal tape trimmed to conform to the plantar skin without reaching into the sulcus.

Plantar cover Lesions commonly arise under the metatarsal heads and an adhesive plantar cover is used in order to provide redistribution of pressure, shock attenuation (cushioning) or friction reduction, depending on the material used.

The shape in foam rubber provides full thickness of material over metatarsal heads 1–5. The top-bevelled distal border follows the metatarsal formula (anterior metatarsal order of length), allowing space between its termination and the webbing area for the application of strapping.

The sides, also top-bevelled, pass proximally in line with the foot, covering the full plantar metatarsal surface without extending towards the dorsum; the bevel allows the pad to curve along the side of the foot at the extreme plantar edge. All borders are singly top-bevelled, except for the proximal edge which uses a double bevel. The plantar cover extends proximally 1.25–2.5 cm distal to the styloid process of the fifth metatarsal.

The felt material version of the plantar cover is designed to have an aperture or modification to its shape; this may take the form of a 'wing' for metatarsal head areas 1 or 5, or a 'U' for areas 2–4. When redistribution is to be combined with cushioning, the 'winged' or 'U-shaped' area may be filled with foam rubber. The same principle may employ a cushioning button within a complete aperture in the felt. An aperture lies over the lesion, thus affording protection from mechanical stress. The use of semi-compressed felt without some aperture is generally considered to be undesirable as it has no benefit to the patient. Where a full, non-apertured dressing pad is used, foam is preferable, at least for its shock-attenuating properties (Fig. 11.9A).

Metatarsal bar The metatarsal bar differs from the plantar cover in that the main bulk of the material lies behind the metatarsals. This design takes up less shoe room as well as redistributing load from the metatarsal heads proximally.

The pad is shaped and bevelled similarly to the plantar cover but does not extend as far distally. The distal border follows the metatarsal formula but has its full thickness lying behind the metatarsal heads. Some use a bevel, while others prefer the full pad thickness without a bevel to allow maximum load distribution from the metatarsal heads to the shafts. A modification to the pad uses a foam apron to cushion a traumatized metatarsal head region (Fig. 11.9B).

Plantar metatarsal pad The plantar metatarsal pad is a traditional pad and it provides a different function to those described above. It is often confused with the plantar cover but has been used to elevate metatarsal heads sufficiently to extend the proximal phalanges at the metatarsophalangeal joint (MTPJ). The effectiveness of this technique as long-term correction is questionable. In flexible deformities, it can be argued that contractures are dissuaded at the MTPJ. The use as a metatarsal brace or for metatarsal alignment does seem to have value with some forms of metatarsalgia and indeed there is some degree of success in treating Morton's plantar digital neuroma in its early stages (Fig. 11.9C,D).

The plantar metatarsal pad is made from felt. The distal edge follows the metatarsal formulae

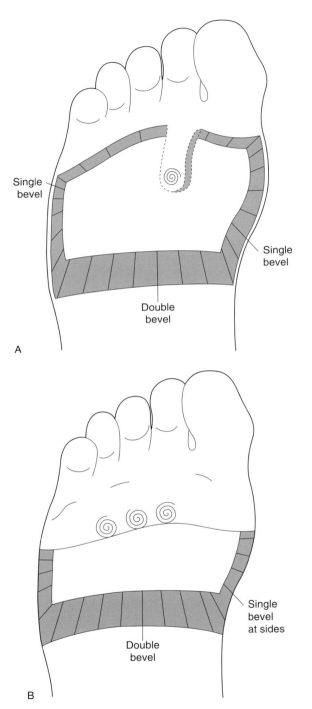

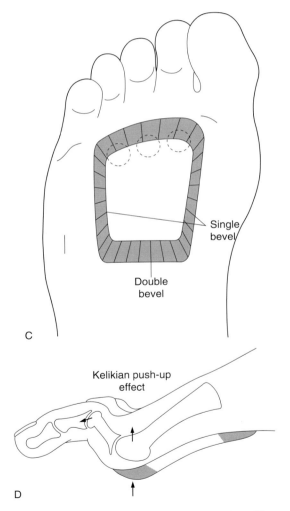

Figure 11.9 Plantar padded dressings. A, Plantar cover, usually has apertures for felt materials. B, Plantar metatarsal bar; the anterior end is proximal to the metatarsal heads. C, Plantar metatarsal pad; the distal bevel elevates and appears to influence the metatarsal alignment at the metatarsal head level (this influence shown in D).

with the width spanning between metatarsals 1–2 and 4–5, the extent of its lateral top-bevels.

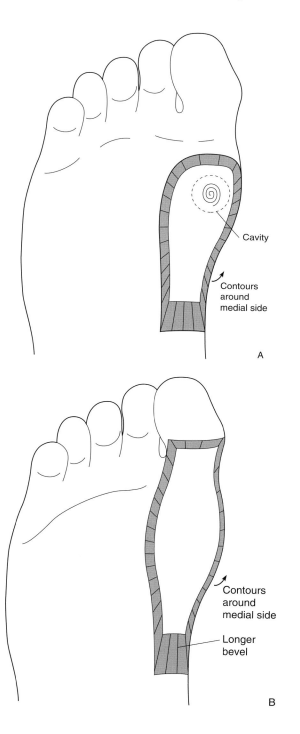

The proximal end is placed, as with other metatarsal pads, 1.25–2.5 cm distal to the styloid process, and the distal top-bevel must have its greatest thickness over the metatarsal heads to provide some lever function.

Shaft pad An unmodified shaft pad attracts a high proportion of load bearing to the underlying metatarsal and, therefore, alters the amount of pressure sustained by the remaining metatarsals. The pad may either elevate the metatarsal or be used to protect it.

The distal edge of the pad, constructed in felt, is rounded and extends over the MTPJ. The sides follow the edges of the metatarsal, the whole width of the bone being covered, and extend its full length. The proximal border is cut squarely across the foot with the edges being top-bevelled. The area covering the metatarsal head may be cut into a cavity or crescent as required (Fig. 11.10A,B).

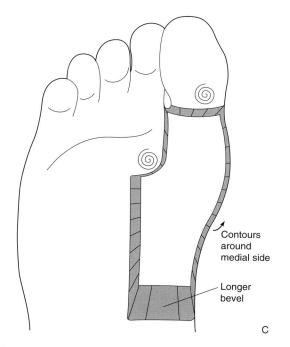

Figure 11.10 Variants on the plantar pad. A, Shaft pad over the first metatarsal. B, An extended first ray shaft is used to completely immobilize the first metatarsophalangeal joint. C, The L-shaped pad functions to protect a distal lesion over the plantar hallux as well as over the second metatarsal head.

Another modification may be employed when there is pain in the first MTPJ. An extended shaft that passes distally to the IPJ of the hallux serves as a splint to the MTP joint, reducing the capacity for dorsiflexion and, therefore, the pain associated with movement. Alternatively, this same pad may be used to redistribute pressure from an IPJ lesion.

L pad   The L pad is a variation on the shaft pad and combines the effect of an extended shaft with a metatarsal bar into one pad. It is usefully employed when significant lesions are present over several metatarsal heads and the IPJ of the hallux. The pad follows the same specifications as the extended shaft, except that it also extends laterally into the described shape of the metatarsal bar, thus appearing like the letter 'L'. If a lesion is present under the first metatarsal head, this may be protected by means of a cavity (Fig. 11.10C).

Padded dressings for the rearfoot

Plantar calcaneal pad   The design of the plantar calcaneal pad follows the shape of the plantar aspect of the heel to the anterior of the calcaneus, where it is cut straight across and proximal to the styloid process by 2.5 cm. A single top-bevel is employed all around to ensure good contact upon strapping into place, except at the anterior border where a double bevel is used. A felt pad may have a cavity or aperture to redistribute pressure from lesions or to contain ointment, using the model already illustrated for the digital pad in Figure 11.2. Unmodified, and in sufficient thickness, it may raise the heel slightly in the shoe and give a degree of rest to a strained Achilles tendon. Foam material in various thicknesses may be applied for shock attenuation in a traumatized heel.

Retrocalcaneal pad   The retrocalcaneal pad is used for redistribution of pressure away from a lesion at the posterior of the heel; it always contains a cavity or an aperture. A pie crust (vertical bevel) all around ensures good conformation around the lesion. The base of the pad follows the line of the weight-bearing aspect of the posterior of the heel, while the vertically ascending

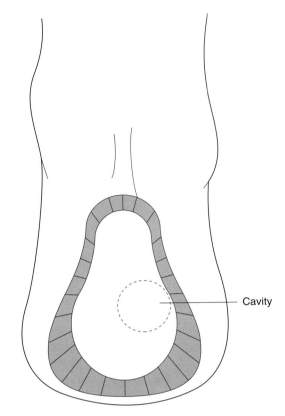

Cavity

Figure 11.11   Retrocalcaneal pad can be apertured for bursae or painful spurs created by Haglund's deformity, or where tissue overlying the heel has become inflamed or sensitive, e.g. perniosis, heel neuroma.

sides curve inwards and complete the shape at the top of the posterior of the heel. In order to achieve comfort and ensure retention, it is essential that the sides of the pad fully embrace the contour of the heel and do not terminate prematurely forming a prominence (Fig. 11.11).

Miscellaneous dressings

Valgus pad   The valgus pad is essentially a space filler and is valuable in a cavus-type foot and in pronated feet experiencing discomfort from fascial strain. In the high-arch foot, tension is removed from the tightly strung fascia, giving some temporary relief.

Sometimes promoted as an antipronatory device, it is unlikely to fulfil this function, partic-

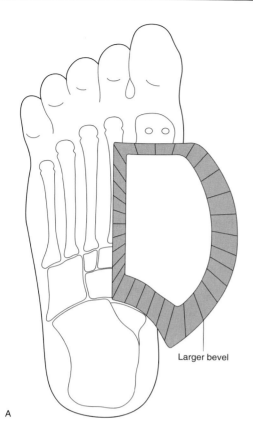

A

Larger bevel

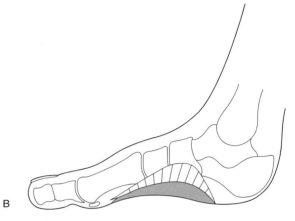

B

Figure 11.12 Adhesive valgus pad. Adhesive pads are shaped somewhat differently from replaceable designs. The pad conforms to the foot with double bevels providing arch conformity (B). This does not provide antipronatory therapy.

ularly in an adhesive form, which has relatively low bulk. However, it does reduce deformation of the foot under load and as such imparts a certain amount of rest to the overstressed foot, reducing strain along the plantar fascia and immobilizing the tarsal joints in the presence of osteoarthritis.

The anterior border of the pad sits just behind the first and second metatarsal heads. From the medial aspect, the pad passes backwards to the tuberosity of the navicular and from there to the medial edge of the weight-bearing aspect of the heel as a cut-away. The lateral border then follows a straight edge in metatarsal space 2–3, bevelled so as not to make shoe fit too bulky. All edges are top-bevelled in order to achieve maximum conformation (Fig. 11.12).

Hallux valgus oval   If cushioning is the aim, Tubifoams or Silipads make the best replaceable dressings. The adhesive dressing is again tempo-

rary, as its main function lies in protecting open wounds, sinuses and ulcers.

Classically, the felt or foam hallux valgus oval pad is ovoid (egg) in shape but tailored to contour the individual foot; this pad has a cavity if redistribution of pressure from the prominent medial aspect of the first MTPJ is required (Fig. 11.13). The main indication for this modality is to protect a lesion over the medial first MTP joint. The exact position of the bony prominence dictates the precise position of the pad, but the following points should be observed: dorsally it should not extend over the tendon of extensor hallucis longus and thus interfere with tendon sheath function; distally it should not extend as far as the IPJ; the full thickness of the pad should not extend plantarly under the foot, although it is acceptable if the bevelled area does so for a short distance. If footwear accommodation does prove a problem, a viable alternative is the hallux valgus crescent. This has the same shape as the oval, except that the anterior portion is crescented to the bony prominence. As with the oval, all edges are singly top-bevelled, except for the crescent, which is back-bevelled or left unbevelled. A *'Tailor's bunion' oval* has the same specifications as the hallux valgus oval but is used on the lateral side of the fifth MTPJ.

Tendon or saddle pad The tendon or saddle pad is used for dorsal protection of the extensor hallucis longus tendon. Roughly oval in shape and top-bevelled, it has a central channel of adhesive removed for the tendon and may have a deeper cavity cut within the channel to accommodate a lesion. The pad is placed on the dorsal surface of the first MTPJ, with the lateral edge lying over the first intermetatarsal space and the medial edge lying on the line of the dorsomedial aspect of the first MTPJ.

Summary

Adhesive padding should only be employed for short periods of time. Success is based upon a number of factors, such as patient acceptability and occupational requirements (i.e. some shoe types may not allow sufficient room for the pads). The obstacle presented by padding to good hygiene, the detrimental effect on the skin with long-term use, and the short life of the materials used dictate the need for eventual progression to a replaceable or alternative form of orthosis or footwear adaptations.

LIMITING FOOT AND ANKLE MOVEMENT

Adhesive tape may be used to limit function and provide rest to an injured part in an acute condition, or periodically to give support to repetitive strain injuries, for instance in sports enthusiasts. Movement can also be limited by casting the area in question.

Neither adhesive taping nor casting is a long-term solution to relieving foot pain, but they both inhibit movement without taking up too much room in footwear.

Recently introduced products provide splinting by pumping air into plastic air sacs (e.g. Aircast). While rather expensive, these devices are easily removed and replaced by patients with little technical instruction.

Taping

Taping can be used successfully for short periods on the ankle, as low- and high-dye taping, on

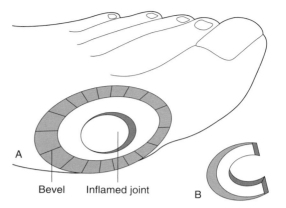

Figure 11.13 The hallus valgus oval (HVO). This can be used on either side of the foot and can be shaped appropriately to conform to footwear and provide protection from cutaneous irritation. A cavity (A) or crescent (B) is provided, the latter being most suitable where the distal end is too bulky.

the arch structure of the foot and on the first MTP joint. Some patients can replace the taping at home to continue the effect, and this is commonplace with sports people. You should note the following points when applying taping to the skin:

- tension should be applied without skin wrinkling
- taping should not encircle parts likely to be vascularly compromised
- taping should be contoured to ensure that it does not ruck up and peel back from socks or shoewear
- a skin tactifier such as tincture of benzoin can be helpful
- hair should be shaved first to avoid damage
- taping should never be used directly on known sensitive skin, infection, or bullous or oedematous tissues
- taping is best overlapped evenly
- the joint position should be corrected before applying the tape.

First metatarsophalangeal joint support

In the case of an acutely painful first MTPJ, strapping can provide rest by limiting dorsiflexion and abduction (Fig. 11.14).

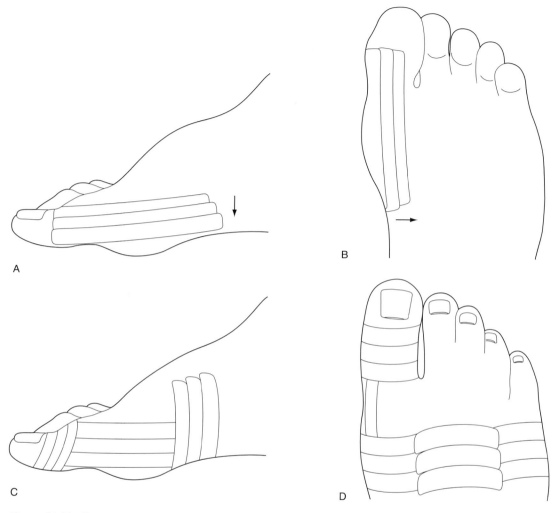

Figure 11.14 Fan strapping is a useful method for painful joints associated with transient synovitis, hallux limitus and acute trauma to the first metatarsophalangeal joint. A–D, 1.25 cm wide strips, usually zinc oxide (ZO) tapes, are placed around the first toe joint, overlapping each other. The proximal ends are left loose until all the ends can be pulled into tension and secured at the base as well as at the distal end around the great toe.

The patient is laid supine with the foot over the edge of the treatment table. If required, the relevant skin area may be prepared with a tincture of benzoin (BPC) or Opsite (Smith & Nephew) to assist skin adherence. The tape used is non-stretchable and 2.5 cm in width. With the hallux placed in the desired position, which is neither dorsiflexed nor plantarflexed, the first strip of tape is placed longitudinally on the superior lateral aspect of the hallux, starting at the mid-portion of the distal phalanx and extending proximally to the base of the first metatarsal. Additional strips are placed to slightly overlap each previous strip in a medial direction, continuing downwards and onto the plantar aspect of the toe and foot. When applying these strips, no traction should be applied in case it dorsiflexes the hallux, but the tape must never be allowed to remain slack because this will decrease the effect.

Anchoring strips are then applied to secure the longitudinal strips. In order to avoid any risk of compromising circulation, the anchoring strips around the toe should never completely encircle it but should terminate at the margins of the interdigital space. In order to avoid tightness, anchoring strips around the longitudinal arches should terminate at either end on the dorsum of the foot.

Low-dye taping

Low-dye taping a form of taping that can be used for symptoms of plantar fasciitis and that has also been found to have an antipronatory effect (McCloskey 1992; Fig. 11.15). McCloskey found a positive effect using low-dye taping with Kistler force plate analysis ($P < 0.05$) for 75% of patients studied ($n = 16$). Again, the same width of tape is employed and the patient lies supine with the foot extending over the table edge and at right angles to the leg. The first of three strips is applied starting proximal to the fifth MTPJ. After the tape is secured on the outside of the foot, the end is grasped in one hand and wrapped around the heel while simultaneously inverting the heel slightly. The end of the tape is then attached to the medial side of the foot, terminating just proximal to the first MTPJ.

This is repeated twice, each subsequent tape overlapping the previous by two-thirds. Finally, transverse strips of 5 cm width should be placed without dragging the skin and causing discomfort. They are placed across the foot from dorsolateral to dorsomedial and should extend from the base of the fifth metatarsal to just proximal to the first and fifth MTPJ.

False fascia taping (for fasciitis)

Tapes applied from the toe sulci to the posterior heel support the three bands of fascia when discomfort has been clearly identified. Figure 11.16 illustrates rigid zinc oxide taping supported with Mefix to ensure good skin attachment. Elasticated plaster rolls provide additional support and are ideal for limiting tensile stresses.

Smaller feet will require two tapes of 5 cm width, whereas large feet will require three.

Ankle support

Support for the ankle (Fig. 11.17) may be necessary in the following cases:

- following inversion sprains, where taping is needed to support the lateral ligament of the ankle without unduly restricting joint motion
- following eversion sprains
- as a general support for the structures of the ankle in an attempt to prevent sprains.

In the first two cases, two types of tape are needed: a 3.75 cm wide non-stretchable and a 5 cm wide elastic adhesive bandage. Two gauze 'diamonds' are positioned, one on the anterior of the ankle to prevent undue constriction from the tape upon ankle dorsiflexion, and one posteriorly to protect the Achilles tendon and prevent undue skin shear. An assistant may be needed to maintain these in place initially. Strips of non-stretch tape are used at first. With the lower leg extended over the edge of the table, the first strip is placed on the medial side of the lower leg and then is taken vertically downwards under the heel and up onto the lateral side of the foot and lower leg as a 'stirrup'. Further strips are added, each slightly overlapping the previous one, until the final strip finishes well in front of the malleolus.

Using the same type of tape, horizontal strips are now applied. The first starts on the lateral side of the foot and passes behind the heel and along the medial aspect of the foot. Further strips are added in overlap fashion until the malleolus is covered. To complete the ankle support, the elastic adhesive bandage is used to form a 'figure of eight'. This begins with placement on the lateral aspect of the leg above the malleolus and passes downwards and medially across the instep, under the foot, up and over the lateral aspect of the foot, and finally upwards and medially to pass above and behind the medial malleolus and terminate at its origin.

In eversion sprains, the directions are reversed; the vertical strips are applied from

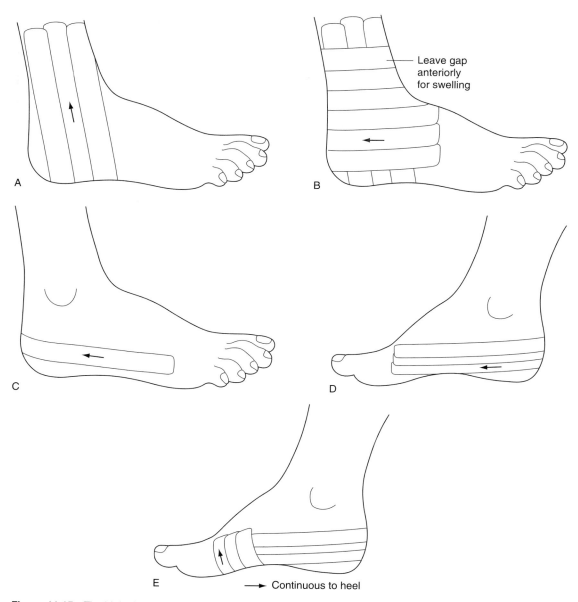

Figure 11.15 The high-dye strapping (A, B) and low-dye strapping (C–E) act as basic orthoses for controlling the ankle and subtalar joint (high dye) and the subtalar joint (low dye), respectively. Taping in an inverted position takes the stress off the fascia and may be applied in a neutral subtalar joint position.

lateral to medial, and the figure-of-eight is applied in the opposite direction.

In order to prevent sprains, a 5 cm crepe bandage is better than a tape. The limb is positioned as before. The end of the bandage is placed on the medial side of the lower leg and encircles it before passing down and over the instep to the lateral side of the foot. The strap is then taken under the foot, up and over the instep, and then under the foot once more. On

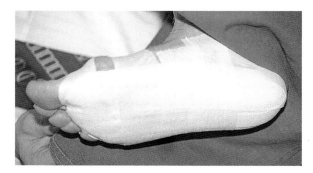

Figure 11.16 False plantar fascia: an alternative system with rigid taping used in longitudinal strips to support the fascia. Elasticated taping is preferred but the principal direction of application is the same and follows the main bands of fascia. Transverse 5 cm taping with Mefix (a hypoallergic tape) supports the zinc oxide-based false plantar fascia tape.

emerging at the medial side, the bandage forms a heel lock by passing obliquely backwards and around the heel to the front of the leg. It then encircles the leg, passes over the instep in a medial direction and under the heel to form a heel lock on the opposite side. Finally it is secured with a short piece of tape horizontally around the leg.

In some cases, it may be advantageous to incorporate an adhesive pad, such as a valgus pad, to assist with a medial foot influence, stabilizing the midtarsus.

Cautions

There are some disadvantages associated with taping. Plaster allergy dictates that tape cannot be adhered to the skin; it is sometimes possible to overcome this by covering most of the foot/lower leg with tubular bandage, which is adhered at either end with hypoallergenic tape. The taping is then placed on the tubular bandage rather than directly onto the skin. However, the intimacy of contact is lost and the effect is likely to be less than adequate. Occupational constraints allied to limitations of hygiene may make taping therapy inappropriate, but these constraints need to be balanced against the severity of the condition under treatment.

Summary

Taping for the acute condition is but one stage in a comprehensive treatment plan. Once the acute phase has passed, the practitioner must consider the next or adjunctive stage in the plan. This may take the form of physical therapy, such as contrast foot baths, infrared irradiation, ultrasound, injection, imaging for further diagnosis (radiographs) and oral/local medication. Rehabilitation may involve passive stretching or exercises. The success of the taping regimen may suggest that a form of orthosis is indicated; this is particularly the case with low-dye taping. To be effective, taping should only be used for short periods. If there is an obvious benefit, patients can be taught to apply their own tapes.

Casting

Casting is a very useful method for enforcing rest. The following four systems are briefly described, with notes on how to apply the casts safely:

- foot cast
- back slab
- full below-knee cast
- pre-moulded plastic walker.

General indications

Foot pain without a clearly defined source can be assisted once the practitioner is satisfied that there is no specific underlying pathology. Apart from use in fractures, casting techniques can provide a valuable tool in managing acute pain.

Cautions

In each of the cases described, the technique offers rest and alignment of the joints of the foot: the ankle is completely limited if splinting is raised above the malleoli. Once a joint is immobilized, it will stiffen as a result of disuse and will thus need rehabilitating afterwards. Bone and muscle will atrophy, as the tissues are not normally exercised. Deterioration of bone during lengthy periods of casting can be limited by bone

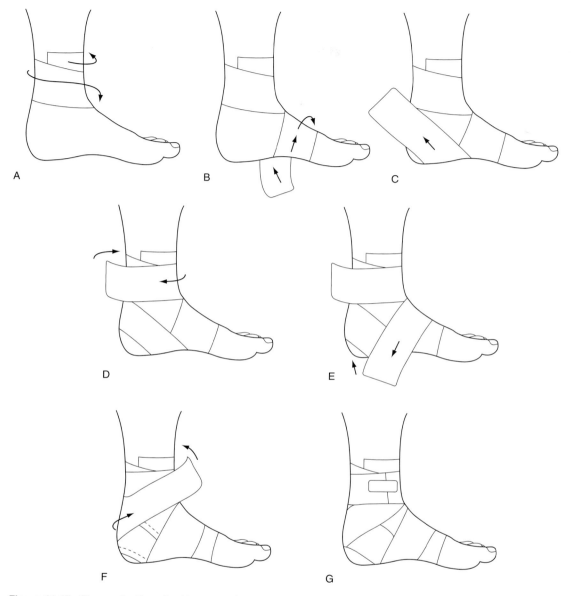

Figure 11.17 The application of ankle supportive taping in order to lock the talocrural and subtalar joints (A–G). The material used should be of a heavy-duty nature, 2.5–5 cm wide and ideally should have a longitudinal stretch. Indications include ankle pain without gross swelling and lateral/medial ankle sprains, especially where bone and joint pathology has been ruled out by X-ray film first.

growth stimulators, which are incorporated within casts to reduce the rate of osteopenia.

Casts applied without sufficient care to protect bony prominences may cause ulcers and erosions of normal skin, blisters and nerve compression. Peroneal compression around the head of the fibula can produce foot drop. Additional padding is required at the heel, digits, lateral joints and malleoli. Patients must be advised to return to the clinic should any unexplained pain or numbness occur. Digits are best left exposed so that their colour can always be inspected. An emergency contact number should be available for use outside clinic hours, or arrangement should be made with accident and emergency departments in advance. It is good practice to give patients a note advising any other practitioners of the reason for treatment. This is particularly helpful if someone else has to remove the cast. Weight bearing is highly desirable to avoid deep vein or pulmonary thromboses following injuries. Patients should be advised that some limb exercise is necessary, by contracting calf muscles and moving the knee joint where the foot and ankle are restricted. Inappropriate casting can also leading to cast disease (wasting and pain from swelling), and sympathetic and ischaemic dystrophy.

All casts are applied in a similar way; a tubular bandage is used as the first layer and this is followed by wool (Velband or similar) to protect the skin. The wool is wrapped around the limb, overlapping at each turn. Additional padding is applied over the prominences highlighted. Finally, synthetic casting material is taken (7.5 or 10 cm) from a sealed packet and firmly unravelled following the route taken by the wool. All casting techniques *must be demonstrated* by experienced practitioners and practice undertaken with supervision.

Foot cast

The application of a slipper cast below the ankle has the advantage of allowing ankle motion and exercise. In some cases, mobility may be undertaken without crutches (Fig. 11.18A) while still protecting the foot. Because the technique used requires a light plastic material, a cast cutter is essential for trimming in front of the ankle, to allow normal dorsiflexion and to remove any potential pressure against the skin likely to cause necrosis or nerve compression (Fig. 11.18B). Sometimes patients find that the roof of the cast

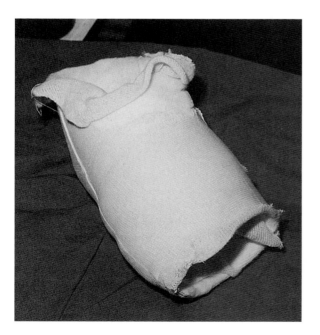
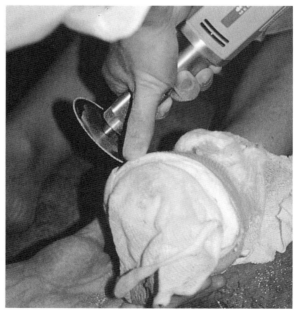

Figure 11.18 Foot cast. A, The foot cast shown should provide support under the toes and not impinge the lateral digits or prevent the ankle from dorsiflexing. The heel should be sufficiently thick to allow weight bearing without premature cracking. B, Removal of the synthetic cast requires an oscillating saw held at right angles to the material. The patient should be warned of vibration and occasionally heat. Soft cast wadding should prevent skin damage. These cast cutters should only be used with appropriate training.

presses, and sometimes swelling is expected; in both cases the cast can be bivalved (cut in half). This adaption allows the roof of the cast to be replaced with additional orthopaedic wool and 7.5 cm bandage such as crepe to prevent the cast slipping or rubbing.

Where a foot cast would not provide sufficient rest and limitation of function, a below-the-knee design might be more appropriate. In both cases, the foot must be over-dorsiflexed to allow normal walking, otherwise patients can be liable to fall over and hurt themselves. Crutches may be used optionally where patients are less steady; however, a walking cast shoe is preferred over the old rubber walkers bound to the bottom of the cast.

Backslab

The backslab technique allows complete rest around and about the ankle, with the potential for removal should any pressure points develop with swelling. This is useful where the patient would be unlikely to seek help early or is going away, or if the practitioner does not have a cast cutter. The practitioner can design this cast for use as a night splint, forming a clinical ankle foot orthosis. Two forms of cast exist: a plaster model (Jones cast) and a synthetic plastic cast. Plaster can be applied in lengths from below the knee to the toes, over padding as described above. Synthetic models are harder wearing but have to be trimmed to remove the anterior portion of the cast following bivalving (Fig. 11.19).

Below-knee cast

The below-knee cast is similar to the backslab except that the cast is not bivalved (Fig. 11.20). Again, plaster or synthetic cast materials can be used over padding. Plaster takes 24 hours to dry thoroughly and is very heavy, causing limb atrophy when left on for long periods. The lighter cast made from polyester, while more expensive, is more popular and much stronger but is not waterproof.

Casts should not be immersed in water and patients should be advised not to use hair dryers to deal with waterlogged casts. There are a

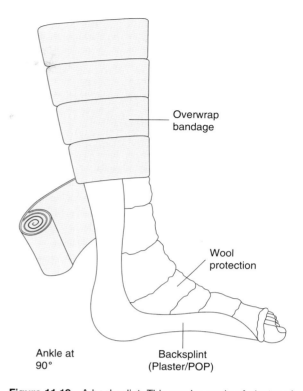

Overwrap bandage

Wool protection

Ankle at 90°

Backsplint (Plaster/POP)

Figure 11.19 A backsplint. This can be made of plaster of Paris (POP) or synthetic material once the anterior part of the cylinder has been cut away. Replacement is not easy at home and only patients who can follow clear instructions should be offered this type of cast. The illustration depicts a backsplint alone, although the Jones splint (POP only) includes a stirrup, which supports the lateral sides of the ankle. Plenty of protective wadding is required, which also absorbs water from the POP. An alternative system is the Pneumatic Walker. (Reproduced with permission from Aircast UK Ltd; see Fig. 11.21.)

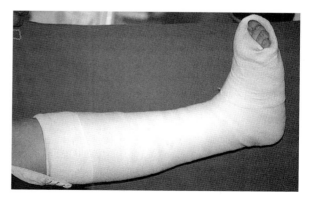

Figure 11.20 A below-knee synthetic cast must be placed on the foot and leg in the correct position. Compression of nerves and soft tissues warrants special caution.

number of products now available that are suitable for limited immersion during showers and baths. XeroSox (Footman) is a waterproof cast, bandage and prosthesis protector developed in the USA; it is a heavy-duty latex bag that conforms to the leg so well that its distributor advertises its use in a swimming pool. Air is removed by sucking via a plastic tube. The advantage lies in its ability to seal without the need for a gasket. It is available in full leg and half leg. Such modalities can greatly assist the practitioner. The inability to bathe remains a major disadvantage of long-term dressings and casts.

Scotchcast boot

The Scotchcast boot is a simple removable boot made of stockinette, Soffban bandage, felt and fibreglass tape. It is effective in redistributing plantar pressure and may be indicated in certain types of diabetic ulceration.

Walking braces

There are a variety of splinting methods that use air in their design. Aircast UK pioneered the functional management of lower leg fractures with the development of the pneumatic walker. The unique support and dynamic compression helps to reduce oedema and promote the healing of fractures (Fig. 11.21). There are several types of walking brace produced by Aircast, including the Foam Walker, the Pneumatic Walker and the Pneumatic Walker Diabetic System. These are bivalved casts joined together with Velcro. The diabetic system is very useful to meet the needs of the higher-risk diabetic patient. The aircast is lined with four air cells that can be inflated with a hand pump (with pressure gauge) through valves to ensure a close fit. This Aircast is supplied with plasterzote insoles, which can be replaced with the practioner's own orthoses if warranted. The Aircast can be removed so the

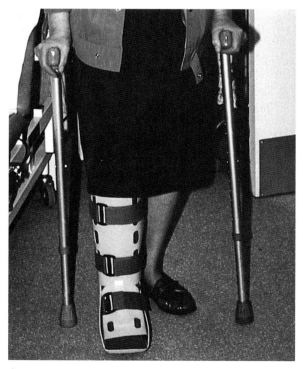

A

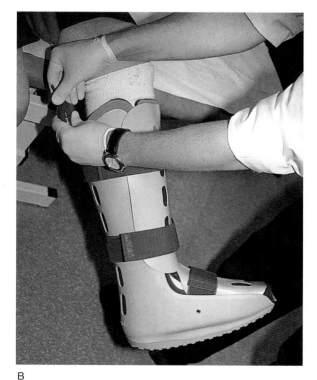

B

Figure 11.21 The Aircast Pneumatic Walker is available in six sizes. (Reproduced with permission from Aircast UK Ltd.)

patient can check their ulcers and it can be removed for sleeping. It may be not suited to certain patient groups such as people with a visual impairment and it makes the disease apparent to everyone.

Summary

Casting offers a valuable tool for dealing with foot pain, provided that infection, tumours and open fractures have been managed appropriately first. The foot cast allows unimpeded ankle motion and walking in a light cast system; above-ankle casts result in a greater level of immobility. For the reasons given above, patients should not use casts, or be immobilized, for indefinite periods.

REPLACEABLE ORTHOSES

Where previously pads as 'chairside appliances' were designed to have a longer effect than adhesive padded dressings, many off-the-shelf materials or stock orthoses are gaining in popularity. The advent of manufactured orthoses has reduced the need to spend valuable time in producing chairside appliances during consulting sessions.

Traditionally, replaceable padding has been made from clinical felt and foam. Handcrafted materials were bevelled using nail drills, and adhesives were on hand during the clinical consultation to manufacture latex or elastic toe and tarsal loops and covers for insoles.

The other form of orthosis commonly made in the clinic was based on an insole design. Wedged insoles with dense felt, and those with plantar pads, are still used, although manufactured pads are available that offer a variety of different functions. Replaceable pads and insoles will be considered separately.

Replaceable padding

If an adhesive dressing has been selected, the next stage of the foot care programme is progression to a replaceable facsimile. While proving as effective as the adhesive form, replaceable padding has certain additional advantages:

- it is far more hygienic and easy removal allows for unhindered bathing
- the non-occlusive effect creates a healthier local environment, avoiding the effects of excessive moisture from heavy perspiration; the pad may be removed at will and allowed to dry
- replaceable padding has a longer life than adhesive dressings
- allergies are far less likely to occur (although it is true that the modern hypoallergenic backing has reduced this problem with adhesives).

Patients generally prefer replaceable padding because it allows them to bathe normally. Those who have used adhesive dressings for years tend to become dependent on them. These patients should be encouraged to convert to replaceable padding in order to improve hygiene as well as to decrease the frequency of clinical visits required. There are, however, some disadvantages of replaceable padding:

- where dressings are necessary for longer periods (e.g. for ulcers), adhesive dressings provide better protection than replaceable padding as less movement will arise on adherence to the skin
- replaceable padding does not conform to the foot as well as adhesive dressing; there is potential for reduced accuracy with replaceable forms because of slight movements of the pad
- the practical problems of removal and replacement by a physically compromised patient negate some of the potential benefits (even so, an alternative to adhesive padding for long-term use must still be sought if detrimental effects to the skin are to be avoided.)

Replaceable padding may be made from clinical materials such as felt and foams or from more durable materials. The advent of products on the market, such as Silopad, is likely to reduce the popularity of chairside manufacture.

The way is open, then, for a staged progression in the foot care programme; just as replaceable padding follows as the next logical step from adhesive, so the results of replaceable padding will indicate the desirability of advancement to more durable orthoses. Most of the adhesive pads described earlier may be converted into a replaceable form. While the range available is very wide, only a few examples are discussed.

Digital pads

Protective function A number of off-the-peg padded 'sleeves' or 'tubes' can be utilized for digital protection; examples of these include tubular foams, sizes A–D (see Table 11.1), and Silipos (Silopad) digital pads, which are thin wafers of gel (Shanks 1991; Fig. 11.22). The

advantage of the gel products lie in their ease of application, their clear effectiveness (as they release an emollient oil softening the keratotic lesion) and good shoe-fit acceptance. Silipos may obviate the need to manufacture IDW, apical and dorsal dressings, although ulcers should first be resolved and any infection cleared.

Semicorrective function Darco and Berkemann have produced a range of soft and hard day and night splints for a variety of digital deformities. Originally designed for the hallux, lesser digits can be splinted during the day with Velcro loops. There now seems to be a place for such modalities, although marked deformity is unlikely to be corrected permanently without surgical intervention first (see Fig. 10.4).

Digital props can also be made from silicone gum (Fig. 11.23) or from preprepared leather-covered foam props. Care must be taken with single toe loops, especially where toes swell or circulation is less than satisfactory.

Forefoot pads

All the forefoot pads previously described may be constructed as replaceable pads. Tubipad offers a method of protection as an elasticated

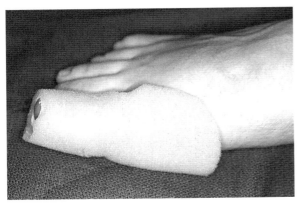

A

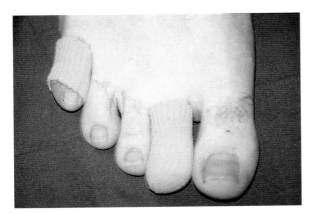

B

Figure 11.22 Protective digital devices. A, Tubifoam for hallux. B, Silopad for the second and fifth digits.

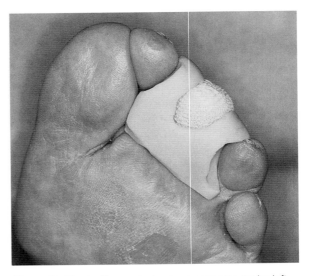

Figure 11.23 A silicone device in seen in situ on the left foot. Toes 2–4 cradle the third toe, which has a tubular bandage dressing underneath.

bandage and can be trimmed from a roll. This is essentially a 'Tubigrip' (Seton) with a polyurethane open-cell foamed uncovered lining. This is a temporary cushioning material and is amenable to adhesive padding additionally attached to its foam surface.

Leather-covered stock pads are available in many shapes as arch fillers, metatarsal pads or domes. Toe and tarsal loops are used to keep the pad securely attached to the foot. Many of these systems have been unpopular amongst practitioners because of their lack of specificity. Foam and felt replaceable pads made in the clinic still have a place (Fig. 11.24). The figure illustrates one of many designs that can be covered by thin leather. Temporary forms may use Tubegauz for toe loops instead of elastic.

Silipos materials are also available as covered and uncovered gels. The benefit is the same as stated above, except that the thin dimensions and potential for compensating for loss of adipose tissue across the metatarsal heads make it highly desirable for a wide range of patients.

A cheap range of forefoot pads is available in the form of a latex foam pad from Scholl. Frequently, these pads are inadequate for the medically compromised foot problem. The attachment relies on a single toe loop and, therefore, is less likely to stay in position. The material used has a limited life and is easily abraded by the shoe. Tight toe loops are a distinct disadvantage and should not be used in patients with poor pedal circulation.

Valgus pads Valgus pads as arch fillers have been found to be valuable for fascial strain, as mentioned above. Where the practitioner wants to use an arch filler for a functional purpose, these are best designed on an insole base. Arch fillers are available with single tarsal loops, although many traditional practitioners still design their own where appropriate facilities exist.

Heel padding

Traditionally the practitioner would adhere foam to an insole template for the treatment of plantar heel pain. Padding designed for the heel may come in the form of a flat or a cupped pad. Figure

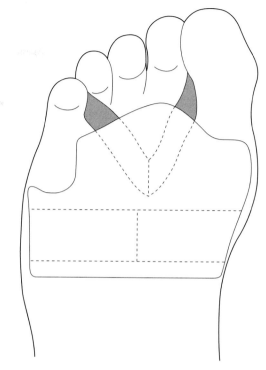

Figure 11.24 Replaceable single-winged plantar cover manufactured in the clinic.

11.25 illustrates some of the stock designs available. The heel may need plantar or retrocalcaneal protection, and appropriate selection must be based on its individual quality. Simple foam inserts exist for the heel and can be found at most large stores, often from the Scholl counter.

Wonderspur (Silipos) or Spenco (Footman) can be used for central heel pain. There is a wide and interesting range of heel cup products and they vary from a simple preformed polyethylene cup to the Tuli pad, which has a waffle network that collapses on pressure. The waffle was designed by a podiatrist in the USA to mimic the fat pad structure.

Complex and much more expensive forms of heel pad are available and these often incorporate Achilles tendon pads, as well as protecting the malleoli; examples of these are the Achilles heel pad (Silipos), incorporating a 4 mm thick gel pad to protect the posterior heel from pressure and friction, and the malleolar sleeve, which

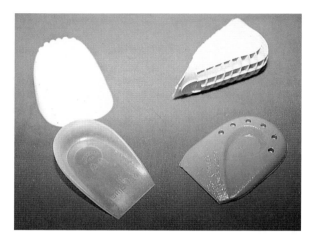

Figure 11.25 Forms of heel pad. Viscolas stippled heel cup (Comed), Tuli heel, and Wonderzorb (Silipos) with variable density centre.

features two large discs of polymer gel placed on the medial and lateral malleloli, reducing pressure and friction to the area (Silipos).

Insoles

The insole starts life as a simple cardboard template taken from the insock outline of a shoe. The advantage of an insole, with a pad adhered under a cover, is that its position is maintained by the shoe, thus avoiding the need for foot straps. The disadvantage of insoles, however, arises from the need to ensure that placement in the shoe is correctly aligned with the foot and the difficulty in ensuring patient compliance. Patients who have more than one pair of shoes need more than one insole.

Template making

The outline of the insock area of the shoe is carefully trimmed in cardboard until it fits accurately. Using a felt-tipped pen, relevant bony landmarks and lesions are highlighted on the plantar surface of the foot (see Fig. 12.6B,C); the complete shape of the pad-to-be may be drawn in this way, if required. The insole is then sprayed with a liquid, such as a spirit-based preoperative skin cleanser. The foot, or feet (if two are being

replicated), is then placed in the shoe(s) and the patient is requested to walk a dozen or so steps. The shoes are removed and the felt-tipped pen markings are observed, having been transferred to the insole. The spirit-based liquid dries quickly and the forefoot pad can now be drawn accurately onto the cardboard template and sent away to a laboratory (as a prescription) or a pad can be adhered directly to the template, which now becomes the insole base. To complete the insole, the pad is covered with non-stretch strapping (e.g. Mefix), which can then be lightly dusted with talcum powder. The foot can now slide into the shoe with the covered padding offering less resistance.

A more accurate method of obtaining a clearly marked base for the insole involves a more dynamic impression. Any base material may be used but 3 mm Plastazote is particularly suitable as it compresses well. This is inserted into the shoe unaltered, and when the patient returns after a period of use, a clear imprint is formed in the soft material, thus indicating precisely the required position of the padding.

Another method of chairside insole construction is described by Kippen (1982a). An impression on a base material is obtained as previously described. A pad is then adhered to this impression using double-sided tape. This method allows the use of those more durable padding materials traditionally associated with the construction of long-term orthoses. Double-sided tape is again used to adhere a covering material such as Yampi. This is a longer-term form of device, which is constructed easily and quickly in a chairside form.

The heel pad adhered to a card base still has a useful place in the clinic, as does the Cobra pad. The latter is illustrated in Fig. 15.10 (p. 370) and serves as a useful short-term antipronatory insole prior to selecting stock or prescription orthoses. High-density (high durometer) felt is used to form a wedge at the heel; this extends forward, incorporating a valgus-type filler. In busy practices, however, the use of the Frelon insole (Footman; Fig. 11.26B,D) offers a cheap time- and cost-effective method for providing similar assistance to the foot. This useful lightweight

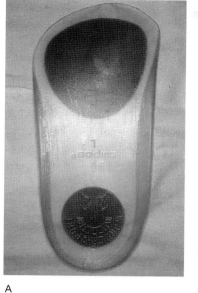

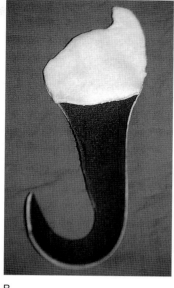

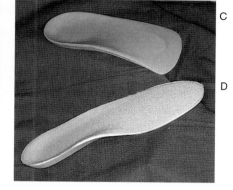

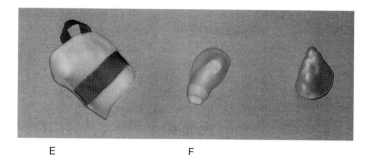

Figure 11.26 Insoles. A, Wonderzorb (Silipos). B, Frelon trimmed to fit shoe, with felt extension added. C, Alphathotic. D, Stock premoulded orthosis. E, Plastazote clinically constructed plantar cover. F, Digital Plastazote cover with padding sandwiched between Plastazote.

moulded insole consists of an upper open cell foam, providing effective cushioning of the foot, combined with a much denser lower foam layer, providing firm support without losing the suppleness of the insole. They are solvent fast so can be lined with postings and paddings (Fig. 11.26B) and are offered in six basic sizes. Unfortunately, no small sizes exist for children. Wedging, now purchased in sheets, can be obtained and tilted in varus, with a 2° and 4° canting (Fig. 11.26D). Once adhered to the Frelon or any similar base, the mechanical effect of wedging on the foot offers considerable orthotic control. Stock orthoses are worth trying as a first-line attempt before turning to prescription orthoses.

There are many stock orthoses available on the market. Formthotics (Procare) are ready-to-fit lightweight, flexible devices that can be heat moulded in seconds. Different densities of material enables a match with the patient's foot pathology, body weight and usage (Fig. 11.27). Formthotics incorporate an intrinsic rearfoot varus post and they contain Ultrafresh, an antibacterial and antifungal agent. Another type of stock orthosis is the Vasyli range (Canonbury). These are heat-mouldable orthotics designed for those patients who need a customized prescription. The Vasyli custom orthoses feature a 6° rearfoot varus angle (2° for the slimfit) and a balance 4° forefoot varus angle; there is a 15 mm

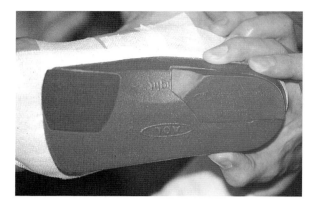

Figure 11.27 The VOL orthosis. A stock orthosis with an in-built 4° varus heel to which forefoot and rearfoot wedging can be added by heat-moulding or adhesive backing. Three densities are available, red, green and blue, red being the most dense and blue the least dense.

heel cup, a Cambrelle cloth cover, a built in first metatarsal plantarflexor and a Poron teardrop shock dot. There are three densities available colour coded as red for high density, blue for medium density and green for low density. The custom orthoses are sold in the following sizes: regular, full length, easy fit and slim fit.

Stock and modular insoles

This section would not be complete without indicating some of the newer orthoses and insoles available. These differ from the previous orthoses in that they have no moulded heel cup and a minimal arch (valgus) filler.

Wonderzorb soft silicone (Silipos) orthoses use a high-quality medical grade silicone. Two different densities of silicone are used in the manufacture of the Wonderzorb range: soft and firm. The coloured area is soft and the surrounding area firm. The firm silicone gives support and the soft offers extra cushioning. Silipos also provide a full-length gel insole with duoflex, a specially designed polymer gel sheet approximately 2.5–3 mm thick The gel insole has an ability to cushion and 'flow' and is ideal for people with diabetes. Spenco (Footman) features a unique cushioning system that provides a soft, environment to help to reduce friction and absorb shock.

They are sold in a variety of forms from standard insoles and heel cushions to a Spenco polysorb cross-trainer replacement insole.

A small number of modular manufacture systems exist, which can be costly to set up initially and time consuming to use in a busy department, unless an orthotist is available to support this activity. Nonetheless, these systems have a particular role to play as they can be used to form an orthosis for each patient's specific foot shape; one of these, the Irving Insole Device (Taylor's therapy), is illustrated in Figure 11.28.

Summary

Where time and resources are available, the practitioner can still offer the patient a chairside appliance. Companies such as Footman make a wide selection of premoulded pads, which can be adhered to a base of the practitioner's choosing. Leather insoles are still available, with valgus fillers and ready-placed metatarsal pads. Experience is the only real basis on which to make a sensible selection.

SILICONES AND MOULDED THERMOPLASTIC ORTHOSES

Silicone moulds

The silicone group of thermoset orthoses gained popularity at the end of the 1970s and they are still a very popular method in the UK for managing digital lesions. Thermosetting plastics, once formed, cannot be reheated. Silicones (polysiloxanes) may also be used for hallux valgus oval shields and for orthoses for the heel; they have even been advocated for forefoot padding on a non-cast insole (Garrow 1979). While silicone can be used to make up full-foot orthoses, the greatest disadvantage lies in its weight. Silicones have rubber-like properties. In effect, this means that they compress without losing their original form, although they are often heavy and bulky in shoes. Silicones have properties that are a blend of the silicates and the paraffins, both of which have a considerable degree of chemical inertness. Consequently,

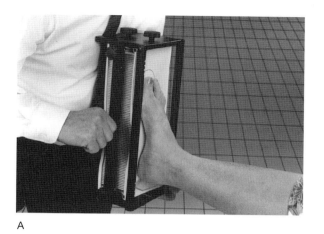

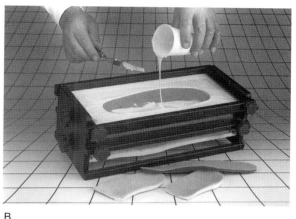

A

B

Figure 11.28   The Irving Insole Device in use. A, Taking the impression. B, Filling with liquid resin. (Reproduced with permission from Taylor Therapy.)

they can be used on the skin without fear of allergic response.

Early products were adapted from dental denture liners and impression materials (e.g. the Verones coloured green and red) in which a catalyst was added to make the product set. Shrinkage following curing was less than 0.8%. While all modern silicones still require an additive, the modern generation of mouldable silicones is lighter and has greater tensile strength. The first silicones to be used in podiatry were fluid in composition and were mixed with a liquid catalyst. Once a hardener paste or catalyst has been added, the silicone forms a thermoset material as the polysiloxane polymer undergoes cross-linking. Silicone devices are usually ready to use immediately, although some practitioners like to wait an hour to ensure adequate curing.

Indications

When adhesive dressings are undesirable because of irritation or because of inability to wash the affected part, a silicone digital device should be considered. The treatment may be curative with some callus and corn-type lesions, where the underlying pathology has not created chronic inflammatory change. The lesion should not be open or have any discharge. Open lesions should be dressed appropriately.

Silicone devices can be used as prostheses following digital amputation. The prosthesis can take the form of a simple toe wedge or a moulded toe(s) copied from the patient's contralateral foot (Ch. 12).

Orthodigita   Correction in younger patients can be applied to flexible deformities, especially those affecting toes 2–5. Black & Coates (1981) suggested that deformities were conducive to manipulation in young children, but this will depend upon the age that treatment commences. Soft tissues can be stretched, as described by Davis's law. This states that as long as a tensile force is applied to the tight structure, some elongation will take effect (Ch. 15).

Protection   This is achieved by building the silicone around the area of maximum pressure and stress (see Fig. 11.23). Continual use can provide impressive results and the treatment is quick and cost effective despite the lack of good scientific research to support these observations. Protective silicones can be used as interdigital spacers and as apical, dorsal and medial/lateral MTPJ protection. Tight extensor tendons can be protected and holes fashioned to help distribute stress away from the traumatized area. Debridement of callus and corns should be undertaken after the mould is applied. The lesion is deemed to be better protected in this way because a natural depression is created.

Clinical application

Silicone elastomers can be applied either during the phase transition (i.e. as the silicone changes from its free-flowing malleable state to an elastic solid) or before the phase transition begins. Whichever method is used, the site of application must be clean and free from debris and the skin unbroken. The amount of paste or putty to be used should be measured. Otoform-K2 is a well-known mouldable putty that, with addition of a red curing agent (Dreve), hardens to form a permanent rubbery appliance. To assess amounts without wastage comes with experience. Generally, it is better to begin with too much material and later discard the excess than to begin with too little. Other silicone putties include Blansil (Canonbury) and Bland Rose (Canonbury). These are hardened in a similar manner to Otoform K2 but tend to feel slightly softer.

The manufacture of hallux valgus oval shields and heel cups require a larger surface area of silicone material. The mix used needs to be more liquid than solid, and this can be achieved before the phase transition begins. The application is easier at this point as the silicone flows more readily than during the phase transition. Application to the foot is made with a spatula in the direction where the bulk of the device is needed.

Summary

While cost effective, silicones will not help every patient. Silicones are not designed to correct hallux deformities; bulky designs are often rejected by patients, while thin designs tear easily. Catalysts and their additives contain colouring; this can be a source of sensitivity in some patients. The practitioner should attempt to use a thin construction, protecting the lesion at the point of maximum stress by increasing the thickness. Correction of long standing problems (e.g. contracted toes such as digiti adducto-varus) is less satisfactory. Silicone material offers poor tensile stretch to tissues but excellent resilience to compression. Often bulk is used to achieve adequate strength. This product has a finite shelf life and careless storage can have an adverse effect.

Thermoplastics

Thermoplastics are materials that can be remoulded and shaped. This group of plastics offers a number of advantages for the production of orthoses, with the potential for clinical adjustment as needed; heat guns are useful when making adjustments.

Low-temperature thermoplastics are particularly valuable in that they do not require expensive ovens. Perhaps the best known of these plastics are X-lite plus (formerly known as Hexcelite) and Aquaplast, which were among the first of this type of material to be given a podiatric application.

X-lite plus is made up of a cotton mesh impregnated with a thermoplastic resin. Initially marketed as a splint material, it can be regarded as a semi-rigid plastic (Smedley 1982) and has been used as heel cups to protect pressure sores (Woods 1982), as functional devices for biomechanical disorders (Smedley 1982), in the management of hallux rigidus (Monaghan 1984) and as resting splints for foot drop (Hicks & McFetridge 1993).

X-lite plus is a light, durable easy-to-use material in the clinic. Although thermally stable up to at least 200°C, it only needs to be heated to 72°C to become pliable. As it is not associated with an exothermic reaction, it can be moulded directly to the foot. The desensitized foot may need to be protected with a tubular bandage. The working time is about 3 minutes, by which time it will have regained its semi-rigid qualities. Modifications are easily carried out by rewarming. Upon heating, it is self-bonding, so that thickness can be increased as required. The mesh construction ensures good ventilation, negating any potential perspiration problems. The only heat source required is a container of hot water. The manufacturer claims that the product has an indefinite shelf life.

Disadvantages associated with X-lite plus include cost. It is made expensive by the fact that construction time is increased with the need to line the device to avoid skin irritation and damage to hosiery.

Aquaplast has similar qualities to Hexcelite. It is solid rather than having a mesh form and is off-white in colour, becoming translucent and workable when heated. It softens at a lower temperature than X-lite plus, approximately 60°C, and takes slightly longer to become rigid, the amount of time varying with the thickness of Aquaplast used. Aquaplast has been compared with rigid high-temperature thermoplastics and was found to be superior in terms of its convenience of construction (Kippen 1982b).

Foamed thermoplastics

Foamed thermoplastics in common use include Plastazote and Evazote. Plastazote is a closed-cell, cross-linked expanded polyethylene. Evazote is ethylvinyl acetate, a closed-cell cross-linked copolymer foam, and is marginally softer than Plastazote.

When preheated to a temperature of 140°C, these materials are readily moulded to contours of the foot. Although they may be directly moulded to the skin, it is wise, initially, to cover the desensitized foot with a tubular bandage. On rapid cooling, the moulded shape is retained. Rapid cooling necessitates a high level of dexterity and swift action in moulding if reheating is to be avoided. The rate of heat loss is dependent on the thickness of the material and the room temperature. Reheating does allow the materials to return to their original shape.

At 140°C, these foamed thermoplastics are *auto-adhesive* upon compression, but below this temperature this quality is lost and an adhesive such as neoprene is required. High-temperature, non-rigid foamed thermoplastics also have a part to play, although only high-density forms last. Two pieces of Plastazote of different densities can be combined by auto-adhesion, as shown in Figure 12.21 (p. 283). In this way, properties of both low- and high-density foams combine to offer a soft contour with a stiff infrastructure to prevent collapse. This type of modification produces an orthosis that lasts longer than one of softer low-density material alone.

Plastazote is chemically inert and may be applied to the foot without fear of skin irritation. As insulators, polyethylene foams are extremely effective in preventing heat loss from the foot. Plastazote material is often prescribed as an accommodative orthosis, which serves to protect against chilblains. This is a disadvantage in patients with hyperhidrosis, necessitating the creation of ventilation holes if an alternative material is not considered.

Orthoses made in the clinic from Plastazote or Evazote are quick to produce and can often be made as chairside appliances; such devices are inexpensive, but resilience is comparatively low and refabrication is often necessary. Both types of material may be used for lining devices constructed from other materials such as X-lite plus. The versatility of Plastazote is demonstrated by the fact that it is used in the construction of orthoses for all areas of the foot. Plastazote may be used to mould arch fillers on simple insoles or to produce orthoses from casts with heel cups. Plastazote has been used for toe props and protection of hallux valgus in the past, and it can be quickly moulded to shape (see Fig. 11.26E,F). Additional material can also be sandwiched between the Plastazote to offer greater protective or functionally corrective properties.

SUMMARY

This chapter has considered the management of foot problems with dressings, pads and a range of available stock orthoses, which offer accommodation, rest, redistribution, stabilization, immobilization and compensation.

The whole area of clinical padding has received scant research and has been relegated to small clinical studies without controls. However, many materials and products have now been made available for easier dispensing, affording greater efficiency in the clinic. Further investigation is warranted if the practitioner is to remain vigilant, as the ever-increasing range of new products requires constant changes in practice.

REFERENCES

Black J A, Coates I S 1981 Silicones: their uses and development in chiropodial orthotic and prosthetic management. The Chiropodist 36: 237–251

Garrow A 1979 The silicone insole: a chairside appliance. The Chiropodist 34: 137–138

Hicks S, McFetridge L 1993 Foot drop resting splint. Orthopaedic Systems promotional literature

Kippen C 1982a The simple insole? The Chiropodist 37: 410–414

Kippen C 1982b Low temperature thermoplastics: application in chairside foot orthotics. The Chiropodist 37: 36–41

McCloskey P J 1992 A study of the effect of low dye taping on the foot. British Journal of Podiatric Medicine and Surgery 4: 6–9

Monaghan M M 1984 The use of Hexcellite in the management of hallux rigidus. The Chiropodist 39: 435–438

Shanks J 1991 Silopad: a clinical trial. The Chiropodist 46: 193–196

Smedley R 1982 The fabrication of a semi-rigid orthosis in Hecellite material. The Chiropodist 37: 338–340

Woods P 1982 The use of Hexcellite splinting material in the prevention and treatment of pressure sores occurring on the feet. The Chiropodist 37: 333–335

FURTHER READING

Coates I S 1979 Silicone orthodigita: principles, aims and prognosis. The Chiropodist 34: 137–138

Kippen C 1989 Insoling materials in foot orthosis manufacture: a review. The Chiropodist 44: 83–87

12

Prescription orthoses

Michael Curran
David Pratt

INTRODUCTION

This chapter provides a broad insight into the principles underpinning prescription orthoses. The practitioner who prescribes orthoses needs to have a fundamental knowledge of mechanics and also of the properties of the materials that are used in their manufacture. In the absence of these, practitioners will have difficulty in providing adequate solutions to the problems they meet.

A practitioner will justify the choice of a particular orthosis in terms of the benefit that is likely to be gained from it. A prescription can be determined once the clinician understands:

- normal lower extremity function (as a basic prerequisite)
- the origin of the biomechanical dysfunction
- the influence of the proximal limb on the foot
- the ideal material properties required of the orthosis
- the role of footwear in relation to the intended orthosis
- the psychological requirements of the patient.

The use of orthoses as part of mechanical therapy in the clinic can complement any programme of treatment. A prescription orthosis is produced from an impression, often on an individual basis. Usually, individual impressions are required because there is no equivalent device available as a stock item or because the problem to be treated does not lend itself to stock materials, as their physical properties cannot achieve the desired effect.

Functional orthoses have already been described in Chapter 10. In this chapter, we will discuss the ways in which the forces applied to the foot are incorporated into their design (Lundeen 1988).

Orthoses described in this chapter fall into three main categories: *digital, foot* and *ankle foot orthoses* (AFO). They may bear some similarity to those described in Chapter 11. For AFOs, there are few stock orthoses available that offer satisfactory functional control. The majority of the principles and designs described in this chapter fall into the 'rigid' category, which refers to the firm plastic shells or orthotic plates that form the basis of control and allow additional material to be incorporated into their design.

The term *prescription* is used to describe the situation where a mould of the foot or of the foot and leg is referred to a laboratory with a written prescription attached from the practitioner or orthotist, and the orthosis is dispensed at a later consultation. No attempt will be made to describe manufacture, partly because this is not the aim of this chapter and partly because the manufacturing process requires a clear manual of instruction, which can best be found in other texts, such as Bowker et al (1993), Wu (1990), Philps (1995), Spencer (1978) and Sgarlato (1971).

The hindfoot or midtarsal components of a functional orthosis are easily modified. The necessary changes may be achieved simply by altering a plaster cast. The incorporation of extensions and posts (the latter are used to pitch an orthosis in an everted or inverted direction) may be best achieved by combining a number of different materials (e.g. ethylvinyl acetate (EVA) and foamed polyurethane) such that their individual properties are used to greatest effect.

Prostheses are introduced in this chapter because they have a clear prescriptive function as well as a contribution to make in controlling unstable feet with poor prognoses. Prostheses can be used to make up for a deficit in foot function, often associated with amputation, as well as

to provide a better foot outline for fitting a standard shoe, thus avoiding the need for bespoke footwear (Fig. 12.1). Of course, many bespoke shoes are made in order to accommodate complicated prostheses, but these fall outside the scope of this book.

DIGITAL ORTHOSES

The number of digital problems that rely upon prescription management are becoming fewer, because of the clinical modalities that are available, as already described in Chapter 11. Tollafield (1985) has discussed the manufacture of latex digita, but these devices are no longer popular because they often cause more problems than they alleviate as the interaction between latex and skin is less satisfactory than that between skin and other materials.

There are two types of prescription digital orthosis worthy of particular mention: the digital prosthetic and the hallux orthosis. Both can be combined with other orthotic designs depending upon their desired function.

Indications

Once the structural integrity and functional efficiency of the forefoot becomes impaired because of digital dysfunction, a variety of pathologies can result that would benefit from orthotic management.

Lesions Dorsal lesions over the interphalangeal joints (IPJ) or apices may develop as a result of hammer toes. Patients may benefit from orthodigita. Redistribution and accommodation are essential to prevent tissue damage over a joint prominence.

Prosthetic function The space left by an amputated toe will allow adjacent toes to deform subsequently into the remaining gap. A replacement digital prosthesis can be made for either single or multiple toes, or, if necessary, a whole forefoot cover can be made. Toes are often

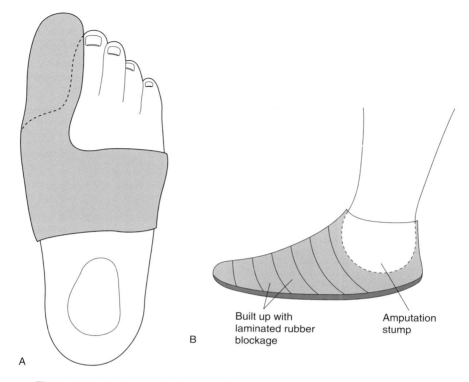

Figure 12.1 Prostheses. A, Prosthesis for amputation in a patient whose foot was injured in a railway accident, affecting the whole first ray. B, Prosthesis for post-Syme's amputation after reconstructive surgery following Buerger's disease of the whole foot.

associated with massive dislocation at the metatarsophalangeal joints (MTPJ) in severe arthritides, and they lose their spring in gait. A prosthesis offers not only a better 'toe-off' action but also improves shoe fit. Metatarsal head areas may require cushioning and the plantar material may be extended back under the foot to improve shock attenuation.

Prophylactic protection The hallux may require a prescription orthosis to prevent recurrence of ulcers in diabetics. A hallux shield can be extended to protect the medial eminence and to deflect shear forces from the plantar IPJ, often associated with a spur or accessory ossicle. Dysfunction from a hallux rigidus can create pressure over the IPJ and MTPJ areas. If footwear cannot be adapted to rock over the great toe joint, a hallux orthosis may provide better propulsion and protection at the same time.

Replication technique

Material

The orthotic laboratory requires sufficient detail to avoid guesswork. The favoured materials include alginate moulding (DeTrey-Dentsply, Zantalgin), as alginate offers greater skin detail as well as making the mould easy to remove because of the material's plasticity (Ch. 10). Plaster of Paris bandage may be used for large areas that need to be captured.

Plaster of Paris bandage is used with alginate to achieve adequate detail around the toes and to support the alginate impression material. A gap must be left for the finished prosthetic toe (Fig. 12.2). The opposite foot provides an accurate impression of the missing toe. If this is deformed or missing, another patient may consent to being casted.

The alginate is mixed according to the instructions provided; some products may vary but each includes graduated scoop spoons and tumblers. Alginate dries quickly and then shrinks, rendering the technique useless if this is not prevented with moisture. A small hole can be made

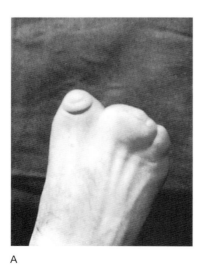

Figure 12.2 A prosthetic toe has been created using a normal toe encased in alginate for detail. The forefoot has been casted separately in alginate and plaster.

at the end of the toe to allow any air to be forced out upon filling with plaster of Paris; in this way the end of the digit is not distorted by an air bubble. Plaster can be used alone but does not offer the same detail as alginate. When it is used alone, greater preparation in the laboratory may be necessary.

This combined casting technique using both plaster of Paris and alginate can be adopted for any part of the forefoot, including the great toe. The practitioner must bear in mind that it is important to have sufficient proximal detail to form a good base for the prosthetic toe. The cast must, therefore, be extended back as far as is reasonable. In the case of replacement toes, silicones are used to obtain greater detail.

Single toes

Replicating digits is achieved by using a 'dummy' silicone toe, which has been cast from a suitable 'donor', usually the opposite foot.

Multiple toe prosthesis

Figure 12.3 illustrates the use of a leather moccasin prosthesis to compensate for the congenital

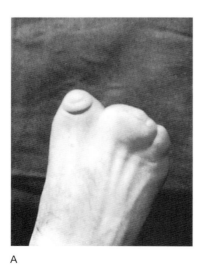

A

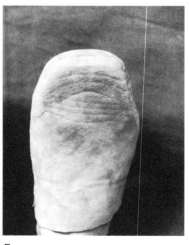

B

Figure 12.3 Multiple toe prosthesis. A, The foot has abnormally shortened toes as a result of developmental failure. B, The finished leather moccasin prosthesis, which has a latex foam infill for the toes.

loss of toes (phocomelia). Although the toes are shorter than in normal feet, foam digital prostheses allow the toe box to fill out adequately. The benefit, as stated above, is that this creates a snug fit for the foot in the shoe, as well as preventing slippage. The laboratory will make these prostheses as leather or half-latex devices. A latex outerskin provides an element of washability. The prescription should state the material preferred and whether the device is to have ventilation perforations.

Hallux and first metatarsophalangeal joint

Paraffin wax sheets for taking bite impressions can be used to make a bunion shield. This thin material only needs to be immersed in water at 40°C before it can be comfortably moulded around the first MTPJ, with no need to protect the skin from heat. The open edges are pinched around the toe and the whole cast is removed, retaining its shape. It is then instantly ready to be filled with plaster powder mix. Bunion shields from thermoplastics, leather and latex can be manufactured after preparing a plaster model.

Foot prosthesis

A whole foot can be made into a moccasin prosthesis (see Fig. 12.1B). This device will provide a block of foam rubber, which often obviates the need for orthopaedic footwear as stock shoes can

be worn. A full foot cast must be taken; the description given here can be applied generally for a number of foot impressions. The impression is taken using either alginate, for easy removal, or plaster of Paris bandage, bivalved or spirally casted (see p. 295). The bivalve technique is very useful where the practitioner wishes to avoid a knife or cast cutter. Two–four ply plaster bandage is applied with the patient lying supine on the couch.

The posterior leg bandage is applied first and an obvious ledge is made, as shown in Figure 12.4. This hardens and the ledge is smeared with a simple emollient to allow separation. The anterior section is placed over the first, marrying the second ledge to the posterior section. Once set, the cast can be split easily along the seam. The seams are then sealed with more bandage, the cast is labelled with the patient's name, date of casting and the practitioner's name, and it is dried naturally. If alginate is selected, it must be stored wet and supported with plaster bandage encased in bubble wrapper.

The cast cannot be sent off to the laboratory until a replica of the in-sock has been cut out of cardboard or regenerated leatherboard. This will provide the laboratory with the width. The girth can be supplied either as the measurements for toe box, height and girth across the metatarsals and midfoot or as a cast of the inside of the shoe. A cast of the inside of the shoe is made with plaster fill, mixing powder with water and placing

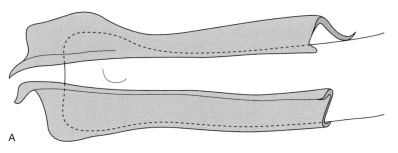

A

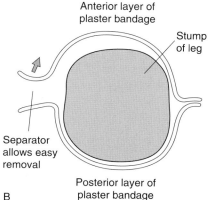

Anterior layer of plaster bandage

Stump of leg

Separator allows easy removal

Posterior layer of plaster bandage

B

Figure 12.4 Stump prosthesis. A bivalve cast (A) can be used for a stump prosthesis (B). This will comprise two separate halves made from plaster bandage layers.

the mix into a strong plastic bag. The shoe replicate gives the laboratory staff an accurate model to follow.

Prescription

In addition to taking personal details from the patient and noting specific points required to provide foot dimensions, the practitioner should decide on the materials and request any additions on the same form. Using an experienced orthopaedic or podiatric orthotist can make a great difference in terms of avoiding problems associated with poor fit.

Prostheses must be made from material that avoids friction at graft sites and scars or in areas that have poor circulation. Where loss of muscle has arisen from injury, the lack of bulk tissue overlying stumps will have to be supplemented with additional hydrogel protection such as second skin (Spenco) or Silipos covers, which are made to fit the lower limb. All materials selected should be light but durable.

After the positive cast preparation, the cast is covered with chamois. Where seams are employed, it is important to ensure that they do not come into contact with amputation scars, as this can cause irritation to the suture line. The seams will be reinforced by the laboratory for added strength. Diagrams and written itemized details are helpful, especially where small variations in design are anticipated.

Summary

Replacement digital prosthetic devices may have a role to play in reducing trauma to adjacent digits and thereby preventing lesion occurrence. New devices should be ordered before any previous prescription deteriorates. Patients will become dependent on their prostheses and they will be unhappy if relieved of them, albeit temporarily, in order to make a copy. Keep all casts and details as necessary unless footwear changes are anticipated. Patients are advised to use similar styles of footwear, wherever possible, to avoid incurring additional costs.

FOOT ORTHOSES

The field of foot orthoses forms a very large part of the foot specialist's work. Here, orthoses are divided into *insoles* and *functional orthoses*. Insoles play a less-important role than functional orthoses and as such they will be illustrated but not described in any detail. Nonethless, insoles do have a role to play, and circumstances may dictate the need to offer patients a range of orthotic designs based on an insole system that uses manufactured pads shaped to the practitioner's requirements.

INSOLES

The greatest advantage of insoles lies in their low cost. Thin 1.5 mm polypropylene sheets have been used for insole bases, with wedges of EVA to reduce base deterioration by decomposition, a common problem associated with insoles. Unfortunately, even these functional designs will fill the toe box of many styles of shoe. Casted orthoses finish behind the metatarsals instead of running the full length and, therefore, fit into more than one pair of shoes more easily.

Designs of insole

Ten insole variations are illustrated in Figure 12.5. Each design comprises a stiff or soft insole base. Materials include a firm neoprene (Spenco), latex foam rubber or polyurethane foam pad (Poron, Cleron).

Composite materials

The use of a combination of different materials offers a variety of properties in a single insole. Firm polyurethane foams can be mixed with foam latex rubber buttons to produce cushioning and compensation, with redistribution or accommodation around rigid deformities on the sole. The use of wedged EVA will provide an element of realignment.

Many of the designs suggested have been described in Chapter 11 and will not be described again.

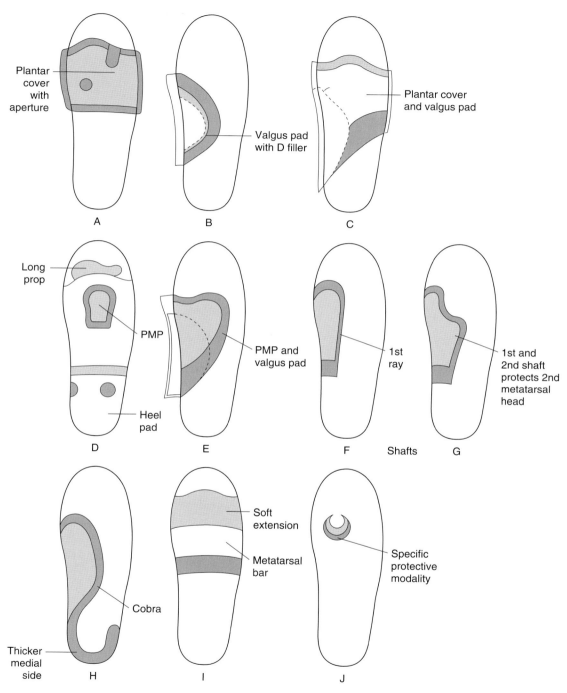

Figure 12.5 Insole designs suitable for manufacture. A, plantar cover; B, valgus filler; C, combined valgus filler and plantar cover; D, long prop and plantar metatarsal pad combined with a heel pad with two point cut-outs for pressure distribution; E, plantar metatarsal pad combined with valgus filler; F, first ray shaft; G, shaft extended as L pad; H, the successful Cobra pad comprising heel meniscus and valgus filler; I, metatarsal bar with soft extension to toe sulci combining cushioning with redistribution; J, insole showing simple crescentic redistribution pad; any shaped design can be used as in (J).

Replication technique

Templates for insoles have already been described for chairside appliances. One problem with taking templates is the poor correlation that is afforded when marking lesion sites. Ink paper systems such as Podotrack (Langer) and mats such as Harris–Beath mats offer alternative dynamic systems of acquiring information for use in bespoke manufacture (Fig. 12.6A). Podotrack impression sheets are a simple clinical tool that provides inexpensive information about pressure distribution and peak pressure on the sole of the foot. The advantages of such a system are that it has a uniform ink layer for accurate measurement of force and pressure can be quantified by a force-measuring colour card provided with every 100 sheets.

Prescription

Specific information should be recorded, as shown in Figure 12.6B,C:

- date, patient's name, practitioner and clinic
- metatarsal head positions
- limits for padded additions, such as styloid process, toe sulci, navicular and central heel point
- lesions (areas of callus, intractable plantar keratoma, verrucae, cysts)
- materials required, thickness, density, pad, insole base and stiffener
- position of materials, drawn onto template
- relevant shoe information.

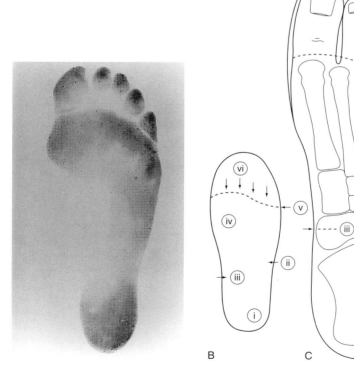

Figure 12.6 Insole template used to manufacture a bespoke orthosis. A, Bespoke orthosis from a patterned and inked rubber mat. B, Information is transferred from the foot onto a cardboard base cut around the inside of the shoe, recording (i) heel centre, (ii) base of fifth metatarsal, (iii) level with navicular, (iv) metatarsal head centres, (v) toe sulci, (vi) interdigital spacing. C, Points (i)–(iv) recorded onto the cardboard template for laboratory manufacture.

Summary

Insoles are formed on a soft or hard base and may have a short life of 6–9 months. Three-quarter length (to metatarsal head) orthoses taken from plaster casts appear to have a greater success rate because of improved shoe fit. As mentioned in Chapter 11, many new stock items have made insole therapy redundant. While some research work has been carried out into the scientific value of this type of orthosis, the greater part of study has involved the shock-attenuation properties, as these are more easily measured. Insoles with redistribution pads rarely remove the long-standing plantar lesion, but they do minimize the load over specific points, thereby reducing symptoms.

CASTED ORTHOSES

The progression from the insole to the casted orthosis is largely dictated by the need to increase foot control, particularly pronation. The cost increases because of the need to take an impression (casting to produce negative plates) and because there are clinical costs and laboratory charges (manufacture). Many types of orthosis exist; two main categories are considered here: the functional orthosis and the accommodative orthosis.

The functional orthosis

The use of the term 'functional' implies that an orthosis will restore the time sequence associated with ground contact by reducing abnormal compensation resulting from foot pathology.

The purpose behind the functional orthosis has been described by many authors, too numerous to cite; suffice to say that this is not a new innovation. The orthosis is produced from a cast or impression of the foot in order to reproduce the contour of the foot in a neutral position. The reason for adopting a neutral position around the subtalar joint (STJ) is associated with the belief that the foot creates an ideal functional platform during *midstance*. Some authors believe that this theory is flawed and that a position of

inversion might be more appropriate during casting. Many different views are held; as long as the laboratory receives adequate instructions, then any orthosis should be able to satisfy the practitioner's prescription requirements. However, one advantage to be gained by taking the impression in STJ neutral is that a useful comparison can then be drawn between the clinical measurement (foot) and the cast alignment after replication, namely the extent of varus and valgus deformity.

Unless there is an obvious valgus or varus, the heel contour will not pick up the minor deformity. The neutral negative plate provides information about forefoot relationship only. Naturally, no rearfoot-to-leg relationship exists once the cast has been removed from the foot. Supinatus, a triplane forefoot deformity similar to forefoot varus, cannot be detected either.

Accommodative orthosis

Accommodative orthoses occupy a position between clinical therapies (Ch. 11) and prescription therapies. The terms so described need clarification: 'clinical' means that the orthosis can be wholly dispensed as part of the patient's treatment at the time of consultation, while 'prescription' implies that the orthosis will be sent away to be fitted on a further consultation.

The Irving Insole Device (Taylor therapy) is an example of an orthosis that can be dispensed within a single clinical visit.

Accommodative prescriptive orthoses are made from casted plaster models, as are functional orthoses, although the practitioner may select a wider variety of techniques than the neutral technique. This type of orthosis usually has a softer design and is made to cushion and protect areas where considerable pressure builds up.

Orthotic designs and specifications

The most common orthotic designs are described below, under general headings: standard foot orthosis, high/low-profile orthoses, heel orthoses and, the latest addition, talar control orthoses. As the selection is very wide, only a few designs will be described to illustrate the varying specifications. Modifications to these orthoses will be elaborated upon later in the chapter.

Standard foot orthoses

The most common types of orthosis are the Root and the Shafer. The Shafer orthosis predated the Root orthosis in the UK. The plate was trimmed to provide a heel cup with sufficient depth to assist rearfoot control, and therefore flared medially with a moderate arch height, although one that was lower than the University of California Biomechanics Laboratory (UCBL) device. The application of a lateral modification or addition prevented any sharp edges sticking into the foot (see p. 285). The Shafer system used extrinsic posts (Fig. 12.7A).

The Root orthosis (Fig. 12.7B) adopted a number of modifications called 'additions' in order to provide a good shoe fit, as well as selecting an intrinsic forefoot post system. Originally, the Root heel cup was lower than its predecessor.

High-profile orthoses

The UCBL orthosis has a very deep heel cup, and the lateral and medial sides of the orthosis extend equally up either side of the foot (Fig. 12.8A–C;

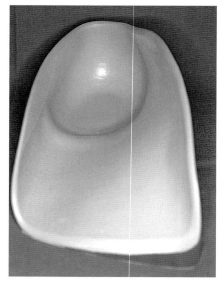

A

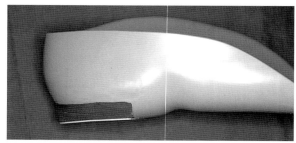

B

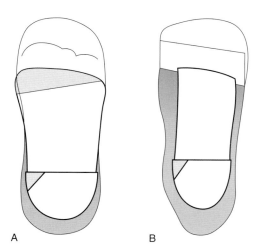

A   B

Figure 12.7 Trims. A, Shafer plate trim shown on casts. B, Root plate trim. (Adapted from Anthony (1991), with permission.)

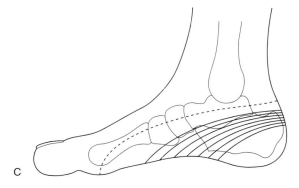

C

Figure 12.8 The University of California Biometrics Laboratory (UCLB) orthosis. A, A small modification made over the cuboid attempts to prevent the calcaneocuboid joint subluxing. B, Outline with rearpost. C, Trim lines conforming around the heel with a high specification to capture and control the sustentaculum tali. (Adapted from Pratt et al (1993b).)

Mereday et al 1972). No medial or lateral additions are used and the device offers the ultimate foot orthotic control for marked pronation. Posts can be applied to the polypropylene plate, although success will depend heavily upon shoe designs accepting this type of orthosis.

The standard orthotic productions follow Root and Shafer designs (see Fig. 12.7). These consist of a plate that is shaped to conform to most Oxford shoe designs, although it may need to be made narrower for Court shoe designs.

Low-profile orthoses

Langer Laboratories has, without doubt, had the greatest influence on the world market and has single-handedly innovated many design changes to assist shoe fit. Their Halfthotic™ has an interesting trim based on the Cobra insole (Fig. 12.9). The lateral portion of plastic is removed, leaving a well-trusted shape proximally, similar to the Rose–Schwartz meniscus. The orthosis is strengthened with EVA and offers an effective design without losing key components for high-heeled shoes and for shoes in which it is difficult to fit the full orthotic plate.

Talar control foot orthoses

Pratt et al (1993a) described an innovative orthosis from the USA. The resulting shape, illustrated in Figure 12.10, is known as a talar control foot orthosis (TCFO) (Brown et al 1987). The difference between this and other orthoses stems from the fact that the arch is not contoured. The orthosis has been designed from the viewpoint that control is better with a total dorsal contact foot orthosis. The cast technique for the TCFO is different from those described earlier. A spiral cast system is preferred, as for AFOs, which are described on page 293.

Heel orthoses

The heel cup has been described in Chapter 11 as being available as a stock item. Where a prescription orthosis is required, mainly to improve heel contour and rearfoot stability, fabrication will be made from a whole foot cast as described above. The heel orthosis is valuable in children,

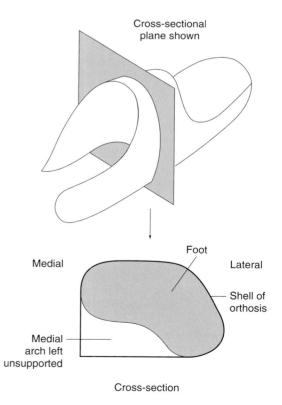

Figure 12.10 The talar control foot orthosis (TCFO) is designed without direct arch contact. It must be taken using a spiral cast technique rather than a slipper-shaped cast. (Adapted from Pratt et al (1993b).)

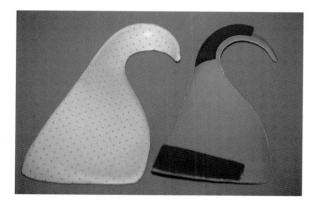

Figure 12.9 Low profile orthosis to allow for fitting in narrow, high-heeled shoes, showing posting on one side.

where the practitioner does not wish to influence the developing forefoot. In adults, it can be used to enhance foot control without compromising the amount of space in the shoe.

Laboratories take the positive cast and can remove the anterior part of the orthosis once the material has been vacuum-formed.

One design involves the use of an extended medial arch, which can extend to either the first ray or the talonavicular joint. As many practitioners have different preferences, no detail is offered here regarding heel cup designs. As with the TCFO, casts can be adapted by having small areas of plaster removed, which in effect creates greater pressure against the foot. This resisting force can help to create further stability, especially around the sustentaculum tali.

Research

Despite the use of many modern materials in the production of foot orthoses, much of the research has been devolved to material sciences rather than looking at specific physical effects upon foot pathology. Tollafield & Pratt (1990a,b) looked at the effects of the Shafer and Root designs of functional orthosis on a normal foot, using pedobarographs, video filming and Kistler force plates (without synchronomy). Acrylic posts were used to angle the pressed plastic plate made from polymethylmethacrylate (PMMA). Little difference between the Shafer and Root plates was noted, except that the Root design offered greater shoe comfort. The trace taken from the Kistler force plate altered between the various angles of tilt, and the sensitivity between $0°$, $4°$ and $8°$ was difficult to interpret with any real significance. The fact that pressure was distributed differently was shown more clearly by the pedobarograph. The rearpost showed some off-loading of the forefoot, presumably because of its larger surface area.

Indications

The influence of the foot on the proximal skeletal structures is now slowly being accepted. It is clear from previous evidence that the STJ has a

profound relationship with the leg and that disruptions in its action do lead to proximal disorders (Inman 1969). The proportional knock-on effect of subtalar frontal plane motion on transverse plane motion within the leg and knee, and vice versa, emphasizes that walking is more than just putting one foot in front of another. Any surface that can change the ground contact relationship will influence rotational movement. These rotations are greater at the top of the leg, reducing movement in a distal direction. However, there are still considerable rotations at the ankle level. If, for example, the STJ is immobile, for whatever reason, these rotations of the leg have to be accommodated elsewhere in the kinetic chain of the leg and trunk. If the ankle cannot cope with the extra rotation, the knee joint is affected next, with a change in the Q angle, causing patella tracking problems (D'Amico & Rabin 1986).

Orthoses function predominantly by reducing the effect of prolonged pronation. The aim of control is to restore the time sequence, i.e. to an acceptable pronation of about 25% of the stance phase when it reaches its optimum pronated position. During midstance, the leg can be influenced by an inlay appropriately balanced to ensure that the STJ is supinated and continues supinating, with consequential external rotation of the leg until final propulsion.

Compensatory pronation at the STJ everts the rearfoot and supination inverts the rearfoot. As the rearfoot moves, the forefoot will also move to remain in contact with the ground. The ability of the forefoot to compensate fully depends on there being sufficient joint motion, requiring inversion during subtalar pronation and eversion during subtalar supination. This midtarsal joint motion takes place largely about the longitudinal axis but is limited by its small range (Root et al 1977).

The effects of foot pathology do not stop at the knee; the hip is able to accommodate some of the rotation but will not then provide the motion needed for normal gait. Therefore, gait changes follow an exaggerated transverse plane body rotation and create the need for shorter stride lengths. Conversely, if there are symptomatic problems in the proximal structures associated with excessive rotations, they may be addressed by controlling subtalar pronation or supination. This is more common in sporting activities, where every possible deficit is examined and treated in an attempt to improve performance.

A sagittal plane relationship exists between the foot and the proximal body structures. Principally, this is reflected in an equinus position of the foot and the ankle joint. If this position is fixed, then the knee and hip must flex sufficiently to allow walking to take place, usually with the toe as the initial contact point between the foot and the ground. This requires an increase in muscle activity in the knee and hip extensors to stabilize the limb, which can tire rapidly. Additionally, discomfort can be experienced at the knee, particularly as a result of the much increased joint loading from the flexed position. This foot position can also lead to hip hiking (lifting up) and circumduction of the leg to obtain ground clearance if knee and hip flexion is not possible. All of these processes consume more energy than normal gait and can lead to arthritic changes later in life. Orthotic contribution can smooth out some of these determinants.

The STJ is the anatomical structure that is responsible for accommodating transverse rotations and it thus enables the leg to rotate on a fixed foot. By tilting the supporting orthotic platform, both midtarsal and proximal joint motions are influenced.

Flexible feet are characteristically easier to control than rigid feet. Nonetheless, the additional effects of abnormal axes within flexible feet can make orthotic control difficult. The foot can easily slip off the inlay despite careful manufacture, because a flexible foot with a high midtarsal joint oblique axis can move over the inlay within the shoe.

Marked rigidity is associated with limited joint movement and may be typified by a forefoot equinus, pes cavus or congenital talipes foot with triplane deformity. A rigid foot with fixed deformities may need to be accommodated with thin foam materials incorporating good shock-absorbing properties and forefoot extensions to

reduce contact pressure. As with any orthotic design, good shoe fit is essential and, as part of good prescribing, both shoe and foot pathology must be considered.

Replication technique

Casts can be taken using plaster of Paris in a variety of ways. Most common methods use non-weight-bearing techniques, with the foot in STJ neutral (the neutral position cast) (Tollafield 1985, Anthony 1991); other techniques have the STJ pronated or weight bearing in a neutral position:

- non-weight-bearing techniques
  - suspension technique, patient supine
  - modified suspension technique, patient prone
  - direct pressure technique, patient prone or supine
  - semipronated technique, patient prone or supine
  - fully pronated technique, patient prone or supine
  - vacuum casting in neutral (in the shoe)
- weight-bearing techniques
  - semi-weight bearing on a foam pad
  - foam impression (Birkenstock).

Suspension technique

The suspension technique is the traditional way in which neutral foot casts are taken. The patient is positioned in a supine (sitting or lying) relaxed position.

The practitioner's forearm, wrist and fingers are held in a straight line and placed over the dorsum of the foot, with the thumb in the sulcus of the fourth and fifth toes (Fig. 12.11). The advantage of the finger position lies in the fact that the cast contour is not deformed by thumb pressure. The foot is extended in order that some weight-bearing lengthening is created. While holding the foot firmly, it is moved through its full range of subtalar pronation and supination, at the same time palpating the head of the talus (Fig. 12.12). When the medial and lateral prominences of the talar head are felt to be equal, the STJ is thought to be in neutral. This can be confirmed quickly by checking that the superior and inferior curves of the lateral malleolus are symmetrical (Root et al 1971).

With the foot held in this neutral position, it is lifted slightly from the couch and a small force is applied to pronate the midtarsal joint and to dorsiflex the ankle joint to resistance (note: this will not necessarily bring the foot to 90° to the leg). During the above procedure, the rest of the leg should be observed to maintain the correct relationship with the foot. In order to avoid dorsiflexion of the fourth and fifth toes, the wrist needs to be rotated to bring them back into alignment with the other toes, as shown in Figure 12.12.

Double or twin-ply plaster bandage is usually used: 20 cm wide for adults and 10–15 cm for smaller feet. The process of applying the plaster bandage is the same for all of the techniques and so will be explained in detail here.

Applying plaster bandage The first length is cut to extend from the first metatarsal head loosely round the toes to the fifth and 15 mm of one long edge is folded over to reinforce it and then immersed in hand-warm water. The bandage is then squeezed of excess water and draped loosely over the toes. It is then positioned to align with the first and fifth metatarsal heads with the reinforced edge running parallel to the first and fifth metatarsal shafts. The plaster of Paris is smoothed onto the sides of the foot then across the plantar surface of the foot on one side then the other. Excess plaster is pushed gently into the sulcus. All air must be expelled from under the bandage before proceeding. A second strip of plaster of Paris is prepared as before, this time just long enough to overlap the first piece when pulled round the heel (Fig. 12.13). The second piece is overlapped with the first and folded over as before. Posteriorly, the plaster of Paris is pulled up to extend to about midway up each malleolus (Fig. 12.14). This ensures a deep enough cast will be produced. The fold at the heel produced by this is pushed to the back of the calcaneus. The foot is now positioned as shown in Fig. 12.14 and held until the plaster sets. A piece of absorbent paper under the thumb can sometimes help the practitioner to hold the position by preventing slipping.

To remove the cast (Fig. 12.15), the skin along the top edge of the cast is carefully eased away from it and then the foot held at the ankle and shaken slightly. The fingers of both hands are then placed along the reinforced edge of the cast at the heel and pulled forward. Patients should not assist with this nor move their toes. Once clear of the heel the cast is pulled up along the

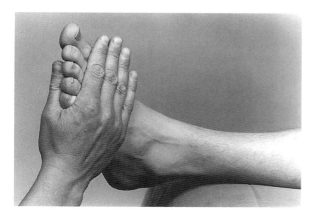

Figure 12.11 Taking a foot cast by the suspension technique. The foot is shown being held in subtalar joint neutral with the midtarsal joint maximally pronated and the ankle dorsiflexed. The leg is suspended over the couch. This is the initial position for holding the forefoot for the suspension technique with the patient supine.

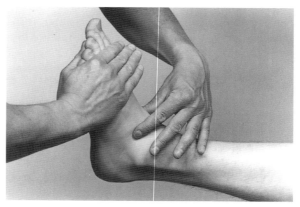

Figure 12.12 The head of the talus can be easily palpated in the supine position.

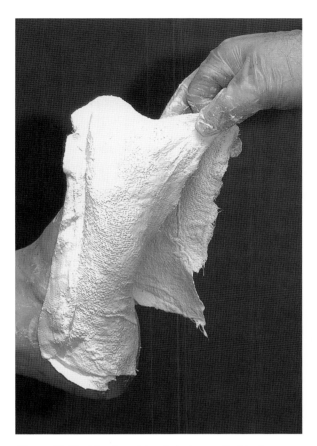

Figure 12.13 The first strip of plaster applied to the forefoot and being smoothed over the plantar surface.

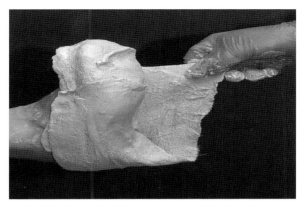

Figure 12.14 The second strip of plaster applied to the rearfoot, overlapping the first and being smoothed over the plantar surface.

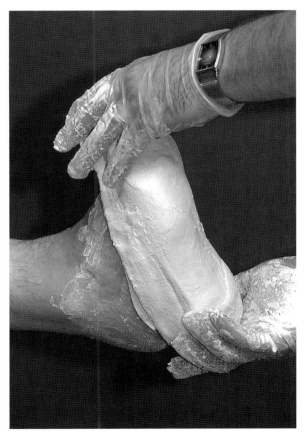

Figure 12.15 As illustrated, the cast removal process has just begun, with the cast clear of the toes and ready to pull up along the plantar surface.

foot and clear of the toes. The cast should now be evaluated before the patient leaves.

Clinical comment This technique produces a good plantar impression without distortion. The supine position allows ready visualization of the extensor tendons to ensure that they remain inactive during casting. The talus is accessible to palpation, which makes detection of the subtalar neutral position simpler. The main drawback of this technique is that it is probably the hardest one to master. Most errors using this approach are a result of the grip used to take the impression; the alignment of the hand and the fingers may be incorrect and, consequently, the resulting cast is easily supinated and the toes can be dorsiflexed.

Modified suspension technique

The modified suspension technique is very similar to that described above except that the subject is prone. The same arm, wrist and finger positions are used as above and the STJ is positioned in neutral much as before. To pronate the midtarsal joint, the leg is not lifted from the couch but pulled downwards and a dorsiflexion force is applied to the ankle joint much as before (Fig. 12.16). Again, the wrist position is checked to ensure alignment of the fourth and fifth toes, and the whole procedure is repeated as necessary as a dry run to become familiar with the position required without the plaster. Plaster is prepared and applied exactly as described above and the foot is repositioned and held until set. Removal is the same as for the supine casting.

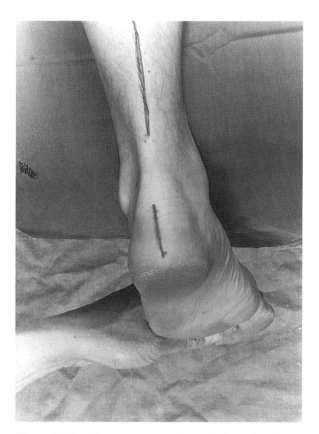

Figure 12.16 The prone suspension technique showing the correct hold.

Clinical comment This technique allows better visualization of the forefoot to rearfoot relationship than possible with the supine position, and the curves above and below the lateral malleolus are easily seen, making confirmation of subtalar neutral simple. The extensor tendons are not visible and so cannot be checked to ensure inactivity, and there is, therefore, greater potential for some distortion of the cast without the practitioner's knowledge. There may also be some discomfort of the anterior leg at the ankle level as it is pulled into the couch during casting. This could result in the subject repositioning themselves and causing unwanted movement; this discomfort can be prevented by using a softer edge on the couch.

Direct pressure technique

The direct pressure technique can be carried out with the patient prone or supine and is probably the most universally used and preferred technique.

The hand position is slightly different from that adopted for the suspension technique; the thumb is placed on the plantar surface of the fourth and fifth metatarsal heads in line with the sulcus of the toes (Fig. 12.17). The foot is moved through its full range of subtalar pronation and supination while the other hand is used to palpate the talar head and identify subtalar neutral. With the STJ in neutral, pressure is applied to the fourth and fifth metatarsal heads to pronate the midtarsal joint fully about both axes and to dorsiflex the foot at the ankle joint to initial resistance.

The plaster is applied as described above. Having a piece of paper or gauze under the thumb during this stage sometimes helps to prevent the thumb slipping on the wet plaster. The cast is removed as described above.

Clinical comment While this is the most common casting technique, it is not without its problems. The forefoot can be forced laterally if the pressure applied to the metatarsal heads is not applied directly in line with the long axis of the leg. Direct pressure can also distort the true position of an unstable fifth ray. A depression

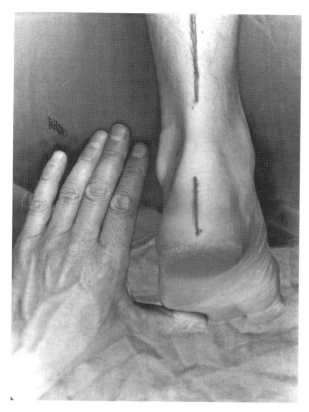

Figure 12.17 The position of the thumb during the direct pressure technique.

created in the cast has to be filled later on unless pushed out at the time of cast removal. In either case, this will introduce some inaccuracy into the forefoot impression, which, for some purposes, may be unacceptable.

Vacuum casting in 'neutral'

The vacuum cast was popular in the USA in the 1980s. A cast is applied as previously described, with a plastic bag wrapped over the foot and a flexible tube placed inside the bag so that the whole foot slips into the shoe easily while the plaster is still wet. The tube connected to a vacuum pump produces compression around the foot, ensuring a very accurate in-shoe impression. Neutral position is selected by talar head palpation and dorsiflexion under the lateral sole of the shoe.

Clinical comment This technique, again developed in the USA, means that sensitive feet, especially following surgery, can be casted in the corrected position without painful manipulation. The vacuum builds up sufficient compression to provide an adequate mould without causing discomfort. Furthermore, patients with court shoes do well with this technique because of a better orthotic fit, although no studies confirm these advantages.

Semipronated technique

Where a neutral STJ position is not indicated, a semipronated cast may be more appropriate. The prone position is preferred as it improves visualization of the forefoot to rearfoot relationship. This is important in eliminating an inverted forefoot by pronating the STJ. The forefoot is held and the whole foot is moved into a sufficiently pronated position at both the subtalar and midtarsal joints. The forefoot should be aligned at 90° to a bisection of the calcaneus and held until the plaster is set.

Clinical comment Different practitioners use different variations on this technique. For example, forefoot supinatus may be reduced by vertical pressure at the base of the first ray or this amount of soft tissue deformity may be left in the cast. The advantages and disadvantages of the technique are similar to those already described.

Fully pronated technique

If the STJ motion is restricted, the foot may have to be maximally pronated during casting. Joint bridging from bony bars, painful sinus tarsi and arthritides are best managed with a pronated cast. The orthosis plays an inhibitive rather than a functional role. The procedure outlined above is still used. In some cases, there may be insufficient motion at the subtalar and midtarsal joints to reduce fully the forefoot supinatus.

Weight-bearing casting techniques

Casts for producing accommodative orthoses can be taken while the foot is bearing weight or by using impression blocks (Fig. 12.18). This technique is clearly unsuitable for any foot that requires significant positioning during casting. The cast is taken with the foot on a foam pad (covered in plastic), maintaining a neutral position (if required) by rotating the leg to obtain talar congruency. In all other respects, the technique is the same as before.

Weight-bearing impression systems Where an accommodative type of inlay does not require a high corrective specification, all that is required is an outline impression of the foot. If the foot is essentially rigid but needs some protection from internal stresses, then it is clearly inappropriate to attempt to position the foot in any particular orientation. It is far better to capture the true position of the weight-bearing foot including the spread of soft tissues. This can be done by getting the subject to stand in putty (Pratt et al 1984), but it is often a messy procedure and the putty needs to be stored in specific conditions so that it remains usable for a reasonable time. A better and cheaper way is to use impression blocks filled with a foam that has no rebound and permanently deforms when an object is pressed into it. The block consists of a box divided into two parts lined with foam. The foam takes up the plantar shape, in a similar manner to 'oasis' used by flower arrangers. By pressing the foot into the foam, a good impression of the plantar surface is obtained quickly and with little mess (Fig. 12.18), from which a plaster positive of the foot can be made.

The Irving (impression) system has been described in Figure 11.28 (see p. 261) and offers the practitioner a weight-bearing orthosis that can be produced immediately from an accurate replication technique.

Summary

Weight-bearing cast techniques have the disadvantage of creating a broader positive cast, which can create footwear-fitting problems. For this reason, the non-weight-bearing cast technique seems, on the whole, to offer a better shoe fit. There are also some doubts about the non-weight-bearing casting procedure. It has been suggested that it does not represent the true forefoot to rearfoot relationship and that it often produces a false inversion of the forefoot (Kidd 1991); this belief arises from the fact that the cast contours the soft tissue rather than the bony structure.

There has been limited research into the effects of neutral foot casting. No controlled studies have been conducted to establish whether variations introduced into casting are significant enough to influence the technique selected. Measured inverted or everted forefoot deformity can be diagnosed. Large variations of deformity are more visible than small changes. Metatarsal sagittal plane deformities cannot be differentiated from frontal forefoot deformities unless the metatarsal can be visibly identified. If an inverted deformity exists, the rearpart of the plate tilts the same number of degrees in an everted direction. Conversely, an everted deformity will cause the plate to tilt in an inverted direction. Some allowance for error, perhaps ±3°, should be made when transposing the values from the measured tilt of the rearpart of the cast.

General cast critique

The practitioner should determine the accuracy and quality of the negative impression before sending the plate to the laboratory.

A clean cast should be produced without lumps or bulges that do not conform to the foot; the plate should appear smooth inside. The more lumpy a cast, the more work a laboratory has to carry out and the more likely it is that there will be inaccuracies in the finished product. Such

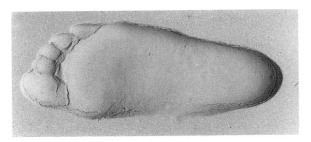

Figure 12.18 A foam impression of a foot, commonly used for accommodative orthoses.

casts should be rejected at the clinical stage. A 12-point checklist can be used to evaluate the quality of a neutral cast taken in the clinic.

1.   Does the cast appear to replicate the same deformity as in the neutrally held foot?

2.   Using the plantar surface as a reference, draw an imaginary line through the heel. A line projected distally should end up between the second and third metatarsals, unless of course there is a transverse plane deformity. If the deformity was soft tissue, this should have been corrected in the cast first.

3.   A 'C' shape along the lateral border indicates either a true metatarsus adductus or the fact that the practitioner has adducted the foot with supination of the oblique midtarsal joint axis.

4.   The inside contour over the calcaneocuboid joint is normally flattened across the lateral furrow. This needs to be seen in transverse perspective (Fig. 12.19). Semi-weight-bearing casts tend to have a flattened area (Tollafield 1985).

5.   When using the suspension technique, the toes should be in alignment, and in particular the lateral fourth and fifth toes should not be dorsiflexed. This type of error would ultimately plantarflex the metatarsals.

6.   The direct pressure technique thumbprint should only cover those lateral metatarsals. It is not unusual to find the plantar surface of the cast rucked up from aggressive and careless casting. In the suspension technique, the lateral side of the cast should not be pinched excessively.

7.   Viewing the lateral arch from inside the cast, one should see a gentle curve in the sagittal plane. A high arch may suggest that the cuboid has been plantarflexed.

8.   The rearpart of the cast should reflect a high lateral and medial side to a point just below the malleolus. A low rear heel part will make filling very difficult and will make a shallow cast for the purpose of vacuum forming.

9.   Excessive pronation, a likely result of using the direct pressure technique, will cause the heel to widen medially. If when looking inside, the talonavicular area is flattened in a 'normal' shaped foot, or a lateral crease is observed under the fibula, then it is likely that pronation has occurred and a new cast should be taken.

10.   The first metatarsal head should leave a clear imprint with skin striae demonstrable. A faint or poor impression suggests that the longitudinal axis has been supinated.

11.   The surrounding rim of the cast should be strong to prevent deformity of the rear section when it is removed. If the rim has been deformed, this means that the cast has been removed carelessly.

12.   The two pieces making up the plate on the inside should have no join. If care is taken, the orthotist is likely to have greater confidence in the practitioner.

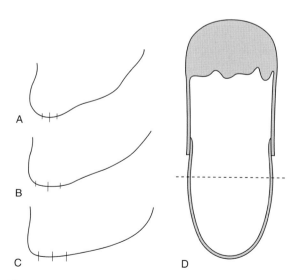

Figure 12.19   The plaster negative shell has been sectioned as shown. A, Supinated; B, correct alignment; C, pronated; D, the position of the cast cross-sectioned. Note the varying widths of the shoulder associated with the fifth ray.

PRESCRIBING CASTED ORTHOSES

All practitioners should routinely undertake a joint and soft tissue evaluation, whether or not orthoses are intended. A more in-depth examination will be necessary to assist with the prescription, particularly in the case of a functional orthosis.

Many claims, particularly emanating from the USA, have been made in support of a variety of prescribing theories. Without doubt, more research is required to assist prescribing decisions. However, in recent years, much interest in the UK has focused on the accuracy of measurements used in prescription fabrication.

Measurement techniques used for prescriptions

Clearly, the techniques required to cast and complete an examination rely on two basic skills:

1. the ability to bisect a limb segment accurately
2. the ability to determine reliably the STJ neutral position.

There are a number of problems associated with these, as both are prone to error. Such errors may be greater than the accuracy with which the measurements are required for any clinical value. Studies have been carried out to examine the ability of practitioners to perform these fundamental tasks.

It is well known that the skin of the body moves as the limbs move. The accuracy of the measurements of skin, determined from lines drawn over joints, limits the accuracy of measurements of motion derived from this activity. Various studies have been highlighted below to illustrate this point.

Subtalar joint assessment

The proportion and range of excursion of the STJ seem to vary widely. Kidd (1991) questioned the accuracy of measurements and bisectors and the validity of the (1/3):(2/3) ratio (Root et al 1971) as a viable technique.

Bailey et al (1984), using radiographic tomography, found a number of subjects with a ratio of 3:1 (3/4:1/4), as did Tollafield & Pratt (1990a,b) using a hand-held tractograph. The wide ranges of STJ movement measured by various clinical authors are well documented, illustrating the variability among the different methods employed: Bailey et al (1984) found a mean of 30°

total motion for those aged 20–30 years; Tollafield & Pratt (1990a) found a mean of 37° in a group aged 19–51 years; Inman (1976) found a mean range of 40° ± 7° with a spherical goniometer; and McMaster (1976) found a total range of 30° with a calcaneal pointer.

Griffith (1988) set out to examine the reliability of measurements. In a large study using nine examiners, he examined the inter- and intraobserver errors associated with the measurements of ankle joint dorsiflexion, STJ motion (in three ways) and the angle of the hallux. The findings of this study revealed the following accuracies:

- calculated neutral position: an average of 2.63° varus (standard deviation (SD) 4.31)
- measured neutral position: an average of 6.02° varus (SD, 3.06)
- stance neutral position: an average of 4.04° varus (SD, 2.59).

When compared with a radiographically determined neutral position, work on the neutral position of the STJ shows that all techniques produced a varus position, with the 'calculated' approach being the most accurate, while the 'measured' technique showed the least variability. Further reference to calculated and measured neutral positions forms part of patient assessment and data can be found in other sources (e.g. Tollafield & Merriman 1995).

There are many reasons for this inaccuracy, which are not a result of observer error. For example, the positioning and lining-up of goniometers with the limb are critical if measurements are to be accurate and repeatable. Add to this the fact that the STJ is triplanar in action, and positioning of the single axis goniometer with respect to the joint is bound to produce some discrepancies in measurement. Ball & Johnson (1993) found errors similar to those found by Griffith (1988) when using a flexible goniometer. In fact, when all of these matters are taken into account, it is surprising that the accuracy is as high as it appears to be.

Phillips et al (1985) used goniometers to measure the calcaneus and lower third of the leg, followed by rigorous mathematical analysis. No allowance was made for the possibility that the measurements used in the equations produced were themselves open to the kinds of error detailed above.

An unreported study carried out in the Orthotics and Disability Research Centre at Derbyshire Royal Infirmary, UK (D. J. Pratt, unpublished work) showed that the most experienced practitioners could not bisect by eye the lower third of the lower leg to an accuracy of better than about 3°. The less able practitioners were even less accurate than this. It was possible to increase the accuracy to about 1.5° if the width of the limb was accurately measured with callipers. However, this took far too long to perform so many of the practitioners said it would not be suitable for use in the clinic.

If the lines drawn on skin are unreliable, then the measurements taken from them will likewise be suspect, and it is these derived angles that have been more often recorded and used to determine the accuracy of the whole approach. Despite concerns about reliability, recent evidence suggests that assessment by eye can produce adequate repeatability and accuracy. A study by Cook et al (1988) examined 138 subjects and measured the neutral position of the STJ in three ways: by palpation of the talus, by equalizing the proximal and distal curves of the lateral malleolus, and by observation of the skin over the sinus tarsi. They found a 95% correlation between the three methods but had assumed that a 2° error was clinically acceptable.

The triplanar motion of the STJ complicates the essentially two-dimensional assessment techniques usually used. This matter was addressed by Engsberg et al (1988) in an in vitro study on nine cadaveric lower legs and feet. They found that the monitoring of the inversion/eversion and abduction/adduction orientations of the talocalcaneal/talocrural complex is more valuable in predicting pronation and supination positions than using inversion/eversion alone.

Components of prescribing

The laboratory requires information that will allow technicians to convert a negative plate into a moulded inlay that conforms to the practitioner's requirements. Any omission of information will lead to further error. The primary aim of the orthosis is that:

- patient symptoms will be relieved
- the foot will feel more stable
- less abnormal shoe wear will be observed
- the patient can use the orthosis in a number of shoes.

The heel shape and skin contours will be affected by different positions adopted when casting the foot. A non-weight-bearing cast should require less plaster work but frequently will need adaptations to allow a weight-bearing simulation, most notably the medial and lateral expansions. Weight-bearing casts may need some surface reduction to improve their shoe fit.

Medial additions

When the flexible foot contacts the ground, the medial long arch descends about the long axis of the MTJ. If the cast is taken while the foot is non-weight bearing, the arch will appear higher than it would functionally when on the ground. In this case, an addition should be ordered to prevent the plastic from gouging the foot. It was Tollafield & Pratt's (1990a) belief (when comparing the Shafer plate (without medial addition) with the Root plate (with medial addition)) that including an addition does not alter the efficacy of an orthosis. The fascial band of the plantar aponeurosis may be prominent and easily irritated. Early concerns with functional orthoses creating fibromatosis have been reported in American podiatric literature. A medial addition, or even an additional channel, to avoid arch irritation may be ordered by asking the laboratory to add plaster to the positive cast. This adaptation will deflect the plastic material when moulded away from any areas of sensitivity. The negative cast must be marked accordingly.

Lateral expansions

An additional ledge of plaster to the cast will prevent the skin becoming pinched. In deciding whether to utilize an expansion, the practitioner will consider the ultimate height of the heel cup first. A high heel cup set at 20 mm (adult foot) is less likely to require a lateral addition than would a low 10–12 mm cup. In the case of the lower specification, an addition is useful and will prevent pinching from the orthotic plate. In other words, when high heel cups are ordered, little additional value is gained from expanding the cast edge, as shoe fit as well as some hindfoot control will be compromised. Medial and lateral additions are shown in Figure 12.20.

Materials

Choosing materials can be problematic because the plastics currently available have very different mechanical properties yet they all look alike

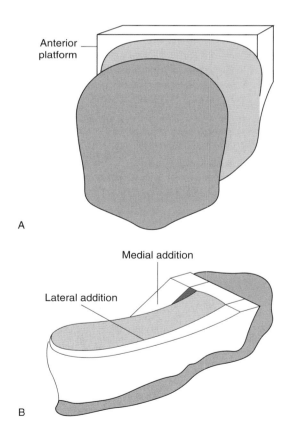

Figure 12.20 Expansions. A, Medial and lateral additions to the positive plaster cast. B, The intrinsic forefoot post. (Adapted from Anthony (1991), with permission.)

(Rome 1990). The acrylics and polythenes are perhaps the most popular, although soft materials for accommodative orthoses vary, from Birkenstock or woodflour (sawdust with latex) to EVA sheets, which are ground by hand to provide a firm but yielding inlay. Leather laminates have fallen from popularity but can be made into acceptable orthoses if the skin type precludes the use of plastics. Top covers can be used to cover surface defects but may lead to the need for early replacement. Top covers are optional and usually depend on the desired cosmetic finish. Polycarbonates, carbon fibre and fibreglass orthoses are less popular. Early polyvinyl chloride (PVC) materials were found to fracture initially (Ch. 10).

Two further matters need to be considered: first, the type of orthosis to be used for the problem, and, second, the required thickness and durability of the material selected for any occupational and additional activities. Orthoses should not break as a result of normal walking cadence stresses. Sporting activities naturally impose forces of greater magnitude in all orthogonal planes. An acrylic device will need to be around 4 mm thick to cope with this stress in the case of an adult, while a polypropylene or high-density polyethylene of 3 mm thickness will be more satisfactory, with less likelihood of fracture, for the same individual.

The patient's weight is a determining factor. Materials can be made thicker, although selecting a material above 4 mm does provide additional shoe fit problems. Arch strengthening can be ordered with foam infills, which are popular additions provided by some orthotic laboratories, particularly those dealing with podiatrists. Lightness has become a serious factor for runners and other athletes. Trainers have become lighter over the years and orthoses have become heavier with the use of elaborate additions and fillers. Ballet shoes often do better with a high-density moulded Plastazote orthosis (Fig. 12.21). The practitioner should study the range of materials on offer to suit the different needs.

Three other factors need to be discussed to fulfil the prescription: elevators, trim lines and addition specifications.

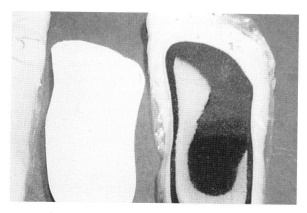

Figure 12.21 Combined high- and low-density Plastazote orthosis indicated for dancers. (Courtesy of Dr Tom Novella.)

Posting

Posting is the method used for controlling an orthosis by tilting the contoured plate against the foot. Two types of posting are currently in vogue: extrinsic and intrinsic. Initially, as with shoes, wedging was applied to the outer surface (extrinsic post). In the 1980s, an intrinsic method was introduced by a number of practitioners in the UK. Little scientific follow-up has been conducted comparing the merits of intrinsic and extrinsic methods.

Intrinsic post An intrinsic post or step is one that is created within the plastic. The forefoot is usually intrinsically posted by adding plaster platforms to the cast (see Fig. 12.20). The plaster additions effectively alter the lie of the positive cast, correcting its valgus or varus position. The anterior platform will create a flat edge to the pressed orthosis. It is usual to order intrinsic posts with medial additions to allow a smoother contour to the finished orthosis. The medial and lateral additions blend better with the anterior platform. Plastic material will be vacuum formed over the anterior platforms. Once a cast is angled intrinsically by more than a few degrees of varus, the control relies proximally on the plate of the orthosis across the position of the metatarsal shafts.

In fact, greater posting angles provide little additional benefit and can cause the patient to slide off the orthosis. The exception to this is that an intrinsic valgus wedge appears to offer more useful control and stability than higher values of varus wedging. Because the fifth metatarsal has minimal contour alterations, any such prescriptive requirement keeps the orthotic plate closer to the surface of the skin.

Selection of the intrinsic post, often associated with the Root orthosis, is particularly beneficial for patients whose shoes cannot accommodate forefoot extrinsic posts. Added to narrow trim lines, the acceptance rate has been found to be much higher. Intrinsic posts can be ground into some plastics more easily than others, particularly under the heel. The laboratory will advise on the most suitable material and technique if doubt exists.

Lundeen (1988) suggested that conventional systems could be used to produce a plaster positive, which can be adjusted by following a series of alterations. By sectioning through the cast at three predetermined points, corrections can be made that influence the position of the foot: *triaxial system*. A screw introduced through the heel along the length of the cast and another screw across the foot are loosened for adjustments. The cast is influenced predominantly through the midtarsal joint and first ray in three planes as necessary. Plaster is smoothed over the adjusted cast to create an orthotic plate. At present this system has not been received favourably in the UK.

Extrinsic post An extrinsic post offers more intimate control against the patient's foot than an intrinsic post. The wedge of plastic PMMA or EVA must be ground to blend in with the anterior edge of the orthosis, offering support to the foot without taking up additional room in the shoe. The proximal part of the orthosis is also blended to sit inside the heel counter and ground down to allow for the heel height. The main prescriptive consideration lies in how much of an angle to order.

The post cannot be balanced to the same number of degrees of deformity established from clinical examination (Fig. 12.22) because it would take up too much room in the shoe. Overposted (balanced) orthoses are uncomfortable and affect the independent first and fifth rays adversely.

Two problems might arise as a result of extrinsic forefoot post design. First, if the deformity in the adult has been present for a long time, the foot will have compensated to some extent, possibly without symptoms. Second, if any material is placed under an independent metatarsal, that ray will become elevated and cause impairment of movement at the MTPJ. If the metatarsal head appears elevated, then some adjustment is necessary.

While practitioners will develop their own preference for either intrinsic or extrinsic posting, both types of system have advantages and disadvantages. A less-common practice of mixing intrinsic and extrinsic posts has been used in the USA. In this prescription, the intrinsic work is carried out first and any additional extrinsic post is added after the plate has been trimmed.

Position of the post   Each orthosis will have either a rearfoot or a forefoot post, or both. Convention dictates, perhaps erroneously, that the rearpost should always have a varus/inverted cant. However, patients who have been provided with valgus/everted rearposts have not always suffered detrimentally. The simple rule-of-thumb that a valgus forefoot deformity be prescribed with a lateral wedge and a varus forefoot deformity with a medial wedge provides a useful place to start. Nonetheless, the absence of problems with everted rearposts does not mean that there should be a sudden change in prescribing fashion: the wary practitioner should use soft valgus wedges first, before converting to a permanent prescription format.

A varus rearpost is used with values of 0–8° as a rule-of-thumb. Posts applied to the anterior and posterior ends of the orthosis appear to offer better control than a single post at one end only (Fig. 12.23).

Varus forefoot posts of values greater than 4–6° create the types of problem alluded to above. Valgus posts can be tolerated until the fourth and fifth toes become irritated; this tends to restrict higher values above 5°.

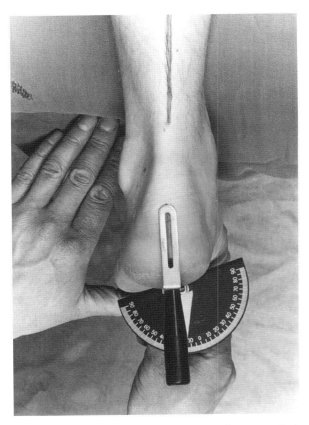

Figure 12.22   The measurement of the forefoot to rearfoot with a special goniometer designed to rest on the plantar forefoot and hindfoot.

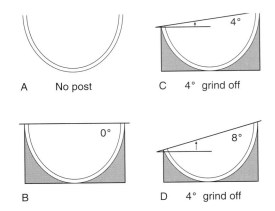

Figure 12.23   Rearposting and heel relationships. A, No post; B, zero post for no motion; C, 4° degree varus post with 4° grind-off (common angle selected initially); D, 8° varus post. If motion is too great, an additional forefoot post is applied, i.e. 3° forefoot varus will limit motion to 5°.

There are only a few studies that consider the scientific basis of posting. Tollafield & Pratt (1990a) commented on the dearth of literature supporting the use of both forefoot and rearfoot posts.

Heel cup heights   Heel cup heights have been discussed above (see p. 287). The height must be selected for the shoe first, and the type of pathology and intended control are considered next. As the post tilts laterally, the heel height on that side may need to be higher than for a lower post angle. This feature is the same for both distal and proximal posts.

Elevators   Ross & Gurnik (1982) pointed out that the stability offered by posts would be affected by variable shoe height. In fact, a point arises where an orthosis offers little benefit to a patient if the heel height is so great that both anterior and posterior posts rock uncontrollably. The adverse mechanical effects from this could cause more harm than assistance. The reasons for such adverse problems relate to the production of unwarranted sagittal or frontal plane rock, reducing the intended stability offered by the orthosis.

An elevator is a piece of plastic of known thickness (4–12 mm) used to account for heel pitch. Given that a shoe has a heel height, an elevator is used to ensure that the orthosis is appropriately balanced such that no adverse movement arises at the back of the shoe. Ross & Gurnick's (1982) main precept considered three bands of heel height: 1.25 cm (0.5 inch), requiring a 4 mm elevator; 2.5 cm (1 inch), requiring an 8 mm elevator; and 3.75 cm (1.5 inches), requiring a 12 mm elevator (see Fig. 12.24). The soft acrylic material or EVA post should be pressed or ground down, respectively, using an elevator to comply with the heel height determined above.

Trim lines   An orthosis made from a plate vacuformed from thermoplastic needs to be trimmed. The use of specific terms will assist the laboratory, although no doubt there is much diversity in the terms used internationally. The practitioner can discuss this with the laboratory, describe the trim lines in detail or specifying a certain type of orthosis, such as a Root orthosis.

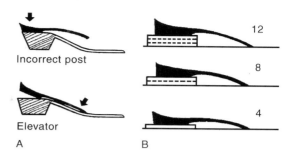

Figure 12.24   Elevator selection. A, Incorrect selection will produce instability where a rearpost should be stable. B, Correct elevator selection is measured in millimetres (see text).

Trim lines also include specifications such as heel height, medial and lateral side heights and additional flares, as in the Robert–Whitman orthosis, where the lateral cup has a flange extending up the calcaneus to grip the heel.

Additions to the orthosis   Part of the prescription is concerned with variations which, when added, have additional benefit upon foot function. In the main, such additions fall into two categories: extensions and adaptations.

Extensions are added to a functional orthosis to enhance further the redistributive, accommodative, stability, compensatory and rest qualities of general therapeutic objectives. Polyurethane foam of thickness 1–3 mm is sometimes added under a vinyl or leather cover (Fig. 12.25). The

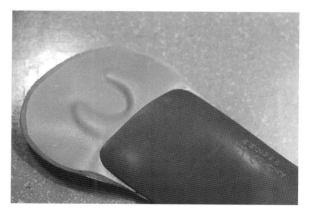

Figure 12.25   An extension placed on a standard orthotic plate offers protection over the forefoot at a specific site of high shear pressure.

extension may be full length, in which case it will be trimmed to the shape of the shoe by the practitioner, or it may be trimmed to the toe sulcus. The latter is favoured, as the toe depth is compromised to a lesser degree. Padded materials in latex foam, neoprene, polyurethane foam, polyethylene foam and PVC foams can all offer redistribution and rest to part of the forefoot, as well as compensating for loss of adipose tissue.

Adaptations are considered to increase surface control. A flared post can be beneficial medially and laterally, to increase pronatory resistance and reduce lateral heel sprain, respectively, by altering moments of force about heel contact. When ordering a flared post, the extent of the flare should be stated (e.g. 1–6 mm) as well as which side (or perhaps both) is to be flared. A Thomas heel, which extends from the medial side anteriorly to fill in part of the long arch, has been used in much the same way as a medial flare. Some anterior posts will need to be trimmed to minimize the vertical forces applied over the independent first and fifth rays.

Many patients, when first issued with rearposts, complain of being lifted out of their shoes. Posts in EVA are capped with thin plastic to prevent material compression, but the capping may need to be removed if the lifting effect is too great. On the whole, an orthosis will bed into the insock and settle after a few weeks. Tollafield & Pratt (1990a) noted that the function of the rearpost provided a large surface area to stabilize the STJ and ankle joint. The varus angle allowed motion to function around a specific STJ axis (low, normal or high).

Posts may be omitted altogether. In this case, the rounded heel cup allows considerable rolling movement at contact. A zero post is a flat post (Fig. 12.23) that will confine the heel (calcaneus) and allow less STJ movement. A zero post may have greater value where patients suffer from arthritic pain in the hindfoot and require limitation of joint movement. If the prescription is likely to work, a higher than normal heel cup should be requested, otherwise the heel will force its way out of the cup with foot rotation. The ability of a foot orthosis to exert this type of control is limited and, if failure is suspected, the practi-

tioner should consider an AFO or a supramalleolar orthosis, which increases heel/ankle control.

The usual initial request for a varus is 4°. The use of a varus tilt of 8° can be equally helpful, creating a greater antipronatory force, and is often made more effective with concomitant forefoot posts. Weed et al (1978) found that the use of a post without grinding off to allow some pronation resulted in back pain. It is probably for this reason that all hard posts made from acrylic have some element of grind-off. EVA posts, being less dense, do not suffer from the same problem. Tollafield & Pratt (1987) found no evidence to support the practice of varying orthotic post prescriptions by single degrees; increments of 0, 4 and 8° are commonly used and work satisfactorily.

Forefoot posts should always be added first and rearposts afterwards; this is because the anterior edge is always used as a reference for rearpost positioning. Rearposts contribute less to the measured values of deformity and predominantly affect heel placement. Any adjustments are best undertaken by a laboratory, as considerable experience is required when working with plastics; furthermore, any warranty that exists may become invalid if this is not done.

The prescription should always indicate how much motion ground into the medial rearpost is required. A summary of the prescription components is included in Box 12.1.

Dispensing a functional device

When fitting a functional orthosis, consideration must be given to the accuracy of plate dimensions, adequate foot-to-orthosis contact and comfort. An optimum fit is essential if the device is to be well tolerated. The orthotic plate and post should conform to the previously examined deformity (Fig. 12.26). The orthosis should be checked during both non-weight bearing and weight bearing. The alignment of the lower extremity is checked while standing on the orthosis, both with and without shoes. Any adjustments for fit, comfort or biomechanical alignment are made at the initial consultation or after a period of acclimatization.

Box 12.1 Prescribing a functional orthosis.

The orthotic prescription comprises many component factors which need to be taken into consideration.

Patient details
- problem, aim, define pathology
- morphology: weight
- occupation/sports activity

Cast (shell) enclosed
- state method used
- pour plaster to perpendicular/inverted/everted
- cast marked: metatarsal heads, lesions, points of pressure

Intrinsic post
- balance to perpendicular
- degrees forefoot varus/valgus

Additions on the positive
- lateral expansion
- medial addition
- fascia

Material
- acrylic, polypropylene, ortholen (high-density poly-ethylene), PVC, foamed high-density polyethylene (Plastazote), carbon fibre, polycarbonate
- thickness: 2–5 mm (stock dependent)
- accommodative orthoses: leather laminate, Levy mould (rubber latex/wood flour), EVA (high or low density)

Orthotic plate/trim lines
- Shafer, Root, University of California Biomechanics laboratory (UCBL), Robert-Whitman, talar control foot orthosis
- modification, width, ray cut-outs, heel cups
- heel cup height (after rearpost applied); state lateral/medial/both symmetrical in millimetres
- anterior edge cut-outs, 'clips' (medial/lateral ray)
- lateral flare (very high lateral edge)

Posting
- forefoot varus or valgus 2–6°
- rearfoot varus 0, 4 or 8°, with 4° grind-off (acrylic), no grind-off (EVA)
- elevator 4, 8, 12 mm (for shoes)
- flare medially/laterally 1–6 mm

Finish (additions)
- vinyl/leather cover/foam cover/perforated
- full polyurethane 3 mm extension
- extension to toe sulcus, polyurethane 3 mm
- polyurethane 6 mm pad as on diagram

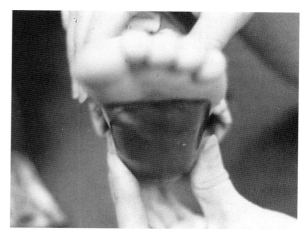

A

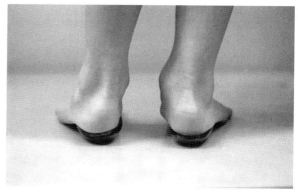

B

Figure 12.26 Fitting an orthotic plate. A, The plate is held against the foot while in a subtalar joint neutral position. The forefoot and rearfoot relationships should conform to the prescribed posting. B, Poor fit, as shown here, only on weight bearing. Insufficient width and poor design have led to an orthosis that has little control over the calcaneus.

Compliance and expectations

Another important consideration is the fitting of the orthosis in footwear; many problems arise simply from a failure to prescribe orthoses appropriate to the patient's footwear. The patient should be told in advance what shoes the orthosis is designed for and ideally should be shown a sample. Confusion over these simple issues can lead to poor patient satisfaction. The side of the shoes should be as high as possible to aid orthotic accommodation and should have a deep heel counter to prevent slippage. Elevators must correspond to the heel height. The patient should be warned about selecting heel heights for the best orthotic function. The patient should be examined while walking to ensure that the device is comfortable and that it controls any abnormal compensation for which it has been prescribed.

All patients should be warned, before they have committed themselves to an orthotic treatment programme, of the damage that orthoses can inflict upon shoes. Post indentation at the heel and forefoot in-sock can cut any delicate material. Because of their width, most trimmed orthoses may protrude medially against the upper, sufficiently to crease and deform this permanently.

In cases where there has been a large degree of correction, the prescription change mentioned may be too great. Patients may complain of aching knees, hips, thighs and back after 3–4 consecutive hours of wear. Pain or discomfort may also be felt on the plantar surface of the foot. Muscle and ligament adaptation particularly affects the leg, while the foot has to cope with the new sensation of an object interfacing between the foot and shoe.

A compromise must be sought to allow a comfortable wearing-in period. When dealing with children and handicapped persons, it is essential that a responsible parent or guardian be informed of the 'wearing-in' process. In these situations, the acclimatization period may need to be longer.

Acclimatization period A suggested regimen for wearing an orthosis, where one has not been worn before, includes use for 1 hour only on the first day of issue. This is then increased by 1 hour each day until the devices are comfortable all day long. The patients are usually asked to return to the clinic 2–4 weeks after the orthosis has been dispensed in order that any problems can be dealt with. If, after 6–8 weeks, the orthosis persists in causing discomfort, the patient should be reexamined, with a view to making adjustments or remaking the foot device.

Production changes

Since the early 1990s, the development of orthoses from computerized analysis has become more sophisticated. Orthotic laboratories can now make use of computer-aided design

and computer-aided manufacture of orthotic devices to eliminate human error from the fabrication process (Stats & Kriechbrum 1989, Michael 1989). Computer hardware has been developed to scan a foot or a negative cast and digitize the information to generate a computerized cast model. An example of this type of production in the UK is provided by Instance Systems, a division of Halo Healthcare. The practitioner finds a suitable orthosis from the Instance Systems brochure, the practioner takes a plaster of Paris cast or foam impression box of the foot and sends this to Instance Systems laboratory. The cast or foam box is scanned by the hardware and an orthosis is milled from the appropriate material.

Summary

The functional prescription orthosis differs from the insole or arch support in two respects. First, the orthosis is commonly taken from a neutral cast. Second, the orthosis is balanced so as to reduce the need for foot compensation via intrinsic or extrinsic posts. The intention behind treatment is, therefore, to improve the ground–foot interface with the shoe and to improve the timing of foot contact so that the foot supinates and pronates in the correct sequence.

The prescription must define the required orthotic design and include, where helpful, a diagram labelling any variations clearly. The practitioner must convey to the patient that the bespoke orthosis is not an arch support and does not function by supporting the arch. All such devices attempt to control abnormal foot function by restoring some of the time sequence to reestablish useful contact and propulsive phases.

Depending upon the design, orthoses will:

- reduce unwanted foot motion at the MTJ and STJ
- create a stable platform
- use materials to apply forces against the sustentaculum tali, calcaneus and lateral border, as well as over the talonavicular complex
- create specific foot influences using handmade cast adaptations.

The medial long arch has not been shown to influence pronation significantly. The concept of creating a painful supinatory reflex offers poor justification for a high-arch prescription, although feet with high arches do benefit from contoured infills. The concepts above are still broadly misunderstood. While the stock orthosis works, few cheap designs can create any of the biomechanical properties inherently incorporated by those prescription orthoses described.

ANKLE FOOT ORTHOSES

The AFO is one of the most commonly prescribed lower limb orthoses. Despite its apparent simplicity, it has proved disproportionately effective in restoring function compared with modalities such as 'callipers'.

Indications

The influence of AFOs can extend beyond the joints of the foot and ankle encompassed by the device to proximal joints; often it is this indirect effect that is being sought. Thus, AFOs may be used to reduce swing phase problems and to influence stance phase characteristics.

The nature of the pathological conditions producing the locomotor functional disorder can be usefully arranged into three groups:

- conditions that result in weakness of the muscles controlling the ankle–foot complex
- upper motor neuron lesions that result in hypertonicity or spasticity of the muscles
- conditions that result in pain or instability through loss of structural integrity of the lower limb and/or foot–ankle complex.

In the first of these categories, weak or absent dorsiflexors, plantarflexors, supinators and/or pronators are included. In the first case, the foot tends to adopt a plantarflexed attitude and the AFO helps to maintain a more dorsiflexed foot to reduce compensatory mechanisms such as excessive knee flexion during swing, circumduction of the leg and hip hiking. It may also prevent the toe from being caught, resulting in trips or falls, and would reduce the energy required to walk. With weak or absent plantarflexors, the swing phase is not affected, but during late stance, excessive dorsiflexion occurs at heel-off, accompanied by a total lack of push-off. Here an AFO has to prevent the excessive dorsiflexion and actively assist plantarflexion, usually via an ankle hinge. However, other techniques, such as the anterior ground reaction AFO (Glancy & Lindseth 1972), can be used.

Subtalar joint instability, resulting in excessive pronation or supination, can be controlled with an AFO in which a stabilizing three-point force system (Ch. 10) is used, with the forces applied on the upper calf, proximal to the ankle and on the border of the foot. Whether these forces are applied medially or laterally depends upon the instability being controlled.

Weak knee extensors, usually unilateral, cause the person to walk with an anteriorly flexed posture of the trunk to induce a knee-stabilizing moment via the anteriorly positioned ground reaction force. In cases of moderate weakness in lighter subjects, an AFO may be able to provide the knee stability without the need for the subject to adopt the ungainly and potentially injurious posture.

In upper motor neuron lesions, such as cerebral palsy, head injury, multiple sclerosis and cerebrovascular accident (stroke), abnormal muscle tone is produced. This may be static or variable and introduces high intrinsic forces and joint moments, which the AFO has to control in addition to those from weight bearing. In addition, if the AFO is not fitted correctly or causes discomfort, it may stimulate reflex activity, resulting in higher tone throughout the body. A well-fitting AFO can reduce whole-body tone (Meadows et al 1980). The function of the AFOs for this category of patient is similar to that mentioned above, although the reason for the prescription will differ (i.e. to resist overactive plantarflexors as opposed to assisting weak or absent dorsiflexors).

Impaired structural integrity takes many forms and can result from trauma or, more commonly, from an arthritic condition. Whatever the underlying pathology, the functional conse-quence of this impaired integrity is pain during essentially normal ranges of joint motions and loading levels. If joint motion causes the dis-comfort, then restriction of the painful motion is the aim of the AFO. Often the pain from joint motion is only part of the problem, which includes discomfort on weight bearing or heel strike. Footwear adaptions can be used to pro-vide shock absorption, as can inserts in the heel (Pratt 1990), but in some cases the foot needs to be off-loaded. This can be achieved using a patella–tendon-bearing AFO (McIllmurray & Greenbaum 1958), which uses the same concept as employed in prosthetics to transfer some limb load to the AFO via the patella tendon, thus bypassing the foot. Only a proportion of the limb load can be redirected, an absolute maxi-mum of 50% having been demonstrated (Lehmann & Warren 1973).

Wapner & Sharkey (1991) reported on the results of the use of moulded AFO night splints for the treatment of plantar fasciitis in 14 patients. All patients had symptoms for greater than 1 year and had previously undergone treatment with non-steroidal agents, cortisone injections, shoe modifications and physical ther-apy without resolution. All patients were pro-vided with a custom-moulded polypropylene AFO in 5° of dorsiflexion to be used as a night splint. In combination with non-steroidal anti-inflammatory drugs, heel cups, shock-absorbing insoles and general stretching exercises, success-ful resolution occurred in 11 patients in less than 4 months. This suggests that the use of night splints provides a useful adjunct to current therapeutic regimens of plantar fasciitis.

AFO designs

There are two main forms of AFO, the older conventional metal and leather 'callipers' and the newer thermoplastic types.

Rigid bracing

The metal and leather AFOs (Fig. 12.27) employ a calf band connected to one or two metal side

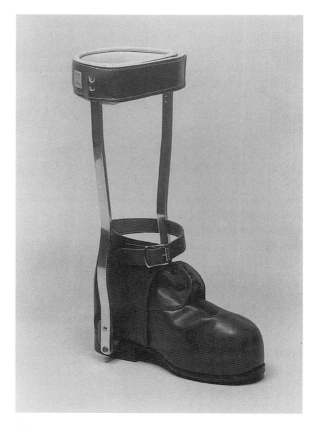

Figure 12.27 An ankle calliper with bespoke shoe is necessary to prevent deterioration of the heel contour. A leather calf band is shown.

bars attached to the shoe, usually at the heel. Variations on the style can include the metal bar connecting posteriorly to the shoe, the inclusion of motion at the heel insert or addition of hinges at the ankle level. These AFOs are made by shap-ing the metal components to a full-sized outline of the limb, drawn by an orthotist, together with details of limb girth. Leather straps are often added to induce or control mediolateral motion, and are called T or Y straps because of their out-line shape. Recent changes to metal alloys and metal production techniques have resulted in the weight of these AFOs being reduced while still maintaining their performance. However, in many instances they have been superseded by the thermoplastic design of the AFO.

Semi-rigid bracing

The thermoplastic design is more complicated to produce than the metal and leather AFO, as a cast of the leg is required (Fig. 12.28). This is taken with the foot–ankle complex held in its corrected position relative to the leg, and from this negative a positive model is made. The positive is modified in line with the orthotist's directions and then a thermoplastic sheet is heated and vacuum formed to the model. Once cooled, the sheet is cut off, producing a plastic shell, which is cleaned and straps added to produce the AFO. The most commonly used plastic for these is polypropylene (homopolymer or copolymer), but polyethylene is also used in some cases (such as night splinting), as are more mechanically weak materials such as Orthoplast.

Thermoplastic AFOs, being a total contact design, are more difficult to fit than the conventional type but offer many advantages such as improved cosmesis, lighter weight, more precise control and less-restricted choice of footwear. However, they are of no value if large diurnal limb volume changes take place or if the patient has anaesthetic skin or peripheral blood flow problems. They are also less successful in treating heavy patients and cost more than the conventional orthosis. In many cases, the advantages of their use outweigh the disadvantages, and improved treatment of lower limb functional impairments has resulted from their development. As development continues, newer techniques are being found to control the foot–ankle complex, and the role of the thermoplastic AFO continues to strengthen (Brown et al 1987).

Replication

A spiral cast is used for the AFO as well as for UCBL and TCFO devices. The plaster of Paris bandage is wrapped circumferentially around the foot and leg and allowed to set. The negative cast should capture the contours of the foot and ankle sufficiently for these orthoses to be made. Unlike the types of cast discussed under foot orthoses, the foot needs protecting before casting to prevent the plaster sticking to hairs on the dorsum of the foot and the lower part of the leg.

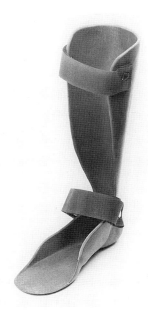

Figure 12.28 An ankle foot orthosis made from thermoplastic material has two points of fastening. In the illustration, Velcro is shown as the most popular system of orthosis/leg retention.

This protection can be either a cream, which is washed off later, or, more commonly, a thin tubular bandage (e.g. Tubifast), extending from the toes to above the height of the finished cast.

As these casts cannot be pulled off like a plantar cast, a strong plastic tube is inserted under the sock, running from one end of the sock to the other and protruding well beyond both ends. Plaster bandage is wrapped around the foot, extending as far proximally as required, usually to above the malleoli for UCBL orthoses or higher in the case of AFOs. A total of about five to six layers of plaster is required, at which point the foot is positioned as required. This may be in subtalar neutral; if so, the foot will need to have been positioned using one of the techniques described earlier in the chapter. Often this is not indicated and the basic requirement is to obtain a specific forefoot-to-rearfoot relationship after a full assessment of the subject. The best position for taking such casts is with the subject seated with their foot at a comfortable height for the practitioner.

Once the plaster has set, it is cut along the tube with a sharp knife and the cast is opened out to remove the foot (Fig. 12.29). The plaster is sufficiently flexible to allow this process and still enable the cast to be closed up afterwards to recreate accurately the full shape of the foot. This is the technique used to cast for an AFO where the upper level of the cast would end just below the knee.

A useful variation of this technique is to use one of the newer quick-setting plaster alternatives, such as Scotchcast, to take the cast. This will set fast enough that the subject can walk in the cast and thus an assessment of the foot position and likely functional result of the orthosis can be readily obtained. Such casts are more difficult to remove, usually requiring the use of an oscillating plaster saw as it is too hard for a knife. In addition, this does add to the cost of the process but may save an inappropriate orthosis being made.

Prescription

Many of the principles described under foot orthoses can be applied to AFOs. Box 12.2 summarizes the steps to be followed when considering taking an impression and prescribing an AFO.

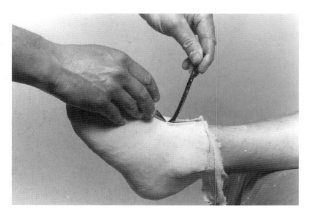

Figure 12.29 A spiral cast for a University of California Biomechanics laboratory (UCBL) orthosis being removed by cutting with a knife onto a dorsal tube. This system of casting can be extended proximally to replicate feet/legs for ankle foot orthoses or talar control foot orthoses.

Box 12.2 The key points considered when taking an impression and prescribing an ankle foot orthosis

Patient details
• biomechanical problem, orthotic aim, define pathology
• morphology: weight
• occupation

Cast taken
• taken weight bearing or non-weight bearing
• mark malleoli, navicular, metatarsal heads, lesions and any points of pressure

Cast rectification
• before filling, check angles
• after filling, set up for additions to be made

Cast additions/modifications
To include some, but not all of the following:
• forefoot intrinsic posting
• rearfoot intrinsic posting
• Carlson modification (Carlson & Berglund 1979)
  – three point pressure
  – calcaneal grip
  – hinging alterations

Material
• polypropylene 3, 4.5 or 6 mm
• polyethylene for night splinting
• foam for padding (often polyurethane foams)

Trim lines
• forward or behind malleoli
• behind or on metatarsal heads or full foot
• include (or not) first or fifth metatarsal heads
• three-point pressure trim

Posting
• rigid or flexible
• forefoot or rearfoot

EEC directive on the manufacture of orthoses From 14 June 1998, Directive 93/42 EEC requires all manufacturers of medical devices who place these on sale to have registered with, in the UK, the Medical Devices Agency (MDA). The regulations require all such devices to display the CE mark of conformity, with the exception of custom-made devices and devices intended for clinical investigation.

Summary

By the very nature of their design, AFOs do not allow normal foot function, as the ankle cannot plantarflex and torque conversion is affected. They are used to provide a larger-scale control over the foot and leg in order to influence such factors as spastic toe walking, knee hyper-extension and excess pronation. As such, the reestablishment of normal foot contact timing sequences is not on the agenda, but the control of potentially damaging abnormal positions of the foot, leg and spine is required.

What is fundamental to the success of AFOs, apart from accuracy of the casting and manufacture, is the correct biomechanical description of the requirements of the AFO. Without this, there is little chance that the optimum orthotic performance will be realized. This takes considerable training and understanding of the practical aspects of the interrelationship between the human being and a plastic orthosis. It should always be remembered that the orthosis should satisfy the three 'S's: straight, stable and symmetrical.

SUMMARY

The process of treating patients has been described on the basis that the practitioner has a clear idea of the products available and their physical and chemical properties (Ch. 10). Mechanical therapy is provided in a variety of ways. In this chapter, the focus has been prescription orthoses as opposed to clinical padded adhesive orthoses or stock devices.

Occasions arise where clinical materials are unsatisfactory. Prescription orthoses may offer materials with better physical properties, made-to-measure designs that should fit shoes more effectively, and prescriptions that can offer a better foot–ground interface for the biomechanical requirements of foot function.

The practitioner is faced with an ever-increasing range of methods to help patients; at present, research has not provided sufficient understanding as to how they work. McCourt et al (1994) undertook a realistic sample size survey and found that all types of orthosis—bespoke, clinical insole and stock designs—showed > 80% effectiveness in each case.

The scientific practitioner must strive to consolidate any process that can offer the most consistent rewards within a cost-effective framework. The aim of treatment is to remove pain, reduce dependency on medication, increase mobility, restore normal function and moderate abnormal footwear patterns.

Too many subdivisions exist to be able to describe all the orthotic designs possible within a text such as this. Readers are, therefore, directed to Bowker et al (1993) for further references to foot orthoses and AFOs. The examples provided in this chapter should assist the new practitioner in selecting orthoses using the basic principles described.

REFERENCES

Anthony R J 1991 The manufacture and use of the functional foot orthosis. Karger, Basel

Bailey D S, Perillo J T, Forman M 1984 Subtalar joint neutral: a study using tomography. Journal of the American Podiatric Association 74: 59–64

Ball P, Johnson G R 1993 Reliability of hindfoot goniometry when using a flexible electrogoniometer. Clinical Biomechanics 8: 13–19

Bowker P, Condie D N, Bader D L, Pratt D J, Wallace W A (eds) 1993 The biomechanical basis of orthotic management. Butterworth Heinemann, Oxford

Brown R N, Byers-Hinkley K, Logan L 1987 The talar control ankle foot orthosis. Orthotics and Prosthetics 41: 22–31

Carlson J M, Berglund G 1979 An effective orthotic design for controlling the unstable sub-talar joint. Orthotics and Prosthetics 33: 39–49

Cook A, Gorman I, Morris J 1988 Evaluation of the neutral position of the subtalar joint. Journal of the American Podiatric Medical Association 78: 449–451

D'Amico J C, Rabin M 1986 The influence of foot orthoses on the quadriceps angle. Journal of the American Podiatric Medical Association 76: 337–340

Engsberg J R, Grimston S K, Wackwitz J H 1988 Predicting talocalcaneal joint orientations from talocalcaneal/talocrural joint orientations. Journal of Orthopaedic Research 6: 749–757

Glancy J, Lindseth R E 1972 The polypropylene solid-ankle orthosis. Orthotics and Prosthetics 26: 14–26

Griffith C J 1988 An investigation of the repeatability, reliability and validity of clinical biomechanical measurements in the region of the foot and ankle. BSc Thesis, Polytechnic of Central London

Inman V T 1969 The influence of the foot–ankle complex on the proximal skeletal structures. Artificial Limbs 13: 59–65

Inman V T 1976 The joints of the ankle. Williams & Wilkins, Baltimore, MD, p 45–66

Kidd R 1991 An examination of the validity of some of the more questionable cornerstones of modern chiropodial diagnosis. Journal of British Podiatric Medicine 9: 172–173

Lehmann J F, Warren C G 1973 Ischial and patella–tendon weight-bearing braces: function, design, adjustment and training. Bulletin of Prosthetics Research 10: 6–19

Lundeen R O 1988 Polysectional triaxial posting. Journal of the American Podiatric Medical Association 78: 55–59

McCourt F J, Bevans J, Cluskey L 1994 Report of a survey on in-shoe orthoses provision. Journal of British Podiatric Medicine 49: 73–76

McIllmurray W J, Greenbaum W 1958 A below-knee weight-bearing brace. Orthotics and Prosthetics Journal 12: 81–82

McMaster M 1976 Disability of the hindfoot after fracture of the tibial shaft. Journal of Bone and Joint Surgery 58B: 90

Meadows C B, Anderson D M, Duncan L M et al 1980 The use of polypropylene ankle foot orthoses in the management of the cerebral palsied child. A guide based on clinical experience in Dundee. Tayside Rehabilitation Engineering Services, Dundee, UK

Mereday C, Dolan M E, Lusskin R 1972 Evaluation of the University of California Biomechanics Laboratory shoe insert in 'Flexible pes planus'. Clinical Orthopedics and Related Research 82: 45–58

Michael J W 1989 Reflections on CAD/CAM in prosthetics and orthotics. Journal of Prosthetics and Orthotics 1: 116–121

Phillips R D, Christeck R, Phillips R L 1985 Clinical measurement of the axis of the subtalar joint. Journal of the American Podiatric Medical Association 75: 119–131

Philps J W 1995 The functional foot orthosis. Churchill Livingstone, Edinburgh

Pratt D J 1990 Long term comparison of some shock attenuating insoles. Prosthetics and Orthotics International 14: 51–57

Pratt D J, Rees P H, Butterworth R H 1984 RTV silicone insoles. Prosthetics and Orthotics International 8: 54–55

Pratt D J, Iliff P M, Ward J B 1993a Talus control foot orthoses. The Foot 4: 31–33

Pratt D J, Tollafield D R, Johnson G R, Peacock C 1993b Foot orthosis. In: Bowker P M, Pratt D J (eds) Biomechanical basis for orthoses. Butterworths, London, p 72–98

Rome K 1990 Behaviour of orthotic materials in chiropody.

Journal of the American Podiatric Medical Association 80: 471–478

Root M L, Orien W P, Weed J H, Hughes R J 1971 Biomechanical examination of the foot, vol 1. Clinical Biomechanics Corporation, Los Angeles, CA

Root M L, Orien W P, Weed J H 1977 Normal and abnormal function of the foot, vol 2. Clinical Biomechanics Corporation, Los Angeles, CA

Ross A S, Gurnik K L 1982 Elevator selection in rearfoot posted orthoses. Journal of the American Podiatric Association 72: 621–624

Sgarlato T E 1971 A compendium of podiatric biomechanics. California College of Podiatric Medicine, San Francisco, CA

Spencer A M 1978 Practical podiatric orthopaedic procedures. Practical podiatric monograph series. Ohio College of Podiatric Medicine, Cleveland, OH

Stats T B, Kriechbrum M P 1989 Computer-aided design and computer-aided manufacturing of a foot orthoses. Journal of Prosthetics and Orthotics 1: 182–186

Tollafield D R 1985 Mechanical therapeutic coursework laboratory I & II. First year Chiropody. Nene College, UK, p 193–202, 210–212, 242–256

Tollafield D R, Merriman L M 1995 Assessment of the locomotor system. In: Merriman L M, Tollafield D R (eds) Assessment of the lower limb. Churchill Livingstone, Edinburgh, p 170–173

Tollafield D R, Pratt D J 1987 An analysis of the effects of posting on casted functional orthoses. In Pratt D J, Johnson G R (eds) The biomechanics and orthotic management of the foot. Orthotics and Disability Research Centre, Derby, UK

Tollafield D R, Pratt D J 1990a The control of known triplanar forces on the foot by forefoot orthotic posting. British Journal of Podiatric Medicine and Surgery 2: 3–5

Tollafield D R, Pratt D J 1990b The effects of variable rear posting of orthoses on a normal foot. Chiropodist 45: 154–160

Wapner K L, Sharkey P F 1991 The use of night splints for treatment of recalcitrant plantar fasciitis. Foot and Ankle 12: 135–137

Weed J H, Ratliff F D, Ross B A 1978 A biplanar grind for rearposts on functional orthoses. Journal of the American Podiatric Association 68: 35–39

Wu K K 1990 Foot orthoses: principles and clinical applications. Williams & Wilkins, Baltimore, MD

FURTHER READING

Anthony R J 1992 The fabrication protocol for the manufacture of a functional foot orthosis. Journal of British Podiatric Medicine 47: 91–98

Bates E H, Chung W K 1988 Congenital talipes equinovarus. In: Helal B, Wilson D (eds) The foot. Churchill Livingstone, Edinburgh, ch 14

Birke J A 1991 Rehabilitation of the diabetic patient. In: Frykberg (ed) The high-risk foot in diabetes mellitus. Churchill Livingstone, New York, p 497–512

Blake R L, Ferguson H 1991 Foot orthosis for the severe flatfoot in sports. Journal of the American Podiatriatric Medical Association 81: 549–555

Blake R L, Ferguson H 1992 Extrinsic rearfoot posts. Journal of the American Podiatric Medical Association 82: 202–206

Brodke D S, Skinner S R, Lameroux L W, Johanson M E, Moran S A, Ashley R K 1989 The effects of ankle foot orthosis on the gait of children. Journal of Pediatrics and Orthopaedics 9: 702–708

Condie D N, Meadows C B 1993 Ankle foot orthoses. In: Bowker P, Condie D N, Bader D L, Pratt D J, Wallace WA (eds) The biomechanical basis of orthotic management. Butterworth Heinmann, Oxford, p 99–123

Diamond J E, Sinacore D R, Mueller M J 1987 Molded

double-rocker plaster shoe for healing a diabetic ulcer. Physical Therapy 67: 1551–1552

Edwards J, Rome K 1992 A study of the shock attenuating properties of materials used in chiropody. The Foot 2: 99–107

Eggold J 1981 Orthotics in the prevention of runner's overuse injuries. Physical Sports Medicine 9: 125–128

Elveru R A, Rothstein J M, Lamb R L, Riddle D L 1988 Methods for taking subtalar joint measurements: a clinical report. Physical Therapy 68: 678–682

Freeman A C 1990 A study of inter-observer and intra-observer reliability in the measurement of resting calcaneal stance position and neutral calcaneal stance position. Journal of Podiatric Medicine and Surgery 2: 6–8

Geary N P J, Klenerman L 1987 The rocker sole shoe: a method to reduce peak forefoot pressure in the management of diabetic foot ulceration. In: Pratt D J, Johnson G R (eds) The biomechanics and orthotic management of the foot. Orthotics and Disability Research Centre, Derby, UK, ch 17

Gibbard L C 1968 Charlesworth's chiropodial orthopaedics. Ballière, Tindall & Cassell, London

Hice G A 1984 Orthotic treatment of feet having a high oblique midtarsal joint axis. Journal of the American Podiatric Association 74: 577–582

Hice G A, Solomon W, Fashada P 1983 The plaster-synthetic cast. Journal of the American Podiatric Association 73: 427–431

Holmes G B, Timmerman L 1990 A quantitative assessment of the effect of metatarsal pads on plantar pressures. Foot and Ankle 11: 141–145

Isman R E, Inman V T 1969 Anthropometric studies of the human foot and ankle. Bulletin of Prosthetics Research Spring: 97–127

Johnson G R 1990 Measurement of shock acceleration during running and walking using the Shock Meter. Clinical Biomechanics 5: 47–50

Lange L R 1990 The Lange silicone partial foot prosthesis. Journal of Prosthetics and Orthotics 4: 56–61

McCourt FJ 1990 To cast or not to cast? The comparative effectiveness of casted and non casted orthoses. Journal of British Podiatric Medicine 45: 239–243

Mann R A 1986 Biomechanics of the foot and ankle. In: Mann R A (ed) Surgery of the foot. Mosby, St Louis, MO, ch 1

Manter J T 1941 Movements of the subtalar and transverse tarsal joints. Anatomical Record 80: 397–409

Milgram C, Giladi M, Kashtan H 1985 A prospective study of the effect of a shock-absorbing orthotic device on the incidence of stress fractures in military recruits. Foot and Ankle 6: 101–105

Novick A, Birke J A, Hoard A S, Brasseaux D M, Broussard J B, Hawkins E S 1992 Rigid orthoses for the insensitive foot. Journal of Prosthetics and Orthotics 4: 31–40

Odom R D, Gaskwirth B 1987 San splint orthoses. Journal of the American Podiatric Association 72: 98–101

Root M L, Orien W P, Weed J H 1978 Neutral position casting technique. Clinical Biomechanics Corporation, Los Angeles, CA

Rose G K 1986 Orthotics: principles and practice. William Heinemann Medical, London

Ross F D 1986 The relationship of abnormal foot pronation to hallux abductovalgus: a pilot study. Prosthetics and Orthotics International 10: 72–78

Schaff P S, Cavanagh P R 1990 Shoes for the insensitive foot: the effect of a 'rocker bottom' shoe modification on plantar pressure distribution. Foot and Ankle 11: 129–140

Schuster R O 1974 A history of orthopaedics in podiatry. Journal of the American Podiatric Association 64: 332–336

Sinacore D R, Mueller M J, Diamond J E et al 1987 Diabetic plantar ulcers treated by total contact casting. Physical Therapy 67: 1543–1549

Sutton R 1989 The thermoplastic elastomer foot orthoses and the thermoplastic elastomer biomechanical foot orthoses. Journal of Prosthetics and Orthotics 2: 164–172

Taillon D M, McCormick D 1992 Tone reducing orthoses: myth or reality? Proceedings of the 7th World Congress of the International Society of Prosthetics and Orthotics, Chicago, p 446

Tollafield D R 1986 A foundation in podiatric orthopaedics. Nene College, UK, p165–166

Tooms R E, Griffin J W, Griffin T P 1987 Effect of viscoelastic insoles on pain in nursing students. Orthopaedics 10: 1143–1147

Volshin A S, Wosk J 1985 Low back pain conservative treatment with artificial shock absorbers. Archives of Physical Medicine and Rehabilitation 66: 145–148

Weatherwax R J 1980 The plaster slipper cast. Clinical Orthopedics and Related Research 154: 327–328

13

Footwear therapy

Marylin Lord
David Pratt

INTRODUCTION

Footwear influences the treatment of many foot problems. For example, no matter how effective an orthosis may be, it will have no therapeutic effect if it cannot be accommodated in the patient's footwear. Conversely, the most effective treatment plan will not achieve its desired results if the patient continues to wear shoes that exacerbate the problem. The use of footwear as a therapeutic tool may involve:

- advice on the purchase of footwear
- prescription of bespoke footwear
- modifications to footwear.

Most patients will benefit from advice about the purchase of suitable footwear. The majority should be able to purchase appropriate footwear from general or specialized retail outlets. For a minority, the only way they can obtain good-fitting footwear is to have it specially made for them (bespoke footwear). Sometimes it is possible to improve foot function by modifying the patient's existing footwear. These three aspects of footwear therapy will be considered in detail in this chapter.

ADVICE ON THE PURCHASE OF FOOTWEAR

Footwear protects the foot from extremes of temperature, moisture, hard surfaces, knocks and scratches. However, for many people its cosmetic value is more important than its functional purpose. The choice of footwear is affected by appearance and current fashion trends as much as, if not more than, by functional purposes. For those with foot problems, however, the choice of footwear may be influenced by supplementary requirements, for example to reduce excessive pressures on sensitive structures, to improve walking ability or to accommodate an orthosis or prosthesis.

This section will discuss the following issues related to the purchase of footwear:

- types of footwear
- where to purchase footwear
- advice to patients on the purchase of footwear.

It is important that the practitioner is familiar with the range of footwear types. The practitioner should also be conversant with the availability of footwear locally, as well as that of specialist footwear, which may only be obtainable from farther afield. Advising patients that they need 'better footwear' is a futile exercise if it is not backed up with specific advice as to what is needed and where to get it from.

TYPES OF FOOTWEAR

Footwear can be classified in a number of ways. For the purposes of this chapter, the following classification will be used:

- mass versus specialist production
- general versus specific purpose footwear.

Mass versus specialist production

Most footwear is mass produced from a statistically determined set of lasts (Fig. 13.1A). The shoe last is not the same shape as the foot that will fit the shoe; indeed, making a shoe directly over a plaster cast of a foot would produce ill-fitting shoes. The last is generally deeper in the midfoot region, has a sharp 'feather edge' where the upper surface meets the sole, is clipped in along the topline (around the ankle) and is faired over and extended in the toe region. This

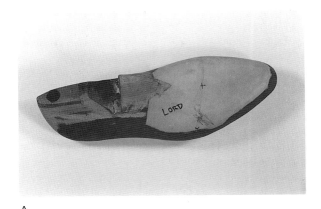

A

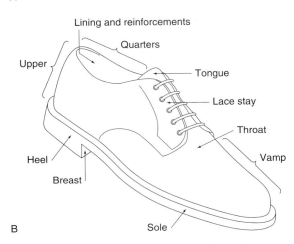

B

Figure 13.1 Footwear manufacture. A, A shoe last. B, Components of a shoe.

provides a shape that applies appropriate tension when the shoe distorts to contain the loaded foot.

It is interesting to note that for female fashion footwear, the tread width across the joint is usually less than the foot outline width by up to 10 mm, and the joint girth may be 10 mm or so less than the foot joint girth. This often results in the sole of the foot spreading outside the shoe insole, and the fifth metatarsal being hammocked on the overhanging upper.

Mass-produced footwear can be produced in *single size/width* or in *half-size/multiwidth fittings*. Most mass-produced adult footwear is produced in single size and width fittings, whereas children's footwear is more likely to be produced in half-size and multiwidth fittings. Inevitably, the cost of producing half sizes and multiwidths is far greater and the additional cost may deter many people. However, as feet come in various shapes and sizes, the use of a range of length and width fittings is more likely to lead to well-fitting footwear.

For those who cannot find well-fitting mass-produced footwear, even when made in half-size and multiwidth fittings, there are a number of alternatives:

- stock footwear
- modular footwear
- bespoke footwear.

Stock footwear   There is now a wide range of footwear targeted at the orthopaedic market that is variously described as stock, off the shelf or ready made. As well as providing depth for a removable cushioning insert, these shoes often have a wider fit than normal, particularly in the forefoot. They may be offered in a range of over-all widths, from normal to extra wide, with a variety of styles and fastenings.

Most companies supplying stock orthopaedic shoes use a limited range of last styles, perhaps up to five different fundamental shapes, which are then produced in a range of sizes. Some companies give details of the lasts and associate these with the styles in their catalogues, which is helpful in making a good choice for an individual patient. Shoes can be bought with confidence if the last shape is known to suit. Lasts can be designed with particular orthopaedic features in mind. For example, the normal straight-edged last can be substituted by a last with the forepart angled with respect to the backpart to provide for supination or pronation (Fig. 13.2). Other lasts are specifically designed to give extra deep toe boxes to accommodate claw toes, or have toe plan shaping to suit hallux valgus.

The use of stock shoes has risen dramatically over the past few years in the UK, spurred on by the increased choice and rapid availability. They cost more than mass-produced shoes but are around a fifth to a quarter of the price of bespoke shoes.

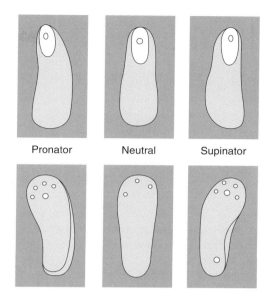

Figure 13.2   Plan views of lasts designed to encourage pronation or supination.

Modular footwear   Modular footwear is fabricated using stock lasts to which minor adaptations are made. The orthotist can conduct a trial fit using the standard stock shoe and then specify a number of fixed modifications to be made. This enables the special shoes to be delivered at the second visit. The John Locke system is one of the well-known implementations of this technique.

Bespoke footwear   Bespoke footwear is custom made for an individual and involves the production of a last specific to that individual's foot. Bespoke footwear can be obtained either privately or via the UK National Health Service (NHS). Because of the production and fitting costs, this type of footwear is considerably more expensive than that purchased in the high street.

General or specific purposes

Ideally, footwear should be purchased with a view to its intended use. Unfortunately, this is often not the case; consider, for example, the habitual wearing of trainers by teenagers in all weathers and for all purposes. Those who wear open-toed, sling-back shoes in the depth of winter are inviting problems with chilblains. Wellingtons, walking boots, safety boots, trainers designed for specific sports, golf shoes and boots are all examples of footwear designed for specific purposes and usually with the intention of protecting the foot in adverse situations. Patients should be encouraged to buy shoes to meet specific purposes.

Where to purchase footwear

Footwear can be purchased from:

- general high street shops
- specialized high street shops
- mail order
- specialist retail outfits.

Additionally, stock, modular and bespoke footwear may be obtained free via the NHS.

General high street shops The majority of people purchase mass-produced footwear from general High Street shops. Such footwear is designed to meet most general-purpose needs but is often only available in single size and width fittings. Much of the footwear is imported and, because of the restriction in sizes, it is usually the most inexpensive type of footwear to purchase.

Specialized high street shops In most towns and cities, it is common to find at least one shop that stocks multiwidth as well as half-size fittings. These shops primarily sell children's footwear, although they often have adult departments where some of the footwear is in multi-width fittings. There are also shops that specialize in the adult half-size/multiwidth market. The cost of this footwear can be up to two or three times more than that purchased in general high street shops.

Mail order Mass-produced as well as specialized footwear can be purchased via mail order. Usually companies produce catalogues illustrating their range. Unfortunately, there is no opportunity to check the fit prior to purchase, although most firms operate a return service. Most of the popular sizes and styles of these shoes are made in bulk and held in stock at the manufacturers;

they are, therefore, available by return of post. Shoes made to order from stock patterns and lasts may have a delivery period of a few weeks.

Specialist retail outlets These cater for specific markets, for example those with very long feet. A wide range of specialist footwear is now available and patients can be guided to those most suited to their needs. Suppliers are listed in the Disabled Living Foundation *Service Handbook*. This encompasses the whole spectrum of special needs: from suppliers of standard shoes in extra small/large or extra narrow/wide ranges, odd and single shoes, rehabilitation and temporary shoes, through to suppliers of orthopaedic footwear. Bespoke footwear can be provided by some specialist footwear retailers.

NHS footwear NHS footwear is usually supplied via a prescription from a hospital consultant. The proposal of direct access for GPs is gaining favour. Under this scheme, patients could be referred directly to a footwear clinic rather than through a consultant. Stock, modular or bespoke footwear may be provided. Stock footwear in the UK must meet standards of construction laid down by the NHS in order to be supplied to NHS patients. Some company orthotists carry their own stock of a few styles, enabling them potentially to fit and supply at the first visit. However, there is a compromise between choice and speed of supply, since holding a stock of more than a few styles would be prohibitive for the normal turnover at most foot clinics.

Bespoke footwear Such footwear is made via a prescription, which is expanded into a full specification either by an orthotist employed by a NHS Trust or by one who works for a private company. Whereas in the mid-1990s, the vast majority of shoes were supplied by contractor's orthotists, it is now more common for hospitals to employ their own orthotist. Other members of the clinical team may be involved in designing the prescription, for example a podiatrist or physiotherapist. Bespoke footwear is usually produced off-site by a contractor for subsequent delivery at a later clinic. The NHS contract normally requires that such footwear is available for fitting 6 weeks after the measurements are taken.

Adaptations and shoe inserts may be made on-site by NHS staff or by the contractor.

ADVICE TO PATIENTS

Whether patients are purchasing mass-produced, stock orthopaedic or modular footwear, the following factors need to be considered:

- fit
- comfort
- cosmesis.

Fit

The concept of a well-fitting shoe involves many factors, which relate as much to characteristics of an individual's foot as to the construction of the shoe. The fit of the shoe should allow for a snug approximation around some areas of the foot, while in other areas a clearance over the skin is required. Excessive tightness and excessive clearance could both constitute poor fit, although these are difficult to determine in any quantitative sense. Additionally, the shoe needs to change shape in concert with the foot during weight bearing and walking.

Because fit is an individual characteristic, a trial fit of footwear is essential when it is supplied for the first time. The assessment of shoe fit is made both subjectively and objectively. For normally sensate feet, the subjective impression is valuable for reporting tightness and discomfort, but where sensory deficits are present this is less effective and the burden of ensuring fit falls to the fitter.

Subjective perception of fit depends on the wearer's preference for tightness and habituation to foot deformation in the name of fashion. It may be necessary to educate some patients to accept a looser fit in the forefoot than that to which they are accustomed. If purchasing from a shoe shop, the patient should be encouraged to walk around to test the fit of the shoe.

Objective assessment by observation and touch is always important in a trial fit. The first requirements for any shoe are those of normal

good sense. The shoe should not compress the joints of the forefoot, should be a good fit, should be capable of secure fastening to prevent slipping, and should be of an appropriate heel height for optimum foot functioning. The following points should be routinely checked (Fig. 13.3):

- location of the metatarsophalangeal joints at the widest part of the shoe
- adequate width across the joint of the foot
- clearance in the toe region
- adequate length for extension of the foot during walking (10 mm)
- snug fit in the midfoot, noting particularly whether the lace panel, when fastened, is too spread out or overlapping
- snug fit at the rear of the heel: excessive space is indicative of a shoe size too large or too great a depth or width across the throat, allowing the foot to slip forward; or an excessive length of the rear part of the shoe
- gaping at the topline of the shoe, which can be caused by inappropriate shaping, incorrect heel height for the shoe or clearance under the malleoli at the topline
- localized tight spots over bunions or other protuberances
- back seam height not excessive to avoid causing irritation over the Achilles tendon
- rearfoot fit in depth and clip adequate to prevent heel slip during walking.

Heel height is important for correct foot function, particularly if it is too high. A steep heel-to-forefoot angle will tend to cause the foot to slip forward and impact against the end of the shoe. Heel heights are generally age related, with up to

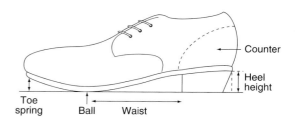

Figure 13.3 Features of a shoe that should be taken into consideration when fitting.

18 mm for children, 37 mm for adolescents and women, and 21–25 mm for men.

Differences in foot dimensions between weight bearing and non-weight bearing vary between individuals, depending on the flexibility and mechanics of the foot (Table 13.1). During walking, the foot flexes primarily at the metatarsal break, that is, approximately along the line of the metatarsal heads (Fig. 13.4). Shoes are also designed to flex in this region. The match of the location of the break and the degree of flexibility are important for correct shoe fit (Chen 1993).

When selecting shoes, the manufacturer's marked size should be treated only as a guide (Rossi 1983). There can be no fixed definitions of shoe sizing because this depends on the shape of the shoe as well as the overall length. The sizing system is graded in length, historically in steps of 8.4 mm per full size in the UK and USA systems, and in steps of 6.5 mm in the European sizing system. The increments in the UK and USA systems are the same, but the sizing systems do not share the same starting point. European sizes cannot be converted exactly into equivalent UK or USA sizes because of the different grading increment.

Because the difference between sizes in the UK and USA systems is quite large, interim half sizes are sometimes used to improve the fitting range. This, however, incurs extra costs in the manufacture and in maintaining stock levels in shops. Cheaper shoe ranges and many of the special orthopaedic shoe ranges are only stocked in full sizes.

Width is usually measured from the forefoot girth, with the increase in one width fitting equivalent to 5 mm for whole sizes up to children's size 13, and 6.5 mm for whole sizes above this. It may also be expressed in terms of the linear width of the shoe across its forefoot.

Special fitting considerations

For certain purposes, problem feet can usefully be categorized into the *hypersensitive* (*painful*) or the *insensate* (*anaesthetic*) foot. In the former, the pressures exerted on the foot by the shoe must be minimized; this can be achieved by underfoot

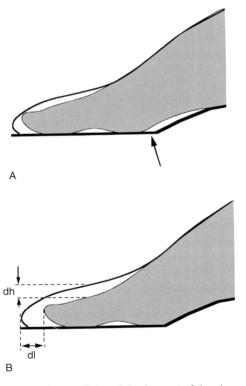

Figure 13.4 Correct fitting of the forepart of the shoe. A, Ill-fitting shoe with ball incorrectly located. B, Well-fitting shoe with the ball correctly located and adequate toe clearance in both length (dl) and height (dh).

Table 13.1 Changes in foot dimension from weight bearing for 26 women in the age range 18–60 years, of average foot size and with normal feet

Foot dimension[a]	Average dimension non-weight bearing (mm)	Change in dimension to weight bearing (mm (%))
Foot length	242	6.8 (2.8)
Joint girth	231	5.4 (2.3)
Joint width	89	5.0 (5.6)
Waist girth	226	5.4 (2.4)
Instep girth	229	3.4 (1.5)
Heel width	59	3.0 (5.1)

[a]The joint is the widest part of the forefoot, the waist is the narrowest part of the midfoot, and the instep is around the highest point of the longitudinal arch.

cushioning, light-weight construction of upper and soles, seamless construction of the upper, use of shock-absorbing heels and sole materials, and perhaps by providing a rigid shoe sole or a boot to immobilize the joints.

Controlling the pressures exerted on the foot is also imperative in the insensate foot. Even though the tolerance of this type of foot to pressure may be normal, excessive pressure from foreign bodies or simply from overuse will not result in the usual pain-avoidance responses. Furthermore, abnormally high plantar pressures are often present in the forefoot with conditions such as diabetic neuropathy (Boulton et al 1983), and these correlate with the location of ulcers. Provision of cushioning and moulded inserts to redistribute pressure can be effective in managing the condition (Cavanagh et al 1987). A study by Chantelau & Haage (1994) showed that the recurrence rate of neuropathic ulcers was considerably reduced in diabetic patients who wore cushioned protective footwear for more than 60% of each day.

The second grouping that can be useful is that of the *hypermobile* versus the *rigid* foot. A hypermobile foot may require a degree of support or correction to maintain the joint orientations. This can be achieved by insole contouring, internal or external wedging and supportive shoe upper design. In extreme cases, the foot may need to be immobilized by the use of a rigid sole, which will require a rockered design to enable roll-off. The rigid foot, by contrast, cannot be corrected and, therefore, must be supported in its fixed position and accommodated. Wedge soles can be used, which result in there being no definite heel breast (Fig. 13.1A). Such a sole will impart intrinsic stability to the waist, which may benefit some foot conditions. It is essential that, of these two – correction versus accommodation – the correct strategy is chosen.

Extra deep footwear may be required to accommodate orthoses or clinical padding. Ideally, if orthoses are being prescribed, the patient should be encouraged to purchase new shoes. The function of an orthosis may be adversely affected if the patient is wearing well-worn shoes that have noticeable wear marks on the heel and sole.

Worn shoes may adversely affect the patient's gait and reduce the therapeutic value of the orthoses.

Comfort

In order to be classed as comfortable, footwear should:

- be as lightweight as possible
- have adequate thermal conductivity
- be permeable to moisture
- not produce excessive pressure or friction
- prevent excessive movement of the foot in the shoe.

Clearly some of these may be mutually exclusive, so it is important to identify which features are most important to assure the patient's foot comfort. Thermal conductivity, permeability to moisture and excessive pressure and friction are considered in detail below.

Thermal conductivity

The temperature inside shoes affects foot comfort. Foot temperature is largely determined by blood flow, as about 10% of the total blood volume exists within 2 mm of the skin surface. When the average foot temperature drops to below approximately 18°C, most people complain of cold feet. Below about 10°C, feet often become painful. This is significant because the foot is generally insensitive to cold: the number of cold receptors on the foot is small (3–6/cm²) compared with the rest of the body (9–13/cm²).

The thermal conductivity of footwear materials varies considerably (see Table 13.2). Patients suffering from vasospastic disorders and poor arterial blood supply need to be mindful of which materials provide the best insulation from external temperatures. The insulation properties of footwear can be improved by the use of fleece linings or thermal insoles. A simple Plastazote insole may be beneficial for some patients.

The feeling of discomfort because of heat is often confused with that from sweatiness, which suggests that the rate of heat dissipation is more relevant to discomfort than the temperature per se. Studies have found that temperatures of approximately 32–35°C are the upper limit for general comfort, and that a temperature of about 45°C is painful (Bunten 1983).

Many people complain of a burning sensation as a source of discomfort. This is a difficult sensation to characterize as excessive shoe tightness and perspiration do not in themselves produce this feeling. It is thought to be caused by activation of type C pain fibres (Rothman 1954). A study by Murray & Peet (1966) suggested a link between temperature and this sensation, but Burry (1956) suggested a number of other possible causes:

- chemical irritation by excess acidity in the insole or allergy to substances from the hosiery or shoes
- poor shoe fit, causing creasing of skin and friction between the foot, sock and shoe
- overheating of the foot as a result of vapour-impermeable materials in the shoe, overly warm clothing or excessive physical activity
- pathological conditions such as Morton's neuroma or fungal infections.

Permeability to moisture

Perspiration within footwear is principally produced by the eccrine glands and is slightly acidic (pH 3.8–5.7). However, as it cannot evaporate quickly within footwear, it decomposes and becomes alkaline. The foot typically perspires about 4 mg/h per cm^2 via insensitive perspiration (water loss without noticeable skin surface moisture). Sensitive perspiration of sweat is dependent upon environmental conditions and the health of the person and varies from approximately 2.5 mg/h per cm^2 to as high as 35 mg/h per cm^2. The water vapour permeability of footwear materials is an important factor to take into consideration (Table 13.3) and varies considerably in the materials used in the manufacture of footwear.

It is doubtful if wetness of the skin from perspiration is itself uncomfortable, but the indirect effects can be very marked. Wet skin, however produced, tends to reduce the cooling effect of the evaporation of perspiration and may stop it completely. Hence, the foot will tend to feel uncomfortably hot. Other indirect effects may arise from the higher heat conductivity of the epidermis if soaked in water and softening of the skin, which could make it more susceptible to damage from friction or pressure. Moisture also encourages fungal growths, which can be irritatingly itchy.

Pressure and friction

Plantar pressure within shoes has been measured by a number of people over the years (Lord 1981, Lord et al 1986, Alexander et al 1990) and now interest is also being shown in the measurement

Table 13.2 Thermal conductivity variation with humidity

Material	Conductivity (W/m^2 per °C/10^2) at relative humidity			
	28%	65%	77%	100%
Microporous PU	7.7	8.0	7.9	8.2
PU-coated non-woven fabric 1	7.7	7.9	8.1	8.1
PU-coated non-woven fabric 2	8.8	9.1	9.6	10.0
Corrected grain leather	9.4	11.2	12.0	14.0
PVC-coated full-grain leather	9.9	11.0	11.2	14.6
PU-coated woven fabric	12.5	13.4	14.1	16.1
PVC-coated woven fabric	17.8	18.1	18.0	18.8

PU, polyurethane.

Table 13.3 Water vapour permeability

Material		21°C, 50% rh	21°C, 100% rh	39°C, 100% rh
	(Inside)	21°C, 50% rh	21°C, 100% rh	39°C, 100% rh
	(Outside)	21°C, 0% rh	21°C, 50% rh	21°C, 50% rh
Sheepskin		1.39	1.25	1.16
Belly leather		0.63	0.80	1.16
Kip leather		0.31	0.23	0.22
Patent leather		0.02	0.01	0.01
PVC on fabric		0.01	0.01	0.02
PVC on polyester		0.08	0.08	0.08
Perforated PVC on fabric		0.05	0.04	0.04

PVC, polyvinyl chloride; rh, relative humidity.

of shear forces (Pollard et al 1983, Warren-Forward et al 1992, Lord et al 1992). There is an established link between excessive pressure/shear and the development of skin damage, particularly in feet considered to be 'at risk' (Bennett et al 1979).

The dorsum of the foot is more sensitive to pressure than the plantar surface. Excess pressure is the most common source of foot discomfort. The extent of foot pathology (e.g. rigid plantarflexed first ray) will dictate the level at which discomfort is felt. In some situations where the disease process may result in insensate feet, such as diabetes and Hansen's disease, patients do not feel discomfort. Damaging pressures may have been acting for a long period of time and may have led to significant damage.

Continued static pressure between the foot and shoe is more likely to cause general discomfort than the high transient pressure associated with walking or running. This is probably because of the static occlusion of blood flow, a subsequent reduction in sweating and an increased perception of discomfort because the foot feels hotter without the cooling effect of the perspiration (Bunten 1983). Hence, a foot will feel hotter when subjected to pressure in a hot environment. The converse happens in a cool climate, as the reduction in blood flow caused by the pressure cools the foot when it is relying on blood circulation to keep it warm. In addition,

soft tissues are compressed by pressure and suffer anoxic damage, which accumulates unless the pressure is removed for sufficient time to allow recovery. A good description of the interface problem is to be found in Bader & Chase (1993).

Repetitive transient pressure, which may occur during walking, can cause localized tissue damage via a more direct mechanism than blood flow occlusion. This involves mechanical injury to tissue and/or formation of callus, leading to skin lesions, which can themselves become the source of discomfort and pain.

Pressure exerted by the shoe upper may be exacerbated by swelling of the foot. Footwear must accommodate the change in foot shape during weight bearing in addition to daytime volume changes associated with orthostatic pressure of the blood and the dynamics of the venous and lymphatic systems. Normal daily changes in foot volume are of the order of 3% (range, 1.5–5.3%), with a further increase of 1–3% caused by increasing foot temperature (Bunten 1983). In those with venous insufficiency and lymphoedema, these increases will be much larger, and the choice of materials and design of footwear become much harder. The ability of footwear materials to respond to the changes in foot shape that occur during the day is an important consideration when selecting appropriate shoes. In particular, the tensile properties of the material will influence the feeling of comfort (Table 13.4).

Table 13.4 Tensile properties at two extensions

Material	Tensile strength (N/cm)	
	2% extension	10% extension
Calf	1.8	4.6
Suede calf	1.3	3.2
Veal suede	4.5	8.2
Grained side	1.6	2.9
Clothing leather	0.15	–
Softee leather	2.0	3.5
Clarino 1 (synthetic)	3.1	2.7
Ortix 1 (synthetic)	2.1	1.9

To reduce friction, all parts of the shoe that contact the foot should be smoothly lined. The vamp should be reinforced by the toe box or toe puff as this helps to protect the toes from knocks and stubbing, and helps to preserve the contour of the vamp.

Cosmesis

The fit of a shoe and its appearance are linked. It is impossible to achieve a satisfactory fit for 'at-risk' feet with high-heeled shoes with pointed toes. However, it is often possible to maximize the cosmetic appeal within the constraints of what is required functionally. The old adage 'beauty is in the eye of the beholder' certainly applies to shoes. What one person accepts as pleasing may be totally abhorrent to another, so an element of individual choice is always necessary. Cultural influences and social patterns can also dictate preferences. Whereas the recent UK fashion for Doc Martens and trainers has provided a welcome temporary remission from the more damaging aspects of some fashions, this will probably not continue.

The psychological effects of the appearance of footwear must not be dismissed lightly. For many, shoes are the item of dress that first marks the person out from their peer group as different. Many a pair of orthopaedic shoes lies unworn in the wardrobe. Conversely, compliant patients often restrict their lifestyles solely because of the appearance of the footwear. Costigan et al (1989) reviewed 82 patients given shoes 2–3 years previously at the General Hospital in Nottingham, of whom 59 were women and 23 were men. Of the 82 original patients, 66 continued wearing the footwear, but 'even patients who still wore their surgical shoes were often dissatisfied, the reasons being the inability to fasten the shoes themselves ... and the appearance of the shoes'. Fisher & McLellan (1989) similarly reported that some patients found their shoes too heavy or clumsy, or of poor appearance.

The balancing of functional needs with aesthetic acceptability is a matter of judgement of the clinical staff. Patient education is advisable.

PRESCRIPTION OF BESPOKE FOOTWEAR

Bespoke footwear is made to fit an individual patient's foot measurements. The process from measurement to delivery usually takes around 2 months in the UK. As already highlighted, bespoke footwear may be purchased privately or obtained free or at reduced costs via the NHS for those referred by a consultant.

Initial assessment

It is essential that a thorough assessment be undertaken, which includes an examination of foot mobility and alignment, presence of sensory neuropathy, skin lesions, prominences and deformities, oedema, alignment and gait. It is also important that the patient's lifestyle requirements and perceived problems and needs are taken into consideration. Additional consideration should be given to educational needs and compliance.

The patient should be shown a catalogue of styles and offered a wide choice of colours, perhaps from swatches of leather. Often the most basic style of shoe can be made more attractive by good colour selection and attention to details such as punch hole patterns on the front part, contrasting topline padding, careful placement of ornamentation or balanced designs (Fig. 13.5).

There are two main shoe styles used in bespoke footwear: the Derby or Gibson and the Oxford (Fig. 13.6). With the Derby shoe, the manner in which the quarters and vamp are cut and attached enables the shoe to be fitted more easily, because the tongue can be reflected completely back and the shoe can be opened wider than with the Oxford style. T-bar styles can be used for certain categories of patients. More recently, trainer styles have been added to the range of many companies, in response to fashion demands, although these usually have a traditional sole construction rather than the moulded soles of the volume shoe. In addition to shoes,

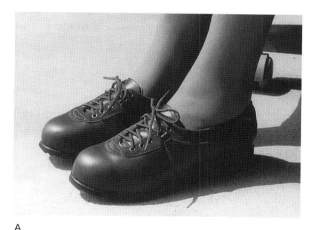
A

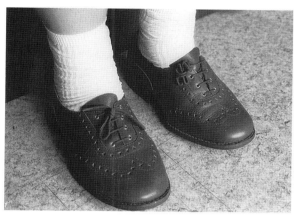
B

Figure 13.5 Well-designed shoes have a traditional shape detailing sufficient toe depth, good quarter fit below the malleoli, facings and tongue, with a small gap not giving rise to pressure over the dorsal midfoot bones. A, Adult; B, child.

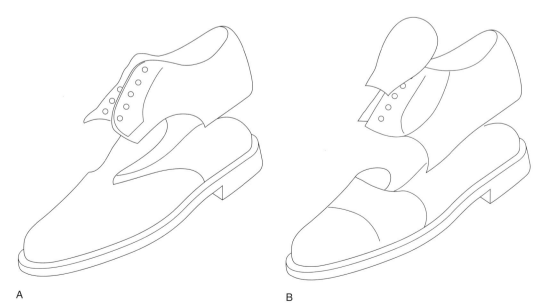
A   B

Figure 13.6 Shoe styles. A, Derby or Gibson style shoe; B, Oxford style shoe.

boots are also available that extend more proximally, to help keep them on in the case of forefoot amputation or to impart extra support around the ankle.

Measurement

Foot measurement can be taken with a pencil of 7 mm diameter, paper and a 6.25 mm wide tape measure (British Standards Institute 1980). The following procedure should be adopted.

1. The outline of the foot with the patient standing should be recorded. The pen should be held vertically but angled in under the longitudinal arch.
2. The height over prominent toes or bony features should be indicated.
3. Sites of skin lesions should be marked.
4. The girth of the foot should be measured while the patient is standing. The tape measure should be slipped under the foot and wrapped over the prominences of the first and fifth metatarsal heads: the tape should be pulled tight then released slightly so as not to compress the tissues. The position of the girth is marked on the outline by dropping the tape flat onto the ground and scoring either side of it (Fig. 13.7).
5. Similarly, the girth at the waist (narrowest dimension) and instep (over the navicular prominence) are recorded and the positions marked.
6. Long and short heel (minimum) measures should be taken. The long heel measure is taken to the same point (navicular prominence) as is used for the instep measure.
7. Foot length should be measured along the medial border with a size stick, with the foot weight bearing or semi-weight bearing.

For more severe cases, a plaster cast of the foot may be taken to represent the overall contours. This is usually done with the foot in its non-weight-bearing neutral position, as described by Root et al (1971), although some practitioners prefer weight-bearing casts.

An impression of the foot bed is required for moulded inserts. This can be taken with a slipper cast, by pressing the foot into a special-purpose

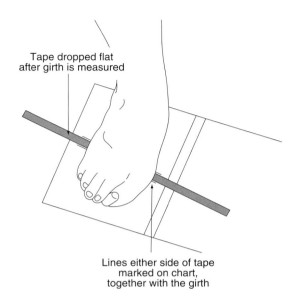

Tape dropped flat after girth is measured

Lines either side of tape marked on chart, together with the girth

Figure 13.7 The position at which girth measurements are taken should be noted on the outline so that the measurements can be matched at the same location on the last.

box of foam or by the use of vacuum bag casting, which is favoured in continental Europe. Other direct methods of making insoles are now available; for example, a device may be used where the foot shape is captured by impressing the sole into a bed of closely packed rods, from which a silicone insert can be directly fabricated. A high-technology approach can also be adopted; for example, the measurement can be taken with the patient standing on a bed of round-ended tubes that are forced up through preshaping templates by a constant, adjustable pressure. The resulting shape is captured on an adjacent computer, where shape compensations can be made before the insert is milled from a preform in a computer controlled machine alongside.

Bespoke lasts

Bespoke lasts are made either by modification of the contours of a stock last, by the addition or reduction of material to suit the individual's measurements, or by producing a custom last.

The dimensions of the custom last do not correspond to those of the foot. The differences in key dimensions are known as the last allowances. There are no hard and fast rules for these, although generally the lastmaker works to a notional standard when making the first attempt at the last. As a general guidance, the values in Table 13.5 are used, although these can be changed in accordance with last shaping and the fit required. For example, it is reported that curvature of the bottom surface of the last can affect the girth allowance and an extra 2 mm of depth above normal is equivalent to an increase in joint girth of 3.5 mm (Browne 1993). Individual allowances may also depend on the foot conditions, for example increased joint allowances for sensitive forefoot and reduced instep girth for supportive footwear.

The allowances do not provide space for inserts, which require further allowances on the forefoot girths of twice the insert thickness (or less if compressible); preferably, the lasts are made to the normal allowance and an equivalent thickness of the insert is blocked onto the bottom of the last before the shoe is constructed.

Construction

Although there are many ways of constructing a shoe, the recommended method for bespoke shoes is by welt construction. This method produces a shoe that is smooth inside, facilitates internal modifications, is simple to repair and retains its shape well.

In a well-constructed bespoke shoe, there are two soles, inner and outer. The outer sole, in contact with the floor, is often leather but is increasingly being made from a synthetic material. The inner sole of leather lies under the foot; between these two soles is a compressible filler.

Patients have complained about the weight of bespoke footwear. This was in the past determined by the standards of leather, and the heavy leather soles and construction dictated by the NHS guidelines. More enlightened interpretation of the guidelines now permits the use of different materials, such as Microlite soles. This allows the possibility of a lighter shoe for patients with occasional or indoor use.

Generally, heel heights for bespoke shoes should not exceed 42 mm and heels should be straight sided and have a low pitch. The heel is nailed to the outsole and the whole shoe is polished ready for delivery.

There is an alternative method for making bespoke shoes called the in-lasted method, in which the upper material is wrapped around and under the last and the sole is attached to the bottom (Fig. 13.8). This produces a close fit but is more difficult to alter and repair, as is so often required for users of special footwear.

Trial fitting

Bespoke shoes provided at the rough finishing stage should have a temporary heel of the correct height attached. It is important to ensure that the

Table 13.5 Suggested average last allowances for orthopaedic shoes

Dimension	Last allowance (mm)[a]
Length	10
Joint girth	10
Long heel	−5
Joint width	0
Heel width	0

[a]Last measurement minus foot measurement.

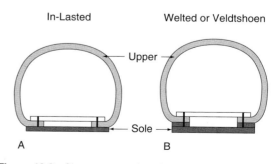

Figure 13.8 Shoe construction. A, An in-lasted shoe; B, a welted shoe.

final versions of any removable inlays are provided with the shoes. These should first be removed from the shoes, and a check made with the patient standing barefoot on the inlay. If satisfactory, the inlays are put back into the shoes. In all cases, the patient should then put on the shoes while wearing the customary hosiery, paying attention to any problems of entry or fastening. With the fastening firmly done up, the patient should be asked to stand. The check list outlined in the section above on fit should be used.

For minor modifications to bespoke shoes or for minor adaptations to the uppers of a stock shoe, positions of local alterations may be marked onto the upper with an erasable pencil. Other fitting observations must be recorded. If the fit requires major modifications, a remeasure should be undertaken, and a further trial fit will be required.

One variant on this process, practised in continental Europe, is the use of shell shoes. At the stage when the last is first made, a plastic shell is fabricated by vacuum moulding over the last and inset (Fig. 13.9). With the addition of a temporary heel of the correct height, this shell is then sent for the trial fitting rather than sending a rough-finished shoe. The advantage of this method is that the shell can very quickly be ready for trial fitting, cutting perhaps 2 weeks off the supply time. More adventurous pattern designs can be undertaken once the last is closer to its final shape.

Delivery

Delivery should be at a clinic where a final fit assessment can be made. Some problems with fit may not come to light until the shoes have been worn. These include creases in the vamp, excessive pressure on the dorsum of the foot, pain from mismatch of foot and shoe function, and rubbing from prominent seams. It is important, therefore, to check the shoes a few weeks after delivery. The lack of any signs of wear on the sole or upper can be quite revealing about usage.

Changes in UK practice

It is hoped that the introduction of computer-aided design techniques will improve the production of bespoke footwear without incurring excessive overheads. It may even allow for the possibility of link-ups with volume manufacturers for subsets of their current ranges (Lord et al 1991). The use of shell shoes to expedite fitting is being introduced into the UK by several contractors. The contractors are also introducing computer-aided design and manufacture for bespoke shoes, which may improve the speed of delivery and quality of the product.

FOOTWEAR ADAPTATIONS

Many adaptations can be made to a patient's footwear. The purpose of such adaptations is to achieve one or more of the following:

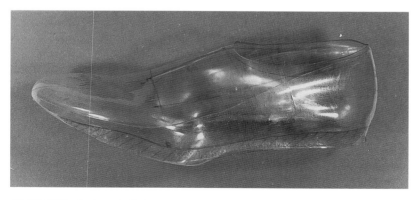

Figure 13.9 A clear shell shoe.

- accommodate fixed deformities
- improve the stability of the foot
- relieve discomfort.

Adaptations may be fitted to the exterior or the interior of the footwear, although most are fitted to the exterior. External adaptations do not usually result in the shoe-fitting problems that often occur with internal footwear adaptations (e.g. insoles and orthoses) nor should they distort the shoe. Any adaptation should be as light in weight as possible so as not to affect adversely what might already be a poor-quality, high-energy-consuming gait.

Before an adaptation is fitted, it is essential to ensure that the footwear is a good fit. To achieve this, the footwear, usually a shoe, needs to:

- extend proximally on the foot to grip the rearfoot and help to control the subtalar joint
- be effectively fastened to the foot by means of laces or straps (elasticated straps or inserts should be avoided)
- have a firm heel counter to help to control the calcaneus

- have a broad heel for overall stability.

Malalignment of the foot joints, plus involvement of the more proximal joints in conditions such as arthritis, may lead to severe pain up through the ankle, knee, hip and spine. It is, therefore, important to consider the whole body alignment when assessing for footwear adaptations. The design of the footwear also needs to take into account the gait. In the typical rheumatoid gait, for example, the foot is placed flat onto the ground and lifted in the same way, without the usual heel strike and rollover pattern of normal gait. The provision of rockered soles can assist in establishing a more normal gait both by pain relief and by reduction of the effort needed from weakened calf muscles (Dimonte & Light 1982).

Any changes aimed at achieving realignment via changes in heel height or wedging must be carefully managed and gradually introduced in order not to induce stresses in more proximal joints.

A range of adaptations can be made to footwear. These are listed in Table 13.6 and discussed below.

Table 13.6 Footwear adaptations for specific conditions as alternative methods to other systems of management

Condition	Objectives	Possible adaptations
Arthritis (traumatic or rheumatoid)	Limit motion, accommodate valgus/varus	Rocker sole, use of boot, ankle stiffener, heel flare, Thomas heel
	Pressure relief	Sach heel, cushioning inserts
Ankle or subtalar arthrodesis	Improve gait pattern	Rocker sole
	Accommodate short leg and equinus	Heel/sole raise
Ankle and subtalar instability	Support unstable joints	Heel flare, boot with ankle stiffener, orthosis with frontal plane control
Diabetic neuropathy	Plantar pressure redistribution and relief	Soft uppers (digits), shock attenuation, moulded inlay or rocker sole
Pes valgus and similar variations	Limit eversion at hindfoot, control forefoot	Use of boot with broad heel, use of long medial stiffened counter, orthotic inlay for forefoot varus/valgus wedge or on outer sole (less control)
	Limit midtarsal compensation	Additional heel adaptations, Thomas heel, extend heel breast, medial flare on orthosis and shoes
	Contour long arch	Longitudinal arch fillers

continued

Table 13.6 (contd)

Condition	Objectives	Possible adaptations
Pes equinus	Assist foot in plantarflexed position (rigid)	Heel raise internal/external to shoe
	Decrease equinus (flexible)	Remove heel or elevate sole
	Hold foot in shoe	Use boots, add collar to shoe
Pes cavus	Plantar forefoot redistribution	Increase heel height
	Foot contour problem	Deeper shoes, use of boot, deep toe puff, soft tongue pad. Inlay to balance heel with forefoot
	Varus heel/valgus forefoot	Heel and sole wedges on shoe
	Metatarsalgia	Insole contoured for arch and metatarsal pressure areas and to cushion shock
Talipes equinovarus	Accommodate deformity	Use of boots for improved control, high heel counters extended forward, breast extended anteriorly, lateral heel extended, lateral heel and sole wedges/flares, shank filler
	Flexible deformity, attempt to assist stretch out deformity	Lower/remove heel, use Bebax design (Ch. 15), use modified (outflared last)
Calcaneal pain	Shock attenuation	Cushion heel material, strong heel counter, Sach heel
	Pressure relief	Insoles/heel pads, heel elevation, remove heel counter
Metatarsalgia and metatarsal depressed transverse arch	Pain relief	Ensure sufficient shoe length for spread forefoot, lower heel height, excavate insole
	Redistribution	External metatarsal bar, add Denver bar, internal metatarsal pads, lower heel to off-load forefoot
Flexion toe deformities	Relief from interphalangeal joint pressure	Deep toe box, balloon patch, soft or Norwegian vamp
	Stabilize metatarsals and hindfoot problems	Attention to valgus/varus as above
Hallux valgus and exostosis	Provide adequate room	Broad last with long vamp, add balloon patch, build adequate depth into shoe design, hindfoot may be narrow (see splay foot); go for snug fit across vamp to prevent movement
	Prevent deformity	Width compression reduced as above; allow room for orthoses
Splay foot	Narrow heel problem	Stiffen and narrow heel counter
	Accommodate Tailor's bunion	Balloon patch over fifth metatarsal or stretch shoe
	Stabilize foot	Use various orthotic modalities or modify heel, elevate heel, use boot and ankle stiffener
Hallux rigidus	Prevent motion and reduce pressure if enlarged	Toe box depth, add rocker sole across metatarsal heads or long rocker sole. Steel sole plate
Foot shortening	Fill room in forefoot	Extra insole, tongue pad, split shoe sizes, filler in toe part with steel sole plate; in extreme cases, use bespoke shoes

continued

Table 13.6 (contd)

Condition	Objectives	Possible adaptations
Leg length discrepancy	Achieve symmetrical posture; additional objectives to improve gait determinants and keep heel in shoe	Internal heel elevation to 12 mm maximum; use collar or boot if fit problems; go for external raise on heel and sole. Metal skate for large discrepancies. More conspicuous extension boot with foot placed in equinus

The sole and heel of the shoe

Heel flares   These can be applied to either side of the heel to provide a correctional moment of force at the heel during heel strike (Fig. 13.10A). They do this by moving the point of initial foot contact medially or laterally such that the moment created by the ground reaction force opposes the deforming moment. They can be used to help to stabilize the subtalar joint in arthritic or unstable foot conditions, which often lead to recurrent ankle sprain. Flares do not alter the resting position of the foot; they only help to correct the foot motion at foot contact. Wedges are used to alter the resting foot position.

Wedges   These can be applied to either side of the heel, over the whole length of the sole, a localized area of the sole (e.g. fifth metatarsal head area) or any combination of these to achieve a tilting of the inside of the shoe relative to the ground (Fig. 13.10B). It is unusual to have a wedge of more than 6 mm, with 4 mm being typical, as higher values than these tend to cause the foot to slide down the incline created without providing any additional benefit. It must be remembered that for wedges to work satisfactorily, there must be the appropriate joint motion in the foot. Wedges can be of value in managing mild pes planovalgus (medial heel wedge) and pes cavus (lateral heel and sole wedges), either on their own or in conjunction with other orthoses; their principal action is to promote inversion or eversion of the foot, particularly via the calcaneus.

Metatarsal bars   These are added to the sole of the shoe, proximal to the metatarsal heads, in an attempt to relieve pain and decrease pressure from the metatarsal heads (Fig. 13.10C). Their effectiveness depends upon the sole material and thickness, with better results found with thinner soles. They are generally less successful than metatarsal pads placed within the shoe.

Sole plates   These are used to stiffen the sole by the insertion of a spring steel shank. They are useful in the treatment of pain associated with hallux limitus, by preventing or limiting flexion at the metatarsophalangeal joints. Rocker soles are used for established hallux rigidus.

Thomas heel   This is an anteromedial extension of the heel that can be used to provide additional support to the medial longitudinal arch of the foot (Fig. 13.10D). Thomas heels may be used in conjunction with a medial heel flare or wedge in managing pes planovalgus or to increase the effectiveness of insoles or foot orthoses in the heavier patient. The use of shoes with a wedge sole has a similar effect.

Heel and sole raises   There are a variety of reasons why raises may be used. Leg length discrepancy is a common factor. Care should be taken when adding raises to footwear, as flexibility of the sole is important for walking. If this cannot be maintained, an additional rocker sole should be considered. Any increase in heel height requires an increase in the amount of dorsiflexion at the metatarsophalangeal joints (i.e. about 1° for each 5 mm of additional heel height). An increase in heel height can also lead to an increase in forefoot loading (Gastwirth et al 1991). Common practice suggests that up to 12 mm may be added to the heel before it is necessary to raise the sole; this could be split by adding 6 mm inside the shoe (providing it has sufficient depth at the heel) and reducing the contralateral shoe outside by 6 mm. The actual prescription must be decided on an individual basis as it is not always advisable to include heel raises in those with neurological damage such as cerebral palsy. It is also necessary to monitor the person with the raise regularly, as not all patients respond in the same way.

Sole rockers These are used to alter the forward progression of the ground reaction force so that loads can be taken off susceptible metatarsal heads. This is particularly relevant in the management of diabetic foot ulceration (Geary & Klenerman 1987; Fig. 13.10E). The reduction in toe dorsiflexion that rocker soles induce often helps to relieve metatarsal discomfort. Rocker soles can also be used as described above to augment other shoe adaptations and orthotic devices, and to replace motion required for gait that has been lost elsewhere in the foot (e.g. through an arthrodesis of the ankle joint).

Cushioned heel These can be used to help relieve the discomfort associated with the shock

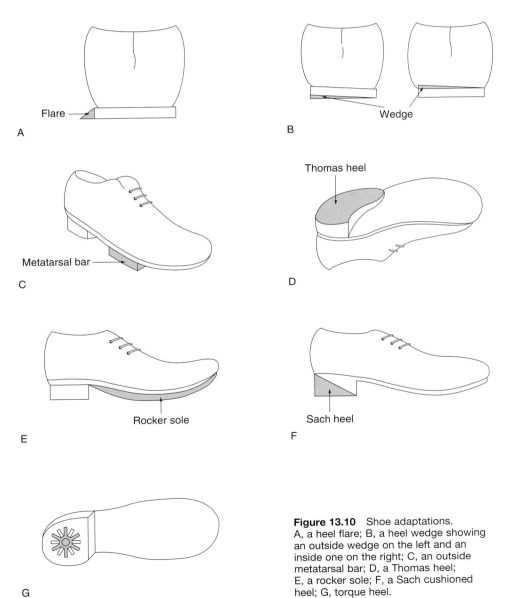

Figure 13.10 Shoe adaptations. A, a heel flare; B, a heel wedge showing an outside wedge on the left and an inside one on the right; C, an outside metatarsal bar; D, a Thomas heel; E, a rocker sole; F, a Sach cushioned heel; G, torque heel.

of heel contact during walking. A compressible material is inserted into the posterior heel as a wedge, which compresses during heel strike and cushions the foot; this is sometimes called a Sach heel (Fig. 13.10F). Heel pain may be caused by a calcaneal spur, and cushioning alone may not be sufficient to relieve symptoms. Here, an excavation in the heel of the shoe can be used to off-load the tender area.

Torque heel   This is a rubber device that can be attached to the heel of a shoe. As the heel is loaded, the rubber wings of the insert are forced over, causing the shoe to twist, usually outwards. This can be used to assist children who walk with their feet internally (or externally) rotated, provided there is no significant spasticity present (Fig. 13.10G).

Calliper   The portion of the sole between the ball and the anterior border of the heel is called the waist. This area is usually reinforced with a metal insert called the shank piece, which must be sufficient to prevent unwanted flexion of this area. This is particularly important if a calliper is to be attached to the shoe, as without this reinforcement there will be too much flexion in the waist and the calliper will not function correctly.

The shoe upper

Stretching and balloon patching   Shoe uppers can be modified to relieve dorsal pressure on, for example, claw toes or bunions. If selective stretching of the shoe does not relieve the discomfort, then a balloon patch may be added. This is a patch of leather, often softer than that of the shoe itself, which is glued over a hole cut in the upper to provide pressure relief. Care has to be exercised to match this to the shoe colour and texture as closely as possible.

Stiffeners   Often shoes can be made more supportive and effective if they are stiffened, particularly around the heel. A more-rigid leather or other material is inserted between the layers of the shoe counter, providing more stiffness and enhanced stability to the foot.

Tongue fillers   If the girth of the shoe is too large, a pad of material can be adhered to the underside of the tongue (in a lace-up shoe). This has the effect of taking up some of the excess room and also serves as a cushion.

Fastening   The means of closure of the footwear can be altered to take account of the clinical need and the ability of the wearer. As well as the usual laces, which may extend down to the toes for easier fitting, there are elastic laces and elastic gussets to accommodate swelling, zips and Velcro for quick easy adjustment, and buckles for extra grip on the foot. There are ways of tying laces one handed that enable those with only one functional hand to still get the benefits of stable footwear (Hughes 1982).

Toe caps   With some medical conditions, such as hemiplegia, the patient may have a tendency to rub the toe end of the shoe because of an inability to dorsiflex the foot. Reinforced toe caps can be added to slow down the shoe wear in such circumstances and prevent irreversible damage to the structure of the shoe.

SUMMARY

It is important that footwear therapy is not overlooked when producing a management plan. This chapter has demonstrated that footwear plays an essential role in the treatment of foot problems. Footwear therapy encompasses a range of activities, from advice to a patient buying a pair of shoes to footwear adaptations aimed at reducing discomfort and improving gait. Appropriate footwear therapy should always result in a reduction of symptoms, and it may sometimes cure the foot problem.

REFERENCES

Alexander I J, Chao E Y S, Johnson K A 1990 The assessment of dynamic foot-to-ground contact forces and plantar pressure distribution: a review of the evolution of current techniques and clinical applications. Foot and Ankle 11: 152–167

Bader D, Chase A 1993 The patient orthosis interface. In: Bowker P, Bader D, Condie D N, Pratt D J, Wallace W A (eds) The biomechanical basis of orthotic management. Butterworth–Heinneman, Oxford, p 68–69
Bennett I, Kavner D, Lee B K, Trainor F A 1979 Shear versus

pressure as causative factors in skin blood flow occlusion. Archives of Physical Medicine and Rehabilitation 60: 309–314

Boulton A J M, Hardisty C A, Betts R P et al 1983 Dynamic foot pressure and other studies as diagnostic and management aids in diabetic neuropathy. Diabetes Care 6: 26–33

British Standards Institute 1980 BS5943: a method for measuring and casting for orthopaedic footwear. HMSO, London

Browne R 1993 Better lasts, better fit. Shoe and Allied Trades Research Association Bulletin April: 57–58

Bunten J 1983 Foot comfort. Shoe and Allied Trades Research Association Report SR 44

Burry H S 1956 Some objective data on a case of burning sensation of the feet. Shoe and Allied Trades Research Association Memorandum TM 1192

Cavanagh P R, Sanders L J, Sims D S, Jr 1987 The role of pressure distribution measurement in diabetic foot care. Rehabilitation Research and Development Progress Reports 54

Chantelau E, Haage P 1994 An audit of cushioned diabetic footwear: relation to patient compliance. Diabetic Medicine 11: 114–116

Chen C 1993 An investigation into shoe last design in relation to foot measurement and shoe fitting for orthopaedic footwear. PhD thesis. London University

Costigan P S, Miller G, Elliott C, Wallace W A 1989 Are surgical shoes providing value for money? British Medical Journal 299: 950

Dimonte P, Light H 1982 Pathomechanics, gait deviations, and treatment of the rheumatoid foot. Physical Therapy 8: 1148–1156

Disabled Living Foundation. Service handbook. Disabled Living Foundation, London

Fisher L R, McLellan D L 1989 Questionnaire assessment of patient satisfaction with lower limb orthoses from a district hospital. Prosthetics and Orthotics International 13: 29–35

Gastwirth B W, O'Brien T D, Nelson R M, Manger D C,

Kindig S A 1991 An electrodynographic study of foot function in shoes of varying heel heights. Journal of the American Podiatric Medical Association 81: 463–472

Geary N P J, Klenerman L 1987 The rocker sole shoe: a method to reduce peak forefoot pressure in the management of diabetic foot ulceration. In: Pratt D J, Johnson G R (eds) The biomechanics and orthotic management of the foot. Orthotics and Disability Research Centre, Derby, UK, ch 17

Hughes J (ed) 1982 Footwear and footcare for disabled children. Disabled Living Foundation, London

Lord M 1981 Foot pressure measurement: a review of methodology. Journal of Biomedical Engineering 3: 91–99

Lord M, Reynolds D P, Hughes J R 1986 Foot pressure measurement: a review of clinical findings. Journal of Biomedical Engineering 8: 283–294

Lord M, Foulston J, Smith P J 1991 Technical evaluation of a CAD system for orthopaedic shoe-upper design. Engineering in Medicine, Proceedings of Institution of Mechanical Engineers 205: 109–115

Lord M, Hosein R, Williams R B 1992 Method for in-shoe shear stress measurement. Journal of Biomedical Engineering 14: 181–186

Murray D L, Peet M J 1966 Summary of work on burning sensation. SATRA Internal Report 219

Pollard J P, Le Quesne L P, Tappin J W 1983 Forces under the foot. Journal of Biomedical Engineering 5: 37–40

Root M L, Orien W P, Weed J H, Hughes R J 1971 Biomechanical examination of the foot. Clinical Biomechanics Corporation, Los Angeles, CA, vol 1

Rossi W 1983 Footwear and the podiatrist: the enigma of shoe sizes. Journal of American Podiatry Association 73: 272–274

Rothman S 1954 Physiology and biochemistry of the skin. University of Chicago Press, Chicago, IL

Warren-Forward M J, Goodall R M, Pratt D J 1992 A three dimensional force and displacement transducer. Proceedings A of the Institute of Electrical Engineers 139: 21–29

FURTHER READING

Shereff M J, DiGiovanni L, Bejjani F J, Hersh A, Kummer F J 1990 A comparison of non weight-bearing and weight-bearing radiographs of the foot. Foot and Ankle 10: 306–311

Snow R E, Williams K R, Holmes G B 1992 The effects of

wearing high heeled shoes on pedal pressures in women. Foot and Ankle 13: 85–92

Tappin J W, Robertson K P 1991 Study of the relative timing of shear forces on the forefoot during walking. Journal of Biomedical Engineering 13, 39–42

Managing specific client groups

14

The adult foot

David R. Tollafield
Tim E. Kilmartin
Trevor Prior

INTRODUCTION

Describing the management of every manifestation likely to arise in the adult foot is notoriously difficult. One of the greatest difficulties in outlining any chapter on treatment is that it relies on a certain amount of common agreement between professionals that certain strategies are effective. The fact that many treatment strategies have unclear outcomes is evident from a paucity of effective audit. Journals dedicated to the scientific study of feet are reluctant to print unsubstantiated work. We have, therefore, been left with the problem of dovetailing historical treatment methods with scientific fact.

This chapter sets out to achieve three aims: first, to provide a summary of common conditions affecting the foot that can be treated by conservative and surgical means; second, to integrate treatment philosophy highlighted in previous chapters with conditions typically seen in adult patients; and finally, to describe common approaches to treatment for foot problems related to articular/bone conditions, deformity, corns and callus, soft tissue pain and some miscellaneous conditions not covered elsewhere in the book.

TREATING THE ADULT PATIENT

Effective management of adult foot problems will only succeed if the following factors are taken into consideration:

- correct diagnosis
- patient compliance
- avoidance of secondary complications
- patient mobility or disability
- economic considerations.

The planned strategy of care will need to be recorded. The type of care selected will depend upon the available resources and the factors listed above. A broad discussion on general treatment planning has already been presented in Chapter 1. The following points will, therefore, have to be considered before treatment commences.

Correct diagnosis Quite often, foot disorders are misdiagnosed or dismissed because there are insufficient clinical signs to suggest the likely trend in pathology. In the USA, financial and legal pressures have created a need for expensive diagnostic centres. Fortunately, in the majority of foot complaints, diagnosis is relatively straightforward, and extensive investigations are unnecessary. Where a condition fails to improve, the practitioner is duty bound to expand the network of investigation, adjust the management plan within moderation or refer to another specialist.

Patient compliance No matter how dedicated a practitioner might be, an unresponsive patient will make management of a problem more difficult. A lack of compliance may relate to one or more of the following:

- limited finance
- misunderstanding
- inability to understand English
- inability to travel to the centre
- poor personal attitude.

In all cases, except the last, supportive help can be given; in the case of language difficulties, translators should be engaged as part of good *Patient Charter* practice.

Secondary complications These creates two problems. First, an associated condition may be exacerbated by treatment for a primary complaint; for example, preexisting metatarsalgia is known to be greatly aggravated by excisional arthroplasty for a painful metatarsophalangeal joint (MTPJ). Second, an underlying disease or concurrent medication or treatment may complicate management or delay treatment response. Cardiovascular disease, diabetes mellitus, medication such as steroids and anticoagulants, malnutrition, alcoholism, drug abuse and preexisting joint replacements or implants will all have significant implications for the success of any treatment. Some of these implications have been described in other chapters.

Patient mobility Disability or immobility affects both young and elderly patients. Treatment is sometimes limited to strategies that are less than ideal. Injudicious management may contribute to a patient's existing disability. The practitioner must select the appropriate treatment, which is sometimes very different from the ideal treatment.

Economic considerations While it is insensitive to ask someone how much he or she earns, a very different question will reveal their status. Do they work? Can they afford time away from work? Many foot problems may be alleviated by changing footwear, but this will usually mean that the patient has to buy new shoes. The practitioner should consider any financial limitations before suggesting that the patient contributes financially to their treatment.

ARTICULAR AND BONE CONDITIONS

This section is subdivided into three areas associated with joint and bone conditions:

- arthritis
- stress fractures
- neoplasia.

ARTHRITIS

Degenerative joint disease may lead to pain, swelling and deformity. In severe cases it will restrict mobility. All joints can be affected and treatment must differentiate between crystal arthritis, rheumatoid arthritis, the seronegative arthritides and degenerative (osteo-) arthritis (OA).

Crystal deposition arthritides

Crystal deposition arthritides can affect the first MTPJ as well as the lesser toes and ankle. The pathogenesis is very different from degenerative arthritis, but there are similarities between the signs and symptoms. Gout and pseudogout (pyrophosphate arthropathy) are the two main members of this group (Klenerman 1991); other variants exist and must be identified.

Principles of management

It is necessary to identify the active process causing inflammation, which should be reversed by systemic medication. Control of the metabolic pathway is usually preferred to using anti-inflammatory drugs alone. Secondary changes associated with the loss of articular surface, soft tissue calcinosis and tophi, synovitis and reduced movement should be managed on the basis of radiographic changes and clinical symptoms. Diagnosis is principally provided by blood assay and joint aspiration.

Gout Hyperuricaemia diagnosed by raised uric acid serum levels does not always provide a positive confirmation of gout, as it may not always precipitate an acute gouty attack. It can, however, lead to kidney stone formation or even cardiomyopathy. X-ray films may be normal initially. Chronic deposition of sodium urate crystals may cause tophaceous gout, where hard nodules or tophi may become apparent subcutaneously and bone erosions are seen on plain radiographs. In gout that appears as an isolated swollen toe, psoriatic arthritis should be considered.

Pseudogout There will be crystal deposition within the cartilage (chondrocalcinosis) in older patients, and calcium pyrophosphate dihydrate will be present. The latter may be associated with a systemic manifestation such as hyperparathyroidism or haemochromatosis.

Hydroxyapatite arthropathy These crystals will cause inflammatory changes in joints, although the pathogenesis of this form of arthri-

tis is controversial (Rees & Trounce 1988). Large quantities of collagenase and neutral proteinase may be identified within the synovial fluid. Deposit over the first MTPJ tendons can mimic gout (Klenerman 1991).

Conservative management

Medical care The use of diuretics causes gout; cessation of their use must be considered appropriate to the condition being treated. Non-steroidal anti-inflammatory drugs (NSAIDs), particularly indomethacin, naproxen, ibuprofen and piroxicam, are valuable as an alternative to colchicine for acute attacks. Corticosteroid injection will abort an acute attack. Where attacks are frequent, hypouricaemic drugs such as allopurinol will block the last stage of the metabolic pathway in urate crystal production. The daily dose is 300 mg, but this will need to be adjusted according to the serum level of urate. Allopurinol is generally cited as the drug of choice and is beneficial where renal disease or stones complicate the picture. Dietary care will have to be considered, moderating excesses of alcohol and offal meats high in purine.

Orthoses and footwear Soft shoe uppers and firm thick soles will reduce the pressure over tender enlarged joints and limit first MTPJ movement. Bunion shields made from latex or foam, or over-the-counter products, may offer some skin protection. These latter products are not tolerated in the acute phase of disease. Tophi can cause ulcerations and the skin will need to be protected by soft redistributive dressings. Low-density, heat-moulded polyethylene (Plastazote) foam may also be used over the joint. Larger shoes will have to be prescribed where the mid-tarsal area is affected. Soft orthoses may be used to protect the medial foot against the shoe, as well as to stabilize the foot where pathology has weakened the foot architecture.

Skin care The skin should be protected at all times and non-viable areas should be prevented from ulcerating. Tophaceous gout can cause considerable shoe wear pressure problems.

Surgical management

Surgery can be used to remove tophi, in order to limit tissue degeneration and inflammation (Case study 14.1). Arthrodesis has been used successfully in psoriatic arthritis, and arthritis caused by tuberculosis and gout (Yu 1992) to limit the extent of movement and secondary changes. Small joints of the toes should be excised and arthrodesed to prevent ulceration. Surgery should be performed between periods of active disease. The gouty patient may have a postoperative gouty attack as a result of local trauma or dehydration, particularly after general anaesthetics.

Degenerative osteoarthritis

OA is not very likely to arise in the young adult unless injury or disease has damaged the joint cartilage. Often the patient complains of toothache-type pain in the joint(s), which is made worse by activity. Frequently, patients will also confirm that the condition is exacerbated by cold or damp weather. When in the advanced stages, crepitus may be noted on examination of the joint. In many joints, synovitis rather than cartilage destruction causes the primary symptoms. Provided that localized heat of an acute inflammation, general pyrexia, sinus tracking and effusive swelling are not present, septic arthritis may be excluded clinically. Aspiration of the joint should be performed under sterile conditions in combination with plain radiographs beforehand (Fig. 14.1).

The midtarsal joint and first MTPJ are perhaps the most common foot joints that present with degenerative OA. The first MTPJ may be damaged by repetitive jamming of the joint secondary to a long or dorsiflexed first metatarsal. Excessive pronation of the foot may malalign the tarsal joints and the subsequent incongruity will predispose the joint surfaces to degeneration. The midfoot may show signs of palpable osteophytes, tenderness and distortion. The misalignment gives the forefoot an abducted, pronated appearance (Fig. 14.2). Osteophytes may rub against soft tissue, causing localized discomfort on specific foot movement. A number of ossicles can become incorporated at joint lines, mimicking osteophytes.

A clinical history may provide evidence of trauma, or the patient may complain of difficult footwear fit without any knowledge of how and

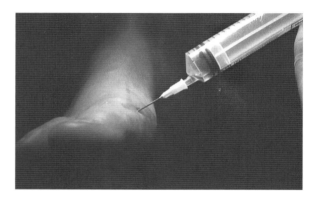

Figure 14.1 Joint aspiration of first metatarsophalangeal joint to rule out gout, infection and presence of blood.

Case study 14.1 Unusual presentation of gout

An 18-year-old wrestler presented with pain in his right first metatarsophalangeal (MTP) joint. There was no previous history of injury. Symptoms included 'throbbing', which was made worse by weight bearing. An examination revealed no swelling. The presence of mild erythema over the plantar aspect of the first MTPJ was noted. There was tenderness over the medial sesamoid, and dorsiflexion elicited moderate pain. Orthoses initially provided some relief from symptoms. Radiographs taken at 10 weeks revealed cystic changes in both the proximal and distal segments of the partitioned sesamoid. An exploratory incision revealed an inflamed capsule and chalky white material that contained monosodium urate crystals; this was later reported to be consistent with gout upon haematoxylin and eosin staining together with Gomori's methenamine-silver stain. These stains were positive for tophaceous gout. The serum uric acid level was 7.8 mg/dl (normal levels 3.5–8.0 mg/dl). History was determined in the family on the paternal side. There was no history of renal disease, nor a use of diuretics or alcohol. This unusual case was reported by Mair et al (1995).

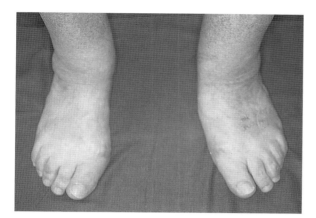

Figure 14.2 Distorted foot shape associated with progressive midfoot arthritis. Note that the left foot looks pronated but that the subtalar joint is not affected.

when the problem started. Radiographs may provide some evidence of degeneration but they often lack the clarity afforded by computed tomography (CT) or magnetic resonance imaging (MRI) scans. Patients admitted to casualty with injury may be dismissed as having simple bruising. Midfoot trauma without obvious radiograph changes can easily mislead the inexperienced casualty doctor. Early discharge may result in failure to achieve a correct diagnosis. This type of problem may well develop active degenerative change several years later.

Principles of management

Once OA has been identified from clinical and radiographic examinations, footwear and general activity may need to be modified. Supportive footwear, particularly above-ankle lace-ups, will reduce pain by controlling joint movement. It is unlikely that footwear alone will resolve the problem without some modification to lifestyle and physical activity.

Analgesics Paracetamol is a useful analgesic that has few side-effects and may be recommended to be taken as necessary. If paracetamol does not help, NSAIDs such as ibuprofen or diclofenac sodium may be used, although gastric irritation arises with long-term use.

Support Strapping will limit joint movement and can be initiated as a short-term measure;

however, it is only a temporary measure as long-term use will almost certainly cause skin irritation. Orthoses may be applied to increase support and further reduce joint mobility, particularly in the subtalar, midtarsal and tarsal joints. The beneficial effect is likely to be reduced where these joints are already subluxed.

Physical therapy Heat is beneficial in acute and subacute stages of the disorder. Infrared and interferential forms of physical therapy should be considered to suppress inflammation.

Corticosteroids Injections are valuable in the joints of the foot but should not be repeated too frequently. The action of the drug is directed at the synovium rather than the cartilage. Corticosteroid given in small quantities will reduce inflammation and relieve spasm and reduce effusion. Reliance on this powerful agent is discouraged and the benefit can be reduced if injections are overused. Certain corticosteroids, such as methylprednisolone (Depo-Medrone) and triamcinolone (Kenalog), may cause a localized flare-up of symptoms in the immediate postinjection phase. Betamethasone (Betnesol) may have a lower propensity to postinjection flare-up as it is water soluble, but it appears to act for a shorter period of time.

Surgery Surgery is indicated where the arthritic condition does not improve with conservative care or medication. Arthritic joints can be approached in the following manner:

- *excisional arthroplasty*: replacement of joint surfaces
- *interpositional arthroplasty*: involves placing soft tissue, usually joint capsule, between the resected bone surfaces
- *osteotomy*: decompresses and realigns the joint surfaces in the earlier stages of arthritis
- *joint replacement*: used for irreversibly damaged joints
- *arthrodesis*: the joint is destroyed by fusion and so is immobilized permanently, thus preventing further pain; restricted footwear height becomes a problem.

While all these measures can be very effective, the foot is a complex structure with interconnecting joints that need to function in equilibrium. There is a high risk that surgery at one joint will have potentially damaging implications for other previously normal or asymptomatic joints. The effects of both conservative care and surgery on the following individual joints are considered below:

- interphalangeal joints (IPJs)
- MTPJs
- midtarsus
- ankle.

Interphalangeal joints

The IPJs are not commonly affected by OA but may develop a fibrous union, limiting movement. The fibrous change creates a fixed flexion deformity due to contraction. Upon dissection, few of these joints show the erosion or damage typical of larger joints. However, the main complaints associated with acquired digital problems are corns and callus caused by footwear irritation. Common sites include the dorsal aspect of the IPJ and, because of weight bearing, the apex of the digit. Joint pain associated with arthritic degeneration is less common.

Conservative management In many cases, the primary cause of lesser digit problems is hallux valgus, which causes crowding of the lesser toes. Definitive treatment involves correcting the hallux valgus in order to achieve an effective prognosis. In the case of lesser digital deformities unrelated to hallux valgus, it is possible to treat individual toes. Protection of pressurized skin areas over the joints will be discussed in greater detail under corns and callus, and surgical correction will be discussed under deformities.

Lesser digit problems may be conservatively treated using silicone props or crescents (see Figs 11.3–11.6, and 11.23).

While excisional arthroplasty or arthrodesis (see Fig. 7.21) has been the traditional surgical approach to painful toe joints in the adult foot, small joint implants have recently become available. These silastic prostheses usually have two stems with a small disk spacer between. While these devices prevent bone-to-bone apposition following joint arthroplasty, they are unlikely to resist deforming forces from muscles or adjacent toes.

First metatarsophalangeal joint

Trauma The effects of acute injury to this joint will reduce with immobilization and ice therapy in the first 2–24 hours. Pain can be managed with analgesics, elevation and ice applied over the affected part every few hours for 10–20 minutes. Forced rest can be assisted with elbow crutches (see Appendix 3 on crutch use). The toe joint may need to be splinted with *fan strapping* for 2 weeks (see Fig. 11.14). The patient can be shown how to replace this every 2–3 days. A foot or below-knee leg cast should be used if pain does not subside, or if the patient cannot rest the foot adequately (see Fig. 11.20). Long-term follow-up may establish the early development of osteoarthrosis (Case study 14.2 and Fig. 14.3).

Case study 14.2 Epiphyseal trauma

A 14-year-old male sustained an epiphyseal injury to the base of his first proximal phalanx following a judo kick. Upon radiograph, the epiphysis showed early closure on the lateral side. While Salter–Harris classification (Salter & Harris, 1963) was difficult to determine, a linear split was probably created across the phalangeal epiphysis, with some distraction away from the main body of bone. Failure of early treatment led to degenerative changes across cartilage of the first metatarsal head. The hallux was limited at the metatarsophalangeal joint, with pain on movement. The joint was exposed and the metatarsal was shown to have tram-line tracks depressed into the soft cartilage. The metatarsal was decompressed to open up the joint line, stabilized with a 2.7 mm screw and the patient was allowed to mobilize at 7 days with crutches.

Conclusion: Epiphyseal injury may settle without treatment but early recognition of such trauma should be followed up. The effects of degenerative arthritis may be reversed and symptoms ameliorated if conservative surgery can be offered as soon as possible. The patient in this case remained pain free at 12 months but required routine monitoring. Joint motion has been improved, establishing normal lubrication (Fig. 14.3).

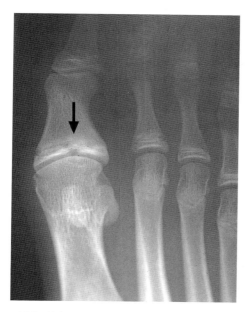

Figure 14.3 Epiphyseal traumea associated with joint changes following a judo kick. Note the irregular proximal (hallux) epiphysis typical of a Salter–Harris fracture.

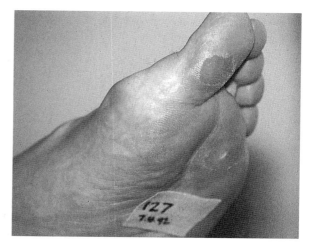

Figure 14.4 An elevated first metatarsal is frequently associated with callus under the hallux.

Hallux limitus In this common condition, extension/dorsiflexion of the great toe (MTPJ) is limited either by a mechanical jamming of the joint or by a large osteophytic projection over both the head of the first metatarsal and the dorsal proximal phalanx. A compensatory ring of fibrocartilage can develop, limiting the first MTPJ further. The exuberant osteophytes will erode the synovial lining and cause the capsule to thin. Radiographs will show diminished joint space and sclerosis (increased density) underlying the cartilage. The presence of lucent (dark areas) suggests synovial/lipid-filled cysts, which occur when bone-to-bone contact forces synovial fluid into the subchondral bone.

Hallux flexus The hallux may flex to gain purchase in the presence of an elevated first metatarsal (metatarsus primus elevatus). In this condition, plantar callus under the IPJ will cause discomfort (Fig. 14.4). Proximal postural symptoms may arise as the patient attempts to compensate by supinating the foot.

Hallux rigidus This presents as a stiff first MTP joint. Because there is no movement within the joint, there is usually no pain other than footwear irritation associated with joint thickening.

Hallux valgus This is commonly associated with hallux rigidus. Degenerative joint disease arises from this condition because it creates incongruity at the first MTP joint. Incongruity affects joint loading. Shear and compressive forces will be abnormally directed over the lateral joint surface. The medial surface becomes atrophied, with thinning of cartilage because of ineffective joint lubrication and reduction of the pressure needed to stimulate normal cellular strength. Where the hallux valgus is associated with an elevated first metatarsal, normal rotation of the hallux over the dorsal articular surface of the first metatarsal head will be impeded. With damage to the articular surface, the joint will become stiff, and new bone and fibrocartilaginous tissue deposited around the joint margin will limit normal motion.

Conservative management In the early stages of OA affecting the first MTP joint, the patient will complain of intermittent toothache-type pain from within the joint. Symptoms are exacerbated by activity, high-heeled footwear and cold, damp weather. On clinical examination, there is slight thickening of the joint and pain on plantarflexion of the hallux; dorsiflexion may be restricted but is rarely painful.

Radiographs will indicate a loss of joint space and possibly the presence of osteophytes on the lateral side of the first metatarsal head (Figs 14.5 and 14.6). At this stage, in-shoe orthoses may be extremely effective in alleviating the joint pain. Any orthotic that extends under the first metatarsal will restrict first metatarsal plantar-flexion, which will reduce mobility of the hallux and thus relieve pain.

In more advanced OA, the joint is enlarged. Pain will arise from damaged articular cartilage interposing against bone or from bone against bone. Footwear may compress the dorsal and medial metatarsal head osteophytes against soft tissue, causing deep tissue shear, inflammation and soft tissue bursae (Fig. 14.7). Radiographs will show an almost complete loss of joint space and prolific osteophytes all around the metatarsal head. In the most advanced disease, osteophytes may also be seen on the base of the proximal phalanx (Fig. 14.8). Joint movement will often be limited to 20° dorsiflexion or less. Orthoses will do little to relieve joint pain at this stage and indeed they may cause further footwear irritation as they fill up the shoe.

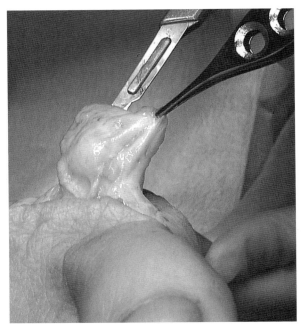

Figure 14.7 Bursal sac removed from an 80-year-old female after aspiration failed to resolve her bunion pain.

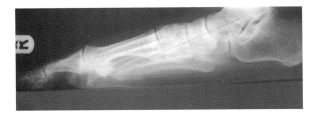

Figure 14.5 The first metatarsophalangeal joint is affected by dorsal lipping with an elevated first metatarsal and this will affect normal first metatarsophalangeal joint function (lateral radiograph).

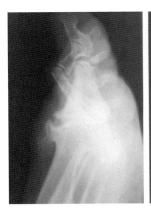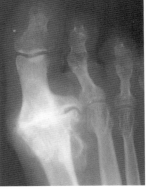

Figure 14.6 Complete loss of joint space and metatarsal lipping form extensive degenerative radiographic changes associated with osteoarthrosis. Two views are required to determine the extent of pathology. Note the parrot's beak effect on the lateral side of the first metatarsophalangeal joint (hallux rigidus).

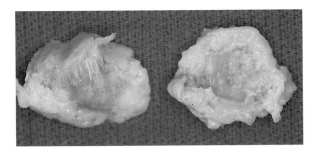

Figure 14.8 Excised joint surfaces of the first metatarsal (left) and the base of the proximal phalanx (right). Pathology shows loss of cartilage, hypertrophic deepening of the base of the phalanx with exuberant osteophytic lipping. The diagnosis is hallux rigidus with gross osteoarthritic changes.

Footwear adaptation Shoe accommodation with balloon patches receives little favour these days but would be valuable in patients unsuited or unwilling to undergo surgery. Alternatively, latex or foam covers can be applied over the first MTPJ to reduce skin irritation. Stiff-soled shoes will restrict movement of the first MTPJ and may relieve joint pain. The application of a rocker bar assists the propulsive phase of gait by allowing the foot to roll over the forefoot. The need to extend the first MTPJ will be reduced.

Injection Synovitis is a feature of degenerative joint disease that often responds to intra-articular corticosteroid injection. A single injection of 0.1–0.3 ml of dexamethasone has been found to be beneficial. A Mayo or metatarsal ring block of local anaesthetic using 1% xylocaine for short duration will remove any spasm from the flexor hallucis brevis. Not only does this allow painless joint injection with corticosteroid medication, but the technique also offers a differential diagnosis in the presence of spasm associated with traumatic change versus true rigidus, where clinical signs are unclear. Loose bodies and marked articular inflammation will cause spasm; some of these symptoms may be reduced by heat therapy. Manipulation of a stiff joint under local anaesthetic will help to break up adhesions after corticosteroid injection. The joint should be physically distracted and circumducted (rotary movements). This exercise can be continued at home or in combination with foot spa baths or hydrotherapy pools. If this technique fails, the practitioner must suspect that advanced stages of pathology have developed.

Surgical management The surgical management of the adult with first MTPJ pain involves a number of different techniques, depending upon the physiological age of the joint and the extent of pathology. The objective of surgery should be the restoration of a normal (45–65°) pain-free range of movement and the removal of dorsal and medial osteophytes. The surgical procedure should be based on the degree of cartilage loss, severity of osteophyte formation, first metatarsal length and sagittal plane position. The patient's age and activity level should also be considered. Where there is still adequate joint space on radi-

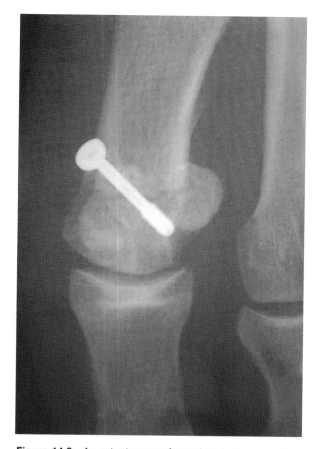

Figure 14.9 An osteotomy performed to decompress the joint, alleviating synovitis and improving joint congruency.

ograph, and only moderate loss of articular cartilage when the joint surfaces are viewed intra-operatively, an osteotomy can be performed to decompress the joint and restore pain-free movement. The osteotomy illustrated in Figure 14.9 shortens the metatarsal length as well as correcting other problems such as hallux valgus.

Gross changes associated with complete cartilage loss and severe osteophytosis can be managed with either a Keller's excisional arthroplasty (see Fig. 7.6) or joint replacement (see Fig. 7.7). In both cases, pain relief should be experienced within the first week following surgery, with reasonable mobility. Casts are seldom required. Joint replacements come in many varieties and opinion varies as to which is most suitable. Hinged silastic implants are probably the most popular (see Ch. 7). Research indicates an average life expectancy of 8 years for an implant. This suggests that they should be avoided in patients much younger than 65 years (Kilmartin & Wallace 1992). The joint implant may well have to be replaced earlier in very active patients.

Arthroplasty without joint replacement does lead to shortening of the toe and is known to cause metatarsalgia. This problem can be limited if the extent of proximal phalanx resection is not very aggressive. No more than 33% of the bone length should be removed in order to avoid marked disturbance of the great toe plantarflexors.

The use of arthrodesis for joint pain depends upon surgical preference. Fusion of the joint has met with success where movement is very painful. A fused first MTPJ can also be very awkward for the patient to tolerate, especially as it limits the range of shoe heel height. In some cases, fusion fails to occur because of inadequate bony compression. An overextended hallux brought about by an arthrodesis can disturb the plantar soft tissue, as illustrated in Figure 14.10.

Lesser metatarsophalangeal joints

Overloading of the lesser MTPJ may occur in hallux valgus or following hallux valgus surgery. If the first metatarsal is dorsiflexed, as it will be in the advanced stages of hallux valgus, or if the first MTPJ has undergone an excisional arthroplasty, the load borne by the first metatarsal will transfer laterally and the second metatarsal will be subject to overloading. This will manifest clinically as tenderness under the metatarsal head, which can be aggravated by direct palpation of the metatarsal head.

Abnormal metatarsal length may also cause painful tenderness on weight bearing. It is usual to find that the second ray has the longest metatarsal in the foot. The first metatarsal is the same length as the third, and the fourth is longer than the fifth. A long second metatarsal or a short first or third is a particularly common finding in cases of plantar tenderness associated with the second metatarsal head. Soft tissue bursae are discussed below under skin/subcutaneous tissues.

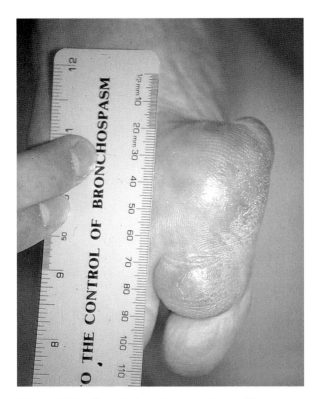

Figure 14.10 The effects on the deep tissues 30 years after a poorly positioned arthrodesis (see Fig. 14.28).

Freiberg's disease, rheumatoid or psoriatic synovitis, painful accessory ossicles, traumatic capsulitis and stress fractures may also cause pain in the lesser metatarsal joints. Any symptoms in this area must always be differentially diagnosed from intermetatarsal neuroma.

Principles of treatment Immobilization of the lesser MTPJs can only be accomplished with below-knee or slipper casting of the foot. It is possible, however, to redistribute some weight-bearing pressure away from the metatarsal heads by using insoles or orthoses.

Corticosteroid injections will have a dramatic effect on synovitis, and often a single injection will bring sustained relief. Repeated injections into the lesser MTPJs can lead to degeneration of the articular cartilage, collateral ligaments of the joint, as well as atrophy of the volar (plantar) plate. Subluxation of the joint is an undesirable side effect of such overuse.

Degenerative arthritic change, often associated with old Freiberg's disease, will only temporarily respond to corticosteroid injections. Excision of the base of the proximal phalanx will, however, eliminate the bone-to-bone contact that causes the pain. Joint replacement may also be considered but tends to act only as a joint spacer. Loss of the load-bearing function of one metatarsal head may cause transfer metatarsalgia of the adjacent metatarsals.

In psoriasis, quite severe erosive changes may destroy the normal metatarsal head. Excision of all the metatarsal heads will reduce joint pain and metatarsalgia but will shorten the foot and destabilize the digits. As with most active forms of arthritis, the disease should be in remission before surgery is considered.

Midfoot arthritis

Trauma to the midfoot is an important cause of long-term disability (Case study 14.3). Any significant trauma, especially from road traffic accidents, should be carefully investigated. Further sequential radiographs should be taken if pain persists. CT and bone scans may be necessary to determine any intra-articular damage.

First metatarsal cuneiform exostosis

Osteophytic thickening at the first metatarsocuneiform joint may present clinically as footwear irritation over the midfoot area (Fig. 14.11). The condition is associated with a hypermobile plantarflexed first metatarsal and develops as a consequence of low-grade but repetitive impaction of the base of the first metatarsal against the medial cuneiform. The osteophytic thickening is best visualized on a lateral weight-bearing radiograph but often looks worse clinically because of the presence of an overlying cartilage cap. In severe cases where there has been considerable footwear irritation, a soft tissue bursa may form dorsomedial to the joint.

Principles of management Footwear advice should be given initially. Certain footwear

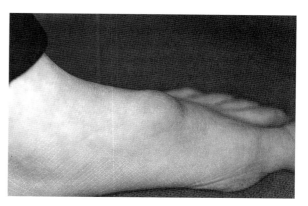

Figure 14.11 Enlarged metatarsocuneiform exostosis and bursa can make shoes difficult to wear. The bursa shown was too established to aspirate and, therefore, underlying bone was flattened by open surgery.

Case study 14.3 Midfoot arthritis

A 46-year-old overweight male caught his foot on a conveyor belt while at work. Initial (plain) radiographs showed no abnormal changes, despite extensive bruising recorded in the medical records. A backsplint cast was applied to the leg and foot, but the period of non-weight bearing was complicated by a deep venous thrombosis, which had to be treated as a medical emergency.

Radiographs taken at 1 year revealed arthritic changes around the second to third metatarsocuneiform joint. Two years following the injury, the patient was still considerably disabled.

Treatment for this form of arthritis initially limited daily pain. Casted orthoses used to splint the midtarsus reduced the effects of movement between the damaged joints. While rest limited symptoms, the patient gained weight. Non-steroid anti-inflammatory drugs (NSAIDs) were helpful but the patient preferred to use them only occasionally. In the long term, arthrodeses of the affected joints may be necessary if symptoms persist.

Conclusion: The prognosis is somewhat unpredictable. Early diagnosis might have used other imaging techniques, such as bone scans and computer tomography, to provide a clearer picture of the damage. A combination of orthoses and NSAIDs will alleviate the symptoms of joint degeneration.

designs will avoid the area; trainers with a soft upper and well-designed lacing system will prevent further irritation of the soft tissues overlying the exostosis.

Protective felt padding can be used to deflect pressure from the area, although the use of felt rings may cause further extrusion of soft tissues. While functional orthoses restrict motion at the first MTPJ (Kilmartin et al 1991), it may be that they could also restrict motion at the first metatarsocuneiform joint and thus prevent further impaction and damage to the joint. To date, however, the role of functional orthoses in this condition remains uncertain. Surgical removal of the exostosis is reserved for recalcitrant problems. Sensitive scarring over the area can be a source of further irritation, especially if the scar becomes thickened postoperatively. Cheilectomy may deal with the prominence but may not deal with the primary mechanical cause. Recurrence does occur.

Ankle joint

Osteoarthrosis of the ankle occurs much less frequently than degenerative joint disease of the knee or hip. Unlike the hip and knee, when the ankle does become arthritic there is usually a history of trauma: repeated low grade injuries, such as recurrent inversion sprains, or a more severe high-impact injury causing fracture of the component bones and derangement of the articular surfaces. In the case of the subtalar joint, intra-articular fracture has a poor prognosis.

Chronic osteoarthrosis of the ankle may be seen on plain radiograph. Acute injuries are better evaluated by CT to account for subtalar involvement and damage to the central mortice of the talus.

The practitioner must exclude tendon inflammation and repetitive strain during examination, as confusion between articular and soft tissue problems may arise.

Principles of management Having excluded a history of trauma, the ankle and subtalar joints should be assessed for motor power, range of motion and specific pain points, which are sought in an attempt to locate the pain over specific anatomical structures, such as the lateral ligaments, sinus tarsi, trochlear surface of the talus and posterior talar process.

Acute pain will be managed as in the case of any joint. Ankle splints can be made or below-knee casts applied. The dorsal (top) part of the cast over the foot and leg can be removed as a night splint. Forced rest and elevation are essential in the early stages to allow repair, assisted by NSAIDs, ice therapy (Fig. 7.27) and the use of crutches. Radiographs may fail to show any early changes and will have to be repeated after 2–6 weeks.

Posterior ankle pain Pain arising behind the ankle is often associated with repetitive plantarflexion of the ankle in soccer or ballet. The posterior process of the talus and the overlying synovial capsule of the ankle become impinged between the posterior lip of the tibia and the calcaneus. The condition occurs more commonly when there is an enlarged posterior or Steida process present, or when the accessory ossicle os trigonum is present. Pain can be elicited by forced plantarflexion of the foot and sometimes by firm palpation of the area. Inversion/eversion of the subtalar joint and dorsiflexion of the ankle prove asymptomatic. Plain radiograph is essential to rule out fracture of the posterior process or separation of the os trigonum from the main body of the talus. Rest and corticosteroid injection into the posterior capsule of the ankle prove to be effective.

Anterior ankle pain Painful limitation of dorsiflexion of the ankle may result from an exostosis on the dorsal neck of the talus. This will impinge on the anterior aspect of the tibia and will present clinically as a painful stiff ankle. The dorsiflexion range of the ankle should be examined with the knee flexed to reduce any soft tissue restriction caused by a tight Achilles tendon/gastrocnemius soleus muscle. Movement will be limited and the range of motion will come to an abrupt bony end. Lateral weight-bearing views of the ankle and a stress view with the ankle dorsiflexed will confirm the presence of a bony block, which can be removed arthroscopically. Tenderness along the plafond of the talus may indicate degenerative pathology, cartilage defects and synovitis. Unilateral, non-pitting oedema is suggestive of any chronic degenerative change, unless an acute injury or disease process can be excluded. Treatment for each of these conditions will depend upon the extent of symptoms and the patient's age, mobility and occupation. The most severe, disabling pain requires subtalar arthrodesis. However, patients find ankle orthoses to be of value, especially where footwear enables higher ankle-conforming orthoses to limit hindfoot motion. The heel seat should have a 0° or flat post, or it should be manufactured to have a flat heel seat. Both modifications will limit subtalar joint movement. The use of ankle splints or braces, along the lines of the inflatable Aircast (Fig. 4.12), offers a useful off-the-shelf semi-immobilization system for the ankle and subtalar joints.

Lateral ankle sprains Ankle sprains are not exclusive to sports persons, but the principles are similar. The principle approach is rest, elevation, ice, analgesia, support, gentle rehabilitation and restoration of activity. Because subtalar damage can arise, patients should be followed carefully for 3 months to ensure that radiographs can be repeated and CT imaging should be used early. Chapter 16 covers recovery from ankle injury in greater detail.

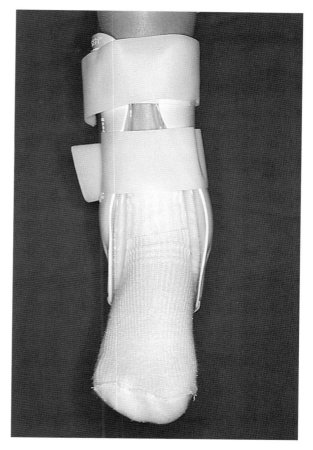

Figure 14.12 Aircast ankle brace can be fitted around the ankle using easy to adjust Velcro straps. The sides can be inflated to improve the fit.

FRACTURES

Stress fractures associated with the foot will most commonly affect the metatarsals (Ch. 16). The patient will present with pain following a history of direct injury or a recent episode of vigorous athletic activity. March fractures were so named because of the high incidence of fractures in military recruits, forced to march while undergoing basic training.

Fractures that extend through the epiphyses are particularly significant because they will disrupt bone growth and, in a long bone, cause premature fusion through closure of one side of the growth plate. As in Case study 14.2, joints may become extensively involved and require fusion.

Conservative management

The principal method of managing any fracture is to limit movement; this will in turn reduce pain and swelling. Stress fractures do not present with any marked deformity, so reduction of the fracture is not necessary. Movement should be reduced initially by using crutches or a stiff walking shoe, and simple analgesics should be used for pain.

Direct application of felt dressings and taping is valuable for central metatarsals. Toes can be taped together but must not be bound tightly, to avoid restricting circulatory flow. This treatment should be continued for 3–6 weeks with a review at that point if progress is satisfactory. A below-knee walking cast or foot cast (below-ankle) should be applied where pain is unremitting, where other soft splinting techniques fail or where analgesia is ineffective. The patient should be counselled to avoid excessive movement and to rest the foot for up to 6 weeks. Bone growth stimulators have been popular in some centres, using a form of piezoelectric field to attract osteogenic activity within the hydroxyapatite salts.

Retention of movement is important for healthy repair of bone but, in rare and unfortunate cases where patients are restricted by long periods of rest, a deep venous thrombosis or reflex sympathetic dystrophy syndrome can arise, both with disastrous effects.

Surgical management

Fortunately, surgery is rarely necessary in stress fractures. Toes may be better pinned with Kirschner wires as a closed technique under fluoroscopy. The Jones fracture associated with the base of the fifth metatarsal is the exception to the rule. Because of the poor blood supply, this fracture may take many months to settle and will cause pain and swelling. Avulsion fracture of the fifth metatarsal must be excluded and not confused with a Jones fracture, which is usually more distally sited. Physiotherapy exercise and manipulation are not indicated and can make the condition worse. A screw to compress the site of the fracture by open reduction provides the most expedient method for young active patients. Casts may assist in the older patient but can cause an element of demineralization.

Displacement and fragmentation should be managed by open reduction, especially where anatomical structures such as nerve pathways and blood vessels are damaged. Joints should be decompressed and deformity corrected as soon as possible. The presence of infection may complicate management, and external fixators may be applied. Bone grafts may also be necessary to replace lost bone, either at the time of injury or as a secondary phase of management.

NEOPLASIA OF BONE

Few bone tumours resolve without surgical intervention. Conservative management relies on monitoring the progress of any swelling and diagnosing the tissue type through radiographs, bone scans and MRI. Aspiration of tumours is generally considered unwise.

Two main considerations must be observed when dealing with tumours after diagnosis has been made. First, the whole lesion should ideally be excised. Second, because removal of bone will leave a weakened structure, surgical planning must include the possibility of bone graft requirements. In bones affected by malignant disease, prosthetic implants are commonly used together with adjuvant chemotherapy.

Treatment must be managed by multidisciplinary cooperation. The principles of management include the following approaches:

- accurate diagnosis
- surgical planning
- surgical biopsy to plan further management/diagnosis
- complete excision
- replacement prosthesis/bone graft/skin grafting
- chemotherapy/radiotherapy
- postoperative prosthesis
- bespoke footwear after resection surgery.

Subungual exostoses

Subungual exostoses cause pain under the nail and, in more severe forms, footwear-fitting difficulties (see Fig. 6.8). Surgical excision provides the most acceptable long-term solution. In order to expose the exostosis, it is usually necessary to remove the nail plate. The tissues overlying the exostosis will be thin, dystrophic, and difficult to reflect. Moreover, once the underlying exostosis has been removed, these tissues are often difficult to close because they are so friable. The area is also somewhat prone to infection because of the presence of a variety of bacterial and fungal elements under the nail. Once a toenail has been removed, it is likely that it will regrow somewhat thickened because of damage to the nail matrix that occurs on avulsion of the nail.

An apical approach has been developed in order to avoid nail removal. This is useful for smaller exostoses, but the technique may lead to temporary skin necrosis at this site. Subungual exostosis excision may cause considerable post-operative pain and tenderness, and a combination of NSAIDs and paracetamol/codeine compounds is advised.

DEFORMITY

The most common deformities seen in the fore-foot are conditions associated with hallux valgus and hammer toes. The most common whole-foot deformity is pes planus; this condition has similarities with pes cavus in that it may be mild, moderate or severe. Classification of digital deformity has been considered in greater detail elsewhere (Merriman & Turner, 2002).

LESSER TOES

Conservative care

Footwear should be evaluated to establish adequate fit and design. Patients are more likely to follow advice if they understand the reason for the problem, realize the limited approaches to treatment and appreciate the long-term effects of unsuitable footwear. This part of management may not be easy if the patient only wishes to have palliative care. Shoe adaptations, as previously mentioned, seldom appeal to patients. Skin and nail management can be provided on a repetitive level and are preferable for elderly patients or patients where surgery would be inappropriate.

Toe deformities respond well to surgery and this form of treatment should certainly be considered, the alternative for many patients being years of palliative care.

Surgical management

A fixed toe deformity can exist at the IPJ or at both the IPJ and the MTPJ. The goal of digital surgery is to return the proximal phalanx to a neutral position (i.e. neither dorsiflexed nor plantarflexed) relative to the metatarsal head. Once this has been achieved, equilibrium will be restored to the digital muscles while simultaneously neutralizing the deforming forces. If the proximal phalanx is left dorsiflexed, the flexor muscles will be kept under tension and the distal and intermediate phalanges will be pulled into plantarflexion. As the intermediate phalanx plantarflexes, a retrograde force will be exerted on the proximal phalanx, forcing it into further dorsiflexion. When the proximal phalanx is in neutral, however, the flexor and extensor muscles are in equilibrium and the digit remains straight.

Hammer toe The single toe with a fixed sagittal plane deformity can be corrected by excising the head of the proximal phalanx. This will relax the passive stretch on the flexor muscles caused by the dorsiflexed position of the proximal phalanx and will also reduce the bony prominence causing corn formation. In younger patients, where there is a chance of long-term recurrence, flexor tendon transfer and arthrodesis of the proximal IPJ may be considered. This procedure will ensure that the flexor tendons, which are transferred into the extensor apparatus, actively contribute to holding the proximal phalanx in a neutral position. Furthermore, a good position of the digit should be retained relative to the relevant metatarsal head and other toes. While most digital surgery will heal within 2 weeks, swelling can sometimes persist for many months.

Retracted toe A toe deformed at more than the IPJ will need to be managed in stages. The toe deformity is corrected by eliminating each deforming factor. The IPJ is dealt with first, then the tendon, then the capsule of the MTPJ and, finally, the flexor surface of the metatarsal. Even using all these stages, the deformity may not be eradicated if the metatarsal is badly plantar-flexed. Metatarsal surgery is then required.

Mallet toes The excisional arthroplasty is also popular for single toe deformities. Excision of the head of the intermediate phalanx is performed through a double ellipse. Insufficient removal of bone may result in only partial correction. Sometimes it is necessary to remove the entire intermediate phalanx. The wound is closed using the double ellipse to draw the distal toe into extension.

Multiple toe deformities The second, third and fourth digits should be arthrodesed simultaneously. Correction of an isolated deformity, where more than one toe problem exists, can be a mistake. This is because the altered vector of forces pulling equally from the shared extensor tendons causes inequality if only a single tendon is transected; furthermore, isolated toe surgery will leave asymmetrical shortening, or uncorrected adjacent digits will continue to underride and deform the remodelled toe. Abnormal digital parabola caused by surgery can lead to buckling of long toes, which will necessitate further surgery. Excessive shortening of single digits may cause plantar metatarsalgia.

Dislocation at the MTPJ Deformity of a toe that has an associated dislocation should be easy to diagnose. The range of motion is unrestricted and the toe sits in an abnormal position above or, less commonly, below other adjacent toes. A second toe deforms either as a result of injury or, alternatively, as a result of pressure from an adjacent hallux valgus pushing the digit dorsally and laterally. Disease processes such as rheumatoid arthritis and psoriatic arthritis can cause multiple digital disturbance at the MTP or IP joints. If a congenitally retracted fifth digit sits too high, rubbing against the shoe can arise. Options available include amputation (see Fig. 7.19), arthrodesis or soft tissue correction. The choice of treatment is influenced by age, occupation, adjacent toe position and likely success.

Amputation This may be considered in a patient who has toe pain associated with shoe-fitting difficulties. An adjacent hallux valgus deformity that is asymptomatic in an older patient may be left uncorrected, instead carrying out a whole or partial toe amputation. The decision must, however, depend upon the patient's preference. If the patient fears losing a toe, then the hallux must be corrected and the second toe brought into alignment with the other toes by arthrodesis. In this case, a pin (Kirschner wire) is passed through the MTPJ and antegraded (or

moved forward) 3 weeks later to avert a stiff toe. An alternative procedure may preserve the toe by excising the base of the proximal phalanx. Care must be taken not to remove too much of the base, and the capsule must be correctly repaired. Failure in either of these methods will lead to a floppy and unsightly toe that is very much foreshortened between the hallux and second digits.

Adductovarus of the fifth toe The fifth toe may adopt various positions of deformity. Adductovarus rotation and overriding (clinodactyly) can be corrected together using a V–Y plasty incision (see Fig. 6.19A), with or without an arthroplasty to the IPJ. The tendon is initially transected to see how much the toe will drop into alignment with the other toes. The capsule is incised (capsulotomy), which again removes tension from a retracted deformity. As a rule, fifth toes are never arthrodesed because they will cause pressure between the skin and the shoe owing to their rigidity. Incisions made around the MTPJ are very important, as lengthening of the contracted skin is required by V or Z incison. In resistant cases, an ellipse of tissue may be removed from the plantar aspect of the toe in the area of the proximal skin crease; this will resist further recurrence.

HALLUX DEFORMITY

Hallux valgus

The deformity of hallux valgus includes a large medial eminence, broadening of the forefoot and dislocation and rotation of the great toe. The condition is often complicated by lesser toe deformity, arthritic changes, splay forefoot or metatarsus adductus. Unfortunately, once developed, little conservative care can be offered; the main choices of care are accommodation and surgical correction.

Conservative management

Bunion The medial eminence frequently produces a bursa overlying fibrous cartilage and bone. The medial eminence is, in fact, the medial metatarsal head made prominent by subluxation of the first MTPJ. *Footwear* may be adapted with balloon patches or a bespoke shoe can be made to accommodate the broad foot. The accommodation of the additional width of the foot is important to limit tissue breakdown and sinus tract formation. A case for prescription footwear is greatest for those high-risk patients suffering from vascular ischaemia, neuropathy or gross arthritic degeneration.

Aspiration   Enlarged bursae are fluctuant sacs that can become infected. Aspiration can be performed using up to 0.5 ml of plain anaesthetic, 0.5–1% xylocaine, and drawing off fluid with a 19G needle and a syringe (20–60 ml) using an aseptic technique. The pressure required is considerable and the fluid should not be allowed to return. The colour of the aspirate can be checked for blood, pus and crystals. In chronic cases, bursae contents are viscous and gelatinous, have a translucent colour and are flecked with blood. If the aspirate is too viscous, it may be difficult to draw off. The effect of aspiration may only last for 6 weeks. The bursa that is too thick for a needle to enter it may prove impossible to aspirate and will need to be resolved by surgery (see Fig. 14.7).

Sinus tracts   At one time it was fashionable to apply phenol or silver nitrate to destroy the organized bursa. However, this is ill-advised because it may lead to tissue breakdown or increased sensitivity. Drainage should be established and swabbed for infection.

Orthoses   The aim of orthotic treatment in hallux valgus must be to:

- prevent further progression of the deformity
- prevent the development of secondary problems, such as lesser digit deformity and related nail and skin pathology
- alleviate pain within the first MTPJ or metatarsalgia of the lesser MTPJs.

A bunion shield can be made from latex dip casts, Plastazote moulded around the enlarged joint or replaceable foam ovals (Fig. 14.13). Protective adhesive dressings offer local protection from potential ulceration but are limited to short-term use only (Ch. 11). Animal wool dress-

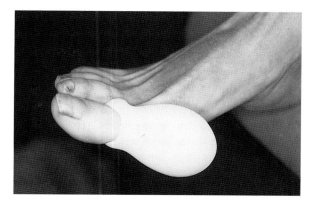

Figure 14.13   Foam to protect a bunion from pressure: available as a stock item.

ings are useful for chilled skin but should not be wrapped around the toe, in order to avoid constriction. The wool nests use fibres running longitudinally. If care is not taken and the wool is haphazardly wrapped 'around' the toes, the fibres will contract when wet, endangering tissue viability.

Hallux deviation   Attempts to wedge material between the hallux and adjacent second toe may alleviate interdigital corns. Prevention of further deviation is limited because the second toe is easily pushed over by the bulky insert. Moreover, the work of Hardy & Clapham (1951) indicated that when the hallux abuts the second toe it forms a retrograde force at the MTPJ, which pushes the first metatarsal into further varus.

In a study of 25 Argentinian children, Groiso (1992) found that hallux valgus night splints could hold the metatarsus primus varus static while correcting the hallux valgus by, on average, 3°. The night splints were used for an average period of 2 years and the hallux valgus showed no sign of further deterioration after 3 years of follow-up. The night splint should, therefore, be expected at least to prevent further deterioration of hallux valgus in the child. It is, however, a treatment that requires considerable patient commitment, because if the device is not worn every night results cannot be guaranteed.

While Groiso's work (1992) on juvenile hallux valgus shows promise, little evidence is available to support the use of night splints in adults, or indeed in advanced hallux valgus. It should, however, be considered as a possible conservative treatment option. The success of night splints can be monitored every 6–12 months with a digital goniometer or weight-bearing dorsoplantar radiographs, which will show the alignment of the first MTPJ.

While casted orthoses have often been recommended for hallux valgus to limit excessive pronation of the foot, longitudinal studies have shown that functional orthoses will not prevent the progression of the deformity in children (Kilmartin et al 1994).

Antipronation orthoses may, however, be used to reduce the first MTPJ pain associated with loss of joint congruity. One reason for this effect is that orthoses have been shown to restrict first MTPJ movement; this relative immobilization reduces irritation within the joint (Kilmartin et al 1991). It is important that the patient is advised that the functional orthosis will not prevent progression of hallux valgus and night splints should, therefore, be used in conjunction with orthoses.

Surgical management

Where night splints have failed to prevent progression of the deformity, or orthoses have failed to relieve joint pain, surgery should be considered as the next appropriate option.

Another important criterion for surgical intervention is the stage when the hallux begins to abut the second toe. At this point, the deformity is likely to progress rapidly (Hardy & Clapham 1951). The condition is no longer just affecting the first MTPJ but is also beginning to deform the lesser digits as well.

Over 150 operations have been described for hallux valgus, but many are simply modifications of original ideas. Essentially, seven approaches exist (Table 14.1), a number of which have been illustrated in Chapter 7.

Hallux valgus surgery must deal with the following components of the condition:

- the first–second intermetatarsal angle
- the sesamoid position

Table 14.1 Approaches to surgical management of hallux valgus

Technique	Example of procedure
Soft tissue	McBride
Excisional arthroplasty	Keller
Exostectomy	Silver
Capital osteotomy	Austin
Phalangeal osteotomy	Akin
Arthrodesis	Various
Proximal osteotomy	Trethowan

- the hallux position in both the transverse and frontal planes.

Failure to achieve long-term correction of the deformity may result from inadequate correction of any one of these components.

Bunion The medial eminence, or bunion, was thought by Haines & McDougall (1954) to be a traction apophysitis caused by movement of the medial sesamoid, and consequently traction on the medial sesamoid ligament's insertion in the metatarsal head. The medial eminence can be safely reduced provided that good capsular repair is achieved. No more than the enlarged fibrocartilaginous bone should be removed, to prevent narrowing of the articular surface ('staking') and the creation of a hallux varus (adductus) (Fig. 14.14). Bursae can be removed at the same time and redundant tissue plicated at both capsular and skin levels. This procedure does not, however, correct the position of the hallux, sesamoids or first–second intermetatarsal angle.

Mild hallux valgus Capital osteotomies are valuable where the toe has not created any pressure against the second digit but the toe (hallux valgus angle) is deviated by greater than 15°. The type of osteotomy selected will depend upon whether the joint needs to be decompressed. In achieving decompression, first metatarsal shortening may arise. Wherever possible, therefore, the first metatarsal length should always be retained relative to the second metatarsal. The act of shortening a metatarsal will slacken tight tissues to assist hallux correction, but the transfer

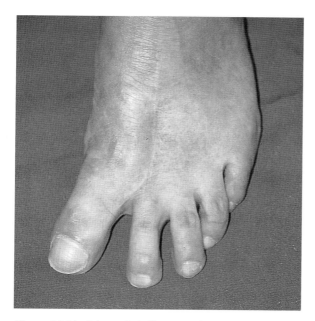

Figure 14.14 Iatrogenic hallux varus from overcorrection of hallux valgus. The metatarsals were splinted together with an internal wire.

of load to a second or third metatarsal is undesirable. Elevatory osteotomies must be used with caution, whether using a capital or proximally placed osteotomy. A number of factors should, therefore, be considered in deciding the appropriate capital osteotomy:

- articular set angle (see Fig. 7.10)
- intermetatarsal angle between the first and second metatarsals is around 10–13°
- soft tissue contracture
- extent of dorsiflexed position.

Severe hallux valgus   Where the characteristic angles that are associated with a large hallux and intermetatarsal position arise, the general approach is to select a proximal osteotomy. Faults lying at the first metatarsocuneiform joint may even require an arthrodesis. In some cases, a capital osteotomy may have to be used to correct the proximal articular set angle at the same time. The association of distal articular set angles within the phalanges may require an osteotomy within the phalanx but should never be used alone to correct this deformity, to avoid failure. The concept of joint congruency is an important

diagnostic feature that must be corrected within the surgical procedure.

Hallux abductovalgus   The presence of a single transverse plane deformity is less complicated to manage than a deformity that has a rotatory twist. Rotation arises when the joint attempts to define a new axis and, consequently, soft tissues shorten. The frontal plane rotation is best corrected by performing a closing wedge osteotomy or Akins operation on the hallux. Double osteotomies may have to be used, and where there is degeneration, a Keller's excisional arthroplasty can be used with a capital osteotomy.

Degenerative hallux valgus   As with hallux rigidus, the options may vary depending upon patient requirements: arthrodesis will correct a moderate angle; Keller's excisional arthroplasty will shorten the hallux and reduce the retrograde force that drives the first metatarsal into varus. A replacement joint cannot be used unless the intermetatarsal angle is small, as too much stress will be placed on the implant.

Postoperative care

Early ambulation is the goal of all foot surgery. First, this lowers the risk of deep venous thrombosis, and, second, weight bearing will stimulate osteogenesis around an osteotomy site. Early joint motion reduces stiffness as it divides adhesions associated with postoperative haematoma formation. However, swelling arises from too much motion in the early postoperative stages. Patients should be asked to rest with their foot elevated as much as possible during the first 2 weeks postoperatively, to allow for normal wound healing.

In older patients with impaired venous return, postoperative swelling can be very long standing. Less-complicated surgery is suggested in order to minimize tissue dissection and to avoid problems associated with bony union failure where poor mineralization is present.

Trigger hallux

The trigger hallux, or retracted great toe, is associated with pes cavus, where plantarflexion of the first metatarsal arises with tightening of the extensor hallucis longus tendon. The patient may complain of footwear irritation on the dorsal aspect of the IPJ and sesamoiditis associated with the plantarflexed position of the first metatarsal. Treatment can, however, be provided to manage the trigger toe in isolation in some cases.

Conservative management

In the early stages of deformity, an insole with a shaft pad extended under the first metatarsal can be used. This is made from a firm foam material such as polyurethane or neoprene rubber. The objective is to dorsiflex and extend the first MTPJ, lessening the dorsal contraction of the capsule and extensor tendons. Conservative management is in most cases aimed at preventing soft tissue damage from footwear over the IPJ and cushioning the plantar surface of the first metatarsal head and sesamoids. Silicone or Otoform putty can be moulded to redirect pressure from the IPJ. Silopos digital sleeves and Cica care gel (Smith & Nephew) can also be used.

As the deformity progresses, the shoe toe box will need to be deepened to accommodate the deformed toe. More substantial plantar cushioning will also be required. A flat 6 mm Spenco insole is most suitable if it can be accommodated within the shoe. However, difficulties do arise when added plantar cushioning fills the shoe and causes further dorsal irritation.

Surgical management

Arthrodesis of the IPJ with a single screw or two wires (sited percutaneously) will prevent the toe from flexing. The joint must be in good condition. The extensor tendon is transferred through a hole made in the metatarsal head in order to elevate the ray. This procedure should not be used in the presence of the following three factors:

- if the metatarsal is rigid in plantarflexion, the tendon cannot be relied upon to provide normal hallux ground purchase
- if the forefoot is everted badly, as in the case of pes cavus, multiple surgery may be needed, affecting the other metatarsals or tarsus

- poorly mineralized bone and marked joint degeneration are unlikely to form a satisfactory union; here, an excisional arthroplasty can be performed as a salvage procedure in the event of deep ulceration.

Hallux varus

Hallux varus is associated with metatarsus adductus in the younger patient but also commonly arises from overcorrection of the hallux valgus deformity or by staking the head during overzealous bone resection (Fig. 14.14). Abductor hallucis release, and division and resection of the lateral capsule, may be used; alternatively a reverse closing wedge osteotomy of the proximal phalanx may be performed.

FOREFOOT DEFORMITY

Metatarsus adductus is rarely noted in adult feet, compared with children. This may be a consequence of spontaneous improvement or secondary compensations; both concepts are discussed further in Chapter 15. In the adult, significant forefoot deformities include splay foot and plantarflexed metatarsals.

Splay foot

In the normal foot, the angle between the first and second metatarsal is between 7 and 9° (Kilmartin et al 1991). The angle between the fourth and fifth metatarsals is between 4 and 5°. A pathological increase in the angles between the first and second, and fourth and fifth, metatarsals is known as splay foot and manifests clinically as a widened forefoot with hallux valgus and Tailor's bunion.

Conservative management

Footwear fitting is the primary problem in splay foot. Soft wide shoes or trainers are most appropriate, although bespoke footwear is worthy of consideration. Another primary complaint is irritation of the dorsomedial aspect of the first MTPJ and lateral aspect of the fifth. Latex rubber and foam shields may be used to palliate this complaint (see Fig. 14.13).

Surgical management

The objective of management is to reduce the width of the foot. Osteotomies that reposition the distal end of the first and fifth metatarsals toward the midline of the foot are indicated. Whether such osteotomies are performed at the proximal or the distal end of the metatarsal is determined by the degree of deformity. Higher intermetatarsal angles (i.e. greater than 16° between the first and second metatarsals, or greater than 10° between the fourth and fifth metatarsals) require proximal metatarsal osteotomy.

Metatarsal plantarflexion

Normally, load should be distributed evenly across the lesser metatarsal heads. When load becomes focused on one metatarsal head, tenderness, callus or even bursae arise.

Unequal load distribution may cause plantarflexion of a single metatarsal. Shortening of a single metatarsal or dorsal displacement of a metatarsal will also cause overloading of an adjacent normal metatarsal. This situation is particularly common in hallux valgus, where the first metatarsal, which has an independent axis of motion, is dorsiflexed by the force of ground reaction, leading to overloading of the adjacent second metatarsal.

In the cavoid foot, overpull of peroneus longus will plantarflex the first metatarsal and significantly increase loading of the metatarsal head. Painful callus of the fifth metatarsal head is also commonly seen in pes cavus. This is caused by the tendency for rapid supination of the foot after forefoot loading, when the plantarflexed first metatarsal makes ground contact first. Forefoot load then rapidly moves laterally. This is, of course, the reverse of the normal situation where the lateral border of the foot and the fifth metatarsal usually make ground contact first.

Conservative management

Metatarsalgia from plantar pain should initially be managed with shock-attenuating orthoses. Alternatively, depressed metatarsals may be accommodated inside the shoe with an insole. A cut-out using a cavity or build-up around the metatarsal will achieve the same effect. The load placed over the metatarsal will be distributed across the remaining metatarsals. Symptomatic relief is very successful and will depend on good shoe design to accommodate the extra material. Plastazote material makes a useful temporary substitute for loss of adipose tissue, as well as forming a natural depression. For long-term use, this is not appropriate. The best result often comes from trial and error (Pratt et al 1993).

More complex prescriptions can be considered with off-the-shelf orthoses such as AOLs, Alphathotics and MBS (Multi Balance System), which are mentioned in more detail in Chapter 12, or by taking a neutral cast to balance the effect of the metatarsals. Contemporary philisophy emphasizes the need to control the hindfoot to influence the forefoot about the midtarsal joint. The converse philosophy may be true as well.

Forefoot varus In the case of forefoot varus, a medial forefoot wedge will prevent the hindfoot from compensating by leaning in medially. The medial long arch is improved by placing a rearfoot wedge or post on the orthosis so that both wedges act to create a reactionary force during forefoot loading (Tollafield & Pratt 1990). Talar and cuneiform alignment are improved while the orthotic is worn. This type of orthotic modification will reduce the strain created in the tibialis posterior and anterior tendons by actively supinating the hindfoot about the midtarsal joint to counter pronation. The use of posting above the deformity value will have deleterious effects on the first ray. Tollafield & Pratt (1990) found that two-thirds of the deformity could be accommodated without elevating the first metatarsal excessively.

Rearfoot posting often commences with a 4° post. Footwear fit and patient tolerance often dictate alterations necessary. The MBS off-the-shelf system (Langer Biomechanics Group) provides an interchangeable posted orthosis without the need for glue or heat guns. This aptly named (Multi Balance System) product allows practitioners to move between 2 and 4° posts by using a press-stud fit, for both varus and valgus wedges (Fig. 14.15).

Forefoot valgus   This deformity arises when all the metatarsals are everted in the same plane. A high-arch foot may be apparent, but the typical plantarflexed first and fifth metatarsals seen in pes cavus are not present. A lateral wedge or post is provided on the orthosis to prevent the foot supinating around its midtarsal and subtalar joint axes. Unfortunately, if toes are already retracted on the lateral side of the foot, they can easily rub against the shoe upper, making tolerance less practical. An intrinsically posted orthosis may fare better.

First ray involvement   The first ray may be dorsiflexed (metatarsus primus elevatus). Metatarsus primus elevatus is quite common and has already been described as part of the

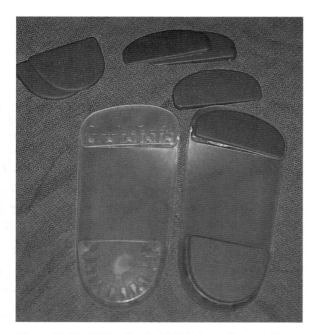

Figure 14.15   MBS orthosis (Multi Balance System). The wedging (posting system) clips on, making this easy to adjust and dispense. (Courtesy of Langer Biomechanics Group UK Ltd.)

contributing aetiology in hallux rigidus and hallux limitus. The first ray may be plantarflexed in three different positions (plantarflexed first ray, PFFR): rigid, semi-rigid or flexible. Each has a slightly different management when prescribing orthoses:

- *Flexible.* The first ray is cast out as much as possible by pushing the first metatarsal dorsally while the negative cast is being taken. Pain at the first MTPJ associated with use of the orthosis may indicate that the first metatarsal has been dorsiflexed too much and that the joint has begun to jam because the hallux can no longer rotate around the metatarsal head.
- *Semi-rigid.* The first ray should be dorsiflexed to reduce any marked plantarflexion in the cast. An extrinsic or intrinsic forefoot post is used along the lateral anterior edge. The aim is to limit compensation through the long axis of the midtarsal joint and subtalar joint, and to prevent abnormal dorsiflexion of the first ray.
- *Rigid.* The first ray is casted as it is assessed in a plantarflexed position. A cut-out in the orthosis can be used at the anterior–medial first ray edge and a bar can be used from the second to the fifth metatarsal to bring the forefoot surface to a level position. Alternatively, a lateral anterior wedge (full or tip post) is prescribed on a firm casted orthosis. Another variation involves the use of softer orthoses with a depression to allow the first ray to find its own level.

Many of these orthotic concepts were developed by Root and his coworkers in the USA during the 1960s. Experienced practitioners find that they prefer their own variations and frequently develop new concepts in casting and orthotic prescription on the basis of experience.

Surgical management

Plantarflexed metatarsals can cause significant pain from bruising, bursae, sesamoiditis, nerve entrapment or keratomata. Osteotomy or excision of the metatarsal head has a part to play in relieving symptoms. There are a number of operations for managing this problem; essentially, the principle involves elevating the metatarsal. This can be done at the base or head of the metatarsal by an osteotomy. The incidence of pain following operations for metatarsal elevation is high and is commonly associated with non-union of bone and with skin transfer lesions (Grace 1993). Where the deformity is rigid, the plantar pressure is greater. In the presence of microangiopathy or neuropathy, ulceration can arise. The views held by foot surgeons vary, but many believe that all three central metatarsals should be operated on simultaneously, as they tend to act mechanically as one unit. This might be less true for an obvious isolated plantarflexed metatarsal.

Rheumatoid patients have the additional problems of forefoot ulcers and large bursae with nodules on the plantar surface. The multiple excision metatarsal was originally described in 1912 by Hoffman. The approach to removing the metatarsal heads may utilize the plantar surface or the dorsum. The plantar approach allows repositioning of the distal fat pad proximally and allows easier removal of the metatarsal head. This type of surgery has had good results according to Grace (1993).

Removal of the metatarsal heads is, however, a very drastic operation with immense implications for forefoot mechanics. Excision tends to be used for sedentary patients, those with extreme forefoot pain and those with digital deformities resistant to other forms of surgery. Where some digital function can be retained, excision is less appropriate.

A lesser metatarsal osteotomy through the cartilaginous head may appear to be inappropriately placed but has been recorded as being highly effective for a wide range of patient groups, including those with rheumatoid deformity. The metatarsal head is elevated by the thickness of the power saw blade. The metatarsal can be shortened and displaced transversely. This type of osteotomy has become very popular with podiatrists and orthopaedic surgeons in France because it is more predictable; non-union is unrecorded and the movement is controlled. The success also lies in the fact that, unlike many elevatory lesser metatarsal osteotomies, this type of procedure is fixed with a wire or screw (Fig. 14.16). When

used for plantar corns, many of the common complications associated with osteotomy do not appear to arise (Barouk 1994).

HINDFOOT DEFORMITY

Serious deformity is rare, but when it does present, as in the case of congenital talipes equinovarus (CTEV), treatment is highly specialized. The adult foot is less amenable to correction because of completed growth and serious contracture. Specialized footwear plays a very large part in accommodating problems. Plantar pressure points can be reduced by orthoses.

Haglund or retrocalcaneal bump

A prominent calcaneal bone may cause significant problems at the posterior dorsolateral edge of the heel. Radiographically, the picture is unclear unless the lateral contour is affected, causing a spur to form (not to be confused with the plantar spur).

Conservative management

The heel bump can be protected by felt and foam dressings in the early stages of the problem. Gel

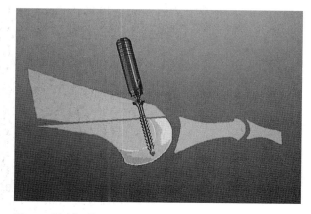

Figure 14.16 Osteotomy associated with Barouk/Weil. Because internal fixation (screw in situ) is used, failed bone union has not been reported in the literature at present. The osteotomy allows decompression of the lesser metatarsophalangeal joints and lateral displacement if required. This technique has distinct advantages over freely displaced osteotomies.

pads such as Silopos of Cica Care (Smith and Nephew) will protect the skin overlying the bone.

The heel counter should be soft, but during flare-ups patients should use open-heeled shoes. High heels should be avoided, especially those with a deep heel counter, which have the effect of cutting into the skin. Soft heel lifts placed in the shoe will elevate the calcaneus above the heel counter. Socks should always be worn to minimize direct pressure and friction against the skin. High ankle training shoes will also help to redirect pressure from the posterior lateral corner of the calcaneus.

The rearfoot condition is often associated with a rigid plantarflexed first ray or partially compensated rearfoot varus. The movement created by these foot problems is thought to act in causing shearing stresses over the skin and periosteum as the heel moves from inversion through to eversion. An orthosis that uses a rearfoot varus wedged post can limit this movement and provides an acceptable treatment regimen. Posted orthotic therapy is often started at a varus cant of 4°. The heel cup should fit the shoe and, if prescribed, should be moderately deep (15–18 mm).

Surgical management

Heel bump surgery should not be entered into lightly. Recurrence, sensitive scarring, damage to the sural nerve, weakening/rupture of the Achilles tendon and prolonged swelling are all possible complications (Fig. 14.17). The procedure may only require the bone to be levelled; unfortunately, because of the bone contour and the poor preoperative value of radiographs, the surgeon can easily continue to resect bone until the area around the calcaneus has been weakened. This can lead to Achilles tendon rupture. Because surgery is often performed close to the tendinous insertion of the Achilles tendon, pain related to movement is not uncommon afterwards. A below-knee cast is required for 6–8 weeks.

Retrocalcaneal exostectomy may require a period of rehabilitation of up to 3–6 months. The position of the incision line is very critical for

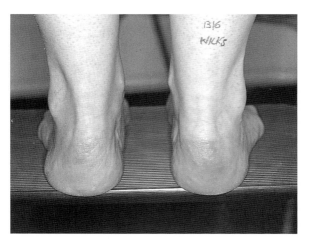

Figure 14.17 Sensitive scar lines affecting both heels following transverse incision. Both scar lines are flat and soft, but the hyperaesthesia leaves the patient with few solutions other than soft shoe counters and heel pads. Incisions placed lateral to the heel may avoid this problem.

limiting nerve damage of the sural and calcaneal branches of the tibial nerve. An alternative procedure is used for dorsal spurs. A V-osteotomy is performed in the sagittal plane to move the proximal superior edge closer to the main body of the bone; this is known as the Keck and Kelly procedure.

DEFORMITIES ASSOCIATED WITH ARCH SHAPE

Pes planovalgus, pes cavus and congenital talipes equinovarus are rare and are helped considerably by footwear modifications and orthoses in adults. These deformities are often associated with hindfoot pathology but may be complicated by forefoot pathology. There is further discussion on this subject in Chapter 15.

Conservative management

Soft tissue problems arise because of hypermobility affecting a less-mobile structure or because the foot is rigid. The hindfoot may be structurally abnormal but it is often the midtarsus that takes the brunt of the pathology through compensation.

Pes planus The talus, navicular and medial cuneiform may all become involved with compensation (Fig. 14.18). The hindfoot should be stabilized early by varus posted casted orthoses. The medial side of the heel cup may be made high to limit the effects of the talus declining and adducting by influencing the sustentaculum tali. The cast should be marked appropriately so that the laboratory technician knows where to increase the heel cup effect.

A University of California orthosis (UCBL) should be considered for ultimate control for the flexible flat foot, providing that no neuromuscular disease is present (see Fig. 12.8). Proximal weakness is likely to require an ankle foot orthosis to stabilize the ankle and the subtalar joint. Supramalleolar orthoses occupy a position midway between ankle foot orthosis and foot orthoses (Fig. 14.19). Control is offered around the ankle, providing ultimate stability to a foot with postural strain. Assessment of the flat foot deformity may require simple forefoot and rearfoot posting to bring the ground up to the foot, as mentioned above with forefoot varus. The more significant modifications, such as UCBLs and supramalleolar orthoses will make acquisition of shoes more difficult, a point that should be discussed with the patient before casting.

Simple orthoses based on insoles, such as the Cobra design, have a place in flexible and rigid flat feet. A trial using compressed felt is worthwhile, or premoulded foamed orthoses such as Frelon, AOL, Alphathotics and MBS, to name but a few, can be selected as economical orthoses (Ch. 11). Stretching exercises should be used in all but the very contracted cases of ankle equinus to ensure that the patient does not lift out of the shoe.

Shoe stiffeners, heel cups and Thomas wedges designed to reduce pronation have found favour in the past. The practitioner will find that an orthotic prescription for inside the shoe is more economical and easier than adapting footwear.

Cavus type feet The conservative approach to problems associated with cavus foot types will

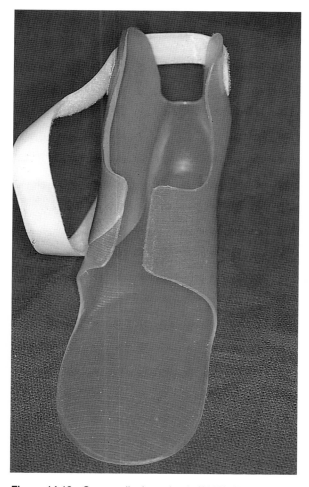

Figure 14.19 Supramalleolar orthosis (SMO). (Reproduced with permission from David Pratt, Derbyshire Royal Infirmary.)

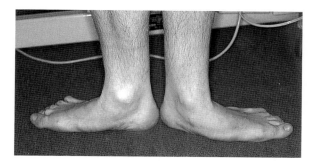

Figure 14.18 This male patient had six pairs of simple insoles, which failed to maintain foot comfort for his pes planus. Because the foot is flexible, UCBL (University of California Biomechanics Laboratory) or supramalleolar orthoses may be considered more appropriate.

depend upon the rigidity of the foot. Shock attenuation will relieve major pressure areas under the first/fifth metatarsal. Flexible cavus feet are treated similarly to those feet with forefoot valgus or plantarflexed first ray. In some feet, Haglund's deformity will have to be protected or operated on, depending upon the symptoms. Retracted digits are difficult to deal with, although some patients find plantar metatarsal pads incorporated into insoles to be of some value. Rigid and semi-rigid toe deformities can easily become forced into shoes if insoles are made too bulky. The secondary iatrogenic corns that develop are not an uncommon problem.

Rigid foot problems Conservative management has been considered for flexible feet. Rigid feet should be treated differently, in that no orthosis will correct an established deformity, and this is particularly the case if the deformity is not corrected in childhood. Shoes may have to be soft along the medial border and patients must be warned that early replacement is expected because of the marked pronatory forces. Heel wear will cause a problem; repair is easier in bespoke footwear than in off-the-shelf shoes because of the construction design. However, some UK manufacturers, such as Clarks, will replace the polyurethane soling unit. This is worthwhile where the uppers are still in good condition.

Soft foamed orthoses will protect skin and offer some relief from foot strain and will hopefully limit proximal stress problems in the leg and knee.

Surgical management

Mixed deformities affecting different parts of the foot may be better dealt with in stages. The reason for this is to allow one part to settle and return to adequate function before another part is dealt with. The best example of mixed deformity is club foot (CTEV), but problems such as pes valgus and pes cavus tend to be more common.

Club foot There is a tight Achilles tendon, which needs to be lengthened by a tendon lengthening procedure. Surgery on the other tendons is designed to restore equilibrium to the evertors and invertors of the foot as well as the dorsiflexors and plantarflexors. Surgery can be quite major in older established deformities or where they have recurred over time, but it is less problematic in a younger child where soft tissue that has contracted can be released before degeneration is reversible.

Pes valgus Surgery is only required if there is pain that cannot be controlled with conservative measures, and there is evidence of progressive deformity and joint degeneration. Again, a combination of tendon-balancing and osseous correction is indicated. With regard to osseous correction, an important component of pes valgus is abduction of the forefoot. This may be reduced by lengthening the lateral column of the foot by placing a bone graft in the lateral border of the calcaneus (see Fig. 7.11). The low medial longitudinal arch with subluxation of the talonavicular and naviculocuneiform joints can be corrected by taking a triangular wedge from the medial cuneiform, the apex of the triangle being placed dorsally. Closure of the wedge will plantarflex the forefoot and raise the medial longitudinal arch. If the forefoot is abnormally adducted and the tarsus is not severely affected, the metatarsals will be divided by closing wedge osteotomies. Where the flat foot deformity cannot be resolved with less radical surgery, correction by ankle arthrodesis may be required. This form of fusion immobilizes the ankle at one to three joints (see Fig. 7.8). Pain and disability often provide the main deciding factors for a procedure that is preferred as the last resort.

Pes cavus This is characterized by a high arch. Fascial release and calcaneal osteotomy may be used to lower the arch height (see Fig. 7.12). The tarsus is frequently 'humped', causing an excessive declination of the metatarsals, which cannot be managed without midtarsus osteotomy. Digital deformity may have to be managed by tendon balancing and osteotomies, as described under forefoot deformity.

Pes cavus and CTEV have similarities in that the foot is rigid and experiences pressure points. Treatment of these complex deformities is managed with a mixture of soft tissue and bone techniques. Details of these procedures fall outside the scope of this text.

CORNS AND CALLUS

The types of problem encountered at the skin and subcutaneous levels must be considered carefully as some overlap in management may be required, because the underlying deformity and deeper tissue pathology may be influenced by different forms of therapy. Callus is usually a response to mechanical pressure associated with shear and friction. Remove the physical irritation and the condition will reverse, leaving the skin soft and pliable again.

Underlying deformity, such as exostoses, should be protected with orthoses or removed by surgery. However, while not exclusive to the plantar metatarsal area and IPJ of toes, callus causes fewer symptoms elsewhere. Penetrating injuries associated with foreign bodies such as glass can cause an irritant effect on deep tissues, leading to thick scarring. Neuroma involvement and synovial cysts have been identified in patients with otherwise typical intractable plantar keratoma.

Conservative management

The use of debridement skills (see Ch. 6) is valuable in reducing the irritant effect of thicker layers of epidermis on sensitive nerve endings. Emollient products can be applied when the skin is thin enough to allow effective penetration. Areas of the foot experiencing localized pressure will develop characteristic concentric centres or corns (clavus). Enucleation will temporarily reduce pain sensation, particularly in younger patients. Recalcitrant lesions will manifest, creating subepidermal thickening, bursa formation and even sinus tracking over joints. The most painful form of corn is associated with fibrous infiltration around sweat glands and nerve endings, often involving blood vessels.

Continuous debridement may cause repetitive trauma and, over long periods, offers proportionally less relief and may require more frequent attention. Callus and corns overlying bone areas are, therefore, more obdurate to treat. Surgery of the underlying cause may be necessary. Nonetheless, non-osseous-related lesions (as cited in Case study 6.1) illustrate some of the problems that can be encountered when no direct irritant factor can be identified.

Orthotic management The use of distributive felt padded dressings with apertures and cavities has proved effective in reducing symptoms. A successful outcome might be measured by reducing the need for frequent debridement. Silicone orthodigital splints are valuable in that they are replaceable and easy to mould to toes. Other ready-made devices include digital Tubifoam and Silipos sleeves and a wide variety of insole bases to which felt may be added. The simple insole used for plantar redistribution invariably reduces symptoms but does not eradicate the build-up of callus completely.

Medication Injectable medication such as vitamin B_{12} (cyanocobalamin), sclerosing agents such as alcohol and even steroids have been used to break down the fibrous tissue with some success. Balkin (1972) advocated implants of fluid silicone injection under lesions. This has been shown both to reduce keratoses and to improve ulcers.

Local application of emollients under plastic occlusion in hard vehicles such as firm pastes has been recommended to hydrate lesions. *Keratolytics* such as salicylic acid preparations can be used in solution, collodion or paste. The availability of similar products in corn plasters causes much controversy. Patients often fail to apply these over-the-counter treatments with appropriate caution. Injudicious application can result in tissue breakdown and infection. Professional treatment is always advocated and Lang et al (1994) concluded that the length of treatment relied upon clinical judgement and patient tolerance. Keratolytics can provide a valuable approach to desquamation. The optimum period of application of corn plasters as 40% salicylic acid was studied over 3 weeks in 240 patients. Some adverse reactions were shown, even in controlled conditions (1.3%).

Maceration around the area of application increased with duration of application; only patients with healthy tissue should be selected.

Silver nitrate in varying strengths has been advocated to astringe (dry up and cause contraction) corns. Lack of scientific evidence and audit has meant that the long-term benefits of these products has not been proven, although pyrogallic acid (50%) does appear to be beneficial in reducing the size of lesions when applied and debrided over 4–8 weeks. The telltale brown stain should lead the practitioner to suspect that either silver nitrate or pyrogallol has been used previously.

A combination of topical medicament and redistributive insoles has been valuable. It would appear from empirical experience that success with all the above treatment strategies relies on early management before chronic subdermal tissue changes occur. Silicone sheeting and Silopos products have provided an alternative philosophy in the hydration of lesions. These products still have to be adhered to skin or applied as a replaceable appliance, which may affect the integrity of skin contact. Orthoses to correct underlying pronation should be considered as an adjunct to the above therapy rather than as a cure for the corn or callus; symptom improvement, however, has only been noted empirically.

Seed corns These small plugs of keratin form in the creases of the epidermal surface of the foot. Research has shown little proof of a different aetiology from those lesions found over weight-bearing surfaces. Emollient appli-cations temporarily improve skin elasticity. Orthoses that can improve pressure distribution serve as a useful adjunct to emollient application. E45 and urea preparations are popular, although any lubricant will provide similar properties. With the exception of excision, little has been written on the subject of surgery for this condition. Regular enucleation, while highly beneficial, still risks further damage to the local skin structure.

Surgical management

Surgical management of corns provides an attractive solution and falls into four categories: skin excision, correction of fixed deformity, elevation of metatarsal head and correction of forefoot/hindfoot alignment. Callus can be helped by the latter three surgical methods.

Skin excision Excision should only be considered where an underlying dermal problem such as bursa, inclusion cyst, fibroma or foreign body, has arisen (Case study 14.4 and Figs 14.20 and 14.21). Furthermore, the lesion should ideally be over a non-weight-loading area such as the metatarsal head area. Removal of such plantar lesions should be followed by a period of assisted weight bearing (e.g. with a cast) or non-weight bearing (with crutches). Early forefoot pressure will strain the incision site.

Correction of fixed deformity Digital deformity contributes considerably to skin lesions. If conservative treatment fails to relieve the problem within 6 months, surgical excision of the head of the phalanx will improve the lesion dramatically

---

Case study 14.4 Excision of a corn

A 63-year-old male presented with a corn under his right foot, which had previously been removed by his GP. The appearance (Fig. 14.20) showed the lesion to be a long-standing intractable plantar keratoma with a well-defined border but with minimal callosity beyond the periphery. The lesion measured 1.5 cm and was excised. A large cyst was identified underlying the hyperkeratosis (Fig. 14.21) and was reported by histopathology as having an epithelial lining of cuboidal cells. A blunt seeker shows a central punctum through the dermis. The depth was recorded as 1.5 cm taken from an ellipse measuring 3.5 cm × 0.8 cm. A small drain was inserted into the wound before closure and removed 2 days later.

Conclusion: The occurrence of intense pain, traumatic origin, length of duration of symptoms and lack of biomechanical abnormality may lead the practitioner to have doubts about a simple corn arising. In the case of intractable plantar keratomas presenting with these findings, surgical care may have to be considered. Because the lesion in this case was not directly over a metatarsal, and a definitive subdermal cause could be found, the wound healed uneventfully.

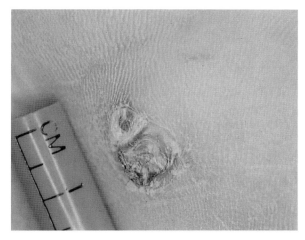

Figure 14.20 Corn overlying a synovial cyst. The appearance is atypical of a corn as this had already been excised once 3 years previously.

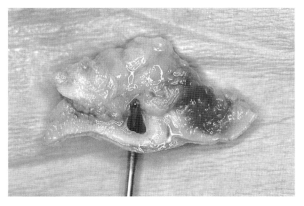

Figure 14.21 Cyst removed from tissue (shown in Fig. 14.20). The central punctum communicates with a cavity in the dermis. Histology shows acanthosis and hyperkeratosis. The cyst was lined with cuboid epithelium surrounded by fibrosis. The diagnosis was a synovial cyst.

in those patients suited to surgery. The dermal changes have often been found to be seriously altered upon excision, with small bursae/cysts present. Without ameliorating the cause, patients are often destined to retain persistent corns in perpetuity.

Apical and interdigital lesions respond equally well to arthroplasty or arthrodesis. Hallux valgus correction and exostectomy should be appropriately selected for medial or phalangeal problems associated with the great toe.

Elevation of metatarsals The metatarsal head that lies below the other four adjacent metatarsals can become overloaded with pressure. Bursa development (see under bursitis) or callus arises as a response of the soft tissues to mechanical stress. Single elevation osteotomies can be undertaken. Some controversy exists concerning the view that the bone should be fixed once divided, since a single non-union can have devastating effects and, on the whole, fixation stabilization is safer (see Fig. 14.12). Overelevation will create two problems. First, the adjacent metatarsals may become overloaded, with new callosity forming within a few months, if not weeks; second, the MTPJ may become stiff, as an elevatus will reduce joint range excursion.

Where very severe lesions exist, metatarsal head excision may be preferred because symptom relief is immediate. However, transfer lesions may still arise and should be anticipated using an insole to protect the other metatarsals. Excision is usually a last resort associated with multiple toe deformities and digital retraction and forms a salvage type of operation.

Forefoot/hindfoot alignment The splayed forefoot, pes cavus and club foot will all give rise to metatarsal callosity. Surgical correction may need to be staged, but these tend to involve both forefoot and hindfoot deformities. Some of these surgeries have already been discussed earlier.

SOFT TISSUE PAIN

Many inflammatory soft tissue problems relate to stress and strain episodes and are associated with repetitive injuries following sporting activities. The adult patient frequently presents with such problems with no recollection of injury. Conservative management is called for in the majority of soft tissue injuries.

Complete rupture of tendons may require surgical repair rather than immobilization in a soft splint or cast. Chapter 16 considers tendon injuries in greater detail.

HEEL PAIN SYNDROMES

Heel pain is responsible for a high proportion of podiatric referrals. Pain on the plantar aspect of the heel is a common problem that has a number of aetiological factors (Sunberg & Johnson 1991). Most heel pain relates to soft tissue.

Accurate history taking should rule out less-common conditions such as gout, Reiter's disease and ankylosing spondylitis. Back pain and referred S1 nerve pain can be excluded by careful examination of the hip and lower back. Haglund's deformity has been described above. Tendo Achilles pain and problems associated with calcaneal and Achilles bursitis/tendinitis are usually located at specific points; these conditions are dealt with in Chapter 16.

Calcaneal tumours are rare, but radiographs are required to rule out unicameral bone cysts, osteoid osteomas, fractures, radioopaque foreign bodies and metastatic tumours. Radiographs should be taken only when no other history fits the symptoms. Nocturnal, non-weight-bearing pain that does not resolve with aspirin or paracetamol may, in rare cases, suggest a malignant tumour.

Although nerve entrapment is dealt with as a separate subject, recent evidence suggests that the practitioner should be aware of variations in the branches of the tibial nerve, which might contribute to heel pain (Campbell & Lawton 1994, Davis & Schon 1995). Nerve entrapment, as with tarsal tunnel syndrome, can be associated with a frequently found anomalous nerve branch supplying the abductor digiti minimi. If the branch divides proximally and close to the medial calcaneal tuberosity, compression can easily arise.

Plantar heel pad pain

Heel pain most commonly affects the plantar surface. Generally, the pain may present as sharp burning or an intense ache, which is reproducible on direct pressure. Pain is increased on walking and standing, and eased by rest. Pain is worse on activity, after a rest period, or when first getting out of bed. There are several factors associated with the cause of plantar heel pain; each needs to be considered and rectified where possible within the treatment plan. Common causes include increased activity, inappropriate footwear design (Fig. 14.22), sudden increased weight, as in pregnancy, and abnormal foot function.

While a calcaneal spur may be diagnosed, asymptomatic spurs may be found on the contra-lateral heel. Unilateral heel oedema suggests chronic heel pad strain, although this can be confused with a bursa. Plantar fasciitis and heel pain syndrome must be distinguished from S1 referred pain, infection and osteoid osteoma.

Conservative management

Heel pain, especially on the medial aspect, is often related to excessive pronation although a supinated foot type may influence symptoms through inadequate shock absorption. Care should be taken to control the rearfoot and forefoot with appropriate orthoses to allow first ray plantarflexion, particularly if there is a tight medial band of the fascia. Rigid orthoses should have a groove or indent to accommodate tight fascial bands. There is a range of heel orthoses available, and no one product has been shown to be superior. Foot or even below-knee leg casts have been used to limit strain or as night splints designed to rest the foot.

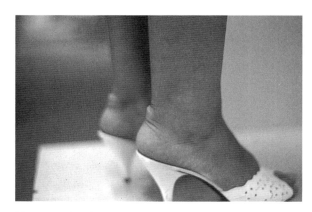

Figure 14.22 Fatty heel bumps in a patient with highly unsuitable shoes. Note that the soft calcaneal tissue is allowed to hang over the edge of the sling-back shoes, leading to further problems: fissuring and hard skin.

Muscle stretching should be included in the management plan and may typically include the calf and hamstring muscle groups. Flexibility exercises for the former will stretch both the muscle and the plantar structures. If a fracture is suspected or ultrasound over the site causes pain on treatment, a radiograph is indicated. Physical therapy has a part to play in rehabilitating the patient with heel pain. Heat, ultrasound, laser and transcutaneous nerve stimulators all have a role.

Chronic heel strain does not resolve with analgesics and NSAIDs as successfully as acute strain. Many patients attend the clinic once the chronic stage has developed, some 7–18 months after symptoms were first recognized. Footwear, insoles and heel cup advice can afford much improvement with occasional analgesic use.

Specific sites of pain with swelling and balottement point to the diagnosis of a plantar *bursa*, which some call policeman's heel. The bursa can be infiltrated with 0.25–0.5 ml corticosteroid such as methylprednisolone or triamcinolone hexacetonide. Cut-outs within heel pads and insoles can provide some relief, as can injection therapy. Flare-up is not uncommon in patients, accounting for 1–2% of cases (Tollafield & Williams 1996). Patients should be warned about this side-effect, which usually lasts for no more than 2 days.

Elasticated support stockings or compressive heel pads are valuable if worn before placing the foot on the floor first thing in the morning (Fig. 14.23). The elasticated support compresses the heel and improves the venous return to alleviate congested tissues. Where orthoses and all the other conservative measures fail, the patient may require walking casts or Aircasts to retain mobility while ensuring that rest continues. Crutches are not recommended, as the patient should maintain weight bearing wherever possible (see Appendix 3). If rest therapy fails, surgery to release the fascia may have to be undertaken.

Heel pain will generally respond well to conservative management. However, no single isolated treatment must be relied upon. It is often a combination of therapies that is most effective. Heel pain may resolve unaided, often after a prolonged period of 2 years.

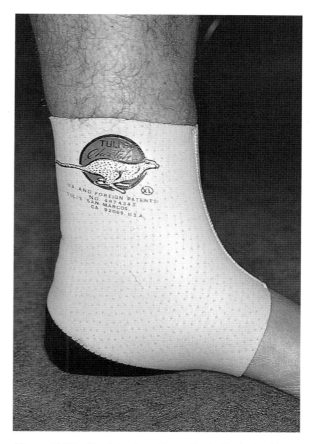

Figure 14.23 Stock heel cushion with elasticated ankle sock (bright green; Tuli pad design).

Fasciitis and plantar spurs

Tenderness along the medial and central bands of the fascia can be located at the insertion point of the calcaneus (associated with an enthesis or projection), although spurs are generally deeper to the insertion. Current literature is divided over the origin of the spur; some take the view that spur resection is the only answer. The tenderness produced by dorsiflexing the toes, dorsiflexing the ankle and palpation will reveal one or more specific areas of pain. While obesity is not the only factor involved, weight loss is to be encouraged, although exercise may not be possible because of the fasciitis; the cycle of events must be broken.

Rupture of the fascia should be ruled out if clinical examination identifies a gap in the fascia or if the patient reports a history of a sudden snap along the band. Injudicious use of steroid injections has been known to cause weakness.

Conservative management

Physical therapy, fascia strapping and single injection therapy with a corticosteroid medication offer an approach to reversing inflammation, resting the fascia and limiting swelling and pain (Fig. 14.24). Relief is usually very rapid, with patients reporting up to 70% relief within 2 weeks. If the pain does not resolve quickly, the practitioner should seek further diagnostic investigation or supplement treatment with varus canted heel cups, heel pads and orthoses, much as for heel pad strain. Repeated steroid injections should be used cautiously; lack of improvement implies that steroid treatment is unhelpful and provocative of further pain. NSAID analgesics have an unpredictable effect and rarely ameliorate a long-standing problem. Ibuprofen or diclofenac sodium may offer valuable supportive therapy in assisting reduction of swelling and inflammation, but complications as a result of long-term use are well recognized (see Ch. 8).

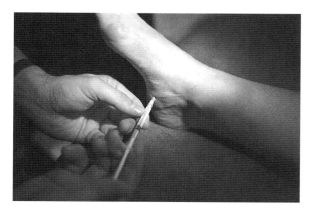

Figure 14.24 Corticosteroid (methyl prednisolone) in heel given from the medial side with a 3.75 cm 27G needle (Sterican, Braun). Patients should be warned to rest and told that 'flare-up' can occur.

Fasciitis may involve the heel fat pad and can complicate the clinical picture. Patients should monitor the association of symptoms at work or at home to rule out exacerbating factors. Heel lifts in felt and foam can reduce Achilles tendon tension. As mentioned earlier, stretching is an important strategy in resolving fasciitis.

Orthotic management of pronation is essential in order to prevent recurrence of the condition. Pes cavus feet require shock attenuation because the taut band is easily traumatized. Plantar fasciitis associated with pes planus requires antipronation (orthoses/strapping) to prevent the fascia lengthening and causing strain.

Surgical management

A small percentage of patients with heel pain will require surgery; most will respond to conservative measures. Surgical intervention is determined by the diagnosis:

- plantar fasciitis is dealt with by division of the plantar fascia from its insertion into the calcaneus (Barrett & Day 1993)
- heel neuroma is dealt with by releasing and decompressing the medial calcaneal nerve as it passes under the abductor hallucis muscle belly; surgery to release nerves and their associated branches has been cited by Campbell & Lawton (1994) to have provided good relief
- plantar bursitis requires excision, although this is very rare (in our practice).

In all cases the surgical approach should avoid areas of stress. The medial side of the calcaneus is often chosen where the plantar and dorsal skin meet. Avoidance of scarring must remain the key objective when selecting incision lines, while still allowing access to tissues involved.

Plantar fibromatosis

Plantar fibromatosis are soft tissue lumps appearing in the medial arch and can arise with nodular lesions associated with subcutaneous tissue. This condition can develop as a proliferative fasciitis in young and old patients. The fibroma forms in the fascia and in the long plantar ligament (Fig. 14.25). In many cases, the condition is an inconvenience. Orthoses must avoid compressing the nodular structure and thus causing irritation. Casted orthoses must take account of the nodular area by marking the negative shell so that the laboratory can add plaster to the positive cast.

Where the digits are affected by marked clawing, or where pain arises, radicle resection is necessary, using Z-skin incisions or curved incisions to avoid inciting further scarring. The fascia and nodules are removed, exposing underlying muscle. Drains inserted into the wound reduce the possibility of haematoma becoming organized into further scar tissue (Fig. 14.26).

TENDINITIS AND BURSITIS

Tendinitis most commonly affects the Achilles tendon, although the posterior tibial tendon can be involved. Overuse can initiate the condition and, therefore, management is largely conservative in nature. Strapping and orthoses are highly effective, although in the early stages heel lifts can be used, providing that the heel cord is not encouraged to shorten and is monitored. Steroid injections are rarely recommended in the early stages of treatment. Stretching and strengthening are discussed in Chapter 16, but active maintenance of controlled tensile stress is essential to prevent contracture.

Bursitis Bursitis around the Achilles tendon shows up as a collection of fluid that can be moved from side to side. A retrocalcaneal bursa may arise from direct irritation from hard or high heel counters; the shoe design should be changed. Aspiration can be attempted to collapse the wall; 20–60 ml syringes should be selected, with large-gauge needles, following infiltration of anaesthetic at the point of injection. The bursa is strapped down afterwards. Steroid injections have been found to be very useful in preventing further swelling. Underlying retrocalcaneal spurs or bumps may need resection.

Plantar metatarsal bursitis This is another condition broadly classified as metatarsalgia. Inflammation of an adventitious bursa arises

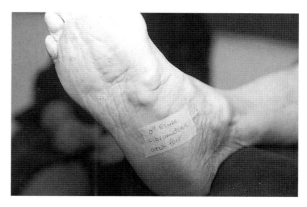

Figure 14.25 Fascia nodules form in plantar fibromatosis as in Dupuytren's contracture. Fibromatosis does not have to be symptomatic.

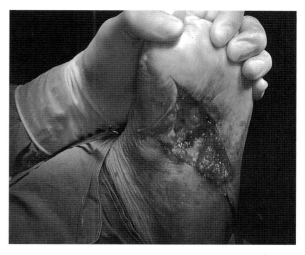

Figure 14.26 Surgery must be aggressive when dealing with fibromatosis. The illustration shows fascial resection following previous surgery. The fascia is stripped away from the underlying muscle. A drain (not shown) is used in situ to prevent haematoma formation.

plantar to the MTPJ and is the result of shearing stress within the tissues. Located under one of the three central metatarsals when prominent, the condition may arise when the first metatarsal is dorsiflexed. An intense pain associated with burning, sharpness and throbbing is present on weight bearing and will reduce on rest. Fluctuant swelling and tenderness provide some idea of the extent of pathology. Figure 14.27 illustrates the type of problem facing the practitioner if a bursa becomes chronically organized under a metatarsal head. Elevated first metatarsals causing plantar overload to second or third metatarsals may be balanced with a metatarsal shaft under the first ray. The disadvantage caused by this technique relates to limiting first MTPJ motion.

Conservative management

Management for bursitis is similar to that for capsulitis. Although conservative measures using physical therapy may be beneficial, the plantar skin is difficult to penetrate. A felt pad for the sole of the foot, with a 'U' cut around the painful area reduces pressure. Corticosteroid infiltration will allow the bursa to shrink unless it becomes chronic.

Surgical management

Surgical excision must avoid the plantar weight-bearing surface. Incision lines must be made between the metatarsals. Displacement of metatarsals by vertical elevation and shortening may alter the weight-bearing balance effectively. The first metatarsal can in some cases be brought into greater plantarflexion.

NEOPLASIA

Skin tumours are far more common than bone tumours (described above). Diagnosis, to rule out infection, should be differentiated by biopsy and microbiological culture.

Principles of management

Conservative management may be appropriate for some lesions. Caustic sticks such as silver nitrate can limit epithelialization. The use of any chemical agent around an undefined lesion may create malignant change; the practitioner should apply the following axiom: 'do not apply any agents to skin that might lead to damage or provoke an abnormal response'.

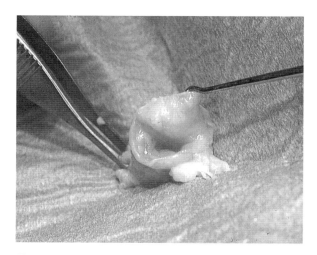

Figure 14.27 Adventitious bursa removed from under the second metatarsal head. The sac was well formed owing to chronic organization of tissue and failed to resolve with steroid injections. There were symptoms of metatarsalgia (burning pain). There was fluctuant presentation underlying skin.

Lesions that discharge, show colour changes, have indistinct borders, show an insidious growth change or are irritant warrant appropriate specialist opinion. Corticosteroids have successfully been used for many inflammatory-based dermatological lesions, such as granuloma annulare (Rasanen & Hasen 1993), but they are not indicated unless the diagnosis is distinct.

Hyfrecation and cryosurgery offer alternative destructive methods but destroy the quality of the lesion for the purposes of biopsy. Where the tumour is small, it is preferable to remove the lesion in one piece together with some of the healthy edge. This provides the histopathology laboratory with better material for analysis and also improves the chances of complete removal. Care should be taken with excisional biopsy surgery to avoid interfering with skin involved with plastic surgery at a later stage. Inadvertent scarring may limit effectiveness of plastic surgery; therefore, careful planning of incision lines at biopsy is critical. Curettage is useful for skin warts (see Ch. 15) and selection of this surgical technique will depend upon the likelihood of scarring and on the site. Keloid or hypertrophic scars (see Fig. 7.27) are undesirable, especially on the plantar surface. Skin tags respond well to amputation by tying a fine thread around the base to cut off the local blood supply.

Surgical management will be determined by the site, depth and likely cause of the lesion. The objective of surgery is to cause limited destruction and, primarily, to allow correct identification. Amputation is used for extensive invasive and malignant neoplasia. Plastic surgery by grafting is considered where a flap cannot be advanced over the defect left by the surgery (see Case study 7.3, p. 141). A skin lesion may need to be traced through fascia and muscle to bone; drains may have to be used and the patient either admitted or appropriately discharged to home.

Ganglionic cysts remain common to the foot as benign fluctuant swellings. If they are closely approximated to joint margins and tendon sheaths, aspiration will fail to achieve lengthy remission. Mucoid cysts over the distal IPJs have a similar appearance, although they are usually much smaller. Surgical excision is the best approach, allowing the foot to be correctly explored and part of the involved joint lining removed. Mucoid cysts affecting toes may require an excisional arthroplasty.

Tumours that cause no pain and remain the same size for years should be monitored. Monitoring consists of measuring the size in millimetres and drawing an outline using the adhesive side of clear tape to mark the lesion. The tape is then stuck securely in the records. An instamatic photograph or digital image will provide visual evidence.

To treat or not to treat?

The reason for dealing with any growth falls into two categories: to identify the taxonomy of the lesion and to prevent space-occupying damage. Large cysts become organized with inflammatory material, cells and cholesterol deposits and damage internal structures (Fig. 14.28) such as tendons, capsules, fascia and muscle. For the latter reason, the patient should have lesions removed that show a steady rate of expansion, even though they show no signs of discomfort,

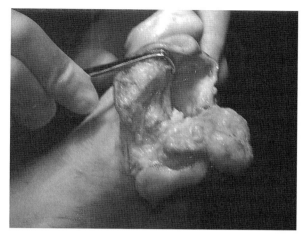

Figure 14.28 Space-occupying lesions may be painless but can cause marked destruction of underlying anatomy if left for years. Where lesions can migrate back in-between metatarsals, the appearance and size are deceptive (see Fig. 14.10). Both lesions come from the same site and patient.

lymphadenopathy, lung, kidney or liver disease. Men should be questioned about prostate problems and women about breast examination and reproductive organ disorders. The patient should be referred to the appropriate specialist if doubt arises.

NEUROLOGICAL PAIN

Neurological pain is difficult to diagnose and may result from back and pelvic problems affecting the nerve pathways that descend into the foot. Pain located to a particular site within the foot may, however, result from local nerve entrapment. Two common sites for nerve entrapment include the intermetatarsal spaces, particularly the third to fourth intermetatarsal space, and the tarsal tunnel, which passes inferior to the medial malleolus; entrapment in the latter is a consequence of tibial nerve compression. Following a thorough examination of the locomotor system and failure of conservative treatment, these specific sites may require investigating and the tissue examined for pathology. The use of ultrasound in diagnosing nerve problems depends upon the available expertise of the radiologist, but as a test may not be wholly conclusive. While surgery should ideally be avoided, procedures are often undertaken as part of the diagnostic process.

Interdigital neuroma

Interdigital neuroma is not a tumour but is associated with degeneration of the nerve caused by stretching and compression. The symptoms associated with it include a sharp, shooting pain radiating into the toes.

Conservative management

A recent study and review of steroid infiltration (Tollafield & Williams 1996) revealed that 30% improvement in neuroma pain was maintained for more than 6 months after therapy and 70% of patients may experience some immediate relief from injection therapy for 2–12 weeks. The use of corticosteroids for adventitious bursae is diagnostic as well as therapeutic, offering a sensible first-line treatment. If the toes part (diastasis), an infiltrated bursa is suggested, as the fluid from the injection causes the separation.

In a report of 21 patients by Kilmartin & Wallace (1994), 50% found their neuroma symptoms relieved by an orthotic (Cobra) insole made from felt. Of the remainder, 30% required cortisone injections, while 20% required surgery. These studies allow us to focus on planned outcomes when advising patients.

Other forms of management include reflexology, osteopathy, plantar metatarsal pad insoles and pads worn with toe loops. A plantar metatarsal pad orthosis is believed to separate the metatarsals by extending the toe with an upward force on weight bearing. Much of the success with conservative therapy is almost certainly related to early intervention and diagnosis.

Sclerosing agents such as alcohol and vitamin B_{12} have both been used for interdigital neuromata. Miller (1992) cites Dockery & Nilson (1986) who used 4% ethanol by mixing 2 ml alcohol with 48 ml anaesthetic. The injection was repeated every week for at least three visits.

Surgical management

Where the nerve has enlarged with fibrotic infiltration, excision is indicated. Pain may, in fact, result from an enlarged bursa. The literature reveals different approaches to removing a neuroma. A plantar approach is easier to undertake but can lead to problems from scarring and seed corn formation. The suture technique is of vital importance to prevent this; skin must be carefully apposed to prevent overlap. The plantar skin approach may vary between patients, but it may result in hyperkeratosis, wound dehiscence and scarring; these features are less common on the dorsum. The dorsal approach is technically more difficult but postoperatively is more reliable. Although loss of sensation is a postoperative feature, this causes little symptomatic concern.

The dorsal- and web-splitting approach is useful if pain from an enlarged mass can be palpated in the intermetatarsal space. Interdigital healing may be slower in patients if the area becomes macerated with sweat; infection is not uncommon with interdigital incisions at 5–7 days.

Histology should always be used to confirm that a neuroma has been identified. It has been suggested that 75–95% of these neuromata can be resolved at operation (Mann 1978). Stumps of nerves can cause painful nodules where scarring has occurred. A repeat operation is often the only recourse, although patients can benefit from manipulative therapy where adhesions appear to respond by being broken up. Revision surgery is more certain to resolve the problem if a plantar approach is made.

Tarsal tunnel syndrome

Nerve entrapment causing pain in the arch and forefoot is attributed to tibial nerve compression. Pain, paraesthesia, dysaesthesia and hyperaesthesia around the ankle and along the distribution of the tibial nerve are common. A positive Tinel's sign, Valleix test (proximal pain along the nerve on pressure) and intrinsic muscle weakness are all suggestive of entrapment.

The use of a sphygmomanometer set at 100–150 mmHg is valuable in determining the extent of pathology. The toes and forefoot become sensitive and painful within 30 seconds of this test if positive. The sphygmomanometer pressure test allows reasonable judgement in referring patients on for nerve conduction and MRI but is not in itself conclusive of tarsal tunnel syndrome.

The nerve conduction test may show altered sensory nerve conduction (i.e. slow or absent), decreased amplitude, increased duration of motor-evoked potential or increase latency of a distal motor nerve. Some patients find nerve conduction analysis quite painful.

Electromyography may show weakness in a muscle, as tarsal tunnel syndrome has been reported by Summarco & Conti (1994) to be caused by an anomalous hypertrophic or accessory abductor hallucis.

An MRI may be warranted to establish nerve and soft tissue entrapment, as in some cases the nerve has to be released at its distal as well as its proximal end. Enlarged or atrophic muscles will also be easier to identify. The patient should be thoroughly reviewed for other differential neurological conditions associated with peripheral sensory and motor disorders.

Conservative management

The foot mechanics should be stabilized with strapping or orthoses early into treatment, provided that temporary orthoses can be shown to resolve some symptoms. Pronatory problems are most likely to cause this condition.

Injection therapy has been used to good effect to reduce the intraneural and extraneural inflammation (Malay & McGlamry 1992). Casting for short periods to rest the inevitable traction along the nerve may reduce symptoms. NSAIDs and physical therapies may be tried to reduce fibrosis and improve movement around the nerve.

Surgical management

Intractable symptoms can lead to a disabling condition. The nerve in this case is not removed but released from scarring causing tethering to adjacent tissues. Nerves must have the freedom

to elongate with foot movement. The tibial nerve runs through the tarsal tunnel and is involved with the tibialis posterior tendon, flexor digitorum longus, neurovascular bundle and flexor hallucis longus. Surgery to expose these tissues should take care not to damage the vascular tissue or nerve (Fig. 14.29). The nerve is traced distally where it will divide into a medial and lateral portion. The medial portion is larger and runs between the abductor hallucis and flexor hallucis brevis, having passed through a fibrous opening between the abductor hallucis and spring ligament. Any fibrous constrictions are released, preserving nerve motility. Symptoms should be relieved once the tibial nerve is no longer compressed. Tarsal tunnel surgery may not always be successful as scarring can recur.

Cutaneous neurological pain

Any nerve close to the surface can be damaged, especially on the dorsal surface of the foot where it can become impinged by compression between shoe and bone. Pain from the superficial peroneal nerves may radiate onto the dorsum of the foot. The practitioner should initially exclude all medical causes, but surgery may provide assistance where all other forms of management fail and where diagnosis casts a high degree of suspicion on a neurological problem.

Surgery certainly cannot assist with nerve problems unless a physical cause can be shown

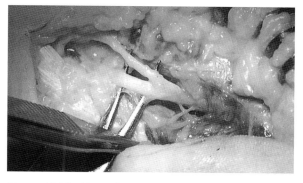

Figure 14.29 Nerve decompressed in the tarsal tunnel showing lateral and medial branches of the tibial nerve. (Reproduced with permission from Scott Hosler, Fifth Avenue Residency Program.)

to have initiated the problem. Neuritic bunion pain has been described in the absence of fixed deformity (Rosen & Grady 1986). Symptoms were associated with shooting pain into the big toe. Diagnosis of medial dorsal cutaneous neuritis was established when, at operation, a fibrous band was shown to compress the nerve.

Miscellaneous nerve entrapment

While entrapment may arise above the ankle, tarsal tunnel is considered the most common form of foot entrapment after Morton's neuroma. In some cases, metatarsalgia may relate to a plantar nerve entrapped under the metatarsal head. The nerve becomes tethered to the metatarsal and is continuously traumatized. Case study 14.5 and Fig. 14.30 emphasizes the need to keep an open mind during examination.

MISCELLANEOUS PAIN

Differentiating pain

Rarer forms of pain arising in the foot and lower limb include reflex sympathetic dystrophy (see Ch. 7) and compartment syndrome (see Ch. 16). Associated neurological pain with evidence of local swelling should be ruled out, and compartment syndrome, localized nerve compression

from a tumour and localized damage to the nerve with fibrosis should be differentiated.

Acute vascular problems arise with disease processes such as diabetes mellitus and peripheral vascular disease, and these patients need to be urgently assessed and sent for appropriate investigations. Differentiation between vascular ischaemia and neuropathic ischaemia is important, and sensory, vibration and pressure testing can be performed in clinic.

Anatomical variation arises in the foot. Venous malformation can arise causing the same symptoms as tarsal tunnel syndrome (Julsrud 1995). More commonly, the types of structure likely to appear in some but not all patients are accessory ossicles. The pain produced by such

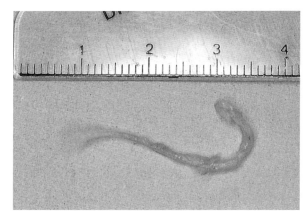

Figure 14.30 Entrapped nerve from under sesamoid bone (see Case study 14.5).

Case study 14.5 Nerve entrapment

A 75-year-old female had been suffering for many years with pain under her first metatarsal. More recently, the symptoms had become more distressing. Examination of the foot provided a diagnosis of plantarflexed first ray causing sesamoiditis. Insoles and careful footwear selection had all been tried, but to no avail. Lateral radiographs were taken and a large medial sesamoid confirmed the suspicion that the first metatarsal pain was related to the ossicle. The surgical plan included planing of the sesamoid to trim it back, or removal if it was too large. Planing provided a less than satisfactory result. Once the sesamoid had been removed, the skin flattened sufficiently to diminish the accentuation of the first ray with its enlarged sesamoid. The interesting point about this case involved the identification of a thickened plantar nerve, which had become invested within the tissues underlying the medial sesamoid (Fig. 14.30).

Conclusion: Trapped nerves must be excluded from foot pathology. Because the anatomical pathway of nerves varies, some of the symptoms associated with nerves may not be that obvious. Removal of the sesamoid was felt to be prudent because of significant pain, although in this case disruption of the flexor pull against the hallux must always remain a concern.

structures varies, causing dysfunction, fracture, inflammatory change or contributing to arthritis.

PAIN FROM COMMON ACCESSORY OSSICLES

Accessory ossicles of the foot are often clinically insignificant as a radiological finding. While as many as 15 accessory ossicles have been documented within the foot (Rowanowski & Barrington 1991), it is the ossicles affecting the tarsus that most commonly give rise to symptoms. The *os trigonum* is one of the largest and most frequently encountered accessory ossicles; it lies posterior to the lateral tubercle of the talus and may be bipartite. Symptoms may arise from compression of the soft tissues between the talus and tibia when the foot is frequently plantarflexed in activities such as ballet dancing or soccer.

Diagnosis is made with lateral radiographs of the ankle, although bone scans may be helpful in confirming increased inflammatory activity.

The accessory navicular situated medial and posterior to the main body of the navicular is another commonly encountered ossicle. It can take several forms, the most common being the ossicle united to the navicular by a synchondrosis of 1–2 mm width. Symptoms are often related to the insertion of the tibialis posterior tendon. Contraction of the tendon causes displacement of the ossicle and stress on the synchondrosis. Eventually, the synchondrosis will fuse to form the corniculate navicular. Symptoms may subside at this point or the prominent navicular tuberosity will continue to be subject to footwear irritation.

Another form of accessory navicular is a sesamoid bone within the tibialis posterior tendon. This sesamoid is quite separate from the navicular and is best referred to as *os tibiale externum*. Apart from increasing the prominence of the navicular, which may cause footwear irritation, this form of accessory navicular is often asymptomatic.

Diagnosis of accessory navicular may be made clinically in the presence of an enlarged navicular tuberosity. Plain radiographs will allow a more accurate assessment. Excision of the ossicle is the definitive treatment for symptomatic occurrence. Careful planning is required in order that the mechanical advantage offered by the insertion of tibialis posterior is not affected as it inserts into the navicular tuberosity.

Os talonaviculare dorsale is worth mentioning as it can present an irregular appearance on a lateral radiograph, appearing as arthritis. Many different ossicles are apparent within the foot. Pain and dysfunction suggest that removal is required. Well-made conforming orthoses and sensible footwear selection play a primary part in managing problems associated with tarsal ossicles.

INFECTION

Infection has been described in Chapter 7 in relation to postoperative management. The principles of management do not differ when infection arises outside of surgery. Infection of the foot without an obvious cause may pose a different dilemma.

Surface infection may arise from fissures of the skin, paronychia, dermatomycosis, deepseated abscess tracking to the surface or focal infection from another part of the body. In children, haematogenous osteomyelitis can cause long bone pain. In adults, more often than not it is an injury that brings about osteomyelitis.

The principles of infection management remain straightforward: identify the signs, take a good history and rule out the less obvious causes of non-specific infection. Furthermore:

- establish drainage
- treat infection
- debride necrotic tissue
- protect with a dressing against further infection
- prescribe rest and elevation.

Conservative management

Drainage is not easy to establish unless access can be gained. Protein-digesting enzymes create a sinus. This can be assisted with a sterile scalpel.

Low-strength antiseptic flush or 0.9% saline can be used to clean out the wound. Where the infection is localized, the wound is left to heal with the aid of a surface antiseptic and dressings. Antibiotics should not be used in this instance unless evidence of cellulitis, distressing pain or vascular damage is present. If the patient can cope with low-grade analgesics, the wound should settle with rest.

Rest may involve casts, crutches and short bed rest. Suitable absorbent dressings should be changed, depending upon the nature of discharge and whether the wound needs regular lavage.

Problems do, however, arise with wounds that do not establish drainage, particularly in patients who are compromised. Their health status must be checked to assess the best form of management, which will undoubtedly include antibiotics.

Surgical management

Once infection shows signs of tracking or bone destruction, or surface necrosis takes place, surgery is indicated. Debridement and drainage will improve the chance of healthy granulation (Case study 14.6 and Figs 14.31 and 14.32). Surgical exposure will ensure that deep tissue is decompressed from swelling and pressure to avoid additional necrosis. The body's defence mechanisms are allowed to reach the site of infection. Antibiotics will be given intravenously to provide high tissue levels of antimicrobial

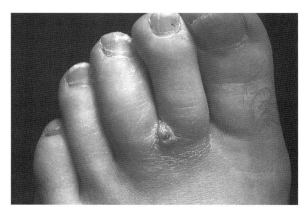

Figure 14.31 A granuloma is apparent between this man's left second and third toes. This is an example of a cutaneous infection that was maintained by antibiotics.

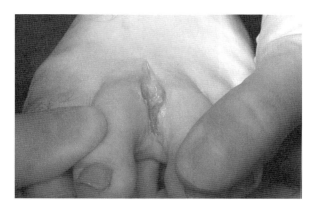

Figure 14.32 Infection being managed. The lesion shown in Figure 14.31 has been opened up and drained, resulting in a complete resolution (see text). The granuloma was removed and shown to be unremarkable. The organism was *Staphylococcus aureus*.

Case study 14.6   Surgical drainage

A 46-year-old male factory worker developed an interdigital problem. Antibiotics were used by his GP, but the lesion did not clear (Fig. 14.31). The lesion presented as a granulomatous mass that had been present for 8 weeks. Access to the site was not possible and surgical drainage was required (a) to establish drainage; and (b) to identify the organism (Fig. 14.32). Deep tissue inflammation with a thin collection of pus was removed. Light sutures only were used with a vacuum drain. Flucloxacillin 250 mg four times a day was continued for a further 10 days. Postoperative resolution was immediate, within 7 days, with return to work at 3 weeks.

Conclusion: The diagnosis was an infection without an identifiable cause. The organism was *Staphylococcus aureus*. The lesion was a granuloma and there was strong suspicion of a secondarily infected interdigital dermatomycosis associated with athlete's foot. Interdigital clefts pose problems from secondary bacterial infection. The cleft is moist, warm and able to sustain bacterial growth well. Once through the epithelial tissue, the spread of infection can travel between the metatarsals quickly. In this case, the patient was fortunate enough to be healthy and maintained from cellulitic spread by his GP.

activity at the time of surgery. The patient will be maintained on oral antibiotics specific to the organism. Heavily infected wounds are always left to drain. Closure may not be necessary, although further debridement may still be required. Clean open wounds may even be grafted over once the swelling has subsided and infection abated.

SKIN DISORDERS

While many texts on dermatology exist, the principles of management involve a multidisciplinary approach, which includes the GP or dermatologist. Psoriasis, eczema and dermatitis are the commonest conditions. Other conditions that are treatable include disorders of keratinization and nail disorders. The principles behind the treatment of nails are discussed in Chapter 6.

Inflammatory conditions associated with psoriasis are difficult to manage because of the underlying abnormality of keratinization, which at best can be suppressed rather than treated. Blisters and fissures may complicate other skin problems, and concern for primary or secondary infection may arise. The patient usually becomes concerned when any skin problem on the foot becomes irritated by shoes. Interdigital spaces, paronychial tissue and the skin around the long arch, heel or ankle may cause pain and itching, or simply ooze, as in the case of varicose eczema. In the latter, ulcers may form around the ankle and medial side of the foot (Ch. 17).

Principles of management

- Keratin disorders may need debriding regularly. Caution should be taken with plaques because small bleeding points can be exposed. Reduction of tissue will maintain comfort.
- Inflammatory bases of hyperkeratosis should be dampened with corticosteroids when highly active.
- Keratolytics are valuable to soften areas, particularly around the heel and plantar metatarsal area in lieu of mechanical debridement.

- Creams and ointments can maintain suppleness and deliver various medications, e.g. allowing penetration of corticosteroids or assisting preparations such as urea, dithranol, antiseptics and antifungal agents.
- Cleansing agents: aluminium acetate 0.65% in water provides an effective astringent; Permutabs (Bioglan) can be used for weeping ulcers.
- Antiperspirants such as aluminium chloride hexahydrate in an alcohol base reduce excessive sweating.
- Barrier creams such as dimethicone or zinc and castor oil will help to protect sensitive skin.
- Antipruritics will help to keep patients comfortable and prevent excoriation of skin from scratching. Calamine and crotamiton are equally effective.
- Agents known to cause irritation should be removed. Footwear and socks/stockings /tights should be evaluated to ensure that component materials do not cause specific site dermatitis.

SUMMARY

The management of pain or deformity in the adult foot requires a quite different approach from that used in a child's foot. Deformities in a child are often flexible and liable to spontaneous improvement. Deformities in the adult, however, are usually rigid and often aggravated by footwear fitting or occupational demands.

Pain is a rare feature in the child, whereas pain may present in a variety of forms in the adult. Most patients are unable to recall specific injuries and so the practitioner must approach the problem systematically.

Where treatment is instigated, it should usually begin with conservative measures, because these methods generally carry fewer potential problems than surgery. A central tenet of conservative treatment is the use of foot orthoses. The high value placed on orthoses reflects the fact that most foot pain occurs on weight bearing, and orthoses have the capacity to enhance the efficiency of weight bearing. Drugs should only be used for short periods. They often work best in combination with other treatment regimens. Surgery should not be considered until all conservative options have been exhausted. When surgery is used, the foot surgeon needs to apply the most appropriate procedure to retain/restore the dynamic function of the foot. For every practitioners, the primary goal must be *first do no harm*; it is only with an understanding of the unique requirements placed on the human foot that that intention can be realized.

REFERENCES

Balkin S W 1972 Plantar keratoses: treatment by injectable liquid silicone. Clinical Orthopedics 87: 235–247

Barouk L S 1994 Weil lesser rays osteotomy. Medical Chirurgie Pied 1: 22–23

Barrett S L, Day S V 1993 Endoscopic plantar fasciotomy: two endoscopic surgical techniques: clinical results of 65 procedures. Journal of Foot and Ankle Surgery 32: 248–256

Campbell P, Lawton J O 1994 Heel pain: diagnosis and management. British Joural of Medicine 52: 380–385

Davis T J, Schon L C 1995 Branches of the tibial nerve: anatomic variations. Foot and Ankle International 16: 21–29

Dockery G L, Nilson R Z 1986 Intralesional injections. Clinics in Podiatric Medicine and Surgery 3: 473–485

Grace D L 1993 Surgery of the lesser rays. The Foot 3: 51–57

Groiso J A 1992 Juvenile hallux valgus. A conservative approach to treatment. Journal of Bone and Joint Surgery 74A: 1367–1374

Haines R W, McDougall A 1954 The anatomy of hallux valgus. Journal of Bone and Joint Surgery 36B: 272–293

Hardy R H, Clapham J C R 1951 Observations on hallux valgus based on a controlled series. Journal of Bone and Joint Surgery 33B: 376–391

Julsrud M E 1995 An unusual case of tarsal tunnel syndrome. Journal of Foot and Ankle Surgery 34: 289–293

Kilmartin T E, Wallace W A 1992 Update on hallux valgus surgery. A review of results in the recent literature. The Foot 2: 123–134

Kilmartin T E, Wallace W A 1994 The effect of a pronation and supination orthosis on Morton's neuroma and lower limb function. Foot and Ankle International 15: 256–262

Kilmartin T E, Wallace W A, Hill T W 1991 Measurement of the functional orthotic effect on metatarsophalangeal joint extension. Journal of the American Podiatric Medical Association 81: 414–417

Kilmartin T E, Barrington R L, Wallace W A 1994 A controlled prospective trial of a biomechanical orthosis in the treatment of juvenile hallux valgus. Journal of Bone and Joint Surgery 76B: 210–215

Klenerman L 1991 The foot and its disorders, 3rd edn. Blackwell Scientific, Oxford, p 134–135

Lang L M G, West S G, Day S, Simmonite N 1994 Salicylic acid in the treatment of corns. The Foot 4: 145–150

Mair S D, Coogan A C, Speer K P, Hall R L 1995 Gout as a source of pain. Foot and Ankle International 16: 613–616

Malay D S, McGlamry E D 1992 Acquired neuropathies of the lower extremities. In: McGlamry E D, Banks A S, Downey M S (eds) Comprehensive textbook of foot surgery, 2nd edn. Williams & Wilkins, Baltimore, MD, p 1095–1123

Mann R A (ed) 1978 DuVries' surgery of the foot. Mosby, St Louis, MO, p 466–468

Merriman L M, Turner WA (eds) 2002 Assessment of the lower limb, 2nd edn. Churchill Livingstone, Edinburgh

Miller S J 1992 Intermetatarsal neuromas and associated nerve problems. In: Butterworth R, Dockery G L (eds) A colour atlas and text of forefoot surgery. Wolfe, London

Pratt D J, Tollafield D R, Johnson G R, Peacock C 1993 Foot orthoses. In: Bowker P, Condie D N, Bader D L, Pratt D J (eds) Biomechanical basis of orthotic management. Butterworth–Heinemann, Oxford, p 86–87

Rasanen L, Hasan T 1993 Allergy to systemic and intra-lesional corticosteroid. British Journal of Dermatology 128: 407–411

Rees P J, Trounce J R 1988 New short textbook of medicine. Edward Arnold, London

Rosen J S, Grady J F 1986 Neuritic bunion syndrome. Journal of the American Podiatric Medical Association 76: 641–644

Rowanowski C A, Barrington N A 1991 The accessory ossicles of the foot. The Foot 2: 61–70

Salter R B, Harris W R 1963 Injuries involving the epiphyseal plate. Journal of Bone and Joint Surgery 45A: 587

Summarco G J, Conti S F 1994 Tarsal tunnel syndrome caused by an anomalous muscle. Journal of Bone and Joint Surgery 76A: 1308–1314

Sunberg S B, Johnson K A 1991 Painful conditions of the heel. In: Jahss M H (ed) Disorders of the foot and ankle, medical and surgical management, 2nd edn. Saunders, Philadelphia, PA, ch 47

Tollafield D R, Pratt D J 1990 The control of known triplanar forces on the foot by forefoot orthotic posting. British Journal of Podiatric Medicine and Surgery 2: 3–5

Tollafield D R, Williams H A 1996 The use of two injectable corticosteroid preparations used in the management of foot problems: a clinical audit report. British Journal of Podiatric Medicine 51: 171–174

Yu G V 1992 First metatarsal phalangeal joint arthrodesis. In: McGlamry E D, Banks A S, Downey M S (eds) Comprehensive textbook of foot surgery, 2nd edn, pp 545–565. Williams & Wilkins, Baltimore, MD

FURTHER READING

Bayliss N C, Klenerman L 1989 Avascular necrosis of lesser metatarsal heads following forefoot surgery. Foot and Ankle 10: 124–128

Laing P 1995 The painful foot. In: Merriman L M, Tollafield D R (eds) Assessment of the lower limb. Churchill Livingstone, Edinburgh

Skalley T C, Schon L C, Hinton R Y, Myerson M S 1994 Clinical results following revision tibial nerve release.

The Foot 15: 360–367

Spooner S K, Kilmartin T E, Merriman L M 1995 Pathologic anatomy of the first metatarsophalangeal joint in hallux valgus. British Journal of Podiatric Medicine and Surgery 7: 35–40

Turbutt I F 1995 Radiographic assessment. In: Merriman LM, Tollafield D R (eds) Assessment of the lower limb. Churchill Livingstone, Edinburgh, p 255–256

15

The child's foot

Paul Beeson
Patricia S. Nesbitt

INTRODUCTION

The treatment of children's foot problems should not be instigated without careful thought as to whether treatment is necessary. Many paediatric complaints are simply normal stages of development, which, in time, may resolve spontaneously. The practitioner's first aim should always be to reassure the parents with a sound explanation of the presenting complaint and the likely prognosis. In view of the fact that many foot and leg complaints are developmental in nature, review and monitoring often provide the basis of treatment. Objective measurements may facilitate this.

The following chapter will describe a range of treatments used in children, some of which are supported by scientific evidence. This chapter is divided into the following areas:

- common foot pathologies
- pain in the lower limb
- gait problems

COMMON FOOT PATHOLOGIES

METATARSUS ADDUCTUS

Metatarsus adductus has an incidence 1:1000 live births. 4% is hereditary. If one child is affected, the incidence increases to 1:20 that the second sibling will be similarly affected

(Wynne-Davies 1964). In the series of cases collected by Thomson (1960) and Rushforth (1978), the condition appeared to be slightly more common in females.

Not all metatarsus adductus requires treatment, as spontaneous resolution is common. Ponsetti & Becker (1966) found that only 12% of their patients required treatment, while Rushforth (1978), in an 11 year follow-up of 83 children, found that 4% retained severe deformity and another 10% displayed moderate deformity. The feet that are unlikely to resolve spontaneously can be identified on examination (Fig. 15.1). Rigidity within the foot makes manual correction difficult. A deep skin crease running along the medial plantar side of the first metatarsocuneiform joint generally indicates a more severely deformed foot.

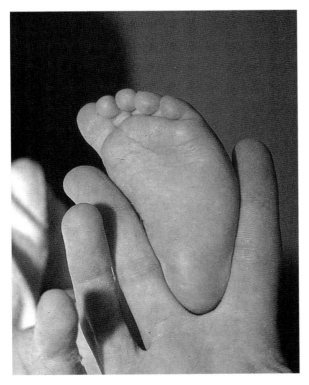

Figure 15.1 Metatarsus adductus. 'C'-shaped curvature of the lateral border of the foot is the key diagnostic feature.

Treatment

Manual manipulation and stimulation It is important to involve the parents in active treatment for this condition. The use of regular manual manipulation is valuable, attempting to maintain a rectus alignment for several minutes at each repetition. It is often useful to undertake this process several times a day. A useful method is to cup the heel with one hand while applying passive medial forefoot correction with the opposite hand.

A useful technique of manual stimulation is to stimulate the lateral border of the foot from heel to toe with your little finger followed by stimulation of the lateral compartment of the leg from heel to head of fibula. This encourages the foot to adopt a more rectus alignment. Suggested times to undertake this is during nappy changes.

Strapping Strapping is a traditional treatment, which can be demonstrated to the parents. The tape is wrapped around the forefoot, pulled proximally over the lateral malleolus and wrapped around the leg, as in Figure 15.2. This should be undertaken with care and attention to principles of strapping. It is important to prevent replacing one deformity with another. Potential complications should be explained to parents.

Reverse footwear Reverse footwear is an outdated and contraindicated treatment modality that renders the foot at risk of further deformity.

Serial casting Serial casting was popularized by Kite (1950), who considered that using constant corrective force was preferable to 'corrective manipulation' (Case study 15.1 and Fig. 15.3). A constant pressure could be better provided by a plaster of Paris cast placed above the ankle (Box 15.1).

Not all such deformities are totally corrected by serial casting. It is, however, noteworthy that where feet have achieved only 60% correction of the deformity, they often correct spontaneously. Whether this is the result of greater flexibility created by corrective casting is uncertain. In addition, manipulation of the foot by the parents prior to casting seems to shorten the length of treatment.

It is preferable to use serial casts before the child walks. Because of the child's activity level,

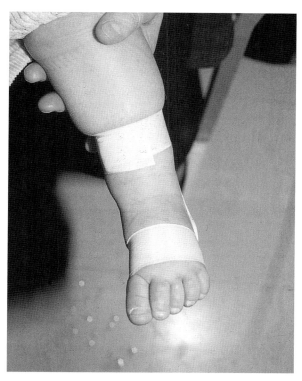

Figure 15.2 Strapping for metatarsus adductus. The strapping is wrapped around the forefoot; the forefoot is pulled into correction and the strapping is secured around the leg.

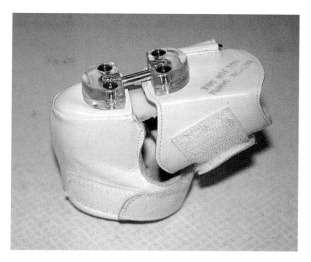

Figure 15.3 The Bebax boot. Triplane adjustment is possible; the ball-and-socket hinge allows the forefoot to be gently pushed into correction while the rearfoot is held in neutral.

weight, height and increasing musculoskeletal rigidity, serial casting is probably not appropriate after 20 months of age. Follow-up treatment to prevent recurrence is often required. In some cases, however, children will not tolerate the plaster of Paris cast and alternative measures

---

Box 15.1 Plaster of Paris casts

Plaster of Paris casts are applied using the following approach. A precast tubular bandage (Tubifast, Seton) is slid over the foot and leg, ending above the knee. Orthopaedic wool (Velband, Johnson and Johnson) is used to wrap over the bandage in order to protect the bony prominences and overlying soft tissue. Two 7.5 cm rolls of wet plaster of Paris are applied from the subtalar joint to just below the patella. As the cast dries, the rearfoot is held very slightly supinated at the subtalar joint, with the ankle at 90°. By dealing with the anatomy in this systematic manner, the possibility of replacing one deformity with another (i.e. valgus rearfoot or ankle equines) is limited. When the first section is dried, another roll of plaster of Paris is extended as far as the toes. The rearfoot is then cupped with the practitioner's dominant hand while the forefoot is pushed into correction using the soft thenar eminence of the other hand. The index finger is placed underneath the forefoot to ensure that the metatarsals do not overlap one another, offering a false impression of correction. The ends of the tubular bandage should be rolled down, having first incorporated sufficient wool packing to prevent chafing of the skin or adverse circulatory compression.

The cast is kept in place for 7 days. The parents are then asked to remove it by soaking it off prior to the next visit. Three to six successive weeks of this treatment constitute the maximum period of time appropriate for this form of therapy. Longer than 6 weeks and it becomes almost inevitable that the leg muscles will atrophy and the skin will start to show rub marks or indeed frank ulceration. The most vulnerable site is the junction of the plantar and dorsal skin at the posterior heel. If ulceration occurs, casting can continue if necessary, although it is important to leave a window in the heel area of the cast.

Extension of the cast above the knee is required if the child has concomitant pathology such as medial genicular position or tibial torsion. Occasionally, the infant will manage repeatedly to push the cast off. This can be overcome by extending the cast above the knee. Extension above the knee should be dealt with only when the foot and leg section is dry and applied in two sections.

Case study 15.1   Metatarsus adductus treated with serial casting

A mother was concerned that her 13-month-old son was pigeon-toed. Shoe fitting was difficult because of the 'banana' shape curve of the child's foot.

On examination, a severe metatarsus adductus was noted with a pronounced medial first metatarsal–cuneiform skin crease. The adducted position of the forefoot could not be reduced with manipulation. On standing, the rearfoot was everted with notable dorsal humping of the midtarsal joint (Fig. 15.3). The complex variant of metatarsus adductus (skewfoot) was diagnosed on the basis of the rearfoot eversion in the presence of metatarsus adductus (Berg 1986).

Treatment consisted of serial casting. The child tolerated this well. After 7 weeks of casting, muscle atrophy of the leg was noted and the child had developed a painful preulcerative lesion on the posterior surface of both heels. The adductus deformity of the foot had improved by some 60% but the heel remained in eversion on weight bearing. Although far from corrected, the foot was much more flexible and could now be corrected by manipulation, which, according to Pentz & Weiner (1993), is an important prerequisite for spontaneous correction.

A suspension cast of the foot was then taken non-weight bearing and a functional orthosis was made with a high medial flange and a deep heel seat to create a corrective abduction force on the forefoot while restricting excessive pronation of the rearfoot. Vitrathene clogs were also provided for night-time wear.

The child was reviewed every 2 months and improvement was noted at each follow-up; by the time the child was 4 years old the metatarsus adductus had corrected. The foot, however, remained excessively pronated, with a low arch and medial bulging associated with the talonavicular joint. Orthotic management would be continued to control the excessive pronation.

Comment: Manipulation or casting under tension in an inappropriate manner can cause severe damage to the mesenchymal precursor to bone and hence can lead to further deformity once the deformed cartilage has matured. Cartilage is easier to deform than tight ligaments or tendons and will yield without the inexperienced practitioner realizing, causing such problems as rocker-bottom flat feet.

---

must be sought. Failure is often inevitable where casts are applied to children who are too old.

Adjustable shoes   Bebax boots are split into forefoot and rearfoot sections, connected by a ball-and-socket type hinge (Fig. 15.4). The multiaxial connector enables the forefoot to be moved in any of the three body planes independently of the rearfoot position. Although expensive, the boots can be supplied in a number of different sizes and provide an excellent medium for correcting forefoot deformity. These are a non-weight-bearing mode of treatment.

Corrective orthoses   Clogs manufactured from heat-mouldable material (e.g. Vitrathene) may be fabricated for the individual; these maintain the foot in a rectus alignment during gait (Fig. 15.5). While the forefoot is held in a corrected position, a neutral suspension cast is taken. A

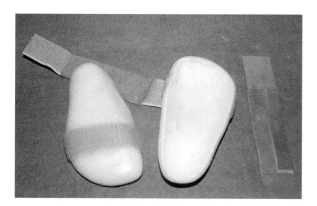

Figure 15.4   Vitrathene orthotic clogs for metatarsus adductus, shown with separate velcro straps.

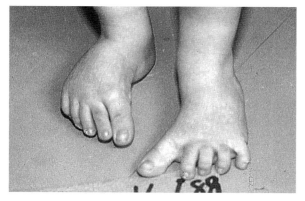

Figure 15.5   Skewfoot: where metatarsus adductus is complicated by rearfoot eversion.

high-sided Vitrathene clog is then vacuum moulded around the positive cast. The inside may be lined with a material of choice to increase comfort. The base of the device may then be finished with a layer of non-slip material such as ethylene vinyl acetate to ensure the child can ambulate safely. From experience, it has been found that it is beneficial to attach the Velcro straps at fitting. This ensures that the foot is securely held within the device.

An alternative therapy may be provided with the use of the child's previous size footwear. If a child has grown out of the footwear in length, then the distal toe box of the shoe can be removed, leaving the complete sole intact and exposing the toes. Bevelled material of appropriate thickness is applied over the cuboid and along the medial aspect of the first metatarsophalangeal joint on the upper of the shoe. This gives a contralateral pressure to the medial forefoot and lateral rearfoot to promote rectus alignment. A very simple effective ambulatory device is produced.

TALIPES EQUINOVARUS

Talipes equinovarus (CTEV), often referred to as clubfoot, is a deformity where the ankle is plantarflexed, the rearfoot supinated and the forefoot adducted. The complex nature of this triplanar deformity make it a challenging condition to treat successfully. Early treatment is indicated, and the nature of management is largely determined by the extent of the rigidity of the deformity. The deformity is assessed by manual manipulation of the ankle, subtalar and midtarsal joints. If each of these joint complexes is found to be flexible, then application of a plaster of Paris cast that extends above the knee may be used to correct both the tibial and foot components of the deformity. Classically, the deformity is treated serially, adductus, varus then the equinus components in sequence. However, in practice with small limbs, practitioner's tend to correct all components of the deformity together. A commonly utilized technique is to hold the forefoot parallel to the rearfoot while the frontal plane bisection of the heel is held parallel to the

leg. At the same time, the foot is dorsiflexed to a 90° angle with the leg. Casts should be changed weekly and the position of the three involved joints and their ranges of motion assessed. If casting fails, then early referral for surgery is indicated. In the surgical management of CTEV, soft tissue division of tight tendons and ligaments is the initial treatment, followed at a later date with bone and joint surgery if appropriate. A recently developed surgical treatment utilizes the Ilizarov technique and has demonstrated promising results.

ARCH HEIGHT

The arch height is a common concern for parents and practitioners. A thorough assessment should be undertaken to establish whether the foot reflects normal developmental parameters (Fig. 15.6). Assessment findings should be related to clinical features to confirm whether the foot arch is normal or otherwise. Low medial longitudinal arches probably attract more concern than high arches. Afro-Caribbeans have a low calcaneal inclination angle, commonly resulting in a low arch profile without symptoms. Careful examination and family history must be undertaken. It is important not to forget the influence of neuromuscular conditions and systemic conditions such as juvenile idiopathic arthritis, which can have a profound effect upon the foot.

Flexible flat foot

In the prewalking child or toddler, the medial longitudinal arch of the foot is poorly developed, largely because in the early years of life the calcaneus lies parallel to the ground (Wenger et al 1989). By 4 or 5 years of age, the calcaneus inclines to form an angle of 13–18° with the ground through developmental ontogeny. Low, or indeed absent, arches are, therefore, not a reliable sign of abnormal foot position or function. Subluxed talonavicular joint demonstrated as medial bulging, everted relaxed calcaneal stance position and forefoot abduction are more significant findings indicating excessive pronation of

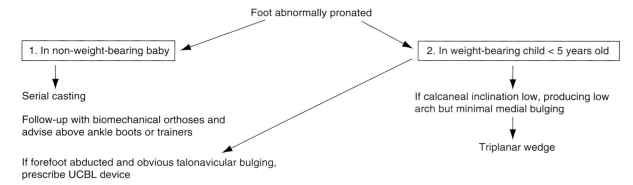

Foot abnormally pronated

1. In non-weight-bearing baby

Serial casting

Follow-up with biomechanical orthoses and advise above ankle boots or trainers

If forefoot abducted and obvious talonavicular bulging, prescribe UCBL device

2. In weight-bearing child < 5 years old

If calcaneal inclination low, producing low arch but minimal medial bulging

Triplanar wedge

Follow-up every 6 months, checking arch index and vagus index. Discharge when foot within normal values

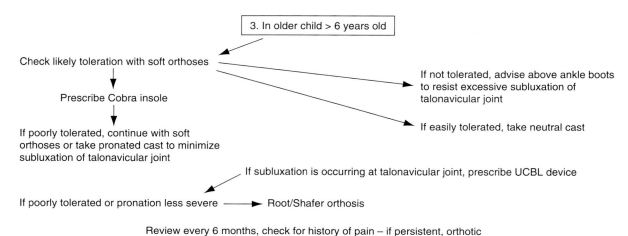

3. In older child > 6 years old

Check likely toleration with soft orthoses

Prescribe Cobra insole

If poorly tolerated, continue with soft orthoses or take pronated cast to minimize subluxation of talonavicular joint

If not tolerated, advise above ankle boots to resist excessive subluxation of talonavicular joint

If easily tolerated, take neutral cast

If subluxation is occurring at talonavicular joint, prescribe UCBL device

If poorly tolerated or pronation less severe ⟶ Root/Shafer orthosis

Review every 6 months, check for history of pain – if persistent, orthotic control inadequate. Also review shoe wear, Rose and Staheli index values

Figure 15.6 Flat foot algorithm. UCBL, University of California Biomechanics Laboratory orthosis.

the foot (Fig. 15.7). In the newborn, observation may reveal asymmetry and absence of normal motion. In the child who is not yet walking, observation with the limbs hanging dependent may demonstrate an abnormal foot position. If the prewalker's foot is pronated, and manipulation of the foot fails to correct this position, mild calcaneovalgus may be suspected and treatment should be considered (Fig. 15.8).

Treatment of calcaneovalgus in the newborn child aims to restore the foot to a plantar grade position without adverse effects on the talocrural and midtarsal joint complex. Flexibility of the

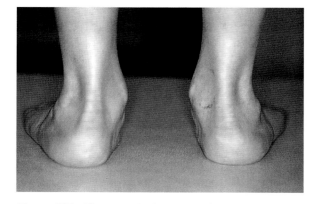

Figure 15.7 The excessively pronated foot.

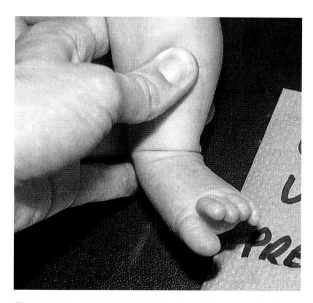

Figure 15.8 Mild calcaneovalgus in a 12-week-old infant.

foot is probably greatest in the younger child. Therefore, the earlier treatment begins, the easier it will be to achieve correction. In very mild flexible feet, manipulation of the foot by the parents may be helpful. Manipulation involves placing the parent's hand on the dorsum of the child's foot and asking them to push the foot down into plantarflexion. Plantarflexion force will supinate the foot, bringing it into a neutral position while freeing up the ankle range of motion. The parent should hold the foot for several minutes at a time, regularly repeating the exercise. Manipulation therapy should be closely supervised by the practitioner; if the foot fails to respond, serial casting may be considered.

Applying plaster of Paris to the limb and then manipulating the foot into maximum plantarflexion is more effective than parental manipulation. The duration of casting may be several weeks.

Once the episode of serial casting is complete, the parents should be encouraged to continue with manipulation of the foot in the prewalker. In the toddler, an orthosis should be used to maintain the corrected position of the foot and prevent it from relapsing into pronation. An orthosis with a deep heel seat of 20–30 mm is vital to resist pronatory forces. Continuous monitoring is advised until the child is at least 6 years of age.

Orthotic treatment in paediatrics remains controversial. The neonate has a normal varus foot position, which reduces with normal ontological changes of the talus. In a study that independently measured talar neck rotation and then the angle of forefoot varus in cadaver specimens, it was disputed whether there was any correlation between the two (McPoil et al 1987).

In situations where prescription orthoses are indicated, the practitioner must prevent abnormal compensation without hindering normal development.

Orthopaedic research has seriously questioned the value of the orthosis because a number of studies have found that the medial longitudinal arch is not raised after sustained wear (Mereday et al 1972, Penneau et al 1982, Wenger et al 1989). It must be emphasized, however, that the exponents of functional orthoses have never claimed that they would improve the arch. Orthoses are prescribed to prevent progressive subluxation of the midtarsal joint complex by reducing the need for compensatory motion.

Ironically, there is also support in the orthopaedic literature for the prescription of orthoses in the treatment of flat feet. Rose developed a 'pronatormeter', which determined the effect of a Rose–Schwartz meniscus on the frontal position of the rearfoot by measuring external rotation of the tibia. The meniscus orthosis was found to produce much greater external rotation of the leg than the simple medial heel wedge (Rose 1958, 1962). This effect forms the basis of orthotic prescription by using antipronatory in-shoe devices to prevent progressive subluxation of the midtarsal region through subtalar joint control (Fig. 15.9).

Orthoses of the Shaffer and Root types assist rearfoot control by means of both forefoot and rearfoot posts (Tollafield & Pratt 1990). The arch area of the orthosis is important for no other reason than that it connects the rearfoot and forefoot posts. Indeed in the Root orthosis, the arch is deliberately lowered during fabrication of the device in order to improve tolerance.

The Cobra insole is a useful extension of the Rose–Schwartz meniscus incorporating a valgus filler (Fig. 15.10). It can be fabricated in felt material as a temporary measure, during consultation, to determine the potential efficacy of prescription treatment. A satisfactory outcome of the temporary device will influence the prescription. The choice of materials will be determined by the amount of control required.

The child receiving orthotic treatment should be reviewed periodically. Details of any aches or pains should be documented. Orthotic fit should be reviewed, as should signs of 'bottoming out' of the orthotic materials. Tools such as Staheli's arch index (Staheli et al 1987) and Rose's valgus index (Rose et al 1985) may have a use in monitoring the patient. These evaluations are made from ink prints of the contact area of the foot using a Harris mat. The Staheli technique records the height of the medial longitudinal arch, while the Rose valgus index determines medial displacement of the medial malleolus, which will occur as the rearfoot everts. Both techniques provide an objective means of recording the foot's abnormality that are useful when reporting the effect of treatment. The decision to discontinue treatment may be influenced by a significant improvement in the arch and valgus index values (Case study 15.2). These techniques must be used in combination with sound clinical observation and interpretation.

Rigid flat foot

Not all flat feet respond to orthoses. Failure to achieve an arch form when the hallux is extended (Jack's test) or when the patient is asked to stand on tiptoe implies that some resistance is present within the tarsus. This resistance can often be associated with spasm or articular limitation, for example various tarsal coalitions with or without peroneal spasm, congenital vertical talus and certain neurological conditions.

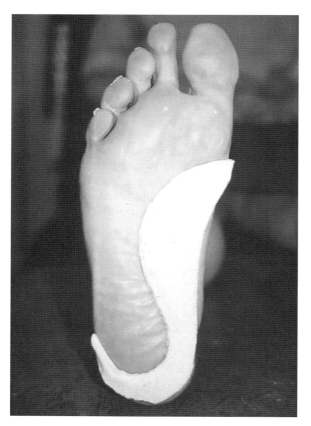

Figure 15.10 The Cobra pad is based on a valgus pad with a meniscus heel.

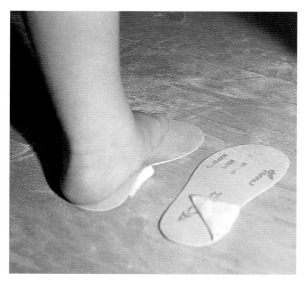

Figure 15.9 The triplanar wedge for limiting of excessive pronation of the foot in a child under 5 years of age.

Case study 15.2   Flexible flat foot

A 7-year-old boy complained of pain in the area of the tibialis anterior muscle belly and the medial longitudinal arch of both feet. His family history was significant in that his father had severely pronated but asymptomatic feet. The patient's foot had marked talonavicular bulging, forefoot abductus, a positive Helbing's sign and absent medial longitudinal arch. Excessive medial heel wear was noted in the shoes. Staheli arch index measurement was 1.4 (normal value for this age group is 0.5–1.2) and the Rose valgus index was 27 (normal is 0.20). The boy also had recurvatum of both knees and elbows. While standing with knees fully extended, he could touch the floor with both palms, and his thumb and fifth fingers could be hyperextended past 90°, indicating ligamentous laxity.

The symptoms were considered to result from overuse and an aphasic tibialis anterior muscle, which failed to decelerate excessive pronation of the forefoot. Chronic soft tissue strain of the structures of the medial longitudinal arch was also diagnosed in association with tissue tenderness.

A Cobra insole was prescribed as the first line of treatment. The patient returned 4 weeks later. The insole was easily tolerated and the pain in the anterior tibia had resolved, although the child still complained that the feet ached after standing.

A neutral cast was then taken and a UCBL (University of California Biomechanics Laboratory) device was fabricated from polypropylene. When supplied to the patient, this device could not be tolerated because of irritation in the arch area of the foot. The positive neutral cast was then modified with plaster in the longitudinal arch to lower the orthotic plate. A Root orthosis was manufactured and this time the medial longitudinal arch pain responded to treatment as the orthosis was tolerated.

Review should continue every 6 months; arch and valgus indices are measured at each follow-up. The objective of treatment is to prevent further subluxation of the talonavicular joint and alleviate all soft tissue strain. Neither child nor parents expect correction of the foot, only prevention of further symptoms.

Radiographs may be indicated to exclude bony pathology.

Tarsal coalitions

Pain in the region of the subtalar and midtarsal joints may, in rare circumstances, relate to tarsal coalition. This may present as a fibrous, cartilaginous or osseous union of two or more tarsal bones and is of congenital origin. The union or bar that bridges joints is not visible on plain radiographs until ossification is complete. Talocalcaneal and calcaneonavicular coalitions are the most common forms of coalition and their presence can lead to peroneal spasm. Other types of coalitions are rarely reported (Fig. 15.11). The coalition is bilateral in approximately 50% of those affected.

The symptoms often present in the second decade of life with mild deep pain in the subtalar joint and stiffness of the foot. The onset of pain is determined by the age at which the cartilaginous coalition begins to ossify. Complaints of foot pain may be aggravated by activity and relieved by rest.

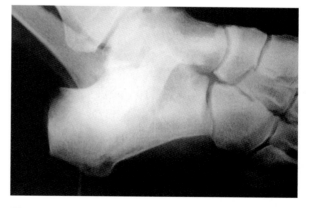

Figure 15.11 A talonavicular coalition. This is a very rare form of tarsal coalition, with few cases having been reported in the literature.

A middle facet talocalcaneal coalition is more likely to lead to severe pronation of the foot than any other coalition. Concomitant spasm of the peroneal muscles may occur intermittently or continuously. This may result from intra-articular effusion within the subtalar joint, causing a protective reflex spasm of the peroneal tendons. This is thought to occur because the posterior subtalar joint intra-articular pressure is less in eversion than in inversion. Alternatively, spasm may be a consequence of adaptive shortening of the peroneal tendons secondary to the pronated position of the foot, or the result of synovial irritation caused by the disturbed mechanics of the foot irritating the peroneal tendons. The use of a local anaesthetic to block the common peroneal nerve just below the neck of the fibular is useful in relieving muscle spasm and will assist with diagnosis. Any residual pain can be resolved by an injection of local anaesthetic directly into the sinus tarsi.

If pain persists, surgical resection of the coalition is indicated. Resection of the bone with soft tissue interposition is suggested for a calcaneonavicular coalition. This is easier to manage surgically than the talocalcaneal coalition, which requires an arthrodesis because the joint cannot be salvaged. Severe unremitting pain may require a triple arthrodesis.

Congenital vertical talus

Congenital vertical talus involves extensive mechanical derangement. It is often known as 'rocker-bottom foot' because of the medial convex shape along the medial border, creating the most severe form of flat foot. Another condition associated with this foot shape is a severe equinus deformity. Both foot shapes, once developed, can cause significant management problems.

Complications associated with this condition may arise with concomitant problems such as spina bifida with myelomeningocele, neurofibromatosis, arthrogryposis and unilateral limb shortening. Multiple defects have been noted, which may include congenital dislocation of the hips. The presence of such problems means that a multidisciplinary approach is desirable. Poor walking ability as a result of skeletal dysfunction may require the input of other disciplines such as physiotherapy and occupational therapy.

In congenital vertical talus, the foot will have the characteristics of eversion and abduction of the forefoot in addition to some forefoot rotation. The heel will appear smaller and rounded prox-

imally. The medial arch will have full contact with the ground because the talus will have adopted a vertical position. Because much of the pathology arises during development, the soft tissue structures are contracted laterally and stretched medially.

There are a number of treatment approaches. First, manipulation will assist to stretch the soft tissues and is most effective at 3–8 days after birth (Becker-Anderson & Reimann 1974). Second, bespoke shoes incorporating custom-made moulded insoles may be required to provide protection. Finally, surgical reduction will prevent long-term cartilage damage and growth disturbance.

Conservative treatment   The objective of conservative treatment is to reduce the talonavicular dislocation, concentrating on the following areas:

- the equinus factor
- pronation of the hindfoot
- stretching the peroneal muscles
- adduction of the forefoot
- toe extensors and ankle dorsiflexors.

The technique involves dorsiflexing the calcaneus with the triceps surae (tendo Achilles) stretched for the count of 10. The calcaneofibular ligament is also stretched by pulling the calcaneus distally. The ankle dorsiflexors are stretched by plantarflexion of the forefoot with adduction.

Manipulations are performed for 15 minutes each, to the count of 10 before release in the newborn child. Tincture of benzoin is painted on the skin and the deformity placed in a cast for maintenance of correction. A thermoplastic splint can be used to continue tension on the contracted structures.

Specialized footwear will be required to accommodate the deformity. It is essential that the shoe has no shank. Severe deformities will shorten the life of the shoe. A soft orthosis ranging from foamed polyethylene (Plastazote) to polyurethane foam (Poron) will protect excessive pressure along the medial structures associated with the vertical talus and navicular, and should be ordered with bespoke footwear.

Surgery As with CTEV, surgery succeeds if undertaken early, and before 2.5 years. Beyond 6 years of age, the deformity will become rigid, and cutaneous pressure problems will start to occur. Soft-tissue release is preferred without articular interference; the forefoot is corrected first and the rearfoot last. Excision of the navicular has been used with some success, the talus being pinned through to the first metatarsal (Clark et al 1977). Casting is essential to maintain correction. Tight structures such as the tendo Achilles must be lengthened and the medial structures must be shortened by plication. The use of the above procedure, however, can lead to shortening of the medial side of the foot. Any aggressive disturbance of the blood supply to the head of the talus will result in avascular necrosis.

Juvenile idiopathic arthritis

The problems and risks associated with juvenile idiopathic arthritis, a systemic autoimmune disorder of collagen, will be dealt with in Chapter 17. All the joints of the lower limb can be affected by this disabling condition. Management of this disease requires a multidisciplinary approach. Podiatric treatment of foot deformities with both digital and functional orthoses is paramount in order to control soft tissue, bony and joint deformities. Regular monitoring and follow-up is essential to prevent deterioration of foot pathology.

Foot orthoses are worn during the day, and specially designed splints are required at night to prevent the development of a fixed frontal or sagittal plane deformity.

Excessive abnormal pronation is a common problem and requires orthoses with high heel cups to provide sufficient control. Where orthoses cannot be used to correct fixed subtalar and ankle joint deformity, patients will undergo either a process of serial casting or manipulation under general anaesthetic. This will then be followed by the use of orthoses. Deformities of the great toe can be corrected by custom-made night splints. Exercise is maintained together with any drug regimens and gentle manipulation. During active phases of the disease, when joint effusion is greater, weight bearing should be reduced; however, younger children will be encouraged to use tricycles to retain independence in addition to maintenance of muscle strength and function. Surgical correction is only indicated when conservative treatment has failed.

Rigid high arch (pes cavus)

Pes cavus may be asymptomatic until adolescence. A high percentage of cavoid feet are related to neurological conditions (e.g. Charcot–Marie–Tooth disease, a relatively common disease affecting the motor and sensory peripheral pathways). In pes cavus, the foot becomes progressively higher arched and rigid. The usual presentation is when the forefoot is everted in relationship to the rearfoot, which may be more pronounced if the first ray is plantarflexed. The need for supinatory compensation results in the arch becoming progressively higher. This compensation leads to instability of the lateral ankle and may result in inversion sprains. With progression of the deformity, the soft tissue structures contract to claw the lesser digits and dorsal humping is evident over the metatarsocuneiform area of the foot. Treatment may be palliative; however, in the early stages of the deformity, a lateral forefoot wedge to reduce supinatory compensation may reduce problems associated with this foot type and slow down progression.

Footwear that is shock absorbing and has adequate room to accommodate the deformity is desirable. Fabrication of orthoses to protect the foot and ankle from damage are essential. Appropriate footcare advise for the age of the child should be given, which may include the use of emollients and pumice to prevent hyperkeratoses. Exercise therapy is advisable to maintain available ankle joint range of motion as pes cavus is always associated with a tight heel cord. In neurological conditions, it is important to maintain function in affected muscle groups (e.g. peroneal muscles). Appropriate massage and stretching programmes may be advocated.

HALLUX VALGUS

Hallux valgus is the most common first meta-tarsophalangeal joint deformity. The condition progresses and ultimately involves the whole of the forefoot with splaying and lesser digital deformities.

Screening and monitoring

It is in recognizing the progressive nature of hal-lux valgus that the practitioner can be most use-ful. Monitoring the progress of the condition is imperative and should be undertaken annually by measuring the first metatarsophalangeal joint angle with a digital goniometer while the child stands in their angle and base of gait (Fig. 15.12).

Radiographs are indicated only when pre-surgical evaluation is required. They are useful in demonstrating the first metatarsophalangeal joint angle, first–second intermetatarsal angle and sesamoid position, all of which need to be corrected in hallux valgus surgery (Fig. 15.13). The above radiological features also correlate directly with the severity of the hallux valgus angle (Mann & Coughlin, 2001). The metatarso-phalangeal joint space will reduce with the onset of degenerative joint disease, an important cause of pain in the condition and almost certainly a consequence of maltracking of the joint.

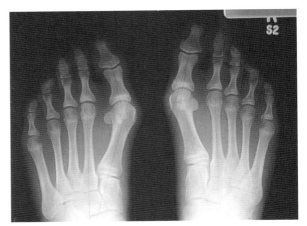

A

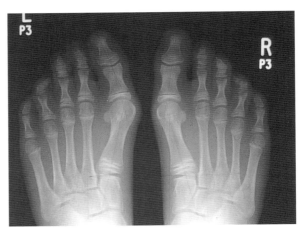

B

Figure 15.13 Weight-bearing radiographs of hallus valgus. Deterioration in juvenile hallux valgus between open (B) and closure of the epiphyses (A). Note the changes in first–second intermetatarsal angle, first metatarsal sesamoid position and first metatarsal–phalangeal joint space.

Figure 15.12 Measuring the first metatarsophalangeal angle with a digital goniometer.

Orthotic management

The aetiology of hallux valgus is multifactorial. If all factors were taken into account, there is no reason why treatment would not be more successful. The concept of abnormal pronation being a factor in the development of hallux valgus is controversial. However, if a plantarflexed first ray is subjected to ground reaction force and does not have an adequate range of dorsiflexion to compensate, then mechanically the movement of the first ray will follow the line of least resistance. The metatarsal will move medially as the hallux moves laterally. The hallux abductus angle would, therefore, increase. If orthoses play a part in the treatment of hallux valgus, then the child and parent should be informed of the progressive nature of the condition and that the orthoses are to improve overall foot function with a possible desirable effect on the pain associated with hallux valgus. Night splints have shown to be an effective treatment for hallux valgus (Groisso 1992); however, they do not prevent progression but may slow the overall process down.

Commercially made night splints are readily available and may have a role in conservative management. Regular review of treatment and continued monitoring are essential. Surgery may be considered where the deformity has advanced and the hallux abuts against the second toe. It is at this point that the condition progresses rapidly. The first–second intermetatarsal angle widens as the proximal phalanx of the hallux begins to act like a wedge to drive the first metatarsal into varus. As the deformity advances, the lateral pressure of the hallux may cause deformity of the lesser toes.

Surgery

The use of surgery to manage hallux valgus may be appropriate to improve footwear fit and prevent secondary problems. The selection of the appropriate procedure is critical to preserve epiphyses and blood supply in the growing foot. The decision to undertake surgery should be carefully considered. It is best left to those conditions in which the deformity is marked, where the child is experiencing continual pain and where secondary changes arise, such as significant clawing of the lesser toes or subluxation of a second toe at its metatarsophalangeal joint. The appropriate surgical management of this condition is discussed in Chapters 7 and 14.

LESSER DIGITAL DEFORMITY

Toe abnormalities associated with the second to fifth toes are very common and can affect very young children. They cover a spectrum of deformity from mild burrowing of the fifth toe to adductovarus of the lateral three toes, or dorsal displacement of the second toe (Fig. 15.14).

Slight malalignment of the fourth and fifth digits may be considered innocuous. Treatment, however, should be instigated if the digital deformity meets the following criteria:

- apical weight bearing with clawing of the lesser toes
- transverse plane deformities of adjacent toes; this can lead to loss of the buttress effect, particularly concerning the second toe, and lateral deviation of the hallux.

Toe deformity is difficult to treat in young children because the toes are small and difficult to hold in a corrected position. In mild deformity, the toes will often improve through the influence

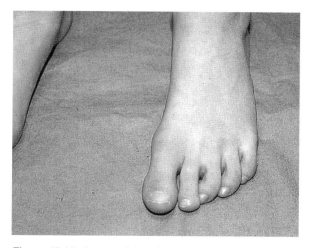

Figure 15.14 Lesser digit deformity in a 7-year-old child.

of the intrinsic muscles when the child establishes a heel-to-toe gait. These muscles primarily function during midstance and propulsion. With advancing age of the child, compliance with treatment improves. If treatment is appropriate, toes may be splinted into a corrected position by taping, silicone devices or using a rubber dam (latex band) (Fig. 15.15).

Deformity in the sagittal plane corrects earlier than other planes, which may resist correction. The objective of treatment must be to restore toe purchase and realign the sagittal position of the three phalanges. Once the proximal phalanx is restored to a neutral position, splinting should be initiated for 1 month and the child should be encouraged to wear the device day and night. Progress should be reviewed and treatment continued if correction is identified.

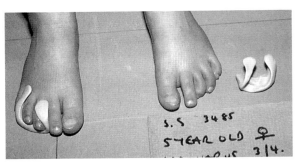

A

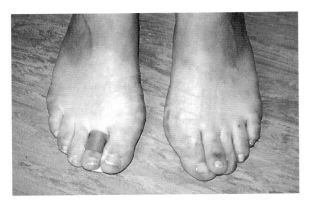

B

Figure 15.15 Treating digital deformity. A, Silicone splints for lesser digit deformity. B, Rubber dam for correction of a dorsiflexed digit.

Polydactyly and syndactyly

Polydactyly and syndactyly are less common. Polydactyly is best dealt with in the infant. Surgical excision of the accessory digit is required in most instances, although in poorly formed digits, devoid of bony or cartilaginous structures, the tourniquet amputation, where a tight thread is drawn around the base of the digit, works well.

Syndactyly is rarely a significant problem in the foot, unlike the hand where it will affect dexterity. The most common presentation is syndactyly of the second and third toes up to the level of the proximal interphalangeal joint; this is known as *zygodactyly*. The concern is usually cosmetic only and reassurance should be given. Desyndactylization can only be achieved surgically and carries a high risk of interdigital necrosis because of the proximity of the syndactyly to the neurovascular bundle of the digit.

Surgery

Surgical correction of digital deformity appears to be highly effective (Ross & Menelaus 1984, Hamer et al 1993). Flexor tenotomy or transfer is performed when the digits are flexible and easily corrected by manual manipulation. Arthrodesis of the distal or proximal interphalangeal joint is indicated when the deformity is rigid. Painful apical weight bearing is a reasonable justification for such intervention. Arthrodesis is considerably more complicated than a flexor release performed alone. The simple flexor release is very successful if undertaken before the joint becomes ankylosed. Flexor stab incisions can be performed through a plantar approach. Splinting with silicone devices may be used as an adjunct to surgery.

PAIN IN THE LOWER LIMB

FOOT PAIN

Foot pain is relatively rare among children. In most cases, the history of the complaint will often provide the diagnosis; however, other investigations such as radiographs may be indicated to exclude other pathology. Many causes of juvenile foot pain are developmental abnormalities of bone and joint. Unremitting pain of a non-specific nature must be considered seriously, with early referral to the appropriate specialty.

Sever's disease

Heel pain in children is seen in Sever's disease, which is a traction apophysitis of the tendo Achilles at its insertion into the calcaneus. This characteristically affects children between 8 and 15 years. Treatment involves reducing the traction that may be created by a tight tendo Achilles acting at the developing calcaneal epiphysis.

The child should be encouraged to wear training shoes with a shock-absorbing insole or heel pad, with rearfoot medial wedging if indicated. Materials used should enable functional reduction of traction. Rehabilitation of the posterior leg muscles may involve massage and stretching of the muscles. Physical modalities (e.g. rest, ice, compression and elevation) may be indicated initially. The child should be reassured that the pain will resolve once the calcaneal epiphysis closes (Case study 15.3).

The result of a severe apophysitis may result in Haglund deformity.

Osteochondroses

Avascular necrosis can occur at various sites in the skeleton of the growing child.

Kohler's disease

Localized tenderness and swelling over the navicular bone in children aged between 3 and 5 years of age should lead the practitioner to suspect Kohler's disease. The onset of the pain in the midfoot can coincide with unusual physical activity or trauma to the area. If Kohler's disease is suspected, the foot should be radiographed. The characteristic radiographic features of increased density of the navicular bone with sclerosis and flattening help to confirm the diagnosis.

Simple insoles to reduce excessive pronation and protection over the navicular may be indicated to reduce symptoms. The application of strapping to reduce excessive pronation and rest the navicular may be warranted (e.g. 'J', low-dye and high-dye strapping). If pain is acute then immobilization may be indicated, but with extreme care. Removable splints may facilitate graded exercises to prevent wasting of soft tissues. Prevention of complications caused by immobilization must be avoided (e.g. reflex sympathetic dystrophy). While in some children the navicular may settle in shape and density within 3–7 months; in others it may take 2–4 years

---

Case study 15.3 Apophysitis

A 12-year-old boy presented with pain in his left heel after games. As a keen footballer, he had already consulted another practitioner, who considered the problem to be caused by the studs on his football boots. Subsequently, the patient had been playing football in normal shoes but found the problem was no better. Although the parents had at one time thought that the problem was nothing more than growing pains, they were becoming increasingly concerned about the chronic nature of the condition.

Examination revealed poor flexibility of the posterior calf muscles, with restricted ankle joint dorsiflexion. Upon palpating the calcaneus, the pain produced was similar to that brought on by activity.

The patient was advised to embark upon regular but gentle gastrocnemius stretching exercises. He was also advised to wear running shoes as much as possible. A functional insole with a heel raise was placed in the shoes. Four weeks later, the child was reviewed. He reported that while the pain had improved considerably, the heel still ached after football. The patient was advised that complete resolution would occur in time.

Comment: Unresolved pain in the heel will require further investigation to exclude bone cysts and avulsion fractures. Casting is reserved for intractable apophysitis for 6–8 weeks. Extended periods of immobility may benefit from bivalved casts or stock prefabricated casts (Air Cast).

(Ferguson & Gingrich 1957). What is significant is that the navicular always returns to its normal shape and density.

Freiberg's disease

Freiberg's disease is a degenerative aseptic necrosis of the secondary ossification centre of a lesser metatarsal head. It commonly affects children in the second decade, with slightly higher incidence in females. The condition frequently causes chronic pain; in the long term, it causes degenerative changes within the metatarsophalangeal joint (Fig. 15.16). The second metatarsal head is most commonly affected, followed by the third. This condition in the fourth metatarsal head is rare, while involvement of the fifth is unlikely (Gauthier & Elbaz 1979).

Freiberg's disease presents as a history of aching or sharp pain localized to the metatarsal head, which is aggravated by physical activity and characterized on examination by a palpable thickening of the metatarsal head. Radiographic examination shows a square, flattened metatarsal head sometimes with evidence of loose bony fragments. Range of motion at the joint is restricted.

Immobilizing the metatarsophalangeal joint motion may reduce symptoms. Immobilization may be in the form of extended polypropylene orthoses to reduce the motion at the metatarsals and provide rest. The outcome depends on the time elapsed until diagnosis and the resultant joint changes. Small cartilage and osseous fragments may produce synovitis as they become compressed with movement of the metatarsophalangeal joint. Smith et al (1991) found that some 50% of those examined improved with conservative treatment. The remainder required surgery. Current procedures may include cheilectomy or a decompression osteotomy. Smillie (1967) recommended the use of autogenous bone chips grafted into the damaged metatarsal head, recreating the articular dome. Often the surgeon sees Freiberg's disease too late for this to be effective, as radiographic changes are poorly identified on plain radiographs. Gauthier & Elbaz's (1979) procedure has proven

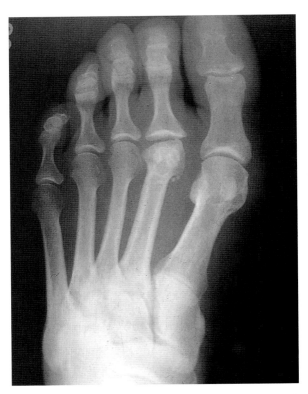

Figure 15.16 Freiberg's disease of the second metatarsal head. Note the classic flattened head compared with the other metatarsals.

successful where the disease has developed. A dorsiflexory osteotomy can restore joint function, remove diseased and deformed bone and decompress the joint (Fig. 15.17). Early recovery is one of the greatest benefits of this approach, and internal fixation is not necessary provided that close attention is paid to capsular repair (Tollafield 1993).

Other osteochondroses of the foot and ankle can include Treves disease (sesamoids), Buschke disease (cuneiforms), Mouchet syndrome (talus), Haglund disease (accessory navicular) and Iselin disease (styloid process). The last has been reclassified as a traction apophysitis.

LEG AND KNEE PAIN

While the diagnosis and treatment of the foot may appear isolated, the influence of the leg,

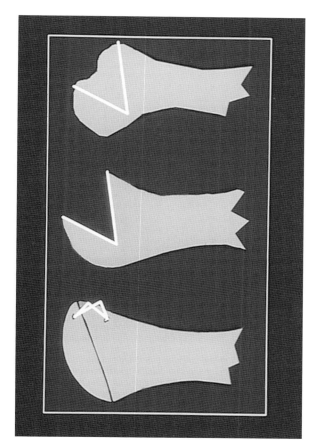

Figure 15.17 Dorsiflexory osteotomy. Removal of a wedge of bone from the metaphyseal area of the metatarsal will rotate the articular surface of the metatarsal head so that the healthy cartilage-covered plantar condyles articulate with the base of the proximal phalanx. The wedge of bone resected from the metatarsal neck is triangular in shape, with the apex of the triangle directed plantarly (Reproduced with permission from Tollafield (1993).)

many conditions that affect the leg are outside the scope of this book. Pain in a child's legs should always be taken seriously. A detailed assessment of the main body systems will elicit the cause of the pain. In many cases, the problem is discomfort during periods of growth.

Pain during periods of growth

Commonly, patients between the ages of 6 and 12 years present with symptoms of pain. In many cases, the pain is the result of poor muscle flexibility, as bone has a tendency to grow at a faster rate than soft tissue, which lags behind. This produces periodic transient tightness of muscle groups (e.g. hamstrings and gastrocnemius).

Tight hamstrings will often lead to nocturnal discomfort in the posterior knee. Stretching exercises shown to the parent, to be performed on the child, will help to alleviate the complaint. Massage and warmth may provide relief from spasm.

If pain presents with fever and general malaise then further investigations are indicated. The possibility of soft tissue or bony infection must be excluded. The tests may include urinalysis, blood tests and radiographs. Blood cultures may not show raised leucocytic activity initially. Erythrocyte sedimentation rates and C-reactive protein assays should be undertaken together with plain radiographs and bone scans. A C-reactive protein blood test is more sensitive in the early stages of inflammatory processes (Lodwick et al 1995).

Osgood–Schlatter disease

Osgood–Schlatter disease is a traction apophysitis of the tibial tuberosity, typically seen in the 10–15 year age group. There is higher incidence in males because of their greater participation in sport. Conservative care comprises moderation of sporting activities, reduction of inflammation with cold modalities and rehabilitation of the quadriceps. In severe cases, a knee brace together with an intensive course of physiotherapy is recommended. The use of anti-inflammatory drugs, including hydrocortisone, is controversial.

acting superiorly to the foot and ankle, cannot be excluded from treatment. Common conditions affecting the leg and knee will be discussed, together with differential diagnostic considerations. Orthoses are commonly used to manage non-specific disorders of the leg successfully, but a judicious approach is always important and a second opinion is suggested if doubt arises with the primary diagnosis. The reader is, therefore, recommended to refer to texts dedicated to the lower limb for further details of treatment, as

Surgical options are not generally recommended. A tell-tale sign of a previous incidence of Osgood–Schlatter disease is an enlarged tibial tuberosity.

Anterior knee pain

Anterior knee pain is very common among mid-adolescent girls (Case study 15.4). Treatment will aim to:

- improve patella position
- restore normal muscle equilibrium to the quadriceps and hamstring muscles.

A high Q (quadriceps) angle (Fig. 15.18) is thought to result from internal femoral position. A high Q angle can be reduced when an orthosis is placed beneath the foot (D'Amico & Rubin 1986). The orthosis is thought to supinate the subtalar joint, producing external rotation of the leg. With reduction of the Q angle, the patella may be positioned more satisfactorily in the intertrochanteric fossa of the femur. This will alleviate the shearing of the patella against the femoral condyles, which is associated with patel-

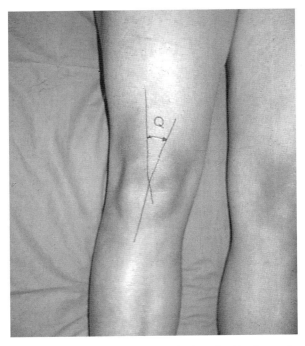

Figure 15.18 The quadriceps angle described by the angle between two lines: one drawn from the anterior superior iliac spine to the centre of the patella and the other drawn from the tibial tuberosity to the centre of the patella.

Case study 15.4 Anterior knee pain

An overweight 14-year-old girl complained of aching behind her knee caps. The pain had been present for at least a year and appeared to be deteriorating. She had been excused from all field games because the knee kept 'giving way' and was made more painful by activity. Since developing the knee pain, she had also missed many days from school because she had found that climbing the school staircases aggravated the pain. Ibuprofen had been prescribed by her GP in order to keep her pain free at school.

On examination, both knees were very sensitive to patella compression; flexing the knee and lateral pressure aggravated the symptoms. Palpation of the posterior medial facet of the patella indicated no fissuring, suggested by the absence of crepitus. The patient was asked to stand and squat; she flexed the knees slowly but only achieved half squat position because the pain became unbearable.

On standing, marked squinting of both patellae were demonstrated. The thighs were thin with little muscle definition of the quadriceps. The Q angle was 30°. Walking revealed a tendency to walk with the knee slightly flexed. The hamstrings were tight when the 90:90 or straight leg raise test was performed; knee was recorded at 40° flexion at maximum extension.

Treatment was planned to deal with the high Q angle, muscle imbalance (i.e quadriceps weakness and hamstring tightness) and obesity.

A neutral suspension cast was taken of both feet, and functional orthoses were prescribed. The patient was asked to perform hamstring stretching exercises by simply touching her toes. Straight leg raises were also recommended to improve the tone of the quadriceps muscles. An appointment was made for her to see a dietician. The orthoses were fitted in her shoes some 2 weeks later and good reduction in the Q angle was noted. At subsequent follow-up, the knee pain was greatly reduced by the use of the orthoses and exercises but had not resolved completely. The patient was referred on for knee arthroscopy or release of the lateral patella fascia.

la malalignment. This shearing is thought to be an important cause of pain (Fox, 1975).

Poor alignment of the patella can also be treated more directly by strapping the patella into a correct position. The *McConnell technique* seeks to realign the patella in the transverse, sagittal and frontal planes. This technique involves the application of rigid strapping to the patella and around the side of the knee to correct any medial or lateral deviation of the patella. Tilting of the patella, which may increase compression on the medial and lateral surfaces, is also dealt with in this manner (Hilyard 1990).

The vastus medialis muscle provides an important stabilizer for the patella. If the muscle is weak, as a result of injury, inherited tendency or biomechanical dysfunction, the patella will be pulled laterally and superiorly by the dominant vastus lateralis. Shearing of the patella against the lateral condyle will result. The vastus medialis must be strengthened by exercises that seek to increase muscle bulk. Straight leg raise (SLR) assessment is useful when the knee is acutely painful. SLRs can be performed by exercising the vastus medialis, without the need for any knee flexion, thus reducing shearing behind the patella. SLRs, however, will not exercise the vastus medialis muscle in isolation from the quadriceps muscle group. The vastus medialis muscle only comes into effect in the last 20–30° of extension. A soft ball/rolled towel is placed behind the semi-flexed knee with the patient seated on the couch/floor; the patient then compresses the ball/towel while extending the knee from its semi-flexed position. This will tone the vastus medialis and assist patella tracking.

GAIT PROBLEMS

Gait variations associated with in-toeing and out-toeing tend to be a concern for parents. The child appears unstable and may trip.

IN-TOEING

Abnormalities in the foot and lower limb may manifest as in-toeing. These anomalies become apparent when walking is established (Fig. 15.19). Svenningson et al (1990) remarked that 30% of 4 year olds in-toe whereas only 4% of adults do. This signifies that there is an overall good prognosis. Spontaneous resolution may occur between 4 and 11 years. This should be considered when deciding upon a course of treatment. Where children are tripping and injuring themselves, treatment should aim to improve gait angle. This reduces the incidence of tripping.

The type of treatment instigated will be largely determined by the cause of the in-toeing. One of the most common causes is hamstring shortening. Simple diagnosis of this is by the 90:90 test or the SLR (Fig. 15.20). In children up to 12 years of age, it should be possible to extend the knee fully when the hip is flexed to 90° as the child lies supine. In many asymptomatic children, however, this test may reveal some tightness as

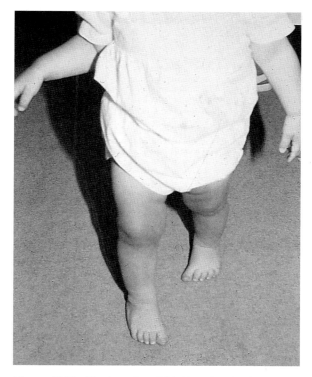

Figure 15.19 The in-toeing child. Note that the feet here are severely adducted while the knees face forwards; therefore, the cause of in-toeing is below the knee.

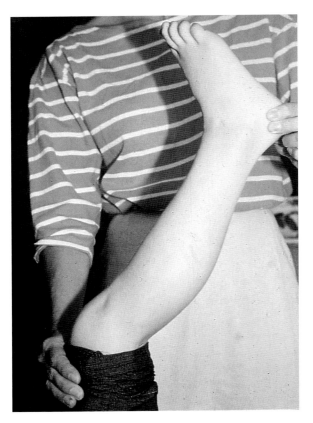

Figure 15.20 The straight leg raise (SLR) or 90:90 test to establish hamstring flexibility.

normal bone growth between the ages of 9 and 12 can outpace muscle lengthening. Where there is a history of problems and the knee will not extend beyond 70°, stretching exercises should be instigated to improve hamstring flexibility.

Treatment

Treatment can be directed at soft tissue, osseous and articular relationships, which cause the adducted position of the foot (see the treatment algorithm in Fig. 15.21).

Soft-tissue relationships

Compliance from young children is poor when asked to undertake stretching regimens. It is more appropriate to ask the parents to perform the exercises on the child. The stretching exercise is quite similar to the diagnostic test. The child lies flat on their back and the hip is flexed to 90°; the parent stabilizes the thigh and, while grasping the back of the child's heel, extends the knee. The child counts to 30 and then the leg is allowed to relax. A minimum of 10 repetitions for each limb is advised. Thirty days of intensive hamstring stretching are usually recommended. The child is then reviewed. If full extension of the knee upon repeating the SLR test is still not achieved, then another 30 days of stretching should be considered. The practitioner should be aware of whether or not the child has recently been through a growth spurt as this may influence treatment decisions.

Reeducation Even when the hamstrings are stretched out, the child may continue to in-toe. In such cases, the parents should be reassured that there is no structural reason why the child should not walk straight; they are simply assuming a habit. The habit may be broken by reminding the child to walk straight or encouraging them to play games that will help them to improve their angle of gait. A useful exercise that can be played out by the child involves placing footprint shapes on the ground and tracing their own feet onto the footprints while walking.

Gait plates Abduction of the foot can be encouraged by limiting toe-off from the lateral side of the forefoot (Fig. 15.22). The gait plate alters the natural metatarsal break at the fourth/fifth metatarsophalangeal joint where flexion takes place. Propulsion from the lateral side of the foot is thwarted so that the child will rotate the leg to offer foot contact from the medial side. In order to achieve propulsion, the child must abduct the foot and roll off from the medial forefoot. This effectively alters gait and produces a straighter alignment. Gait plates cannot treat rotational problems; they can only realign the foot at contact whilst in use. The gait plate is fabricated in much the same way as a Root or Shaffer orthosis. The anterior edge of the orthosis, however, is extended distally to a point just short of the fourth/fifth toe sulci. The gait plate can be prescribed in 3–4 mm polypropylene or 3 mm acrylic. A deeper heel seat can be made

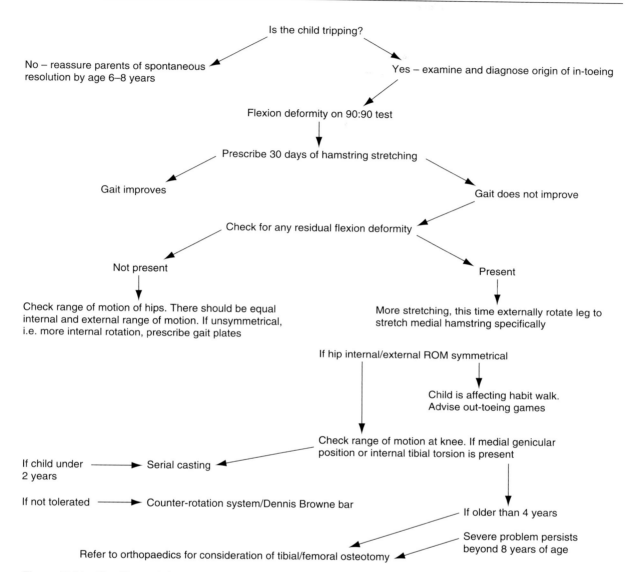

Is the child tripping?

No – reassure parents of spontaneous resolution by age 6–8 years

Yes – examine and diagnose origin of in-toeing

Flexion deformity on 90:90 test

Prescribe 30 days of hamstring stretching

Gait improves

Gait does not improve

Check for any residual flexion deformity

Not present

Present

Check range of motion of hips. There should be equal internal and external range of motion. If unsymmetrical, i.e. more internal rotation, prescribe gait plates

More stretching, this time externally rotate leg to stretch medial hamstring specifically

If hip internal/external ROM symmetrical

Child is affecting habit walk. Advise out-toeing games

Check range of motion at knee. If medial genicular position or internal tibial torsion is present

If child under 2 years ⟶ Serial casting

If not tolerated ⟶ Counter-rotation system/Dennis Browne bar

If older than 4 years

Severe problem persists beyond 8 years of age

Refer to orthopaedics for consideration of tibial/femoral osteotomy

Figure 15.21 Algorithm to help determine the most appropriate treatment strategies for in-toeing gait. The practitioner is particularly interested in managing foot problems associated with recognizable developmental variations. Any suggestion of hip or knee disease warrants a different management. Orthoses are strictly contraindicated until an accurate diagnosis has been undertaken. ROM, range of motion.

from polypropylene and a high medial flange fabricated. Gait plates are not recommended for the apropulsive gait seen in children under 4 years of age, as the device will not work as effectively as in older children. Muscles in the child should be continuously stretched during development in combination with gait plate prescription. Repeat stretching programmes are indicated, although a long-term programme is likely to result in non-compliance.

Osseous and articular relationships at the hip

In-toeing may also be a consequence of limited external rotation at the hip joint. Torsion within the proximal head and neck of the femur must be excluded, although diagnosis is difficult from clinical examination alone. Recent diagnostic aids now include ultrasound scanning. Serious torsion should be referred on to the orthopaedic specialist. Osteotomy of the femur is still the main treatment for these conditions. This is an option that must be very carefully considered. Corrective osteotomy is far from being a minor procedure and is known to carry important complications such as postoperative compartment syndrome as well as recurrence of the original condition.

Articular, soft-tissue limitations and minor torsions may still benefit from a prescription gait plate. In some cases, a gait plate will produce no obvious benefit and alternative treatment must be considered. In the past, twister cables and Dennis Browne bar and boots have been used (Fig. 15.23). These devices are worn at night and hold the legs in an externally rotated position. Their value has been seriously questioned by Fabry et al (1973), who found that these devices actually retarded the rate at which children grew out of the condition.

Holding the legs in external rotation with a device worn on the feet primarily exerts a corrective force on the foot but it also exerts a force on the knee joint. If the cause of the in-toeing is proximal to the knee joint, the corrective force is obviously not being applied at the appropriate level.

Knee and tibial relationship

The effect of treatment on the knee joint may, however, be useful in the treatment of medial

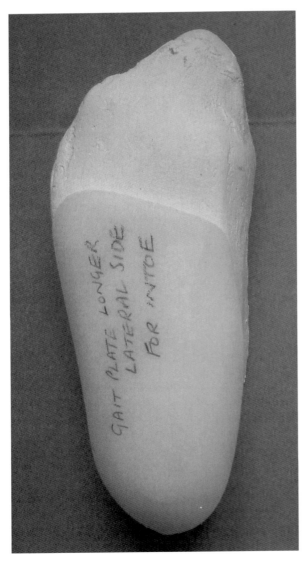

Figure 15.22 A gait plate for in-toeing children.

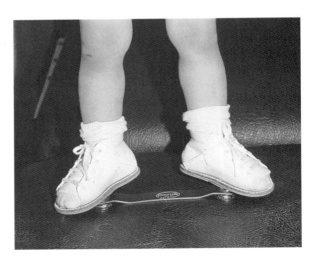

Figure 15.23 The Dennis Browne bar and boots.

genicular position or internal tibial torsion, both of which are causes of in-toeing. Medial genicular position occurs when the entire tibia is internally rotated at the knee joint. Internal tibial torsion, however, is caused by a lack of normal external torsion of the distal end of the tibia relative to the proximal end of the tibia.

The prognosis without treatment for medial genicular position has not been determined. However, it is a condition rarely seen in adults. Both medial genicular position and internal tibial torsion have been successfully treated by above-knee serial casting. A treatment approach commonly used in the nineties.

Serial casting   In applying a plaster of Paris cast, the area should first be protected from irritation with a pre-cast wrap of green line Tubifast covered by orthopaedic wool. The Tubifast should extend 25 cm (10 inches) beyond the distal ends of the toes and up as far as the groin. Special attention should be paid to protect the malleoli, extensor retinaculum, posteroplantar calcaneum and the dorsum of the toes. Double-thickness orthopaedic wool may be applied to those high-pressure areas or alternatively silastic sheeting can be used.

Once the limb has been protected, the first section of the cast is applied. The cast is applied as three cylinders, the first from the foot to just below the knee joint and the second around the thigh. When these are set hard, they are joined together by a third cylinder that encircles the knee. As the third cylinder of plaster sets, the knee is extended and the tibia rotated externally. Two 7.5 cm rolls of plaster of Paris are applied from the foot to the tibial tuberosity. Rather than smoothing out the end of each roll, the ends are turned over, forming a convenient tag (Fig. 15.24). In this way, the end of each roll can later be found and the plaster unravelled by the parents. While the first section of the cast is drying, the foot is held at 90° to the leg to prevent any accommodative shortening of the triceps surae muscle group. The rearfoot is also held in neutral or very slightly supinated to prevent the foot adopting a pronated position. The second cylinder is then applied around the middle of the thigh. Once dry, the two sections of the cast are

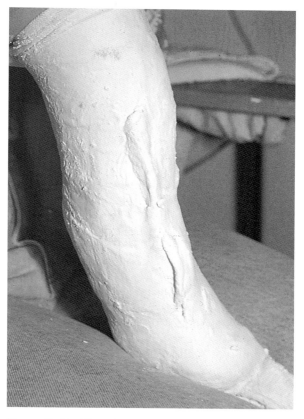

Figure 15.24   Above-knee plaster of Paris serial casting, with plaster tags to allow parents to remove the cast.

then connected by a third cylinder. Once this is applied, the tibia is externally rotated on the knee joint, the corrected position being maintained while the knee section of the cast dries.

Once the cast is complete, the ends of the Tubifast are pulled down over its proximal and distal edges. Sharp edges of the cast can be protected by the overturned Tubifast; this can be assisted by placing an adult's sock over the cast to protect it further from damage with walking. The cast should be left in place for 1 week. The parents should be advised that if the child is overly distressed, they should not hesitate to remove it. The cast is removed by placing the child in a bath of warm water and soaking the plaster of Paris for at least 20 minutes. The tags at the end of each roll are then found and the rolls of plaster unwound. Cutting the cast off with a cast cutter is not really appropriate for young children and should be avoided.

Three weeks of casting is usually sufficient to correct the in-toed gait, although another 3 weeks of casting is often employed to guard against recurrence. Use of the Dennis Browne bar and boots may also prevent recurrence, although many children will not tolerate having both feet secured by a single bar (see Fig. 15.23). The counter-rotation system is better tolerated because it allows independent movement of both legs and is used when the child is non-weight bearing.

Serial casting and counter-rotation devices can be employed to good effect in inferopatellar in-toeing. Their value in the treatment of conditions originating above the knee is questionable, because it is difficult to achieve a corrective effect at this level. In suprapatellar in-toeing, gait plates and hamstring stretching forms the mainstay of intervention. The prognosis for most children with an abnormal angle of gait is good, with clear evidence that this developmental problem is outgrown by the age of 6 to 8 years. However, if problems persist beyond 8 years of age, referral to an orthopaedic specialist is appropriate.

OUT-TOEING

Out-toeing or markedly abducted feet may also be a cause of parental concern because of the cosmetic appearance and the apparent clumsiness. Causes of out-toeing may include excessive amounts of:

- external femoral position
- external tibial torsion
- subtalar joint pronation

Out-toeing may respond to orthotic treatment that seeks to supinate the foot and thus create adduction. The forces that are to be resisted by the orthosis require very effective control of the foot: in particular, a deep heel seat and high medial flange are indicated. Shoes must be adequate to accommodate the dimensions of the orthosis.

SUMMARY

Abnormal foot shape may have the potential to cause pain. It is important that early developmental problems are recognized as these may have a profound effect on foot position and gait. In some cases, monitoring of the condition is all that is required; however, where treatment is indicated, this must be commenced early. Treatment should facilitate normal development. It is with this in mind that treatment should only be provided where necessary. In some situations, treatment may fall outside the remit of the podiatrist, despite the ability to diagnose the condition. In these cases, its important to recognize and refer to the appropriate discipline.

REFERENCES

Becker-Anderson H, Reimann I 1974 Congenital vertical talus. Reevaluation of early manipulation treatment. Acta Orthopaedica Scandinavica 45: 130

Berg E E 1986 A reappraisal of metatarsus adductus and skew foot. Journal of Bone and Joint Surgery 68A: 1185–1196

Clark M W, D'Ambrosia R D, Ferguson A B 1977 Congenital vertical talus. Journal of Bone and Joint Surgery 59A: 816

D'Amico J C, Rubin M 1986 The influence of foot orthoses on the quadraceps angle. Journal of the American Podiatric Association 76: 337–340

Fabry G, McEwan G D, Shands A R 1973 Torsion of the femur (a follow-up in normal and abnormal conditions). Journal of Bone and Joint Surgery 55A: 1726–1738

Ferguson A B, Gingrich R M 1957 The normal and abnormal calcaneal apophysis and tarsal navicular. Clinical Orthopedics 10: 87–95

Fox T A 1975 Dysplasia of the quadraceps mechanism. Surgical Clinics of North America 55: 199–225

Gauthier G, Elbaz R 1979 Freiberg's infarction; a subchondral bone fatigue fracture. A new surgical treatment. Clinical Orthopaedic and Related Research 142: 93–95

Groisso J A 1992 Juvenile hallux valgus. A conservative approach to treatment. Journal of Bone and Joint Surgery 74A: 1367–1374

Hamer A J, Stanley D, Smith T W D 1993 Surgery for curly toe deformity; a double blind randomised prospective trial. Journal of Bone and Joint Surgery 75B: 662–663

Hilyard A 1990 Recent developments in the management of patellofemoral pain: The McConnell programme.

Physiotherapy 76: 559–565

Kite J H 1950 Congenital metatarsus varus. Journal of Bone and Joint Surgery 32A: 500–506

Lodwick D, Tollafield D R, Cairns J 1995 Laboratory tests. In: Merriman L M, Tollafield D R (eds) Assessment of the lower limb. Churchill Livingstone, Edinburgh, p 311

Mann, R A Coughlin, M.J. 2001 Surgery of the foot and ankle, 6th edn, vol I. Mosby, St Louis, MO

McPoil T, Cameron J, Adrian M 1987 Anatomical characteristics of the talus in relation to forefoot deformities. Journal of the American Podiatric Medical Association 77: 77–81

Mereday C, Dolan C, Lusskin R 1972 Evaluation of the University of California biomechanics laboratory shoe insert in 'flexible' pes planus. Clinical Orthopaedic and Related Research 82: 46–57

Penneau K, Lutter L, Winter R 1982 Pes planus: radiographic changes with foot orthoses and shoes. Foot and Ankle 2: 229–330

Pentz A S, Weiner D S 1993 Management of metatarsus adductovarus. Foot and Ankle 14: 241–246

Ponsetti I V, Becker J R 1966 Congenital metatarsus adductus, the results of treatment. Journal of Bone and Joint Surgery 48A: 702–711

Rose G K 1958 Correction of the pronated foot. Journal of Bone and Joint Surgery 40B: 674–683

Rose G K 1962 Correction of the pronated foot. Journal of Bone and Joint Surgery 44B: 642–647

Rose G K, Welton E A, Marshall T 1985 The diagnosis of flat foot in the child. Journal of Bone and Joint Surgery 67B: 71–78

Ross E R S, Menelaus M B 1984 Open flexor tenotomy for hammer toes and curly toes in childhood. Journal of Bone and Joint Surgery 66B: 770–771

Rushforth G F 1978 The natural history of the hooked forefoot. Journal of Bone and Joint Surgery 60B: 530–532

Smillie I S 1967 Treatment of Frieberg's infarction. Proceedings of the Royal Society of Medicine 60: 29–31

Smith T W D, Stanley D, Rowley D I 1991 Treatment of Freiberg's disease. A new operative technique. Journal of Bone and Joint Surgery 73B: 129–130

Staheli L T, Chew D E, Corbett M 1987 The longitudinal arch. Journal of Bone and Joint Surgery 69A: 426–428

Svenningsen S, Tierjesen T, Auflem M 1990 Hip rotation and intoeing gait. Clinical Orthopaedic and Related Research 252: 177–182

Thomson S A 1960 Hallux varus and metatarsus varus. Clinical Orthopedics 16: 109–111

Tollafield D R 1993 Freiberg's infarction: surgical management by osteotomy; a forgotten technique? British Journal of Podiatric Medicine and Surgery 5: 2–5

Tollafield D R, Pratt D J 1990 The control of known triplanar forces on the foot by forefoot orthotic posting. British Journal of Podiatric Medicine and Surgery 2: 3–5

Wenger D R, Mauldin D, Speck G 1989 Corrective shoes and inserts as treatment for flexible flat foot in infants and children. Journal of Bone and Joint Surgery 71A: 800–810

Wynne-Davies R 1964 Family studies and the cause of congenital clubfoot, talipes equino-varus, talipes calcaneo valgus and metatarsus varus. Journal of Bone and Joint Surgery 46B: 445–456

FURTHER READING

Banks A S, Downey M S, Martin D E et al (eds) 2001 McGlamry's comprehensive textbook of foot and ankle surgery, 3rd edn. Lippincott Williams & Wilkins, Philadelphia, PA

16

Management of the sports patient

Ben Yates

INTRODUCTION

The management of lower limb sports injuries can be both very challenging and rewarding. The vast majority of injuries seen by the podiatrist are chronic in nature and caused by overuse of a specific part of the musculoskeletal system. These represent a diagnostic challenge, as both the actual injury and its aetiology are often difficult to identify because of the length of time the injury has been present and potential compensatory changes. Without a specific diagnosis, management of the injury is often difficult or inappropriate, rendering success less likely. With correct diagnosis, the management can be targeted both to treat the condition and to address the potential aetiological causes.

It is not possible to discuss all of the common lower limb sports injuries a podiatrist is likely to treat in a single chapter. The chapter is, therefore, divided into the principles that should guide management, the common treatment modalities used in sports injury management, and the common injuries that affect the different tissue types: skin and nails, bursae, tendons, muscle and fascia, ligaments, joints, bone, nerve and vascular tissue.

GUIDING PRINCIPLES

Before embarking on treatment it is important to identify short- and long-term treatment goals and discuss both the practitioner's and the patient's expectations of the proposed management. Some athletes may have unrealistic expectations of treatment, expecting a miracle cure or to be able to continue their exercise schedule during treatment. In either situation, treatment is likely to fail. Similarly, the practitioner may have unrealistic expectations of the patient in terms of adhering to advice on activity modification, stretching programmes, self-treatment with physical therapies, etc. Effective communication is key to preventing misunderstanding between the practitioner and athlete. The practitioner must explain to the athlete the nature and severity of the injury and be realistic regarding the likely outcome if the athlete adheres to the suggested treatment. Many athletes are knowledgeable about injuries associated with their sport and respond positively to a practitioner who demonstrates knowledge and understanding of both the injury and the needs of the athlete.

In identifying treatment options it is important to consider who will be providing the treatment. This may be straightforward if the practitioner is working as part of an interdisciplinary or multidisciplinary sports medicine team, with established referral protocols to physiotherapists, physicians, surgeons, etc. However, the podiatrist may often be working in isolation or is hampered by lengthy time delays when referring on to other health care practitioners. In such a situation, the podiatrist may need to incorporate a number of mechanical, physical, and pharmacological treatment strategies into the management plan.

Choosing a treatment strategy for the condition should be based upon evidence-based practice. This is often difficult as empirical evidence to support one treatment strategy over another for a specific condition is frequently lacking. In such a situation, the clinician should manage the patient based upon the best available evidence integrated with clinical experience. In the past, sports medicine literature, similar to other newly developing fields, has been criticized for its lack of scientific rigour (Hart & Walter 1990, Hart & Meeuwisse 1994). However, the quality of the research is undoubtedly improving as our knowledge of the aetiology and treatment of con-

ditions is enhanced. More recent studies have identified current sports medicine literature as comparable to other medical specialties (Bleakley & MacAuley 2002). Practitioners regularly treating athletes should keep abreast of the current literature to ensure they employ the most effective treatments.

Regular evaluation of the management plan is important to ensure overall treatment success and maintain patient motivation. This can be achieved by regularly recording a number of factors such as:

- pain levels with visual analogue pain scales
- activity diaries
- improvements in flexibility, strength etc.
- improvements in functional tests
- improvements in athletic performance.

By regularly assessing the outcome of the management plan, new treatment options may need to be considered. If the patient is progressing beyond expectations then the treatment plan can be accelerated or modified as appropriate. If little or no progress is being made, then the practitioner must reflect on a number of issues. Was the diagnosis and grading of the injury correct? Are there other aetiological factors present that were not initially considered? How closely has the patient adhered to the management plan? If the management is proving unsuccessful, then the practitioner should consider requesting further investigations to clarify the diagnosis or referring on to other health care practitioners who could provide a second opinion or offer other treatment options.

COMMON TREATMENT OPTIONS

Before considering specific injuries, it is worth appraising the treatment options available to the podiatrist. These can be broadly classified into mechanical, physical and pharmacological therapies. These therapies are discussed in detail elsewhere in this book. What follows is a discussion of their application in the management of sports injuries.

Mechanical therapies

The two main aims of mechanical therapies in the treatment of sports injuries are to rest an injured structure or to facilitate improved function. Frequently both aims may be needed in the management of the same condition, where resting an injured structure can enable recovery and improving function can help to prevent recurrence of the injury. There are a number of mechanical therapies available to the podiatrist including activity modification, padding, strapping, commercial braces/splints, footwear modifications, prefabricated orthoses, custom foot orthoses, walkers, fiberglass casts, etc.

Activity modification

Resting an injured structure may involve absolute rest through bed rest or immobilization in a non-weight-bearing cast. However, for the majority of injuries this is unnecessary and relative rest through activity modification or other mechanical therapies is used. Activity modification may include complete rest from all sporting activity or modifying the exercise schedule by reducing the training volume, intensity or types of activity. Where possible, the practitioner should try and avoid advising complete rest from all sports, as many athletes will be unwilling to adhere to such a programme. Modification might include advising non-weight-bearing sports such as swimming or alternatively exercising on softer surfaces. In the majority of chronic overuse lower limb injuries, modifying the training programme rather than complete rest can be achieved without detriment to the injury rehabilitation.

Padding

Padding materials such as felt can be very useful as an initial mechanical support to alter function and off-load a painful structure. It is readily shaped and adheres directly to the foot, orthoses or the sock of the sports shoe, so it can enable immediate treatment. Also as the material is cheap and short lasting it can be useful as a trial

mechanical treatment to see if more permanent orthoses would be beneficial.

Strapping

Strapping has become an integral treatment modality used by physiotherapists, podiatrists, athletic trainers and sports physicians alike. Its main advantages lie in its cheap cost, immediate treatment, ease of application and adaptability to any body part. Patients can often be taught how to apply the strapping themselves prior to sporting activity. The main disadvantage is that it is short lasting. Occasionally, patients may develop skin reactions or allergies to the tape, although this can be reduced by applying pre-tapes or occlusive sprays such as Opsite.

One of the most contentious issues regarding strapping is the mechanism of action. It was previously thought that strapping worked by limiting joint movement. A more probable explanation for the positive effect of strapping is through proprioceptive feedback improving muscle function. Whether the effect is mechanical, proprioceptive or both is also dependent upon the strapping technique. For example, with McConnell taping for patellofemoral pain, any mechanical effect is very short lived (Larsen et al 1995) or absent (Gigante et al 2001). High-dye strapping is more mechanically effective in limiting frontal plane subtalar joint motion than low dye (Keenan & Tanner 2001). Ankle strapping is likely to work by a combination of both mechanical support and by increasing proprioceptive acuity and muscle activation (Manfoy et al 1997). Table 16.1 lists the common lower limb strapping techniques and their indications. Examples of two of the strapping techniques can be seen in Figures 16.1 and 16.2.

Braces and splints

There are a number of commercially available sports braces and splints. Braces have been shown to have significantly greater mechanical effect than taping in limiting ankle joint range of motion (Safran et al 1999a, Verhagen et al 2000). The commonest lower limb braces are used in

Table 16.1 Common strapping techniques of the lower limb

Technique	Indications/injuries	Comments
Flask	Acute hallux rigidus, turf toe, Sesamoiditis	Mechanically limits first metatarsophalangeal joint motion
Campbells rest (false plantar fascia)	Plantar fasciitis/plantar fascial tears	Can help determine if heel pain is mechanically induced. Often combined with low-dye taping
Heel lock	Anterior/posterior ankle impingement	Shown to have strong mechanical effect
Low dye	Excessive foot pronation with intrinsic foot injury	May be combined with Campbell rest or J strap
High dye	Excessive foot pronation/tibialis posterior dysfunction	Resists foot pronation greater than low dye
Figure of 8 or basketweave	Lateral ankle sprain, functional or mechanical ankle instability	Mechanical and proprioceptive effect
Stirrup	Achilles tendonopathies/calf muscle tears	Limits ankle dorsiflexion. Often with felt padding as a heel lift
J strap	Tibialis anterior or tibialis posterior tendonopathy	Combined with low or high dye; J shape follows path of muscle origin
McConnell	Patellofemoral pain syndrome, patella mal tracking	Proprioceptive effect increases vastus medialis muscle action

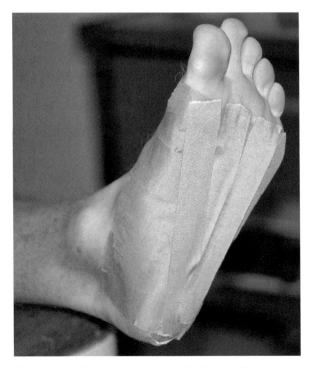

Figure 16.1 Low-dye strapping with Campbell's rest.

the rehabilitation of ankle sprains or ankle instability. However any brace that can limit frontal plane ankle movement also limits subtalar joint motion (de Clercq 1997) and could, therefore, be used to treat injuries associated with excessive pronation, such as tibialis posterior dysfunction.

The style and material of the brace are important. Elasticated braces such as those made of neoprene have little mechanical effect. Tubigrip, commonly used for acute ankle sprains, has been shown to have no effect on functional recovery following ankle sprains and actually increased the need for analgesia (Watts and Armstrong 2001). Braces made of semi-rigid thermoplastic, such as the Aircast airstirrup, the Donjoy ALP, the Malleolarloc or the reinforced canvas Swede-O-universal brace with sliding plastic struts, can all significantly reduce frontal plane movement and, therefore, provide excellent mechanical support to an injured ankle. Their disadvantages are the relative expense and they often appear too bulky or restrictive to patients.

The use of braces in anterior knee pain has been studied to determine any preventive effect.

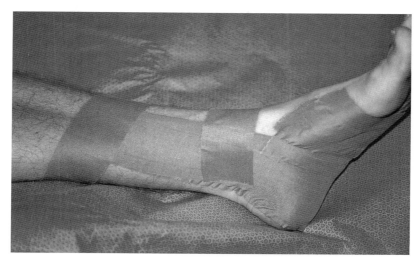

Figure 16.2 High-dye strapping.

Bengal et al (1997) demonstrated that a knee brace with a silicone patellar ring reduced the incidence of anterior knee pain (relative risk 0.35). Similar findings for the incidence of ankle sprains with ankle braces have also been demonstrated (Sitler et al 1994). The prophylactic use of braces to prevent a common injury or reduce the risk of reinjury is often questioned by athletes as to whether the brace will limit performance. The results of studies in this area would suggest that there is a very small effect upon both vertical jump and sprint performance when wearing an ankle brace (Burks et al 1991, MacKean et al 1995). This should not prevent the average athlete from wearing a brace, especially in those with a history of a chronic or repetitive injury. Prophylactic use of braces in the elite athlete is more contentious and should be discussed on an individual basis.

The use of splints worn at night in the treatment of plantar fasciitis has now become commonplace. The splint is used to stretch both the plantar fascia and the calf muscle. The splints are cumbersome and many patients discontinue treatment because of interrupted sleep patterns. However, for those who persist, the night splints have a relatively high success rate and are particularly good at preventing post-static dyskinesia (pain upon first rising) (Martin et al 2001).

Walkers

Walkers are very useful in the acute management of a sports injury or when a chronic injury has become severe enough to significantly limit function. They allow a structure to rest while still enabling the patient to remain relatively mobile. They provide excellent protection from further injury and are removable, allowing the patient to wash and undertake range of motion exercises. Another advantage is the relatively low cost, as the walker can be reused for other patients by either washing or replacing the in-sock.

The main disadvantage is the cumbersome nature of the device (Fig. 16.3). They are bulky and much heavier than conventional footwear. They also create an artificial limb length discrepancy because of the thickness of the sole, which may be an issue if used for a prolonged period. The common uses of walkers and below-knee casting in sports medicine can be seen in Table 16.2.

Below-knee casting

When complete rest and immobilization of an injured structure is required, then the patient should be placed in a fibreglass below-knee cast. Such a functionally limiting treatment is reserved for severe acute injuries or when a significant chronic injury is not responding to other mechanical treatments. The patient will require crutches to remain either completely non-weight bearing or partially weight bearing. The use of a postoperative shoe is required if the patient is to bear weight through the cast. Most patients report a dramatic improvement in symptoms almost immediately or within the first week. The period of time the cast should remain on is dependent upon the condition but for most it is between 4 and 8 weeks. As a general rule, the patient should have been partially or fully weight bearing through the cast and pain free for 2–3 weeks before contemplating removing the cast. This period may be less if the patient is going into a cam-walker or brace.

There are obviously disadvantages to placing a limb in a cast. Muscle atrophy starts within 48 hours of immobilization. Prolonged immobilization can result in joint stiffness, significant muscle atrophy and osteopenia. Reversing these changes takes time and requires committed rehabilitation by the patient.

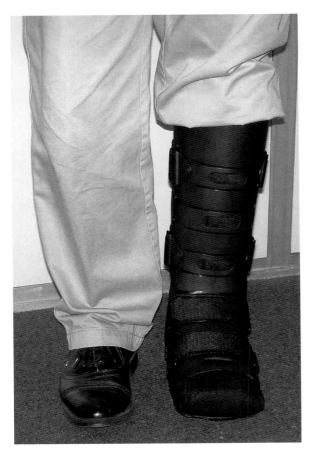

Figure 16.3   Walker.

Footwear modification

Athletes will often seek advice from podiatrists about the suitability of their athletic footwear. Assessing the athlete's shoe can assist both the diagnosis and the treatment of the condition (Yates 2002). In terms of management, the podiatrist may recommend a complete change in footwear. This may be based upon the style, such as changing from a neutral running shoe to one with more pronation control. The athlete must also be wearing a shoe that is appropriate for the sport and the exercise surface. Novice

Table 16.2   Common indications for the use of walkers or below-knee casting in the injured athlete

Condition	Walker	Below-knee cast
Bone pathology	Acute stress reactions, stress fractures, non-displaced fractures	Displaced fractures, stress fractures; talus, navicular, fifth metatarsal, sesamoid, anterior tibial crest
Cartilage pathology	Tarsal coalition, osteochondroses (Freiburg's, Iselin's, Kohler's)	Osteochondral defects of the talus grades I and II
Ligament pathology	Grade II or III ankle sprains	Syndesmosis tears
Tendon pathology	Acute tendonopathies; Achilles, tibialis posterior/anterior, peroneals	Conservative management of Achilles rupture
Fascial pathology	Acute plantar fasciitis, retinacula tears	Acute plantar fasciitis

athletes will often wear the same shoes to play several different sports. Occasionally, the footwear may need to be modified, such as a lateral heel float to prevent ankle sprains, addition of further cleats to increase traction, cushioning the tongue or heel counter, etc. Case study 16.1 illustrates footwear modification as a management technique.

Prefabricated and custom-made foot orthoses

The use of both prefabricated and custom-made foot orthoses has become widespread in the management of lower limb sports injuries. Prefabricated orthoses are dispensed by a number of health care workers, including physiotherapists, podiatrists, osteopaths, chiropractors and sports physicians, and are also readily available in chemists and sports shops. Custom-made foot

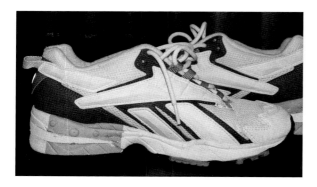

Figure 16.4 Running shoe with 1 cm ethylenevinyl acetate heel raise built into the heel.

orthoses are prescribed by either podiatrists or orthotists. Comparison of the efficacy of these two types of device is a contentious issue and beyond the scope of this chapter. Both types of device have been shown to be successful in the management of sports injuries and also as a prophylactic measure to prevent injury. Both types are becoming more sophisticated as technology develops. An example of this is that some prefabricated orthoses now come in multiple styles, densities and shapes, armed with further additions that can be utilized by the practitioner.

This widespread use of orthoses in the treatment of sports injuries has been criticized because of the lack of rigorous research studies showing their positive effect (Kilmartin and Wallace 1994, Yeung and Yeung 2001). However, similar claims could be made about the use of a number of other treatment modalities. From the literature, it would appear that custom-made foot orthoses can improve symptoms of lower limb overuse injuries in approximately 80% of cases. Resolution of symptoms, to the point where the athlete can return to previous levels of activity, has been reported as 70% (Donatelli et al 1988; Gross et al 1991). These were for a variety of foot, ankle, shin and knee complaints. Research studies on the use of prefabricated orthoses have mainly used military recruits as subjects. Schwellnus et al (1990) conducted a randomized controlled trial on 1500 recruits and found that contoured neoprene insoles reduced lower limb injuries by a third and common injuries such as medial tibial stress syndrome by 50%.

Case study 16.1   Footwear modification

A retired international cricketer was running a marathon to raise a lot of money for charity. He started training 10 weeks before the race in a pair of racing flats donated to him by a sponsor. He immediately tore the medial head of his gastrocnemius muscle and could not run for 3 weeks. He was jointly managed with the physiotherapist, who treated the soft tissue injury daily, and the athlete tried to maintain fitness by swimming. He was determined to run the race so his sponsor was contacted and a more appropriate running shoe was provided. These were modified by sectioning the shoe sole from the upper, avoiding the rearfoot cushioning device and inserting 1 cm high-density ethylenevinyl acetate heel raises (Fig. 16.4). Orthoses with a full-length cover and a further 7 mm heel raise were manufactured to reduce the stretch and eccentric load through the medial head of the gastrocnemius. The orthoses and shoe modifications were made for both feet to prevent an artificial limb-length discrepancy. Video analysis demonstrated that he was a midfoot striker and he was educated to alter his stride to become a rearfoot striker to minimize calf muscle activity further. He was able to complete the race in just over 4 hours without further tearing his calf muscle.

The choice of material may also be significant with specific injuries. Finestone et al (1999) demonstrated that soft custom-made foot orthoses were more effective than semi-rigid custom-made orthoses in prospectively reducing stress fractures among military recruits. They demonstrated that the soft orthoses reduced the stress fracture rate to 11%, compared with 16% for the semi-rigid orthoses and 27% for the control group receiving neither type of orthosis. Similar findings were reported by Larsen et al (2002), where soft custom-made foot orthoses reduced the incidence of shin splints among army recruits from 38% to 8%.

The rationale for prescribing orthoses to an athlete may include:

- improve skeletal alignment
- reduce levels of tissue stress
- improve sensory feedback
- provide extrinsic shock absorption
- increase shoe comfort.

If any of these goals are achieved, then specific injuries may be prevented or resolved. Different materials may be better at achieving different goals. Also specific injuries are thought to be linked to specific biomechanical aetiologies. An example of this is repetitive ankle sprains, where improving sensory feedback would be more important than providing extrinsic shock absorption. The opposite would be true for preventing or treating stress fractures, where increasing extrinsic shock absorption should be the main aim of any orthosis.

It is important that, whenever mechanical therapy use is contemplated, that the practitioner is clear on the rationale for prescribing that particular type of mechanical treatment. It is often worthwhile utilizing temporary materials or strapping to see if symptoms are reduced before embarking on prescribing braces or orthoses. This is especially true if the diagnosis or aetiology is unclear.

Physical therapy

The initial goals of physical therapy in the treatment of sports injuries are to reduce the levels of pain and inflammation and to accelerate the natural healing process. The acronyms of RICE, NICER, and PRICE have all been advocated in the initial management of an acute injury. The individual letters stand for:

- *r*est
- *i*ce
- *c*ompression
- *e*levation
- *n*on-steroidal anti-inflammatory medication
- *p*rotection.

All of these are aimed to assist in the reduction of swelling and pain and a combination of them should be used for the first 48–72 hours following an injury. The use of interferential stimulation has also been advocated in the early management to help to minimize swelling. Ice can also be used in the management of long-term or chronic injury where the reduction of swelling or pain is recommended. This can be particularly beneficial just after activity. Examples of chronic injury where ice has been recommended are tendonopathy, plantar fasciitis or medial tibial stress syndrome.

The application of heat can be used in the management of sports injuries after the first 48 hours. The hyperaemia produced can accelerate the absorption of inflammatory mediators, reduce muscle spasm and increase the extensibility of collagen. A combination of hot and cold treatment is contrast baths. This form of treatment can be very effective in reducing residual swelling by alternating vasodilatation and constriction. Common sports injuries treated in this way include delayed-onset muscle soreness (Kuligowski et al 1998), and the post-acute management of ankle sprains and fractures.

Electrotherapy

The beneficial effects of electrotherapeutic modalities in the treatment of sports injuries is less certain. Ultrasound is widely used in a variety of sports injuries, although there is little evidence as to its beneficial effects. Cochrane reviews on the use of ultrasound for both ankle sprains and patellofemoral pain syndrome found no beneficial effect (Brosseau et al 2002, van der Windt et al 2002). Advocates of ultrasound claim it can accelerate the healing process and reduce muscle spasm and pain. Several of these claims have been proved in laboratory studies but remain unconfirmed in clinical trials (van der Windt 1999). Non-conventional low-intensity, pulsed ultrasound has been used successfully in the treatment of delayed fracture healing of the tibia (Heckman et al 1994).

Transcutaneous electrical nerve stimulation (TENS), the localized application of an electrical current, can be used for pain relief in sports injuries. One of the main advantages of TENS is its size and its transportability, allowing patients to take it with them and use it as required. The effect of TENS is patient specific, with some achieving considerable pain relief while others find no benefit (Ellis 1998). Interferential stimulation is a form of TENS that has the added advantage of being able to produce muscle activity or vasodilatation depending upon the frequency used. It is commonly used in acute management to minimize pain, swelling and muscle spasm.

Laser therapy is becoming more widespread as a therapeutic modality for sports injuries. Results from studies on its use are often conflicting (Belanger 2002). As with ultrasound, this may be because of differences in the type of laser used and the wavelength applied. For lower limb injuries, laser is most often used for superficial tendonopathies, ligament injuries and the stimulation of trigger points. It has not been found to be beneficial in plantar fasciitis (Basford et al 1998).

Manual therapy

Manual therapy involves the application of force to joints, muscles and neural tissues to facilitate improved function. This may be achieved by increasing the range of motion of joints, reducing swelling or enhancing skeletal alignment. Manual therapy can be applied during and following the acute phase of the injury. Joints can be mobilized or manipulated to increase the range of motion, improve alignment, or reduce pain and swelling. Various mas-

sage techniques can be used including petrissage, effleurage, transverse frictions or gliding, digital ischaemic pressure and vacuum cupping. Massage techniques in sports injuries are used to aid drainage, increase localized blood flow and breakdown scar tissue.

Exercise therapy

Exercise therapy is a key component in the rehabilitative phase of an injury. The core components are to restore range of motion and to improve flexibility, strength and proprioception of the injured structure. Once these have been achieved, then the athlete can progress to increasing their fitness through both general and sport-specific functional exercises before making a return to their sport. Such a programme is likely to involve collaboration with a physiotherapist and the athlete's coach. Podiatric involvement is primarily centred on the core components and Table 16.3 outlines these for four common injuries the podiatrist is likely to encounter.

A variety of exercise techniques can be used including isometric, isotonic and isokinetic exercise patterns performed either in the closed or open kinetic-chain position. Isometric are used in the early phase of an injury or when trying to stabilize a structure. Isotonic exercises involve both concentric and eccentric contractions against a known load through a known range of motion and have been shown to be very successful in the management of many lower limb injuries such as Achilles tendonopathy and patellofemoral pain syndrome.

Isokinetic exercises are performed on specific machines where the speed, resistance and range of motion can be determined on an individual basis. The main advantages are being able to produce numerical data that can help to determine rehabilitation progress, compare agonist–antagonist muscle strength ratios and injured and non-injured side strength ratios. The exercise is also controlled so reinjury is less likely. The main disadvantages are the cost and that the exercises are not functional. The main lower limb injury where isokinetics play a significant rehabilitation role is in anterior cruciate ligament injuries.

Table 16.3 Common injuries and the exercise therapy used in their management

Injury	Flexibility exercises	Strength exercises	Proprioceptive exercises
Patellofemoral pain syndrome	Gastrocnemius, soleus, hamstrings, iliotibial band, quadriceps (especially vastus lateralis), lateral retinaculum	Vastus medialis, gluteus medius	Vastus medialis obliquus (often with biofeedback machine), gluteus medius and core stability exercises
Achilles tendonopathy	Gastrocnemius, soleus, hamstrings, plantar fascia	Soleus, gastrocnemius	–
Plantar fasciitis	Gastrocnemius, soleus, plantar fascia	–	–
Repetitive ankle sprains	Gastrocnemius, soleus, tibialis posterior	Peroneus longus and brevis, tibialis posterior	Peroneals and lateral collateral ligaments

More advanced stretching techniques are available, such as proprioceptive neuromuscular facilitation. This exploits the normal physiological stretch reflex to increase the muscle stretch and achieve a greater level of flexibility. Stretching of neural tissue can be very important in both the prevention of reinjury and the treatment of an existing injury. Injuries that are initially thought to be muscular in origin may in fact be caused by nerve trauma or altered neural dynamics. Common examples include altered neural dynamics of the sciatic nerve, causing pain in the hamstrings or calf muscles, or of the saphenous nerve, causing medial knee pain. Controlled stretching of these nerves can help to breakdown the intra- or extraneural adhesions causing the pain. Figure 16.5 demonstrates the slump position used both in the diagnosis and management of altered neural dynamics of the sciatic nerve. Case study 16.2 further demonstrates this point.

Pharmacological therapy

Pharmacological agents used in sports injuries are taken orally, injected or applied topically to the skin. The absorption of topical agents can be enhanced by the application of occlusive dressings or by using ultrasound (phonophoresis) or electrical current (iontophoresis) to drive the medication across the epidermal barrier to deeper structures. Pharmacological agents are primarily used to reduce pain and swelling. They should be seen as a component of the

---

Case study 16.2 Altered neural dynamics of the sciatic nerve

A 23-year-old female was referred by a sports physician with a 1 year history of atypical exercise-induced leg pain. She complained of pain in the anterior aspect of the shin that was induced by exercise or wearing heeled footwear. The pain was described as a cramping, tearing sensation that occasionally radiated distally. Chronic anterior compartment syndrome was diagnosed by the physician, but exercise intracompartmental pressure tests were negative. The physician referred her to a physiotherapist, who diagnosed tibialis anterior myositis and treated her with electrotherapy and manual therapy techniques. When this failed to alleviate symptoms, she was referred for a second opinion and biomechanical evaluation. A thorough history revealed a grade 2 ankle sprain on the affected side 3 months prior to the anterior compartment pain. This coupled with the symptom of pain occasionally radiating distally warranted further testing of the superficial peroneal nerve. With the patient sitting and the knee fully extended, the foot was maximally plantarflexed and then slowly inverted. This reproduced her symptoms as the superficial peroneal nerve was stretched. The pain could be exquisitely reproduced by further compression of the nerve as it pierces the superficial fascia on the anterior aspect 10 cm proximal to the ankle. It was, therefore, apparent that the previous ankle sprain had resulted in trauma and impingement of the nerve, resulting in altered neural dynamics. She was prescribed daily exercises to stretch the nerve, which quickly resolved her pain.

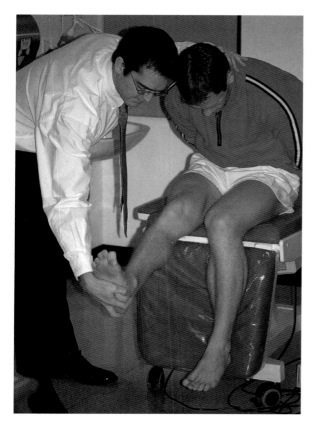

Figure 16.5 Slump test for altered neural dynamics.

rehabilitation programme and not used in isolation or to mask symptoms to allow an athlete to continue to exercise or perform.

Analgesics

Common analgesics used in sport include paracetamol, aspirin and codeine. Codeine is often taken in combination with paracetamol or aspirin and is no longer a banned substance by the International Olympic Committee (IOC). The use of aspirin in sports injuries is generally not recommended because of its antiplatelet effect, which can increase the bleeding associated with an acute injury. Also, the aspirin dosage required to reduce inflammation is associated with the potential side-effect of gastrointestinal bleeding. Paracetamol is an analgesic and antipyretic agent but has no effect on inflammation. It is safe to use in any phase of an injury when mild pain relief is required. Codeine is a more potent analgesic and as a narcotic agent may be used when more significant pain relief is needed.

Non-steroidal anti-inflammatory drugs

The use of non-steroidal anti-inflammatory drugs (NSAIDs) in the management of chronic and, particularly, acute sports injuries is very common. NSAIDs are analgesic and also anti-inflammatory when taken regularly. It is the anti-inflammatory effect that has promoted NSAIDs above analgesics in sports injury management. Despite this widespread use, there is actually little evidence to support this practice. There have been a number of trials but most simply compare one anti-inflammatory drug with another. The lack of placebo-control groups, grading of injuries, the subjective nature of pain and the lack of appropriate outcome measures make designing a robust research project in this area difficult. Some randomized controlled studies are underway and include the use of the newer safer cyclooxygenase-2 (COX-2) inhibitors.

NSAIDs are relatively safe drugs, with a small number of known side-effects. Their use in a generally healthy athletic population for short periods of up to a week is usually uncomplicated. Long-term use should be avoided because of the potential for gastric bleeding and ulceration. NSAIDs can also be applied topically for superficial injuries such as bursitis and can achieve similar local levels to those achieved with systemic administration without the potential side-effects.

Corticosteroids

Corticosteroids are usually administered via injection. Localized injection into an inflamed structure avoids potential systemic side-effects, which are common when oral corticosteroids are taken in high doses or for a prolonged period. Corticosteroids are the most potent anti-inflammatory medication and concern over their use in treating sports injuries has been raised both because of the systemic complications and because of their localized effect on tissue healing. Corticosteroids are known to inhibit collagen synthesis and can decrease tendon load to the point of failure. Despite these issues, many patients express considerable relief following a single injection.

Corticosteroid injections should only be administered where the condition is not responding to other measures. Repeat injections should be spaced at least 4 weeks apart to enable the effect of the injection to be gauged and also to allow some systemic absorption of the drug. Conventional wisdom suggests no more than three injections, as further injections risk tissue degeneration and it is unlikely that further injections will improve the clinical outcome. The injection should contain a 50:50 ratio of corticosteroid and local anaesthetic. The benefit of the anaesthetic is to reduce the pain from the injection and also to assist in the diagnosis. If the pain is relieved for a short period then it is likely to confirm the diagnosis, as the anaesthetic has blocked the painful stimuli from the injured structure.

Within the lower limb, corticosteroid injections have been used successfully as part of the treatment of plantar fasciitis, Morton's neuroma, hamstring injuries, bursitis and retrocalcaneal and intra-articular pathologies. Their use in the management of tendonopathies is very controversial because of the increased chance of tendon rupture and recent evidence suggesting that tendonopathy is not an inflammatory process (Khan et al 1999). Despite this, corticosteroid injections are still commonly administered directly into or around tendons and their sheaths. Intra-articular injections are also controversial because of the potential damage to articular cartilage. However, when synovitis or arthritic pain is severe, they can produce dramatic results. A common condition within the foot that benefits from such an injection is sinus tarsi syndrome (Fig. 16.6).

When administering a corticosteroid injection, it is important to discuss potential complications with the patient. By far the commonest is post-injection flare or 'steroid flare'. This is characterized by intense localized pain with occasional erythema or swelling. It occurs shortly after the

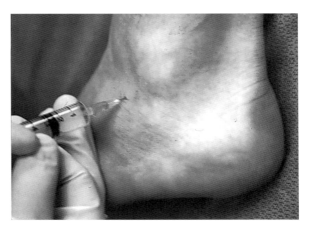

Figure 16.6 Injection of corticosteroid and local anaesthetic into the sinus tarsi.

injection and usually subsides within 48 hours. The cause is unknown but some believe it is a sign of the effectiveness of the injection. It is seen more often with the phosphate steroids and when injecting close to a nerve, such as for Morton's neuroma. The frequency of the reaction is unknown but experience suggests that up to 30% of patients undergoing an injection for Morton's neuroma may experience it. The other main complication is tissue damage leading to failure and then rupture. It has been demonstrated that when rupture of the plantar fascia occurs, it has often been preceded by a corticosteroid injection (Acevedo & Beskin 1998). Similar results have been found in Achilles tendonopathies progressing to rupture (Astrom & Rausing 1995). Infection following corticosteroid injection is extremely rare, less than 1 in 160 000, as long as appropriate aseptic guidelines are followed (Seror et al 1999). Corticosteroids can also be administered orally or topically. Short oral courses of moderate dosage (<50 mg) have become popular to limit swelling and pain following acute injury and do not appear to be associated with adverse side-effects.

Local anaesthetics

Local anaesthetics can be used to assist in the diagnosis of a condition. The ability to anaesthetize a specific structure such as a joint, tendon, bursa, accessory bone or single nerve branch can help to isolate the source of pain. This can be useful when the diagnosis is uncertain, such as in metatarsalgia or posterior ankle pain. Evidence is also emerging that repeated injections of long-acting local anaesthetics can also have a therapeutic effect. Positive results have been achieved in Achilles tendonopathy (Johnston et al 1997) and plantar fasciitis (Pavier & Liggins 2001). The mechanism of this effect is unknown. It may be by mechanical 'brisement' (distension and separation of adjacent tissues), by breaking the pain cycle or by the vasodilatory effect of the drug. This form of treatment is still being investigated but appears encouraging. The frequency of injections differs from that with corticosteroids, with injections administered weekly.

Other substances have also been injected for the treatment of Morton's neuroma, tendonosis or arthritis. Hyaluronic acid is a natural occurring polysaccharide occurring in synovial fluid and cartilage. Genetically produced forms have been injected into arthritic knees, with considerable success in reducing symptoms (Altman & Moskowitz 1998). Ethanol and vitamin B_{12} injections have been used in the management of neuromas. The therapeutic action of vitamin B_{12} is unknown but success has been reported with this technique (Miller & Nakra 2001). Dilute (4%) ethanol solutions have been used as serial injections for their sclerosing effect on the perineural fibrosis associated with neuromas (Dockery & Nilsson 1986). A sclerosing agent, pilidocanol, has recently been shown to be effective at removing the neovessels associated with Achilles tendinosis. The agent is injected under ultrasound guidance directly into the neovessel. Not only did the neovessels disappear with the treatment but 80% of patients were pain free at 6 month's follow up (Ohberg & Alfredson 2002).

Surgery

Despite the best efforts of clinicians and patients, many sports injuries do not respond to conservative care. In these situations, surgery is often required to improve function and provide pain relief. The goal of surgery in sports medicine is to allow the athlete to make a full uninhibited return to their previous levels of activity. The ability of the surgeon to achieve this goal is largely dependent upon the injury type, the procedure selected and the postoperative rehabilitation. The surgery performed can be broadly classified into four categories:

- repair of fractured, torn or ruptured tissues
- excision of pathological tissue
- soft tissue reconstruction
- osseous realignment.

Table 16.4 lists common lower limb injuries and their surgical management grouped in these categories. Figures 16.7 and 16.8 show examples.

In the majority of cases when surgery is considered, the injury has not responded to conservative care and the athlete is unable to perform normal daily activities without pain (Case study 16.3). In such a situation, there is little alternative but to undergo surgery.

Surgery may also be considered when it will accelerate the return to sport or improve the function of the injured structure postoperatively beyond that achieved with conservative care. Examples of these would include surgical repair of a Jones fracture of the fifth metatarsal and surgical repair of a ruptured Achilles tendon, respectively. However, when the surgical out-

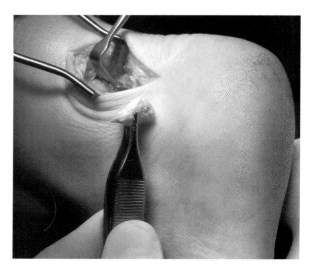

Figure 16.7 Excision of an os trigonum.

Table 16.4 Common surgical procedures for lower limb sports injuries

Surgical repair	Surgical excision	Soft tissue reconstruction	Osseous realignment
Stress fractures: anterior tibia, navicular, fifth metatarsal	Fascial release or excision: chronic compartment syndrome of the leg or foot, plantar fascia, medial tibial stress syndrome (with periosteal excision)	Anterior cruciate ligament instability (reconstruction with tendon graft of hamstring or patella tendon)	Osgood–Schlatter: realignment of tibial tubercle
Tendonopathies: Achilles, tibialis posterior, patella tendon, flexor hallucis longus	Accessory bones: os trigonum, os tibialis externum, os peroneum	Mechanical instability of ankle (reconstruction with peroneus brevis tendon)	Haglund's 'pump bump': calcaneal osteotomy
Ligament: lateral ankle ligaments, medial collateral knee ligament, knee cruciate ligaments	Hypertrophic bone: posterior or anterior ankle impingement, Haglund's 'pump bump'	Tibialis posterior dysfunction (Youngs' tibialis anterior suspension, or flexor digitorum longus transfer)	Tibialis posterior dysfunction: talar navicular fusion or calcaneal osteotomy
	Morton's neuromas		Hallux valgus: metatarsal osteotomies
	Bursae: retrocalcaneal, sub first metatarsophalangeal joint		Hallux rigidus: metatarsal osteotomies, fusions or implants
	Tarsal coalition		
	Intra-articular loose bodies		

come may be uncertain in terms of the athlete being able to return to sport, or the athlete is only incapacitated when exercising, the decision to operate becomes more contentious. The athlete must carefully consider how important the sport is to them and whether they are prepared to take the risks associated with the surgery. It is essential that the referring practitioner and surgeon properly counsel the athlete about any proposed surgery.

Miscellaneous therapies

Several other therapeutic techniques can also be used in the management of the injured athlete. These include trigger point therapy, acupuncture, extracorporeal shock wave therapy (ESWT) and hyperbaric oxygen.

Trigger points are points of maximum tenderness, causing reflex pain proximally and distally. They can be found in myalgia, myositis and fascial pain syndromes, where a fibrous nodule is often palpable. Trigger points are associated with a cycle of pain causing muscle or fascial spasm, which then causes more pain. Manual compression, dry needling or injecting small quantities of local anaesthetic directly into the trigger point interferes with the sensory feedback and can break the trigger point cycle. At the

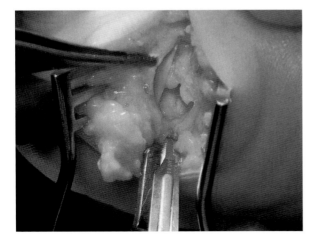

Figure 16.8 Tear of the plantar capsule of the second metatarsophalangeal joint.

Case study 16.3   Decision to undergo surgery

An 18-year-old female was referred by a local podiatrist with a 1 year history of bilateral medial longitudinal arch pain. The pain was initially induced by running and described as cramp like and fullness in the proximal part of the arch. It would resolve within 30 minutes of stopping exercise. It had initially been diagnosed as plantar fasciitis but had not responded to stretches, ultrasound, icing, topical NSAID gel and several different types of orthosis. The condition had deteriorated to the point where the patient was unable to run and the pain was induced by fast walking. The patient had a normal body mass index and was otherwise healthy. There was an absence of neurogenic symptoms. It was suspected that she had chronic medial compartment syndrome of the foot and this was confirmed by a 5 minute postexercise intracompartmental pressure reading of 35 mmHg. Both normal and pathological intracompartmental pressures of the foot are the same as found in the lower leg (Mollica & Duyshart 2002). She underwent bilateral medial compartment fasciectomy, where a section of the fascia was removed. Six weeks later she was able to return to exercise without pain.

---

point of contact of the needle or compression on the trigger point, the patient will experience increased pain, which is then followed by relaxation of the tight structure. Several treatment sessions may be required to remove the trigger point and cure the pain. There are specific sites where trigger points can occur with common injuries such as iliotibial band friction syndrome, Achilles tendonopathy, tibialis posterior dysfunction and plantar fasciitis.

Acupuncture is a medical tradition dating back 5000 years. It is based upon the philosophy that the body and mind are one unit and that symptoms are an indication of an imbalance of this unit rather than an illness to be cured. Central to acupuncture is the person's 'chi', which means life force. This life force flows through the body through a network of channels called meridians. Acupuncture points are found along these meridians and can be manipulated by the application of 34 or 36 gauge needles to 'rebalance' the body. Acupuncture has been used to treat a number of sports injuries throughout the body. Advocates have claimed a lot of success when treating tendonopathies, patellofemoral syndrome (PFS) and plantar fasciitis.

ESWT has been used in the medical treatment of renal stones since the 1980s. It is only since the mid-1990s that it has been used in the management of sports injuries. This was initially for calcific tendonopathies such as the supraspinatus tendon in the shoulder (Haake et al 2002), and in fracture non-union (Haupt 1997). Its most recent application is for insertional plantar fasciitis associated with a heel spur (Ogden et al 2002,

Rompe et al 2002). ESWT can cause significant pain and many patients discontinue treatment for this reason. For those who persevere, success rates are generally high, especially when bone marrow oedema can be detected on magnetic resonance imaging (MRI) (Maier et al 2000). Because of the pain associated with the treatment, ESWT is generally reserved for recalcitrant cases where more conventional conservative treatment has failed. Confirmation of the diagnosis by ultrasound, radiograph or MRI is usually required before commencing treatment.

Hyperbaric oxygen is a form of treatment where the patient breathes in 100% oxygen while the entire body is exposed to slightly elevated air pressure. It has been used medically in the treatment of ulcers, burns, decompression sickness and carbon monoxide poisoning. In sports medicine, its use is controversial because of the lack of scientific evidence. Anecdotal evidence, often involving high-profile athletes, suggests hyperbaric oxygen can accelerate the natural healing process. This is thought to occur by reduction of the inflammatory response and enhanced collagen deposition. However, it has been shown to have little effect on the healing in ankle sprains (Borromeo et al 1997) and delayed-onset muscle soreness (Staples et al 1999).

INJURIES TO THE SKIN AND NAILS

The integumentary system is often traumatized in sport. Abrasions and lacerations to the lower limb are common in contact sports such as football and rugby. They may also be seen when an athlete falls from loss of balance while exercising on uneven terrain or in sudden changes in direction. Such cuts and grazes generally heal quickly and do not require medical attention. Occasionally, treatment may be sought because of infection or the presence of foreign material in the wound. Standard wound management principles should be applied, with extra protection to the wound if the athlete is continuing to exercise. This extra protection should reduce the skin tension around the wound and prevent external trauma.

The most common foot injuries of the skin and nails are blisters, fissures, subungual haematomas and ingrown toenails. Blistering of the skin in athletes follows excessive frictional forces between the layers of the skin. One study demonstrated that the commonest cause of blistering in runners was wearing new shoes (Pharis et al 1997). Blisters are exacerbated by excessive sweating (hyperhydrosis), which causes a reduction in skin tone and can lead to blistering of large areas of the foot (Fig. 16.9). These are more commonly seen in endurance events such as marathon running. More localized blisters are associated with areas of increased forces, which may result from deformity, abnormal function or external footwear pressure. The treatment of painful superficial blisters requires drainage. If the blister is large, drainage should be from

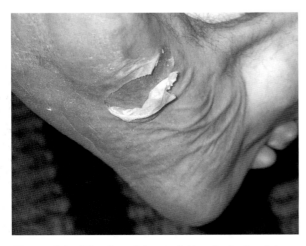

Figure 16.9 Blistering of the medial longitudinal arch in a marathon runner.

several points and is best achieved with a sterile scalpel blade. Removing the roof of the blister should be avoided, as exposure of the immature epidermal tissue is very painful. A sterile dressing should be applied and the athlete encouraged to allow the roof of the blister to peel off naturally. The use of specific blister dressings such as Spenco Second Skin can help to reduce frictional forces around the blister while providing protection. Deeper blisters involving the dermis are usually seen under the metatarsal heads or heel. They are too deep to be drained and should be treated with rigid strapping to encourage resorption and padding to redistribute pressure away from the site. Long-term management requires addressing the aetiology through reducing hyperhydrosis and frictional forces.

Skin fissures are splits in the skin, usually to the point of bleeding. They can occur interdigitally, especially between the fourth and fifth toes, and are caused by hyperhydrosis or prolonged sweating in endurance events. Fissures are also seen with reduced moisture content of the skin (anhydrosis) around the heels. Treatment for both requires sterile dressings that draw the skin edges together, such as Steri-strips. Once the fissure has resolved, the aetiology should be addressed through appropriate topical treatment.

Athletes are also prone to the development of corns, callus, fungal and viral infections of the foot. Corns and callus may develop naturally from the increased forces associated with the sport. They may also be caused by ill-fitting or inappropriate footwear or biomechanical dysfunction. If the corns and callus become symptomatic, the practitioner should address these issues through appropriate footwear advice and mechanical therapies. Athletes are more prone to foot infections because they use communal changing rooms and have chronic perspiration from exercise and footwear. Treatment requires eradication of the infection and advice on hygiene and reducing foot perspiration.

Nail disorders in athletes are usually caused by incorrect footwear, digital deformity or direct trauma. Footwear that is too small will result in trauma and cramping of the toes. This is often seen in kicking sports, where the athlete claims to get a better feel for the ball if the boot is very tight. Footwear that is too long can cause the foot to slide repetitively inside the shoe, also leading to nail trauma. Digital deformity such as claw or mallet toes, where the distal phalanx is plantar-flexed, can result in continual pressure on the proximal nail fold and matrix. Direct trauma is usually from a stubbing injury or the toe being trodden on.

Any of these situations can lead to a subungual haematoma (see Fig. 16.10). The immediate treatment for subungual haematomas is to establish drainage. How this is achieved depends upon the location under the nail. If the haematoma extends beyond the margin of the nail, this is easily achieved with a scalpel blade. If the haematoma is in the distal half of the nail, then a section of nail is removed and the nail bed pierced with a scalpel blade. If the haematoma is

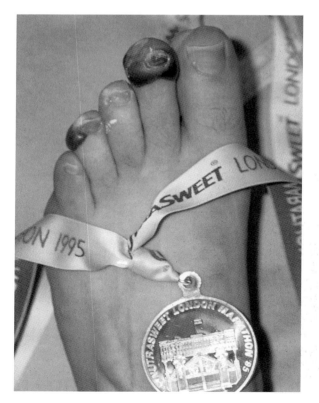

Figure 16.10 Subungual haematoma.

in the proximal half, then the nail plate and bed should be pierced with a sterile 16 or 19 gauge needle. Once the blood has been drained, a sterile compressive dressing is applied to prevent infection and refilling of the haematoma. The compression may also help to rebind the layers of the nail apparatus.

Ingrown toenails may occur at any age among athletes but are most often seen in adolescents. They are associated with an involuted nail, poor nail cutting technique or both. They can be exacerbated by hyperhydrosis or the factors mentioned above. Treatment depends upon the level of pain and deformity, the athlete's schedule and the aetiology. Removing the ingrown spike of nail, applying an antiseptic dressing and educating the athlete on nail cutting may be all that is required if the condition is mild. If the pain or deformity is severe, or there have been repetitive bouts of the problem, then surgery should be advocated. This should be by chemical matrixectomy or surgical excision. Both techniques have similar success rates although surgical excision may be advocated if the time taken to return to sport is crucial, as healing is faster. However, this needs to be balanced with the greater postoperative pain and increased cost of this technique.

Chronic nail problems can also occur in the athlete from repetitive trauma. The two commonest examples are thickening of the nail plate (onychauxis) and partial separation of the nail plate from the nail bed (onycholysis). The treatment of these is discussed in Chapter 6. It is also important to consider the possible presence of osseous pathology with a painful nail. Subungual osteochondromas are thought to be caused by repetitive trauma and will cause elevation of the nail plate and pain. Treatment usually requires surgical excision.

BURSITIS

Inflammation of an anatomical or adventitious bursa in athletes is relatively common. This is not surprising given the close proximity of anatomical bursae to tendon attachments and that both anatomical and adventitious bursae develop at sites of increased force or friction.

With muscular overuse, these bursa can become enlarged and inflamed. Poor biomechanics is often present, especially tight musculature causing greater compression of the bursa against the underlying bone. Table 16.5 details common sites of bursitis in the lower limb and the potential biomechanical cause.

Treatment of bursitis involves the application of ice and NSAIDs in the acute stage. Topical NSAIDs can be used for superficial bursitis such as retrocalcaneal or pes anserinus bursitis. A short oral course is required for deeper lying bursae, such as below the first metatarsal, or in the iliotibial band friction syndrome. Crucial to the success of any conservative treatment of bursitis is stretching of the tight structures. This should begin as soon as pain allows. It is important to note that fascial structures such as the iliotibial band require prolonged stretching for several minutes to achieve any noticeable lengthening. Addressing other biomechanical causes such as excess pronation is also important to the long-term success of treatment. If the pain has not resolved with this form of treatment, then a corticosteroid injection is warranted. Prior to the injection of the steroid, an attempt can be made to aspirate fluid from the bursal sac using a 16 or 19 gauge needle and large syringe. The skin should be anaesthetized first to reduce discomfort from the large needle. It should be noted that aspiration is usually unsuccessful because of the viscosity and organized nature of the bursal fluid. Finally, if pain persists despite repeat injections, isolated removal of the bursa may be advocated. Soft tissue reconstruction such as tendon lengthening or osseous remodelling of prominent underlying bone may also be required at the same time to guarantee long-term success.

TENDONOPATHIES

Tendonopathies represent the commonest type of overuse injury in the lower limb. Tendon pathologies usually occur at specific well-recognized sites along the tendon path. Certain factors are usually present that predispose that specific part of the tendon to injury. These factors are:

- reduced blood supply (hypovascular or watershed area)
- section of the tendon adjacent to a bony prominence
- section of the tendon that changes direction
- section of the tendon with reorientation of its fibres.

Awareness of these principles can assist the practitioner in diagnosis of tendonopathies. One or several of these factors are usually present in tendonopathy. Consider tibialis posterior tendonopathy, which characteristically occurs inferior to the medial malleolus about 4 cm proximal to the insertion. This section of the tendon is associated with a change in direction; it lies close to a bony prominence and has the least blood supply. Many factors exist that can predispose tendon injury. Intrinsic risk factors include muscle inflexibility, muscle weakness, joint stiffness, malalignment, increased age,

Table 16.5 Common sites of bursitis in the lower limb with associated sports and potential biomechanical causes

Site of bursitis	Associated sports	Potential biomechanical cause(s)
Trochanteric	Long distance running	Gluteus medius inflexibility, lateral pelvic tilt
Iliotibial band friction syndrome	Running especially long distance/downhill	Hamstring and iliotibial band inflexibility, lateral pelvic tilt, excess pronation
Prepatellar	Wrestling, judo	Quadriceps inflexibility
Pes anserinus	Breaststroke: swimmers, runners	Hamstring and sartorius inflexibility, genu valgum, excess pronation
Retrocalcaneal	Running, basketball, ice skaters	Gastrocnemius and soleus inflexibility, rear foot varus
Sub first metatarsal	Sports requiring studded footwear	Plantarflexed first ray, long first metatarsal, cavus foot

poor technique, inappropriate training schedule, obesity and systemic disease. Extrinsic risk factors include inappropriate or old footwear, exercising on hard surfaces, oral or injectable corticosteroids, and use of fluoroquinalone antibiotics.

Tendonosis

The exact pathological process that causes the pain in tendonopathies is not fully known. The athlete will often complain of stiffness and discomfort before exercise that reduces during exercise and usually returns several hours after exercise. Inflammation of the tendon itself does not occur and, therefore, the term tendonosis (American spelling: tendinosis) has now replaced the term tendonitis, following histological studies most commonly performed on the Achilles tendon (Alfredson and Lorentzon 2000). Inflammation of the tendon sheath or paratenon (paratenonitis) can occur and results in obvious swelling with occasional crepitus and formation of nodules. Fibrous thickening of the tendon sheath can occur in long-standing cases (Fig. 16.11). Histologically, tendonosis represents a degenerative non-inflammatory process characterized by mucinoid fatty deposits and a disorganized collagen structure. Infiltration of neovascular structures has also been noted. Partial tears have been found at the time of surgery in 25% of patients with tendonosis (Astrom and Rausing 1995). Tendonosis is characterized by long-standing (>3 months) pain, with little swelling, that is limiting the athlete from training fully. Discrete areas of tenderness or nodules are palpable. The athlete may recall instances of sharp pain during exercise, which may represent partial tears. It is important to note that both paratenonitis and tendonosis can coexist, giving mixed symptoms.

The treatment of paratenonitis should include the use of activity modification, ice, oral NSAIDs or phonophoresis with topical NSAIDs (Schepsis et al 2002). Once the inflammation has subsided, the treatment is the same as for tendonosis. This should include addressing the aetiological factors along with heavy-load eccentric exercises.

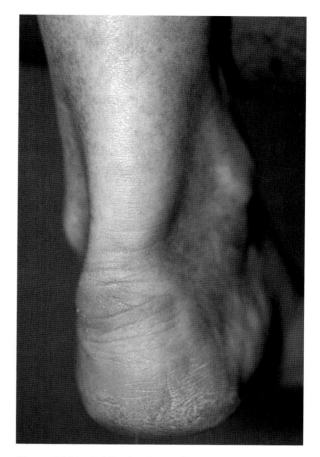

Figure 16.11   Achilles tendonopathy.

These exercises have been used very successfully in the treatment of chronic Achilles tendonosis (Niesen-Vertommen et al 1992, Alfredson et al 1998, Silbernagel et al 2001). The exercise programme uses calf drops where the person bears weight on a stair through the forefoot and lowers the heel below the level of the forefoot, thus eccentrically loading the calf (see Fig. 16.12). These exercises are initially performed with both legs with the knee both extended and flexed. It is normal for the exercise to cause pain and the athlete should be encouraged to continue unless the pain is disabling. When the exercise no longer causes pain, the athlete should progress to single limb stretches and then stretches while wearing a weighted backpack.

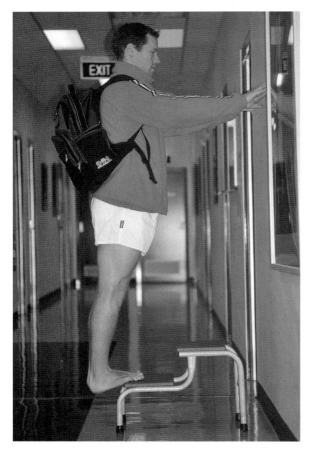

Figure 16.12 Stair-drop eccentric calf exercise with weighted back pack for Achilles tendonopathy.

In a large study involving patellar tendinopathy, Panni et al (2000) demonstrated good results using a combined conservative regimen of a short course of NSAID followed by 6 months of isometric lower limb exercises and eccentric exercises of the quadriceps. Four years later, 33 of the 42 subjects were asymptomatic. The remaining nine subjects underwent surgery. Surgical intervention for any tendonosis involves incising the tendon and removing the area of degeneration. If the defect is very large, then the tendon may need to be strengthened by the augmentation of a section with an adjacent tendon or allograft tendon. Surgical management of paratenonitis involves debulking the paratenon and removing any adhesions between the paratenon and the tendon. Results of surgery vary depending upon the technique used, the degree of pathology and which tendon is affected. Surgery for paratenonitis is successful in about 90% of cases. For tendonosis, the success rate is lower with approximately 70–80% of subjects able to return to previous sporting levels (Paavola et al 2000, Tallon et al 2001). These figures are based on the Achilles tendon. There are no large studies of surgery for the other lower limb tendonopathies with the exception of the patella tendon, where symptomatic improvement is seen in 80–90% of surgical cases but only 50% make a full return to sport (Coleman et al 2000).

Tendon rupture

Acute tendon ruptures are generally managed surgically in the athlete as rehabilitation is faster and the re-rupture rate is much less. In a recent multicentre trial, Moller et al (2001) demonstrated a re-rupture rate of 21% for subjects treated conservatively compared with 2% for surgical repair of a ruptured Achilles tendon. Interestingly there was no functional difference between the tendons surgically repaired and those that healed by conservative treatment at 2 years follow-up. The decision to operate when the rupture is not promptly diagnosed is less clear cut because of the atrophy of the tendon ends that may have occurred. Case study 16.4 demonstrates this point.

The diagnosis of acute tendon rupture is generally straightforward because of the level of pain, the swelling and the lack of function of the torn tendon. However, in long-standing tendonosis that progresses to rupture, the diagnosis often requires imaging for confirmation as these signs and symptoms are already present from the tendonosis. Surgical repair of ruptured tendonosed tendons or acute ruptures that are not diagnosed early requires augmentation with sections of adjacent tendons. Examples include Achilles tendon rupture repairs with peroneus brevis grafts, and tibialis posterior ruptures that are augmented with grafts from the flexor digitorum longus or tibialis anterior tendons.

Case study 16.4 Treatment of ruptured tendon

A 43-year-old male who was a recreational runner presented to the clinic with a 6 week history of right heel and calf pain. He had stumbled on some stairs and woke the next day with severe pain and swelling in his heel. He suffered from severe gout and both he and his GP believed it was a gout attack. He was, therefore, placed on colchicine as was customary when he had a flare up of his gout. He walked with a limp from the pain and was unable to run. When the pain and swelling did not resolve, he self-referred himself to the clinic. On examination, there was swelling present with an obvious tendon defect and calf atrophy. With the patient lying prone, the right foot was less plantarflexed than the left, indicating a ruptured Achilles (Fig. 16.13). The rupture was confirmed by an MRI scan, where the tendon ends were 2.5 cm apart. The conservative and surgical options were discussed with the patient and he elected for conservative treatment, which consisted of 8 weeks of below-knee casting. The ankle was casted in maximal plantarflexion for 4 weeks and then gradually dorsiflexed and recasted each week for a further 4 weeks. An MRI scan confirmed union of the tendon ends. He then underwent an extensive physiotherapy programme for 6 months to increase calf flexibility and strength and reduce joint stiffness. He was prescribed foot orthoses with heel raises before returning to running. Two years later he is still running regularly without pain.

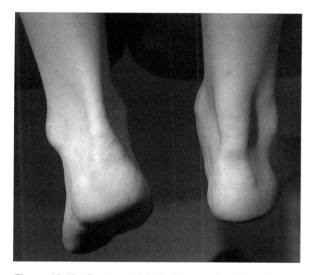

Figure 16.13 Ruptured right Achilles tendon. Note the lack of ankle plantarflexion on the right side compared with the left.

Tibialis posterior tendon dysfunction

Tibialis posterior tendon dysfunction requires special mention as tendonopathy is often accompanied by significant structural changes affecting the midtarsal, then subtalar and finally the ankle joints. Changes to the tibialis posterior tendon have been classified by Conti et al (1992) based on MRI appearance:

- *grade 1*: accumulation of fluid and longitudinal micro-tears

- *grade 2*: attenuation with frank tears and intramural degeneration
- *grade 3*: partial or complete rupture of the tendon, marked swelling and scar tissue.

As the tendon changes progress, the foot becomes more pronated, with lowering of the medial longitudinal arch, inversion and abduction of the forefoot and eversion of the rearfoot. These changes result from the loss of supinatory power of the tibialis posterior and are exacerbated by ankle equines, which is invariably present. In long-standing cases, the rearfoot joints become fixed in this position and significant arthritis develops. Athletes are generally affected by the early stages, where treatment involves activity modification, high-dye strapping with J straps, ankle braces, physical therapies and rearfoot controlling orthoses incorporating a Kirby skive, Blake inverted technique or a University of California Biomechanics Laboratory (UCBL) orthosis. If the pain is severe, then a below-knee cast or walker is required for 3–4 weeks. When the pain and swelling have subsided, then calf stretches and eccentric strengthening exercises of the tibialis posterior should begin. It is important that orthotic control is maintained especially when the athlete returns to sport.

In the later stages of the condition, it is unlikely the person will be exercising because of the pain and the apropulsive gait that has developed. At this stage, management comprises orthoses designed to enhance extrinsic shock absorption or ankle foot orthoses (AFOs). Chao et al (1996) demonstrated good success with an AFO or UCBL in patients with stage 2 or 3 posterior tibial tendon dysfunction. Footwear that gives support to the ankle and rearfoot is essential in the later stages of the condition.

Tendon dislocations

Tendon dislocations are not common injuries. The two sites where they can occur in the lower limb are the medial and lateral malleoli, affecting the tibialis posterior tendon, and more commonly the peroneal tendons. There have been only 20 cases reported in the literature for tibialis posterior tendon dislocation, compared with several hundred for the peroneal tendons. The dislocation occurs because of tearing of the flexor or peroneal retinacula, which then allows the tendon to dislocate back and forth over the malleoli during gait. This invariably causes pain, and some swelling may be evident posterior to the malleoli. The athlete will often develop gait compensation to avoid the recurrent dislocation, such as walking with the foot everted for peroneal dislocation.

Diagnosis is straightforward as the athlete usually remembers the time of the injury and may recall a popping or snapping sound. Peroneal tendon dislocations are caused by forced dorsiflexion with the foot in an everted position. This can occur in any sport, although experience suggests it is more common in skiing, basketball and rugby. The dislocation is readily visible by resisted eversion for the peroneal tendons or inversion for the tibialis posterior. This test is best performed with the athlete prone and the knee flexed to 90°. Conservative care is only appropriate for acute cases where non-weight-bearing cast immobilization is performed for 6 weeks. This achieved 50% success rate in a small case series of peroneal dislocations (McLennan 1980). Surgical treatment is generally very successful for both acute and chronic dislocations (Safran et al 1999b). It involves repair of the retinacula and any tendonosis with additional deepening of the fibular malleolar groove or osteotomy to prevent redislocation if required.

MUSCLE AND FASCIAL INJURIES

Acute muscle strains can be graded:

- *grade 1*: a minimal tear with no loss of strength
- *grade 2*: a macroscopic tear with some loss of strength
- *grade 3*: a complete tear with no function.

Immediate treatment is designed to reduce bleeding and swelling and involves following the principles of NICER. Electrotherapies and manual therapies are then used to minimize the formation of scar tissue. Finally, the cause of the strain should be addressed through correcting muscle inflexibility, imbalance or poor biomechanics. Muscle strains most commonly affect muscles that cross two joints, such as the hamstrings or gastrocnemius, and occur during eccentric contraction.

Contusions can occur in any contact sport. Their acute management is identical to that of muscle strains and full healing occurs rapidly. They are most often seen in the lower limb in the thigh or calf muscles. Occasionally, a large contusion may fibrose and then calcify. This is termed *myositis ossificans* and can lead to a delayed return to sport and prolonged treatment involving manual therapies and electrotherapies.

Delayed-onset muscle soreness occurs 1–2 days following an unaccustomed bout of exercise such as the beginning of a season or starting a new exercise programme. The exact aetiology is unknown but it is much worse following eccentric muscle activity and is probably caused by microscopic tears and the body's attempt to heal them. Delayed-onset muscle soreness is treated with manual therapies, heating the tissues, contrast baths, whirlpools or spa baths. Emphasis on proper stretching techniques before and after exercise is essential.

Minor repetitive trauma to muscle and fascia can lead to chronic inflammation and scar tissue formation. The development of scar tissue reduces the flexibility of both tissues, predisposing further injury and inflammation. This cycle can continue to the point where more serious injuries occur to the muscle and fascia, or to adjacent structures as a result of the myofascial inflexibility. Treatment consists of trigger point therapy, acupuncture and myofascial release through manual therapy.

Chronic compartment syndrome

Chronic compartment syndrome (CCS) occurs when the intracompartmental pressure within a myofascial compartment is abnormally high. During exercise, muscle volume increases by up to 20%. The muscles within the lower leg and foot are surrounded by inelastic fascial boundaries. If these boundaries cannot accommodate the increase in muscle volume, then the intracompartmental pressure rises and interstitial fluid accumulates. The exact cause of the pain that ensues is not known at present. It may be that the increased pressure inhibits muscle blood flow, causing ischaemic pain. It may also be that there is increased pressure on the pacinian corpuscles (pressure receptors) within the fascia, causing pain.

CCS most commonly occurs in the anterior compartment of the lower leg, followed by the deep posterior compartment and then the lateral compartment. CCS of the foot has been diagnosed more frequently in the recent literature but still remains a rare condition. When present it usually occurs in the medial compartment. Whichever compartment is affected, patients complain of a cramping aching pain that is induced by exercise. The athlete will have to reduce the intensity of exercise or stop exercising before the pain disappears. Pain usually resolves with 5 minutes to 1 hour of stopping exercise. Occasionally, the athlete will complain of numbness distal to the affected compartment because the elevated pressure inhibits sensory nerve function.

The aetiology of CCS is also not known. Excessive muscle hypertrophy is often present clinically. Turnipseed et al (1995) demonstrated that the fascia in subjects with CCS was twice as thick and twice as stiff as control subjects, but this may have been an effect rather than a cause of CCS. Eccentric muscle activity also increases intracompartmental pressures. Conservative treatment should be designed to reduce eccentric muscle activity during exercise. This may be achieved by addressing muscle inflexibility or imbalance through exercise therapy, orthoses or footwear modifications. Jerosch et al (1995) demonstrated a reduction in intracompartmental pressure of the anterior compartment of the leg through modifying footwear. This was achieved by producing a negative heel in the shoe, therefore reducing eccentric muscle activity of the anterior leg muscles. Rest is an ineffective treatment for CCS as the pain returns as soon as the athlete returns to exercise. If conservative treatment fails, then surgery, through fasciotomy or fasciectomy, is very successful.

Plantar fasciitis

Plantar fasciitis is undoubtedly one of the commonest foot injuries in both the athletic and non-athletic populations. It has been estimated to affect two million people a year in the USA (Pfeffer et al 1999). Obesity and increasing age are two common features in the non-athletic population with plantar fasciitis. Athletes with plantar fasciitis usually report an insidious onset of pain or occasionally recall an instance of a sharp stabbing pain, which may be caused by a small tear in the fascia. In either situation, the injury is nearly always chronic in nature at the time of examination. Poststatic dyskinesia is invariably present and the athlete has usually had to reduce the exercise volume because of the pain. The pain is localized to the medical calcaneal tubercle or more distally along the central or medial bands of the fascia. Imaging may demonstrate a thickened plantar fascia, calcaneal marrow oedema or spur.

Treatment of plantar fasciitis is similar in the athlete and the non-athlete. Ice, topical or oral NSAIDs and rest, though activity modification and strapping are undertaken initially. Once the symptoms have reduced, then stretches of the plantar fascia and calf muscle should be undertaken along with a more permanent orthoses. This may be a custom-made foot orthoses, a prefabricated foot orthoses or a silicone heel cup. The evidence over which type of device is the most effective is conflicting at present (Gill and

Kiebzak 1996, Martin et al 1998, Pfeffer et al 1999, Martin et al 2001). None of these studies was based on athletic populations. The author prefers to treat the athlete initially with strapping and, if this is effective, then proceed to prescribe an orthosis. If there is obvious excessive pronation, then a custom-made foot orthosis is prescribed. If there is none or mild overpronation, then a prefabricated device is prescribed. In instances of reduced fibrofatty padding, a silicone heel cup is used.

If symptoms remain, then a combined corticosteroid and anaesthetic injection or just an anaesthetic injection should be administered. As already discussed, night splints and ESWT can be effective in the treatment of recalcitrant cases. In acute cases, cast immobilization or using a cam-walker should be undertaken initially until the athlete is able to bear weight through the heel without limping. Conservative care is generally successful in 90–95% of cases. If the athlete fails to respond to conservative care, then plantar fascial release, via a plantar incision, of the medial and central bands should be performed. This surgical technique has a very high success rate, although the athlete should be warned that transient lateral midfoot pain is common initially.

LIGAMENT INJURIES

Ligament injuries are very common in the lower limb. The lateral collateral ligament injury to the ankle is the commonest acute sports injury seen today. Other common sites include the anterior cruciate and medial collateral ligaments of the knee, interosseous ligament of the sinus tarsi and occasionally the deltoid ligament, spring ligament, bifurcate ligament and medial collateral ligament of the first metatarsophalangeal joint. Ligament injuries are graded from one to three depending upon the severity of the injury:

- *grade 1*: stretching of the ligament without macroscopic tears or joint laxity
- *grade 2*: partial macroscopic tear with joint laxity
- *grade 3*: complete rupture with excessive joint laxity

Injuries to ligaments are invariably acute in nature and occur when the applied force exceeds the mechanical strength of the ligament. Chronic overuse injuries can follow ligament trauma because of the reduced mechanical stability. An example is mechanical instability of the ankle following a lateral ankle sprain causing peroneal tendonopathy.

Although ligaments are primarily avascular, ligament injuries involve significant swelling because of trauma to the adjacent soft tissues. Therefore, the principles of RICE or NICER are used in the early treatment to reduce swelling and pain. For grade 1 or 2 injuries, this is followed by further physical therapies involving electrical and manual therapies. Grade 3 injuries may require surgical repair of the torn ligaments or reconstruction with tendon augmentation. Grade 3 injuries can also be treated conservatively with protective functional bracing. For all injury grades, the final stage of treatment involves an exercise programme designed to enhance muscle strength and joint proprioception plus a sporting technique to prevent recurrence.

Previously, immediate surgical repair or reconstruction was reserved for elite athletes while non-elite athletes generally underwent conservative bracing and exercises, followed by surgery if this treatment failed. Current evidence suggests that conservative treatment outcomes are better than, or comparable to, surgical outcomes for both medial collateral knee ligament and ankle collateral ligament grade 3 injuries (Lynch and Restrom 1999). Surgical reconstruction of the anterior cruciate ligament involves prolonged rehabilitation and is generally reserved for those athletes whose sport involves pivoting, turning and jumping, or in athletes with recurrent episodes of the knee giving way.

Ankle ligament sprains

The majority of ankle sprains involve grade 1 injuries to the anterior talofibular ligament that heal without complication. However, up to 40% of ankle sprains are associated with persistent pain, that may be caused by mechanical or functional instability of the ankle, subtle fractures, osteochondral defects of the talus or additional soft tissue injuries to adjacent structures (Fallat et al, 1998, Gerber et al 1998). Diagnosis of these additional injuries starts with the clinician having a high level of suspicion that additional pathology can and often does occur with an ankle sprain. Attention to detail of the injury mechanism and location of symptoms is essential in identifying the additional injured structure. Finally, specific tests or imaging techniques can confirm the diagnosis.

Mechanical instability occurs with grade 2 or 3 sprains and is associated with the ankle repeatedly giving way because of ligament laxity. This mechanical instability can affect both the ankle and subtalar joints (Clanton and Berson 1999, Hertel et al 1999). It may be associated with a cavus foot type, weak or dysfunctional peroneal muscles or an ineffective treatment plan following the initial ankle sprain. Examination may reveal these associated factors along with laxity of the anterior talofibular ligament on the drawer test. Tenderness over the ligament and minor swelling are also present. Treatment requires mechanical support through taping or bracing together with strengthening exercises for the peroneal muscles and calf stretches if an ankle equinus is present. Orthoses can be beneficial incorporating a lateral pronatory rearfoot post to prevent respraining the ankle. Supporting the medial longitudinal arch may be required with this technique to prevent overuse of the tibialis posterior.

Functional instability occurs because of impaired proprioception following an ankle sprain. In true functional instability, there is no ligament laxity. It has been demonstrated that the peroneal reaction time is reduced for up to 12 weeks following ankle sprains (Kleinrensink et al 1996, Konradsen et al 1998). This loss of the protective action of the peroneal muscles greatly increases the susceptibility of the ankle to further spraining. An example of this was seen in a study of over 10 000 basketball participations involving 400 players who were followed for a season. A history of a previous ankle sprain

increased the risk of further spraining by five times (McKay et al 2001). Treatment of functional instability is centred on functional rehabilitation through strengthening the peroneal muscles and improving proprioception of the mechanoreceptors. This improved proprioception is achieved through progressively harder balance exercises involving standing on one leg, then repeating this with the eyes closed, using a wobble board or minitrampoline and finally shuttle-run exercises. Proprioceptive retraining can reduce the incidence of ankle sprains in athletes with recurrent sprains to the same level as athletes without a history of ankle sprains (Verhagen et al 2000).

Syndesmosis sprains

Syndesmosis injuries to the anterior inferior tibiofibular ligament are relatively common with lateral ankle sprains. They occur in 15% of ankle sprain injuries and are the commonest cause of persistent pain after ankle sprain (Gerber et al 1998). They can be diagnosed clinically by combined dorsiflexion and external rotation of the foot, which pushes the talus against the fibula, stretching the ligament and causing pain. This can also be achieved by squeezing the fibula against the tibia at the midshaft level. This is called the squeeze test and can be seen in Figure 16.14. Diagnosis can be confirmed by weight-bearing radiograph views or MRI. Grade 1 or 2 sprains are treated similarly to ankle sprains, but prolonged treatment is required as residual pain, stiffness and swelling are always seen with these injuries. In a retrospective study of 50 syndesmosis grade 1 or 2 injuries, a full return to activity required 31 days of treatment and one-third of the athletes complained of residual symptoms 4 years later (Taylor et al 1992). Heterotrophic ossification of the interosseous membrane can be found in up to half of patients with a previous sprain but is generally asymptomatic. Complete rupture of the syndesmosis requires surgical stabilization with a syndesmosis screw to prevent chronic pain, instability and subsequent arthritis.

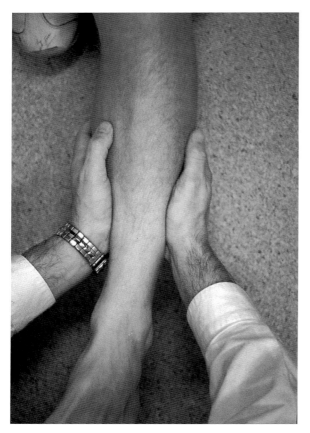

Figure 16.14 Squeeze test for tibial-fibula syndesmosis tear.

Fractures with ankle sprains

The Ottawa ankle rules were developed to identify those subjects with an ankle sprain who required radiographs to rule out the presence of subtle or frank fracture. Patients with osseous pain in the lower 6 cm of the fibula or tibia or inability to bear weight immediately after injury should have anterior–posterior, lateral and ankle mortise views taken. Patients with bone tenderness of the navicular or fifth metatarsal should have dorsal–plantar, medial–oblique and lateral foot views taken. Following these guidelines reduced the need for radiographs after ankle sprain by 30% without missing any fractures (Steill et al 1994, Leddy et al 1998). Patients who present with a painful ankle or foot with a history of a recent ankle sprain with an incomplete or absent radiograph evaluation should be sent for the above radiograph series. Fracture of the lateral, posterior or medial malleoli should be visible on the ankle radiograph series.

Pedal fractures with ankle sprains are not common but can occur to the lateral process of the talus, posterior process of the talus or the anterior process of the calcaneus. The commonest foot fracture with an ankle sprain is an avulsion fracture of the peroneus brevis on the styloid process of the fifth metatarsal. Management of these pedal fractures depends upon the size of the fracture fragment and whether the fracture is displaced. Non-displaced fractures can be treated with 2–4 weeks of immobilization in a below-knee cast. Displaced fractures will require surgical excision if the fragment is small or reduction and internal fixation if large. The other causes of a painful ankle after an ankle sprain are discussed under articular injuries.

ARTICULAR INJURIES

Joint injuries can be caused by both acute and chronic trauma, resulting in pathology of the articular cartilage, synovium, intra-articular ligaments or joint capsule. Joint injuries that are left untreated usually result in arthritis and possible deformity. The commonest articular lower limb sports injury is PFS, also known as anterior knee pain, runner's knee, chondromalacia patella, excessive lateral pressure syndrome, extensor mechanism disorder or patellofemoral pain syndrome.

Patellofemoral syndrome

PFS is the commonest chronic sports injury. It has been estimated to affect up to 25% of the population at some stage of their lives. The exact aetiology of the condition is still not known although structural malalignment causing maltracking of the patella in the trochlea groove is likely to play a significant part. Numerous factors can cause this maltracking, including abnormal alignment from excessive pronation, genu valgum, internal femoral position, internal femoral torsion, patella alta or baja, or a high Q angle. These factors may result from the muscle inflexibility and weakness outlined in Table 16.3. Activities that are known to predispose to PFS include long-distance running, hill walking or running, or descending stairs. PFS is more commonly seen in adolescents and in females. This is probably because of the developing structural alignment and the tendency for muscle inflexibility to be prevalent during periods of rapid growth such as adolescence.

Treatment of PFS involves the initial reduction of symptoms through activity modification, ice and NSAIDs. Following this, treatment should focus on addressing the aetiological factors present. This will include an extensive exercise programme, including stretching, strengthening and proprioceptive exercises. Taping to enhance muscle function and orthoses to improve alignment are also frequently required for successful treatment. Acupuncture has also been used with some success. Surgery is rarely indicated and in the past has not been particularly effective. When required in recalcitrant cases, it involves either chondroplasty or, less frequently, lateral retinacula release.

Osteochondral lesions

A common articular sports injury is an osteochondral lesion or defect. This can be seen in any joint following an injury but is most often seen on the posteriomedial or anteriorolateral aspects of the trochlear surface of the talus following an ankle sprain (Fig. 16.15). Other common sites include the first metatarsal head and

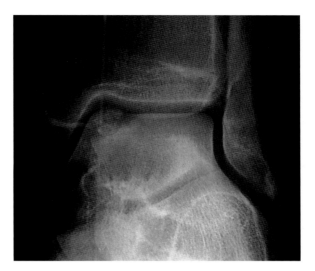

Figure 16.15 Osteochondral lesion of the talus grade III.

the tibial plafond. Osteochondral lesions can be graded 1 to 4 (Table 16.6). Classical symptoms are constant articular pain and stiffness with some swelling. Catching or locking can occur with grade 3 or 4 lesions. The purpose of the grading is to guide management. Grades 1 or 2 injuries are usually treated with a below-knee cast for 2–4 weeks followed by exercises without significant loading, such as cycling or hydrotherapy. Grades 3 or 4 generally require surgical excision with curetting and drilling of the lesion bed. Some residual pain and stiffness is often present and the athlete should be counselled that early arthritis is likely to develop in the joint. Orthoses designed to redistribute pressure away

Table 16.6 Classification of osteochondral lesions

Grade of lesion	Description	Imaging investigation required for diagnosis
I	Subchondral cystic lesion with intact roof (also known as articular bone bruise)	MRI
II	Subchondral cystic lesion with communication to joint surface	CT/MRI (may be visible on X-ray scan)
III	Separate non displaced chondral lesion	CT/MRI/X-ray
IV	Displaced chondral lesion	CT/MRI/X-ray

CT, computed tomography; MRI, magnetic resonance imaging.

from the affected side of the joint may help to alleviate symptoms.

Sinus tarsi syndrome

Sinus tarsi syndrome was first described in 1958 by O'Connor. It involves inflammation and fibrosis of the contents of the sinus tarsi following a sprain of the cervical and talocalcaneal ligaments. This usually occurs as part of an ankle sprain but may also be caused by compression of the lateral aspect of the subtalar joint in severe pronation. The athlete will complain of localized pain with minimal swelling that is exacerbated by subtalar motion or firm palpation of the sinus tarsi. Diagnosis should be confirmed by injection of local anaesthetic into the sinus tarsi. Treatment consists of taping or orthoses to control subtalar motion together with NSAIDs and activity modification to reduce the swelling. Once the pain has reduced, then mobilization of the subtalar joint can be beneficial as can proprioceptive exercises. Frequently, athletes will require corticosteroid and anaesthetic injections to alleviate symptoms fully. If conservative treatment fails, then surgical excision of the sinus tarsi is very successful.

Synovitis

Intra-articular bleeding caused by acute or chronic trauma will cause synovitis. Common sites include the ankle following an acute grade 2 or 3 ankle sprain or the metatarsophalangeal joints after chronic repetitive overloading of the joint. In chronic synovitis, poor biomechanics from functional or structural malalignment are often present, resulting in altered joint reaction forces and abnormal joint movement. The pain is generally provoked by activity, and swelling is usually present. Pain can be reproduced by compression of the joint surfaces and then taking the joint through its range of motion. Excessive motion indicating joint instability is often present.

Treatment involves activity modification, NSAIDs and ice or electrotherapies in the short term. Mechanical treatment such as taping, braces or orthoses to control excessive joint movements or improve alignment should be employed. If these measures fail, then corticosteroid injections may be tried. Conservative treatment is generally very successful but occasionally surgery may be warranted to prevent joint instability or to reduce pain via a synovectomy.

Capsular tears

Tears in the joint capsule are usually caused by an acute injury such as hyperextension of a toe causing a tear in the plantar joint capsule of the metatarsophalangeal joint. They are often misdiagnosed in the acute form, as the symptoms of pain and swelling without deformity or abnormal movement are similar to many soft tissue injuries. Often it is not until constant pain and developing deformity occur that the diagnosis is made (Case study 16.5). The situation is compounded by the inability of MRI or ultrasound to pick up tears in the joint capsule, as these tests are the standard for soft tissue pathology. Tears can really only be seen by injecting a dye into the joint and then imaging the joint with radiograph, MRI or computed tomography. Conservative management of the athlete is aimed at reducing the pain and preventing deformity through splinting the joint in the correct position. If this can be achieved in the acute stage, then the tear may heal without extensive scar tissue or deformity. Surgery is often required to repair the torn capsule and correct any residual deformity.

Plica

Plica are embryological synovial folds. They can be present in numerous joints without causing symptoms. If traumatized, they become thickened and can cause pain and altered joint function. The commonest example in the lower limb is a plica in the medial aspect of the knee, which can mimic the symptoms of PFS. The thickened fold can often be palpated with the knee flexed to 90° and deep palpation against the medial femoral condyle just medial to the patella. Conservative treatment is the same as for PFS; if this fails the plica is removed arthroscopically.

Case study 16.5 Tears in the joint capsule

A 32-year-old international kick boxer self-referred to the podiatry clinic. He had previously injured his right forefoot while kicking an opponent during a match. The forefoot had become swollen following the injury and he was treated at a casualty department with NSAIDs, a tubigrip and crutches, following radiographs that proved negative for a fracture. He was then treated by a physiotherapist, following referral from his GP, with manual therapy and electrotherapy, which significantly reduced the pain and swelling. He returned to kick boxing 7 weeks later but felt there was residual weakness in the two toes. He attempted self-treatment with ice and strapping but the pain soon returned whenever he trained or competed. One year after the initial injury, he complained of almost constant pain and increasing deformity of his second and third toes and was now unable to compete at national or international level. The deformity can be seen in Figure 16.16 and was not manually reducible. He was treated surgically by repairing and plicating the capsules, fusing the proximal interphalangeal joints and retrograding the wires into the metatarsal heads for temporary stabilization. Surgery alleviated his pain and he was able to train again, but he never returned to international competition. This case demonstrates the need for early diagnosis and appropriate early management.

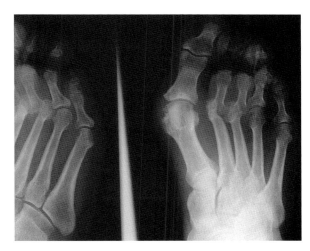

Figure 16.16 Dislocation of the second and third toes at the metatarsophalangeal joints.

INJURIES TO BONE

Stress fractures

Stress fractures are the commonest bone pathology seen among athletes. Repetitive loading of bone causes osseous microdamage and results in the bone remodelling itself to become stronger. Stress fractures occur when these repetitive loads exceed the bones' ability to adapt. The incidence of stress fractures varies between different athletic populations and between athletic and military populations. The incidence among track and field athletes has been shown to be as high as 21% (Bennell et al 1996) while among military recruits it can be as high as 27% (Finestone et al 1999). Lower rates have been shown in other sporting and military populations.

Numerous risk factors have been proposed for the development of stress fractures, with considerable variation in the level of supporting evidence. People with smaller bone geometry are more prone to stress fractures probably because of a reduced ability to resist osseous bending forces (Crossley et al 1999, Beck et al 2000). Reduced bone density has long been suggested as a cause of stress fractures, although only one well-controlled study demonstrated a significant reduction in bone density between those with and without a stress fracture (Bennell et al 1996). Menstrual irregularities increase the risk for stress fracture between two and four times compared with that in eumenorrhoeic females (Brukner and Bennell 2001). Muscle helps to attenuate force and, therefore, reduces the stress applied to bone. This has been demonstrated in stress fracture populations where the muscle mass has been proportionally smaller than in asymptomatic controls (Beck et al 2000), and the maximal muscle strength has also been less (Hoffman et al 1999). Physical fitness also plays a role, as reduced fitness leads to earlier muscle fatigue, increasing the strain to the bone through greater ground reaction forces. In a study by Shaffer et al (1999), reduced physical fitness tripled the risk of developing a stress fracture. Grimston et al (1994) demonstrated increased ground reaction forces at the point of fatigue in subjects with a history of stress fracture but not in control subjects.

Poor biomechanics has long been thought to be a crucial risk factor. A cavus foot type has been shown to be associated with tibial and femoral stress fractures (Giladi et al 1985, Brosh and Arcan 1994) and also for repetitive stress fractures (Korpelainen et al 2001). A low-arched foot type has been associated with pedal stress fractures (Simkin et al 1989). Limb length discrepancy of greater than 5 mm has been linked to the development of stress fractures in both military and athletic populations (Friberg 1982, Bennell et al 1996, Brunet et al 1990).

The location of stress fractures can vary, depending upon the activity. However, the vast majority occur below the knee. In the four largest series, involving over 1100 stress fractures, 38–54% occurred in the tibia, 7–13% the fibula, 9–23% the metatarsals and 2–10% the navicular (Orava 1980, Hulkko and Orava 1987, Matheson et al 1987, Cameron et al 1992). Treatment of stress fractures depends upon the location. Stress fractures can be classified into high and low risk (see Table 16.7). Low-risk stress fractures will generally heal within 6–8 weeks with initial rest followed by a gradual return to activities. The degree of rest depends upon the level of symptoms. If pain is present with normal daily activities, then a short period of 1–2 weeks in a below-knee cast or walker may be required. When normal daily activities are pain free, the athlete should be instructed to resume gentle exercise such as fast walking or aqua aerobics. The exercise can be slowly increased in time to a point when a short jog can be incorporated into the walk. Eventually, the athlete should be able to resume normal sporting activities. Crucial to any management programme is addressing the aetiological factors. Case study 16.6 demonstrates this point.

High-risk stress fractures require prolonged non-weight-bearing immobilization for a minimum of 6 weeks. Immobilization for up to 6 months may be required for anterior tibial cortex stress fractures. Conservative treatment is generally successful as long as the diagnosis is made early and the athlete adheres to the treatment. Stress fractures that become displaced or go on to non-union require surgical fixation and occasionally bone grafting (Saxena et al 2000, Boden et al 2001). Non-healing stress fractures of the sesamoids should be excised.

Bone stress reaction

In some athletes, the normal physiological adaptation by bone to exercise causes pathology. This is termed periostitis, periostalgia or a painful bone stress reaction and is commonly seen in athletes during the first 2 months of an exercise programme. Normal bone stress reactions can be seen in any bone undergoing adaptation where the bone is initially weakened and then becomes stronger than the state before exercise. This is a result of initial osteoclastic activity followed by osteoblasts laying down new bone. This strengthening process usually takes 6 months.

Painful bone stress reaction most commonly occurs in the tibia along the posterior medial border and is termed medial tibial stress syndrome. Poor biomechanics and fitness levels are common among athletes with this condition (Yates & White 2004). Muscle inflexibility of the gastrosoleus complex may also play a part (Yates 1999). Recent evidence suggests that the bone remains osteoporitic in patients with longstanding medial tibial stress syndrome, being 15% more porous than in control subjects and 23% less than in athletic control subjects (Magnusson et al 2001). This osteoporosis was only seen in the painful section of the tibia and was shown to return to normal levels when the symptoms resolved (Magnusson et al 2003).

Table 16.7 Low- and high-risk stress fractures

Low risk	High risk
Metatarsal necks/shaft	Sesamoids
Calcaneus	Metatarsal bases
Fibula	Fifth metatarsal diaphysis
Tibial shaft	Navicular
Femoral shaft	Talus
	Medial malleolus
	Anterior tibial cortex
	Femoral neck

Case study 16.6 Stress fracture

A 23-year-old female aerobics instructor presented with pain under her first metatarsophalangeal joint. The pain had been present for 3 weeks and was deteriorating to the point she was unable to take classes. Prior to this, she had been instructing for up to 18 hours per week. She was eumenorrhoeic with a healthy diet and no history of previous lower limb injury. The pain was located to the fibula sesamoid with swelling evident. She had a plantarflexed first ray with a high-arched foot. She changed her aerobics shoes annually. Radiographs and a bone scan were requested, which demonstrated a stress fracture of the fibula sesamoid (Fig. 16.17). She was placed in a below-knee cast for 6 weeks and issued crutches to keep the foot non-weight bearing. The foot remained symptomatic for the first 10 days of casting and then resolved. Following removal of the cast, the bone was palpated and was found to be pain free. If the bone had still been painful, then further recasting was warranted. She was prescribed orthoses to redistribute pressure away from the tibial sesamoid and increase extrinsic shock absorption. She was also advised on changing her footwear more frequently and a gradual return to exercise and teaching classes.

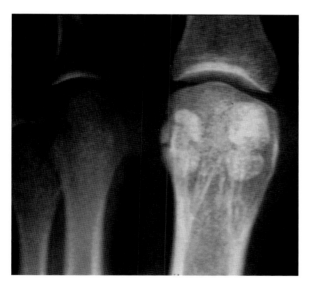

Figure 16.17 Stress fracture of the fibula sesamoid.

In the author's experience, conservative treatment is successful in 80–90% when the diagnosis is made early and appropriate treatment initiated. In long-standing cases, one in three will fail to respond to conservative care. Treatment consists of activity modification to allow the bone reaction to run its natural course. This must include reducing the number of hours of weight-bearing sport. The athlete may cycle or swim to maintain fitness. Addressing biomechanical malalignments through orthoses is often required. Increasing extrinsic shock absorption through footwear, orthoses and exercising on softer surfaces is crucial when the athlete returns to weight-bearing sport. Muscle imbalances should also be corrected through appropriate stretching exercises, especially the soleus muscle. Other treatments that have been used with some success include digital ischaemic pressure, vacuum cupping and neoprene calf sleeves.

Prophylactic treatment can include the use of orthoses or shock-absorbing insoles. Exercises that involve jumping can also significantly strengthen the tibia and, if performed as part of a controlled slowly progressive exercise programme, should lower the rate of medial tibial stress syndrome (Milgrom et al 2000). Surgery is only advocated in recalcitrant cases. In the largest series to date, symptoms were reduced by over 70% but only half made a full return to previous levels of sporting activity (Yates et al 2003).

Bone impingements

The normal response of bone to repetitive trauma is to lay down new bone. When this occurs close to a joint, the osteophytes produced will cause pain at the end range of motion and eventually lead to a reduced range of motion. The commonest site in the lower limb is the anterior and posterior aspects of the ankle and the first metatarsophalangeal joint. Ankle impingements are common in football and the condition is often termed 'footballers ankle'. Posterior impingement can occur in any sport or activity that requires maximal plantarflexion such as football, ballet, yoga or gymnastics. An enlarged posterior talar process or os trigonum becomes impinged against the posterior aspect of the tibia at end range of plantarflexion. Diagnosis can be confirmed by palpation, passively taking the joint to end range, a local anaesthetic injection at the site of pain or a radiograph taken in maximal plantarflexion. Treatment consists of NSAIDs, subtalar and ankle mobilizations, heel-lock strapping to limit motion and evaluation of the sporting technique that produces the pain. If conservative treatment fails, which is not uncommon, then surgical excision is generally very successful.

Anterior impingement occurs at maximal dorsiflexion in football and ballet. It is probably common in football because of the design of football boots. These offer little protection on the anterior aspect of the ankle, and the lack of a raised heel means that greater levels of dorsiflexion are required during propulsion than in other sports. Osseous spurs occur on the dorsal aspect of the talar neck and tibial plafond. As the spurs enlarge, they can irritate overlying soft tissues and eventually lead to a loss of motion. Conservative treatment is similar to posterior impingement, with strapping, NSAIDs and mobilizations. Large spurs often require surgical excision.

Impingement of the first metatarsophalangeal joint is also called hallux rigidus or limitus. This can be seen in contact sports where the joint may be easily traumatized, such as American football, soccer and rugby, or in sports where the athlete frequently lands on the forefoot, such as tennis, athletics and sprinting. Biomechanical abnormalities, including a long or dorsiflexed first metatarsal or excessive pronation, are common contributory factors. Athletes will complain of pain localized to an enlarged joint with dorsal osteophytes. Occasionally, they may complain of neuritic symptoms where the osteophytes are compressing the medial or lateral dorsal nerve against footwear, causing a Joplins' neuroma. Conservative treatment consists of ice, NSAIDs and flask strapping in the acute stages, followed by mobilizations and orthoses. Occasionally, corticosteroid injections are needed or manipulation may need to be performed under anaesthesia. Surgery for hallux rigidus is discussed in more detail in Chapter 6, but maintaining first metatarsophalangeal joint function is paramount for an athlete to be able to continue to exercise at a high level.

Accessory bones

Accessory bones are anatomic variants that are found in tendons. Some are always present, such as the patella or hallucal sesamoids, where they increase the mechanical advantage of the attached muscle by acting as a pulley. Numerous other accessory bones have been documented within the lower limb. The vast majority are asymptomatic but some have been associated with pathology. These include:

- os tibialis externum with posterior tibialis tendonopathy
- os peroneum in peroneus longus tendon (often following an ankle sprain)
- os trigonum causing posterior ankle impingement
- fabella causing posterior lateral knee pain.

Treatment for these conditions varies, but for all a period of initial rest, ice and NSAIDs should be tried. Reducing the stress on the associated tendon is attempted through orthoses and appropriate exercises. Local anaesthetic injections can help to reduce inflammation around the accessory bone but corticosteroids should be avoided. If conservative treatment fails, surgical excision is successful as long as meticulous detail is paid to repair of the tendon and achieving normal physiological tension of the tendon.

NERVE INJURIES

Sports injuries to nerves will result in neurogenic symptoms involving altered sensation or function. The athlete will usually complain of painful tingling that is often diffuse and burning in nature. Complete numbness is rare. The practitioner must be aware that the symptoms may be part of a systemic disease process or distal symptoms from a proximal pathology such as a radiculopathy. Clinical diagnosis of a nerve entrapment starts with exclusion of the more common pathologies. If palpation of the area is painful and percussion elicits distal symptoms

(Tinel's sign) or proximal symptoms (Villeix phenomenon), then nerve entrapment is strongly suspected. Specialist tests such as MRI, ultrasound or nerve conduction may show the entrapment but are often negative. Local anaesthetic injection can be helpful diagnostically if the entrapment is to a small branch of a nerve and well localized, such as for Morton's neuroma. The common sites for nerve entrapments in athletes are shown in Table 16.8.

Treatment for nerve entrapments includes measures to reduce local inflammation, such as ice and NSAIDs. Biomechanical treatment is often essential to prevent further compression of the nerve or reduce nerve tension. This may include strapping, orthoses or footwear modification. Laterally posted orthoses can reduce superficial peroneal nerve tension, while medially posted ones can reduce tibial nerve tension. If scarring is present at the site of the entrapment, friction massage and neural stretches should be performed. If muscle inflexibility or imbalance is present close to the entrapment, then stretching exercises should be performed (Schon 1994). Transcutaneous nerve stimulation has been advocated for neuropathic pain (Smith and Dahm 2001). The use of combined corticosteroid and anaesthetic injections can be very beneficial.

Surgical intervention involves nerve decompression or excision in the case of Morton's neuroma. Surgery may also be performed to improve structural alignment or prevent osseous compression of the affected nerve.

VASCULAR INJURIES

Arterial and venous sports injuries are very rare. As with nerve injuries, a clinician who suspects a vascular cause of the symptoms should consider systemic vascular disease as well as localized pathology. Atherosclerosis may be present in the older athlete or the younger athlete with obvious risk factors. Symptoms of exercise-induced claudication will be present and can be confirmed by pre- and postexercise ankle brachial indices. Vasospastic conditions, such as Raynaud's or Buerger's disease, may be present, causing claudication, pain, numbness and cyanosis of the feet and hands.

Effort-induced deep vein thrombosis

Effort induced deep venous thrombosis has been rarely reported in the sports medicine literature (Ali et al 1984, Gorard 1990). It should be suspected in those with calf tenderness and swelling

Table 16.8 Common sites for nerve entrapments in athletes

Nerve	Pathology	Area of symptoms	Comments
Digital	Mortons' neuroma	Third or second web space	Commonest nerve entrapment; often visible on MRI/ultrasound
First branch of lateral plantar	Baxter's nerve or inferior calcaneal nerve entrapment	Inferior medial heel; occasionally lateral border of foot	Often misdiagnosed as a heel spur/plantar fasciitis; limited fifth toe abduction often present
Medial plantar	Jogger's foot	Medial arch and forefoot	Entrapment from abductor hallucis muscle, often with excess pronation
Tibial	Tarsal tunnel syndrome	Sole of the foot/medial side of ankle	Usually caused by excess pronation; seen in runners
Superficial peroneal	–	Dorsum of the foot and ankle	Occurs after ankle sprain in 25%; also with tight boots, e.g. ski boots
Deep peroneal	Anterior tarsal tunnel syndrome	Dorsal midfoot or first web space	Caused by osteophytic compression or tight footwear
Saphenous	–	Medial aspect of knee or calf	Usually caused by contusion or adductor canal pathology

in the presence of factors known to increase the risk of thrombosis (Virschaud's triangle). It can also occur following a calf strain (Taylor 2002). Confirmation requires duplex sonography or a venogram. Treatment requires anticoagulation and advice to the athlete on reducing the risk factors to prevent recurrence.

Popliteal artery entrapment

Popliteal artery entrapment is caused by an anatomic muscular variant that leads to compression of the popliteal artery by the medial head of the gastrocnemius during exercise. It is also possible for the artery to be compressed by the soleus or plantaris muscles. The symptoms are of intermittent claudication in the calf, foot or anterior aspect of the leg. Diagnosis is by pre- and postexercise ankle brachial indices or duplex sonography. Confirmation may require angiography with the patient performing calf exercises. Treatment is by surgically decompressing the artery.

SUMMARY

The majority of lower limb sports injuries seen by the podiatrist are chronic in nature. Initial treatment usually requires physical, pharmacological and mechanical therapies if symptoms are to be reduced successfully. Long-term management is aimed at preventing recurrence. Similar modalities may be used for this long-term goal but the practitioner must attempt to address both the intrinsic and extrinsic risk factors present to ensure success. This chapter has outlined the common lower limb sports injuries and their management based upon these principles.

REFERENCES

Acevedo J I, Beskin J L 1998 Complications of plantar fascia associated with corticosteroid injection. Foot and Ankle International 19: 91–97
Alfredson H, Lorentzon R 2000 Chronic Achilles tendinosis. Sports Medicine 29: 135–146
Alfredson H, Pietila T, Jonsson P et al 1998 Heavy load eccentric calf muscle training for the treatment of chronic Achilles tendinosis. American Journal of Sports Medicine 26: 360–366
Ali M S, Kutty M S, Corea J R 1984 Deep vein thrombosis in a runner. American Journal of Sports Medicine 12: 169
Altman R D, Moskowitz R 1998 Intra-articular sodium hyaluronate (Hyalgan) in the treatment of patients with osteoarthritis of the knee: a randomized clinical trial. Journal of Rheumatology 25: 2203–2212
Astrom M, Rausing A 1995 Chronic Achilles tendinopathy. A survey of surgical and histological findings. Clinical Orthopedics 316: 151–164
Basford J R, Malanga G A, Krause D A et al 1998 A randomized controlled evaluation of low-intensity laser therapy. Archives Physical Medical Rehabilitation 79: 249–254
Beck T J, Ruff C B, Shaffer R A 2000 Stress fracture in military recruits: gender differences in muscle and bone susceptibility factors. Bone 27: 437–444
Belanger AY 2002 Laser. In: Belanger A Y (ed) Evidence-based guide to therapeutic physical agents. Lippincott Williams & Wilkins, Philadelphia, PA, p 191–221
Bengal S, Lowe J, Mann G et al 1997 The role of the knee brace in the prevention of anterior knee pain syndrome. American Journal of Sports Medicine 25: 1118–1122
Bennell K L, Malcolm S A, Thomas S A et al 1996 The incidence and distribution of stress fractures in competitive track and field athletes. American Journal of Sports Medicine 24: 211–217

Bleakley C, MacAuley D 2002 The quality of research in sports journals. British Journal of Sports Medicine 36: 124–125
Boden B P, Osbahr D C, Jimenez C 2001 Low risk stress fractures. American Journal of Sports Medicine 29: 100–111
Borromeo C N, Ryan J L, Marchetto P A et al 1997 Hyperbaric oxygen therapy for acute ankle sprains. American Journal of Sports Medicine 25: 619–625
Brosh T, Arcan M 1994 Toward early detection of the tendency to stress fractures. Clinical Biomechanics 9: 111–116
Brosseau L, Casimiro L, Robinson V et al 2002 Therapeutic ultrasound for treating patellofemoral pain syndrome (Cochrane Review). The Cochrane Library Issue 2, Update Software, Oxford
Brukner P D, Bennell K L 2001 Stress fractures. In O'Connor F G, Wilder R P (eds). Textbook of running medicine. McGraw-Hill, New York, p 227–256
Brunet M E, Cook S D, Brinker M R et al 1990 A survey of running injuries in 1505 competitive and recreational runners. Journal of Sports Medicine Physical Fitness 30: 307–315
Burks R T, Bean B G, Marcus R et al 1991 Analysis of athletic performance with prophylactic ankle devices. American Journal of Sports Medicine 19: 104–106
Cameron K R, Wark J D, Telford R D 1992 Stress fractures and bone loss: the skeletal cost of intense athleticism. Excellence 8: 39–55
Chao W, Wapner K L, Lee T H et al 1996 Nonoperative treatment of posterior tibial tendon dysfunction. Foot and Ankle International 17: 736–741
Clanton T O, Berson L 1999 Subtalar joint athletic injuries. Foot and Ankle Clinics 4: 729–743

Coleman B D, Khan K M, Kiss Z S et al 2000 Open and arthroscopic patellar tenotomy for chronic patellar tendonopathy. American Journal of Sports Medicine 28: 183–190

Conti S F, Michelson J, Jhass M 1992 Clinical significance of MRI in pre-operative planning for reconstruction of posterior tibial tendon ruptures. Foot and Ankle 13: 208–214

Crossley K, Bennell K L, Wrigley T et al 1999 Ground reaction forces, bone characteristics, and tibial stress fracture in male runners. Medical Science and Sports Exercise 31: 1088–1093

de Clerq D L R 1997 Ankle bracing in running: the effect of a push type medium ankle brace upon movements of the foot and ankle during the stance phase. International Journal of Sports Medicine 18: 222–228

Dockery G L, Nilsson R Z 1986 Intralesional injections. Clinical Podiatric Medical Surgery 3: 473–485

Donatelli R, Hurbert C, Conway D et al 1988 Biomechanical foot orthotics: a retrospective study. Journal of Orthopaedics and Sports Physical Therapy 10: 205–212

Ellis B 1998 Transcutaneous electrical nerve stimulation for pain relief: recent research findings and implications for clinical use. Physical Therapy Review 3: 3–8

Fallat L, Grimm D J, Saracco J A 1998 Sprained ankle syndrome: prevalence and analysis of 639 acute injuries. Journal of Foot and Ankle Surgery 37: 280–285

Finestone A, Giladi M, Elad H et al 1999 Prevention of stress fractures using custom biomechanical shoe orthoses. Clinical Orthopedics 164: 153–156

Friberg O 1982 Leg length asymmetry in stress fractures. A clinical and radiological study. Journal of Sports Medicine 22: 485–488

Gerber J P, Williams G N, Scoville C R et al 1998 Persistent disability associated with ankle sprains: a prospective examination of an athletic population. Foot and Ankle International 19: 653–660

Gigante A, Pasquinelli F M, Paladini P et al 2001 The effects of patellar taping on patellofemoral incongruence. American Journal of Sports Medicine 29: 88–92

Giladi M, Milgrom C, Stein M et al 1985 The low arch, a protective factor in stress fractures. A prospective study of 295 military recruits. Orthopaedic Review 14: 709–714

Gill L H, Kiebzak G M 1996 Outcome of non-surgical treatment of plantar fasciitis. Foot and Ankle International 17: 527–532

Gorard DA 1990 Effort thrombosis in an American football player. British Journal of Sports Medicine 24: 15

Grimston S K, Nigg B M, Fisher V et al 1994 External loads throughout a 45 minute run in stress fracture and non-stress fracture runners. Journal of Biomechanics 27: 668

Gross M L, Davlin L B, Evanski P M 1991 Effectiveness of orthotic shoe inserts in the long distance runner. American Journal of Sports Medicine 19: 409–412

Haake M, Deike B, Thon A et al 2002 Exact focusing of extracorporeal shock wave therapy for calcifying tendinopathy. Clinical Orthopedics 397: 323–331

Hart L E, Walter S D 1990 Critical appraisal of a selection of the sports medicine literature. Medical Science and Sports Exercise 22: S116

Hart L E, Meeuwisse W H 1994 Evaluating methodology in the sports medicine literature. Clinical Journal of Sports Medicine 4: 64

Haupt G 1997 Use of extracorporeal shock waves in the treatment of pseudarthrosis, tendinopathy and other orthopaedic diseases. Journal of Urology 158: 4–11

Heckman J D, Ryaby J P, McCabe J et al 1994 Acceleration of tibial fracture healing by non-invasive, low intensity pulsed ultrasound. American Journal of Bone and Joint Surgery 76A: 26–34

Hertel J, Denegar C R, Monroe M M et al 1999 Talocrural and subtalar joint instability after lateral ankle sprain. Medical Science and Sports Exercise 31: 1501–1508

Hoffman J R, Chapnik L, Shamis A 1999 The effect of leg strength on the incidence of lower extremity overuse injuries during military training. Military Medicine 164: 153–156

Hulkko A, Orava S 1987 Stress fractures in athletes. International Journal of Sports Medicine 8: 221–226

Jerosch J, Castro W H, Halm H, Bork H 1995 Influence of the running shoe sole on the pressure in the anterior tibial compartment. Acta Orthopedica Belgique 61: 190–198

Johnston E, Scranton P, Pfeiffer G B 1997 Chronic disorders of the Achilles tendon: Results of conservative and surgical management. Foot and Ankle International 18: 570–574

Keenan A M, Tanner C 2001 The effect of high-dye and low-dye taping on rearfoot motion. Journal of the American Podiatric Medical Association 91: 255–261

Khan K M, Cook J L, Bonar F et al 1999 Histopathology of common overuse tendon conditions: update and implications for clinical management. Sports Medicine 27: 393–408

Kilmartin T E, Wallace W A 1994 The scientific basis for the use of biomechanical foot orthoses in the treatment of lower limb sports injuries: a review of the literature. British Journal of Sports Medicine 28: 180–184

Kleinrensink G J, Stoeckart R, Meulstee J 1996 Lowered conduction velocity of the peroneal nerve after inversion moments. American Journal of Sports Medicine 24: 362–369

Konradsen L, Olesen S, Hansen HM 1998 Ankle sensorimotor control and eversion strength after acute ankle inversion injuries. American Journal of Sports Medicine 26: 72–78

Korpelainen R, Orava S, Karpakka J et al 2001 Risk factors for recurrent stress fractures in athletes. American Journal of Sports Medicine 29: 304–310

Kuligowski L A, Lephart S M, Frank P 1998 Effect of whirlpool therapy on delayed onset muscle soreness. Journal of Athletics and Training 33: 222–228

Larsen B, Andreasen E, Urfer A et al 1995 Patella taping: a radiographic examination of the medial glide technique. American Journal of Sports Medicine 23: 465–471

Larsen K, Weidich F, Leboeuf Y de C 2002 Can custom made biomechanical shoe orthoses prevent problems in the back and lower extremities? A randomized, controlled intervention trial of 146 military conscripts. Journal of Manipulative Physiol Therapy 25: 326–331

Leddy J J, Smolinski R J, Lawrence J L et al 1998 Prospective evaluation of the Ottawa ankle rules in a university sports medicine center. With a modification to increase specificity for identifying malleolar fractures. American Journal of Sports Medicine 26: 158–165

Lynch S A, Renstrom P A 1999 Treatment of acute lateral ankle ligament rupture in the athlete. Conservative versus surgical treatment. Sports Medicine 27: 61–71

MacKean L C, Bell G, Bunrham R S 1995 Prophylactic ankle bracing vs. taping: effects on functional performance in female basketball players. Journal of Orthopedics and Sports Physical Therapy 22: 77–81

Magnusson H I, Westlin N E, Nyqvist F et al 2001 Abnormally decreased regional bone density in athletes with medial tibial stress syndrome. American Journal of Sports Medicine 29: 712–715

Magnusson H I, Ahlborg H, Karlsson C, et al 2003 Low regional tibial bone density in athletes with medial tibial stress syndrome normalizes after recovery from symptoms. American Journal of Sports Medicine 31: 596–600

Maier M, Steinborn M, Schmitz C et al 2000 Extracorporeal shock wave application for chronic plantar fasciitis associated with heel spurs: prediction of outcome by MRI. Journal of Rheumatology 27: 2455–2462

Manfoy P P, Ashton-Miller J A, Wojtys E M 1997 The effects of exercise, pre-wrap and athletic tape on the maximal active and passive ankle resistance to ankle inversion. American Journal of Sports Medicine 25: 156–163

Martin J E, Hosch W P, Murff R T et al 2001 Mechanical treatment of plantar fasciitis. Journal of American Podiatric Medicine Association 91: 55–62

Martin R L, Irrgang J J, Conti S F 1998 Outcome study of subjects with insertional plantar fasciitis. Foot and Ankle International 19: 803–811

Matheson G O, Clement D B, McKenzie D C et al 1987 Stress fractures in athletes. A study of 320 cases. American Journal of Sports Medicine 15: 46–58

McKay G D, Goldie P A, Payne W R et al 2001 Ankle injuries in basketball: injury rate and risk factors. British Journal of Sports Medicine 35: 103–108

McLennan J G 1980 Treatment of acute and chronic luxations of the peroneal tendons. American Journal of Sports Medicine 8: 432–436

Milgrom C, Simkin A, Eldad A et al 2000 Using bone's adaptation ability to lower the incidence of stress fractures. American Journal of Sports Medicine 28: 245–251

Miller S J, Nakra A 2001 Morton's neuroma. In: Banks A S, Downey M S, Martin D E et al (eds) McGlamry's comprehensive textbook of foot and ankle surgery, 3rd edn. Lippincott Williams & Wilkins, Philadelphia, PA, p 231–252

Moller M, Movin T, Granhed H et al 2001 Acute rupture of tendo Achilles. A prospective randomized study of comparison between surgical and non-surgical treatment. British Journal of Bone and Joint Surgery 83: 843–848

Mollica M B, Duyshart S C 2002 Analysis of pre- and postexercise compartment pressures in the medial compartment of the foot. American Journal of Sports Medicine 30: 268–271

Niesen-Vertommen S L, Taunton J E, Clement D B et al 1992 The effect of eccentric versus concentric exercise in the management of Achilles tendonitis. Clinical Journal of Sports Medicine 2: 109–113

O'Connor D 1958 Sinus tarsi syndrome: a clinical entity. American Journal of Bone and Joint Surgery 40A: 720–729

Ogden J A, Alvarez R, Levitt R et al 2002 Shock wave therapy for chronic plantar fasciitis. Clinical Orthopedics 398: 267–269

Ohberg L, Alfredson H 2002 Ultrasound guided sclerosis of neovessels in painful chronic Achilles tendinosis: pilot study of a new treatment. British Journal of Sports Medicine 36: 173–177

Orava S 1980 Stress fractures. British Journal of Sports Medicine 14: 40–44

Paavola M, Kannus P, Paakala T et al 2000 Long-term prognosis of patients with Achilles tendinopathy. An observational 8 year follow up study. American Journal of Sports Medicine 28: 634–642

Panni A S, Tartarone M, Maffulli N 2000 Patellar tendinopathy in athletes, American Journal of Sports Medicine 28: 392–397

Pavier J C, Liggins W J 2001 The use of 0.5% bupivocaine hydrochloride plain solution injections in the treatment of chronic plantar fasciitis. British Journal of Podiatry 4: 90–94

Pfeffer G, Bacchetti P, Deland J et al 1999 Comparison of custom and prefabricated orthoses in the initial treatment of proximal plantar fasciitis. Foot and Ankle International 20: 214–221

Pharis D B, Teller C, Wolf J E 1997 Cutaneous manifestations of sports participation. Journal of American Academy of Dermatology 36: 448

Rompe J D, Schoellner C, Nafe B 2002 Evaluation of low energy extracorporeal shock-wave application for treatment of chronic plantar fasciitis. American Journal of Bone and Joint Surgery 84A: 335–341

Safran M R, Zachazewski J E, Benedetti R S et al 1999a Lateral ankle sprains: Treatment and rehabilitation with an emphasis on the athlete. Medical Science and Sports Exercise 31: S438–S447

Safran M R, O'Malley D, Fu F H 1999b Peroneal tendon subluxation in athletes: new exam technique, case reports, and review. Medical Science and Sports Exercise 31: S487–S492

Saxena A, Fullem B, Hannaford D 2000 Results of treatment of 22 navicular stress fractures and a new proposed radiological classification system. Journal of Foot and Ankle Surgery 39: 96–103

Schepsis A A, Jones H, Haas A L 2002 Achilles tendon disorders in athletes. American Journal of Sports Medicine 30: 287–305

Schon L 1994 Nerve entrapment, neuropathy, and nerve dysfunction in the athlete. Orthopedic Clinics of North America 25: 47–59

Schwellnus M P, Jordon G, Noakes T D 1990 Prevention of common overuse injuries by the use of shock absorbing soles: a prospective study. American Journal of Sports Medicine 18: 636–641

Seror P, Pluvinage P, d'Andre F L et al 1999 Frequency of sepsis after local corticosteroid injection. Rheumatology 38: 1272–1274

Shaffer R A, Brodine S K, Almeida S A et al 1999 Use of simple measures of physical activity to predict stress fractures in young men undergoing a rigorous physical training program. American Journal of Epidemiology 149: 236–242

Silbernagel K G, Thomee R, Thomee P et al 2001 Eccentric overload training for patients with chronic Achilles tendon pain: a randomized controlled study with reliability testing of the evaluation methods. Scandinavian Journal of Medical Science and Sports 11: 197–206

Simkin A, Leichter I, Giladi M et al 1989 Combined effect of foot arch structure and an orthotic device on stress fractures. Foot and Ankle 10: 25–29

Sitler M, Ryan J, Wheeler B et al 1994 The efficacy of a semi-rigid ankle stabiliser to reduce acute ankle injuries in basketball. American Journal of Sports Medicine 22: 454–461

Smith J, Dahm D L 2001 Nerve entrapments. In: O'Connor F G, Wilder R P (eds) Textbook of running medicine. McGraw-Hill, New York, p 257–272

Staples J R, Clement D B, Taunton J E et al 1999 Effects of hyperbaric oxygen on a human model of injury. American Journal of Sports Medicine 27: 600–605

Steill I G, McKnight R D, Greenberg G H et al 1994 Implementation of the Ottawa ankle rules. Journal of American Medical Association 271: 827–832

Tallon C, Coleman B D, Khan K M et al 2001 Outcome of surgery for chronic Achilles tendinopathy. American Journal of Sports Medicine 29: 315–320

Taylor A J 2002 Deep vein thrombosis following calf strain: a case study. Physical Therapy for Sports 3: 110–113

Taylor D C, Englehardt D L, Bassett F H 1992 Syndesmosis sprains of the ankle. American Journal of Sports Medicine 20: 146–150

Turnipseed W D, Hurschler C, Vanderby R 1995 The effects of elevated compartment pressure on tibial arteriovenous flow and relationship of mechanical and biochemical characteristics of fascia to genesis of chronic anterior compartment syndrome. Journal of Vascular Surgery 21: 810–816

van der Windt D A 1999 Ultrasound therapy for musculo-skeletal disorders: a systematic review. Pain 81: 257–271

van der Windt D A, van der Heijden G J, van der Berg S G et al 2002 Ultrasound therapy for acute ankle sprains (Cochrane review). The Cochrane Library Issue 2, Update Software, Oxford

Verhagen E A, van Mechelen W, de Vente W 2000 The effect of preventative measures on the incidence of ankle sprains. Clinical Journal of Sports Medicine 10: 291–296

Watts B L, Armstrong B 2001 A randomized controlled trial to determine the effectiveness of double Tubigrip in grade 1 and 2 (mild to moderate) ankle sprains. Emergency Medicine Journal 18: 46–50

Yates B 1999 Biomechanical aetiologies and surgical outcome in medial tibial stress syndrome. MSc Thesis, Manchester Metropolitan University, UK

Yates B 2002 Assessment of the sports patient. In: Meriman L, Turner W (eds) Assessment of the lower limb, 2nd edn. London, Churchill Livingstone, p 373–395

Yates B, White S 2004 The incidence and risk factors in the development of medial tibial stress syndrome. American Journal of Sports Medicine 32: 772–780.

Yates B, Allen M, Barnes M 2003 Outcome of surgical treatment of medial tibial stress syndrome. American Journal of Bone and Joint Surgery 85(A): 1974–1980

Yeung E W, Yeung S S 2001 A systematic review of interventions to prevent lower limb soft tissue running injuries. British Journal of Sports Medicine 35: 383–389

REFERENCES

Brukner P, Khan K 2002 Clinical sports medicine, revised 2nd edition. McGraw-Hill, Sydney

O'Connor F G, Wilder R P (eds) 2001 Textbook of running medicine. McGraw-Hill, New York

Prentice W E 2002 Therapeutic modalities for physical therapists, 2nd edn. McGraw-Hill, New York

Subotnik S I (ed) 1999 Sports medicine of the lower extremity, 2nd edn. Churchill Livingstone, New York

17

Management of tissue viability

Kate Springett

INTRODUCTION

A leg or foot that has poor tissue viability is 'at risk' and can cause the individual concerned great distress and pain as well as disrupting their daily living. Having poor-quality skin and other tissues, the at-risk person has a high propensity to tissue damage and infection. With appropriate management, the limb status may be cured, be improved, the status quo maintained or, regardless of the skill of the practitioner, may deteriorate.

Whatever situation arises, management requires involvement of at least one person in the care of the limb; the individual concerned. Others involved in the care of the at-risk limb include the carer, the practitioner, who may be a podiatrist, another allied health professional, specialist physician or surgeon. Interprofessional and multidisciplinary team working is, therefore, essential to optimize management regimens. This requires good communication practices, knowledge of each other's scope of work, knowledge of the local policies, guidelines and infrastructure, and national management guidelines. Concurrent with these skills is the need to develop and apply knowledge- and evidence-based practice, relating this to the whole patient, the chronic wound and any other chronic soft tissue damage.

Skin and soft tissue injury that does not resolve becomes a chronic problem, which is costly to the individual and to society as a whole. Ulcers (chronic wounds) are very common conditions that frequently develop following even the smallest injury in an at-risk person. The aim of this chapter is to introduce methods of management relevant to chronic foot wounds (foot ulcers) and also to consider management relevant to ulcer prevention and recurrence.

There is an almost primitive urge to patch someone up when they have injured themselves; although this characteristic is perhaps more enhanced in some of us than others. We have an instinctive need to stop bleeding and to cover any break in the skin, to reduce healing time, so the injured person has a chance to run away and live to fight another day. Once outside the womb, this is what the human body does for itself; clotting, pouring inflammatory mediators and growth factors into the wound site, creating a prolific source of nutrients and upregulating the immune system to combat invading organisms (Yamaguchi & Yoishikawa 2001). The aim of this tightly controlled (Hart 2002, Stephens & Thomas 2002) complex sequence (inflammation and repair) is to seal the break in the skin and to repair whatever other damage is present as rapidly as possible to allow return to participative living: to minimize 'down time' and reduce risk from predators and infection.

Legs and feet are in contact with a sometimes harsh environment, and can be injured in a number of ways with resulting healing by first or secondary intention (Table 17.1). Generally, an injured but fit, healthy person who has good nourishment (Shetty & McPherson 1997, Williams 2002), will heal readily, though not necessarily to the original structure, function and efficiency. Chapter 9 looks at some management approaches for treating injuries such as tendon or muscle rupture, including use of modalities such as low-level laser therapy and/or therapeutic exercises.

Someone who is frail, is malnourished as a consequence of poor diet or a malabsorption syndrome (e.g. ulcerative colitis) or who has peripheral vascular disease is likely to have skin and soft tissues that are less robust than a healthy person. The likelihood of injury is then quite high subsequent to even minor trauma, and healing will be delayed as the person concerned does not have the 'building blocks' (pro-

teins, vitamins, trace minerals) available for tissue repair. Someone who has a medical disorder such as diabetes mellitus or rheumatoid arthritis is similarly at risk (Box 17.1) of being injured, having delayed healing and developing ulcers. Chronic ulcers are 'holes' or breaks in the skin that heal slowly or not at all. Such problems are costly to the individual concerned in terms of pain, distress and quality of life, and to society as a whole (Williams 1999).

For the purposes of this chapter, it is assumed that a thorough, general assessment of the patient will have been carried out, including note of their lifestyle, nutrient intake (diet), occupation, footwear, etc. Brief reference will be made to specific assessments when this is important to tissue viability management. Management of the at-risk leg and foot will require consideration of all these factors, which forms quite a challenge for the practitioner, who may not have the knowledge, skills or facilities to respond appropriately. The multidisciplinary team is an invaluable resource.

TREATMENT OF ACUTE, UNCOMPLICATED WOUNDS

An acute, incisional wound will heal by first intention with minimal difficulty in a healthy person, while a scooping injury, healing by secondary intention, takes longer. Treatment for wounds of this nature aims at maintaining an infection-free environment, providing protection from mechanical stress (see Table 17.1) and generally optimizing opportunity for the body to heal itself (Moore & Foster 2002). The principles are:

- involve the patient in checking progress, presence of infection, etc.
- maintain an infection-free environment for the wound
- ensure the patient knows when and who to contact if necessary
- protection from mechanical stress.

Be prepared to change treatment (including referral) if the wound deteriorates or is slow to resolve. Some wounds can be considered as at risk (Box 17.1).

Table 17.1 Outline of management for acute, uncomplicated wounds in a healthy person[a]

Size	Management
Acute incisional wounds healing by first intention	
Small incision (approx. <1 cm)	Cleanse with tap water (Griffiths et al 2001) or normal saline
	Dry dressing (low or no adherence)
	If at site of mechanical stress, protect with deflective padding (e.g. holed/aperture felt 3 mm or 5 mm pad), sponge pad (for shock absorption, insulation) or insole with similar function
	Ensure there is sufficient space in footwear for dressings and any padding
	Wound will normally close in 2–3 days, with adequate strength achieved in around 10 days (Centre for Medical Education 1992)
	Patients can check their own wound progress and contact for an appointment as necessary
Long incision (approx. >1 cm)	As above, and additionally: close with adhesive skin closures or sutures
	Patient may shower after 3–4 days; wound should be patted dry with a clean towel/tissue
	Involve patient with checking wound progress
	Check around 10 days and remove any sutures
	Be prepared to manage post-injury scarring if possible
Wounds healing by secondary intention ('scooped' out wounds)	
Small (approx. <1 cm diameter, dermis only involved)	Cleanse (as above)
	Ideally use a primary dressing to maintain a moist environment (Eaglestein 1985) or a low/non-adherent primary dressing
	Protect from mechanical stress (as above)
	Involve patient in wound management (warn them about the wound appearance if a 'moist environment' dressing is used)
	Wound is likely to granulate within 10 days and reepithelialize over the next 2 weeks (Centre for Medical Education 1992)
Large (approx. >1 cm diameter, deep structures involved)	As above, and additionally: refer as appropriate (e.g. via GP to vascular or plastic surgeon for grafting, specialist in tissue viability)
	Consider antimicrobial therapy
	Rest (bed rest), footwear adaptations, orthoses, padding (ensure sufficient space in footwear for these)
	Check nutrient intake, refer to dietitian or GP as necessary
	Discuss with patient the time likely to be taken for healing plus impact on their life

[a]Treatment for burns will vary according to severity, but principles are similar.

Inevitably, scarring occurs, sometimes complicating function once the wound has healed over. This is particularly noticeable in someone who has a history of hypertrophic scarring or who develops keloid. In anyone, scars may have soft tissue adhesions from surface to bone, which pull and cause, at times, marked discomfort. The treatment for scarring is considered below, both to minimize discomfort and to reduce the risk of wound recurrence at a site that is less robust than before it was injured.

HISTORICAL APPROACHES TO CHRONIC WOUND AND INFECTION MANAGEMENT

We have a long human history of tissue repair methods. We have used cobwebs (Moore & Foster

---

Box 17.1 What is an at-risk leg or foot?

The person concerned may:

- be frail (very young or very old)
- have a medical disorder (e.g. diabetes, rheumatoid arthritis, peripheral vascular disease) or surgical complications
- have been injured
- have poor nutrition (poor diet or a malabsorption syndrome, e.g. Crohn's disease)

When the tissues of the limb have poor blood supply and/or poor enervation, then their mechanical strength, immunological capacity and healing potential are reduced. The tissues in that area are then at greater risk of being damaged than normal healthy tissues and are also at risk of having delayed healing. These tissues would show features of poor tissue viability and are at-risk.

2002) to reduce bleeding, unwittingly mimicking the fibrin meshwork occurring during clotting. Svagnum moss was another wound dressing, used in part for its capacity to absorb and retain moisture, as with natural sponges. Bandages of various types have been used to strap or, more recently, adhere dressings in position.

Leeches and maggots (larval therapy) were used to reduce swelling from haematomas and to deal with slough or infection, respectively, and these two organisms have had some favourable return to the injury and wound management portfolio recently (Courtney 1999).

Use of herbals has occurred since time unrecorded regardless of geography and culture, handed down from one person to another, often with accompanying incantation. There has been a considerable resurgence of interest in these substances in recent times (Baker 1998), and the benefit of a positive psychological attitude (in the past achieved through the 'magic' of the healing experience) is now well recognized and should be included in the management approach (Table 17.2). Honey has also returned to the wound management portfolio (Molan 1999).

The concept of providing a moist environment for healing (Eagelstein 1985) has the benefits of reducing pain (nerve endings not dehydrated and irritated), optimizing fibroblast activity, promoting capillary angiogenesis and providing an environment where reepithelialization can occur

Table 17.2 Reflective practitioner's skills essential for the management process

Skills	Example
Ability to recognize abnormality clinically and accurately diagnose its nature, complications and associated conditions	Practitioner can identify an ischaemic ulcer and infection as a complication, and the antalgic gait changes that the patient develops as a consequence
Willingness to consider, with the patient, their perspectives and expectations and to involve the patient in their care (Gripton 2002)	The patient explains that continuing working is more important to them than healing the wound in the optimum time, and management plan incorporates this
Knowledge, self-discipline and ability to apply relevant outcome measures (both patient and clinician centred, if available)	Ulcer dimensions recorded, with pain scale, at each visit, along with description of other relevant clinical features where no quantifiable measure is available or applicable, e.g. volume of exudate
Willingness to recognize the need to apply appropriate knowledge- and/or evidence-based treatments	All assessment information suggests a clear diagnosis and a foray into the literature and review of own existing knowledge recommends a particular treatment
Consideration of the applicability of national and local guidelines to the individual patient	National guidelines are in accord with local guidelines, most of which recommend an approach suitable for this patient; check that recommended approaches have been applied to the patient
Ability to change management approaches and treatments as and when relevant	No benefit has been recorded from the past treatment, so an alternative appropriate treatment is selected from knowledge and further perusal of the literature

more readily. Currently, much wound management is still based around this concept and many wound dressings are active dressings that aim to promote optimum hydration levels at the wound–dressing interface.

Autologous skin grafts can be successful skin substitutes (Ballard & Baxter 2002) to cover a large chronic wound. Recent developments include interactive dressings such as human skin replacements (living skin equivalents, e.g. Dermagraft (S&N); McColgan et al 1998). Research and development costs for these products were high and unfortunately this has spilt over into dressing costs. Biodegradable/bioabsorbable scaffolds (Bader & Bouten 2000, Ballard & Baxter 2002) inserted into the wound are being developed to aid cellular motility and thus repair. Other wound management approaches include negative pressure (vacuum-assisted closure), hyperbaric oxygen and low-level laser.

Considerable interest in the effect of growth factors (e.g. Becalpermin; Wiemann et al 1998) in chronic wound management continues (Cox 1993, Graham 1998). Wound biochemistry (Yamaguchi & Yoishikawa 2001) is also of considerable interest. Promogram (Johnson and Johnson) has been developed to downregulate matrix metalloproteinases, which inhibit local growth factors (Cullen 2002).

PRINCIPLES OF MANAGEMENT IN TISSUE VIABILITY

The basic management of tissue viability involves:

- using all assessment information in developing a management plan
- developing skills in clinical recognition of very early abnormal changes
- being clear about management aim(s)
- involving the patient and/or carer in clinical decision making
- using knowledge and evidence base to select optimum management regimens
- using national and local guidelines as relevant, and adapting to the individual concerned

- recording, monitoring and evaluating treatments and their effects
- being prepared to change treatments as appropriate
- being prepared to refer as appropriate and use the knowledge base and skills of other professions
- continuing professional development and updating knowledge base; this is essential to support clinical practice so that patients benefit.

Using assessment findings to inform management

As in all clinical practice, management of the at-risk lower leg and foot requires the practitioner to derive information from a number of sources (see Table 17.2) including verbal reports and non-verbal cues from the patient and/or their carer, the practitioner's assessment processes, knowledge of the presenting disorder and specific interventions (treatments) (Merriman & Tollafield 1995). Synthesis of information of this nature, coupled with the patient's perceptions and expectations of treatment, and knowledge- and evidence-based practice (Oxford Centre for Evidence Based Medicine) should result in selection of an optimal treatment regimen. When there is lack of evidence for a time-tested approach, this does not mean that the approach should be disregarded (Ryan 1998), but critical skills and knowledge must be applied to assess its value. The selected regimen will also need to encompass change as the condition progresses.

To personalize the assessment process, a patient with an ulcer expects the practitioner to look at it, if not straightaway, then at least near the beginning of the consultation. Because of this expectation on the patient's part, there is a great temptation for the practitioner to concentrate only on this lesion, when in fact this is poor practice. After an initial look at the lesion, it is wise to follow the sequence below in the assessment, which, in turn, will help with developing the management plan.

1. Assess the whole patient first (including any relevant specific investigations)

2. Assess their peripheral state
3. Assess the local and contralateral (opposite side, same site) state
4. Assess the periphery of the ulcer
5. Assess the wound bed.

Aims of management

Assessment findings, knowledge of the literature and guidelines on best practice will inform the management plan, which may aim to resolve the condition. Resolution may not be feasible, especially if there is an underlying medical condition that cannot itself be resolved. In this case, the therapeutic aim of treatment may be to prevent further problems developing or to minimize the effects of peripheral complications, such as odour from chronic ulcers or fungating (malignant) wounds. The patient (and/or carer) will need to be involved in this decision-making process, and it will become apparent that the issues that are most important to the patient are those that the practitioner may need to manage first (e.g. pain reduction, management of odour). The management and specific treatments for preventing deterioration and for treating overt ulceration are discussed later in this chapter.

There are a number of guidelines, information sources, outcome measures and health-gain tools to aid clinical reasoning, decision making relating to management and service provision, and to monitor progress of individuals.

- Internationally and nationally published documentation and guidelines, for example National Service Framework (NSF) for Older People (NICE 2001), NSF for Diabetes (NICE 2001), Scottish Intercollegiate Guidelines Network (1998), the care of patients with chronic leg ulcers (European Pressure Ulcer Advisory Panel 1998ab).
- Health gain tools and outcome measures, for example the Foot Health Status Questionnaire (Bennett & Patterson 1998), the Foot Health Activities Questionnaire (Gripton 2002), the Foot Function Index (EQ 5D; Euroqol; Budiman-Mak et al 1991). Some are specific and sensitive, others are 'broad-brush'.

- Systematic reviews (e.g. on debriding chronic wounds (Bradley et al 1999), on diabetic foot ulcers (Spencer 2000, Smith & Thow 2001), on antimicrobial agents (O'Meara et al 2000)
  - Local guidelines and practices
  - Guidelines from special interest and reference groups.

Good management in tissue viability requires clinical skills that will enable early (and preferably very early) recognition of abnormality (Table 17.3) and suitable treatment for this before it becomes an overt problem. Clinical experience and working with others are two ways of developing this ability. Continuing professional development and referral to others for their clinical expertise is all part of clinical governance and good clinical practice (Bowman 1998, Bradshaw 1999).

Screening practices may be beneficial to identify an at-risk foot or leg. Nursing scores (Russell 2002) to record the patient's status can be helpful but may not transfer readily for use in someone who is ambulant. Instrumentation (e.g. Fscan, Tekscan, USA) to provide quantitative data on foot loading (magnitude and duration) can also be helpful if these facilities are available and accessible.

Synthesis and evaluation of recorded clinical (and instrumented) data with the patient's comments may necessitate change in treatment approaches as time progresses, requiring the practitioner to have a wide-ranging management portfolio, and to work with the multidisciplinary team (Bradshaw 1999). No one practitioner can be expected to have all the knowledge and skills, nor access to all necessary facilities to undertake suitable management for all conditions. It is often valuable to consult a practitioner specializing in tissue viability, for example a clinical nurse specialist in tissue viability or diabetes, or a podiatrist with specialist skills and knowledge (see Table 17.2).

Despite the skill of the practitioner, there are times when the patient and/or their chronic wound(s) deteriorate. It is so important to recognize this trend early and instigate relevant approaches promptly (Foster 2002). These may include involving other specialties (Case

Table 17.3   Clinical features of cutaneous tissues that have poor tissue viability[a]

Mild	Anhydrosis, increased tendency to callus and corn formation possible, superficial fissures around heel and apices of toes
	Skin cool to touch (not always); skin may appear pale (not always)
	Some suggestion of soft tissues overly deforming to routine contact surfaces
	Patches of cyanosis may be evident
	Bony prominences show areas of erythema (reactive hyperaemia)
	There may be signs of previous chronic wound (e.g. scarring, atrophe blanche)
	Patients may remark on sensation of discomfort and skin tightness (providing they have normal sensation)
	Soft tissue changes in tone (e.g. loss of resilience on palpation)
	Some evidence of neuropathy
Moderate	Features noted for 'mild' and anhydrotic fissures may involve dermis readily
	Patients may remark on slow healing rates or increased propensity to cutaneous bacterial infection (e.g. following gardening)
	Areas of erythema over bony prominences readily apparent
	Skin pliability noticeably reduced and tissues feel stiffer on palpation
	Soft tissues appear to deform to routine contact surfaces with no return to normal contours on relief of this mechanical stress (little elasticity in tissues)
Severe	Features noted for 'mild' and 'moderate' plus minimal trauma causes tissue breakdown
	Overt ulceration may be evident
	Skin may be white or red, cool or warm, respectively
	Cyanosis may be marked (or not present at all)
	Patients complain of pain, which can either awake them at night or keep them awake (providing sensation is perceived), i.e. rest pain

[a]This is not a definitive list, and clinical features will be present singly or concurrently. Also the clustering of information under the three headings is for convenience and has not been validated.

Adapted from Edmonds & Foster (2001), MacFarlane & Jeffcoate (1999) and Springett (2002b), with permission.

study 17.1). It does not reflect poorly on the practitioner who has been caring for the patient if it becomes necessary to refer the patient to a colleague. Rather the converse, it demonstrates self-awareness, reflective practice and an understanding of the value of others in the multidisciplinary team; most importantly the patient may benefit from this referral (Box 17.2).

PRACTICAL ISSUES IN TISSUE VIABILITY MANAGEMENT

This section considers the broader, practical issues relating to tissue viability management, and the sections following this deal with specific treatments relevant to the management aims outlined in Box 17.2.

- What are your management aims?

- Have you involved your patient (and/or carer) in the management of their foot problem?
- Have you obtained useful baseline measures or used an existing suitable outcome measure or health gain tool?
- Do you have a diagnosis, or are you working to symptomatic management?
- Do you have the necessary knowledge and skills or do you need to consult, and work with, the multidisciplinary team?
- Is there a specialist in tissue viability you can, or should, refer your patient to?

The management plan, decided upon in consultation with the patient, may highlight issues that are common, or different, for the patient and practitioner. It is, therefore, important to obtain a baseline measure to assess what the patient's status is at the start of the management process,

---

Case study 17.1 Treatment of an ischaemic ulcer

Despite the practitioner's knowledge, skill, care and attention, Mrs B's ischaemic ulcer on her right foot was worsening. The skin surrounding the ulcer was glassy and swollen, suggestive of infection, but antibiotics (amoxicillin and flucloxacillin) had made no difference. The ulcer had enlarged to 1.5 cm diameter and its base was covered in slough. She was in a lot of pain, being woken at night by her throbbing foot. Even cooling it and hanging it out of bed did not help. She was beginning to feel sitting up all night was the best option and she was becoming very tired. Mrs B had been so positive about her treatment at her first visit and felt encouraged by the practitioner's approach, but now she was depressed as things clearly were not being cured; in fact they were not even improving.

Her right foot was warm, bright red, but pulses were monophasic and an ABPI of 0.9 at her first visit, changing to 0.8 today, indicated worsening ischaemia. Earlier referral and results of an appointment for arterial angiogram had not, in Mrs B's view, been at all satisfactory. On rereferral, Mrs B took part in a vascular surgeons' educational conference and as a result was offered a balloon angioplasty and stent distal to the popliteal fossa. Much to everyone's delight and relief, this proved successful and the majority of Mrs B's problems resolved; she could sleep unmolested by pain. Cefalexin proved to be an effective antibiotic. Mrs B elected to follow the nutritionist's dietary advice and also rested and redressed her foot ulcer following information explained by the podiatrist. With the improvement in arterial blood flow, the wound healed within 7 weeks.

Box 17.2 Aims of management

The options can be described as '2Rs, 2Ps, 1A':

- Resolve (heal) the condition
- Relieve symptoms (which may include pain, odour, exudate)
- Prevent recurrence of the condition
- Prevent new complications developing
- Accommodate existing problems/conditions if these cannot be resolved.

In the presence of disease or disorder, resolution of the foot or leg condition may not be possible. Clinical decision making will be influenced by interpretation of the patients' expectations, assessment findings and national and local wound management guidelines.

---

so that the effect of the intervention (treatment) can be monitored and changed where and when necessary (Russell 2002). This allows different practitioners to observe the patient's progress with some attempt at accuracy. The issues that are important to the patient can be monitored also. These baseline measures may be used as an outcome measure or may be part of an outcome measurement tool. However, generally such tools tend to be clinician based and do not encompass the patient's views and expectations (Gripton 2002), and as such their value can be limited. Quantifiable data such as obtained from instrumentation (ankle brachial pressure index (ABPI), in-shoe foot pressure, scaled photo-

graphs of ulcers, etc.) also provide useful information from which to evaluate progress.

Both Edmonds and Foster's (2001) 'simple staging system' and MacFarlane and Jeffcoate's (1999) SAD system included foot status as well as that of any specific lesion such as an ulcer (chronic wound) in management of the diabetic foot. However, both these measures are based on the diabetic foot and may not be transferable to other situations. The Foot Health Status Questionnaire (Bennett & Patterson 1998) allows foot conditions to be monitored generally. The Foot Health Activities Questionnaire (Gripton 2002), when validated for use in the general population, will allow a patient-centred approach as well as using clinically derived data. Scoring systems such as the Waterlow Score or the Bradley system have been used in nursing for a number of years (Waterlow 1985, Russell 2002) to record the at-risk status of patients, but these do not transfer readily to the foot in an ambulant patient.

If a suitable health gain tool applicable to the at-risk foot is not available, useful monitoring measures include (adapted from Merriman & Tollafield 1995, Lorimer et al 2001, Gripton 2002, Russell 2002, Springett 2002a):

- visual analogue scales to assess patient and clinician-derived subjective issues such as pain, appearance of skin texture and tone surrounding a wound

- descriptors to record how much the individual feels their life is affected
- distance walked before pain (or other descriptor) starts
- note of activities patient can undertake at that time, for comparison at a later date
- number and site of lesion(s)
- measurement of lesion dimensions (depth is difficult without appropriate instrumentation)
- quantifiable data from instrumentation, e.g. ABPI, in-shoe foot pressure
- colour change of a wound, its base and margins, and that of surrounding skin compared with the contralateral or more proximal site
- temperature change of tissues around a wound and compared with contralateral site
- nature (colour, smell) and volume of any exudate (in the wound and on the dressing).

Symptomatic management

There are times when it is not possible to make a clear diagnosis of the patient's complaint, and then symptomatic management comes into play. In these instances, clinical features (signs and symptoms) direct the type of treatment, until such times as a diagnosis becomes possible enabling more specific and perhaps appropriate treatment to be undertaken (Case study 17.2). Foot health education and self-help (Box 17.3) is always worthwhile.

Often, it is possible to transfer symptomatic treatments suitable for someone in good health to an at-risk foot. However, this treatment must be thought through for its applicability and suitability to fragile tissues that have a high potential for breakdown (Case study 17.3). For example, in a painful, hyperkeratotic lesion with differential diagnosis of wart, fibrous corn or foreign body, use of a caustic (e.g. salicylic acid >10%, silver nitrate 75%) would be contraindicated in poor tissue viability, but a deflective pad and use of emollients to hydrate and soften the hyperkeratotic tissue can be useful. However, emollient application in an ischaemic foot (especially if secondary to diabetes) may be best avoided to minimize potential for damage through vigorous application and overhydration to an epider-

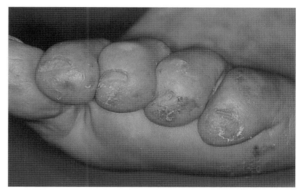

Figure 17.1 Chilling (cyanotic and pink patches) may be indicative of local or systemic state. Diagnosis should be clear before management starts.

Case study 17.2 Symptomatic management of an at-risk foot

Figure 17.1 shows skin changes in Mrs F's feet, which are suggestive of chilling. The diagnosis is not clear. This may be a primary condition or may be secondary to Raynaud's phenomenon, peripheral vascular disease or a collagen disorder such as systemic sclerosis. In the absence of a diagnosis, and given the severity of the clinical signs, it is appropriate to start some form of treatment, but this will need to take into account the possible aetiologies. It is not wise, therefore, to use a rubefacient, as the peripheral vasculature may not be able to respond to the demand for increased blood flow. The skin is already fragile and the act of rubbing an 'antichilblain' cream into the skin may damage it further.

A suitable approach for symptomatic management would be to aim to maintain a constant temperature for the feet using insulating insoles (ensuring there is sufficient space in footwear first), explaining to the patient the need to avoid extremes of temperature, not placing hands and feet next to radiators to warm up quickly but to allow a slow warming. Use of heated gloves and thermally insulated footwear when going out would be valuable. If the patient chooses to use lined footwear, the internal dimensions must allow room for the foot, otherwise areas of ischaemia on the foot, usually over bony prominences, following pressure from footwear will develop.

Box 17.3 Foot care advice in poor tissue viability

The practitioner can advise the person with at-risk feet as follows. Information will need to be adapted with, and for, each person. Many of the specialist organizations (e.g. Society of Chiropodists and Podiatrist, Diabetes UK, Tissue Viability Society) and NHS Trusts have footcare leaflets containing greater detail than that outlined below.

Seek help and advice early
It is advisable to seek help from an appropriately qualified person (e.g. chiropodist/podiatrist registered with HPC, clinical nurse specialist in tissue viability or diabetes, pharmacist or GP).

Check legs and feet frequently (ideally daily or more often).

You will need to look at your skin for changes from normal (e.g. bluish tinge, redness, swelling), and for any specific patches of skin or nail that appear different from normal (e.g. flaky areas, cracks, weeping). You may need help, or you could use a mirror (in good lighting) to check the underneath of your feet and between your toes.

If you find a skin or nail problem, apply a dry dressing (e.g. gauze, low-adherent dressing) to protect it and minimize the chance of infection. Hydrocolloid wafers (e.g. ulcer dressings, blister patches, callus dressings) can be helpful but only if instructions are followed closely (Springett et al 1997). There is contention over the use of hydrocolloid dressings in feet with poor sensation (neuropathy) (Lithner 1990). If your skin is very fragile then the dressing used may need to be bandaged in place rather than adhered with tape.

Good hygiene
Keep feet clean and make sure the skin between the toes is dry before replacing hosiery. Dry feet, especially toes, gently.

Make sure all footwear (shoes, slippers, socks) fits, especially that it has enough girth around the toes. An easy way to check is to draw around your foot and match this against the size and shape of the shoe/slipper. If your shoes, slippers, socks, etc. have any bumps or rough seams, do not wear them. Ideally shoes should have some way of attaching them to your feet (lace or bar) to reduce the potential for rubbing the skin.

Avoid extremes of temperature
If your feet are cold, let them warm up gradually, do not use a hot-water bottle or put them on a radiator. Check water temperature before bathing. Using an insulating insole can be helpful, but only if you have enough space in your shoes or slippers.

Topical applications
If your skin is dry, an emollient (cream to moisten the skin) can be helpful, but massage this in carefully so you do not injure your skin.

Avoid using 'over-the-counter' medicated corn plasters as potential for damage (e.g. ulceration) to skin increases in the at-risk foot.

Ulcer dressings
If you have a foot ulcer, ensure you have information about how to deal with this:

- whether you can get your foot wet
- if you should wear a particular pair of slippers or shoes
- if you must leave the dressing in place or if you can redress it yourself
- when you should return for your next appointment.

---

mis that is trying to stay intact. It is important to know the effect of herbals and essential oils (Baker 1998) on skin and wounds. It is not safe to assume that all 'natural' products are safe to use in all situations.

The team approach to managing the at-risk foot

No one individual can be expected to have all knowledge and skills required to manage an at-risk foot satisfactorily all the time. The practitioner should recognize and acknowledge their abilities and those of others, and refer the patient as necessary (Frykberg 1997, Bowman 1998, International Working Group on the Diabetic Foot 1999). As with all medical conditions, judgement as to when to refer is difficult to develop and experience counts, so if in doubt refer. There are a number of useful specialties such as tissue viability nurses, diabetes nurse specialists, podiatrists to contact for advice.

Case study 17.3   'Routine' treatments adapted to the at-risk foot

Brian T, now aged 32 years, fell off his motor bike 4–5 years ago and sustained extensive soft tissue injuries to both lower legs. His right leg lost much of its muscle bulk and the reconstruction and grafting was complicated by infection. Now there is marked scarring, the arterial supply is limited, venous drainage poor and his lower right leg and foot show signs of skin atrophy (suggesting a similar state in deeper tissues). Brian continues his hectic and active life: where angels fear to tread goes Brian. In a recent instance, Brian had an inversion sprain of his right ankle.

In a healthy person, 'rest, ice, compression, elevation' would be the first aid treatment of choice. However, three of these four routine treatments are inappropriate for Brian's ischaemic right foot and leg. The treatment had to be tailored to his needs and peripheral condition, and gentle compression and rest were achieved through strapping onto tubigrip and Brian wearing his biking boots. These boots were so ungainly that they limited his walking and by default he rested. He could have used a walker (e.g. Aircast walker) instead if there had been concerns about space and fit of his biking boots.

THE SKIN AS AN INDICATOR OF TISSUE VIABILITY

The skin is an easily observable indicator of systemic disorder and is a 'mirror' for the state of deeper tissues, which are not visible on clinical assessment. Usually it is skin that is monitored for change (see Table 17.3), along with other clinical assessments. When carrying out a clinical assessment relevant to tissue viability, the practitioner needs to touch the skin (gloved/ungloved as determined through risk assessment) to evaluate temperature, texture and tone (Springett & Merriman 1995). It is essential to recognize early (preferably very early) changes in skin state so that management to prevent ulceration can be started. Skin changes can also indicate, for example, infection, requiring a change in regimen.

When skin is damaged, the tone of the skin and underlying soft tissues changes. Increased turgidity may be palpable (perhaps caused by glycation of tissues in diabetes (Boulton et al 2000, Hashmi 2000, Levin 2002)), or the tissues may feel more rigid and almost dent, like an old ping-pong ball. Alternatively, tissues may feel more flaccid on palpation when compared with the contralateral side or more proximal sites. If changes of this nature are palpated, then it is best to assume some adverse tissue change is developing and prompt management will prevent further deterioration. The nature of treatment will vary according to suspected or diagnosed cause, site, patient's activity levels, etc.

Colour is also a useful clinical indicator of change. Redness (erythema) may indicate autonomic neuropathy (Frykberg 1998, Boulton et al 2000, Levin 2002) with fast blood flow through arteriovenous shunts (missing out the capillary bed and reducing the opportunity for oxygen dissociation into the tissues). Alternatively, erythema may indicate reactive hyperaemia following compression (Bliss 2000). Erythema may indicate infection (Humphreys 1999), assuming the vascular supply is capable of vasodilatation in response to inflammatory mediator release associated with tissue damage following bacterial toxin insult. Odour (Bowler et al 1999) may also indicate infection. Again, prompt intervention may prevent exacerbation of the condition.

The extent of changes (e.g. how far up the leg) and the nature, size and spread of any lesions also need to be assessed (Springett & Merriman 1995, Dawber et al 2001). Methods of recording this type of clinical information vary. Some are readily quantifiable (e.g. skin temperature) while other methods are feasible but instrumentation may not be accessible (e.g. skin dryness) and therefore these clinical features tend to be subjectively assessed using, for example, visual analogue scales (Merriman & Tollafield 1995, Lorimer et al 2001).

TREATMENT APPROACHES IN TISSUE VIABILITY

The principles for management of poor tissue viability have been outlined above and some of the practical issues explained. Box 17.2 lists management aims, which obviously will need to be adapted for each person. In this section, some specific treatment approaches will be discussed in relation to these aims.

Preventing deterioration and ulceration

The following steps help in the prevention of deterioration and ulceration:

- involve patient and/or carer in clinical decision making
- provide foot health and footwear advice (Box 17.3)
- identify and treat potential and actual at-risk sites
- reduce mechanical stress
- insulate (thermal)
- maintain optimum hydration and thence strength and pliability of the stratum corneum
- treat infection (bacterial and fungal)
- refer as appropriate, and early, involve the multidisciplinary team (e.g. for nutrition or vascular management).

Preventing ulcer formation is such an important aspect of practice, but it is one often forgotten because of pressure of time, facilities and sometimes lack of forethought. There are many factors to be considered concurrently, which can be challenging.

Paramount in prevention of ulceration is the ability to anticipate problems (Table 17.3) that may develop and to treat these before they become overt (Dealey 1994, Flanagan 1997). Bony prominences on the foot are sites particularly prone to tissue breakdown and ulceration (Fig. 17.2), and shoe wear will indicate patterns and sites of high load. Instruments (e.g. Fscan, Tekscan, USA) can be used to demonstrate to the patient, as well as the practitioner, sites of high and/or prolonged loading and change with treatment. Clinical skill in recognition of very early changes at these, and other sites, is invaluable (see Table 17.3).

Involvement of the patient and/or carer in frequent (daily and more often) foot inspections and application of appropriate 'first aid' is also essential (see Box 17.3). Treatments suitable for

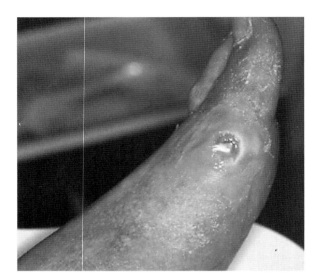

Figure 17.2 Foot ulceration frequently develops over bony prominences where mechanical stresses are highest and most prolonged.

someone who is in good health can be transferred to someone with poor tissue viability but often these need to be adapted considerably in an at-risk foot (see Case study 17.3).

Any breaks that do develop in the skin need to be kept free from infection, both bacterial and fungal. However, prophylactic use of topical antimicrobial drugs is controversial and may predispose to skin sensitivity. It is possible that some essential oils can be beneficial (Baker 1998), promoting both a sense of well-being and an improvement in skin quality.

Good foot hygiene (see Box 17.3) and footwear that fits is an essential part of management (Mantey et al 1999).

Reducing mechanical stress for tissue viability management

Off-loading mechanical stress is predominant in preventing wound development (Jude & Boulton 1998, Bader & Bouten 2000, Cavenagh et al 2000, Levin 2002). The majority of patients will need to be kept ambulant because the nature of their problem does not warrant admission to hospital, they cannot afford to take time off work or from caring for others, or because facilities are not available for bed rest. Therefore, the practitioner will need to devise other ways of reducing mechanical stress on the foot or feet (Colagiuri et al 1995, Armstrong et al 1998, Cavenagh et al 2000, Spencer 2000). This approach also has the advantage of minimizing interference with the patient's lifestyle and gives the opportunity for continued social interaction, which have been shown to be beneficial to healing.

As a temporary measure, holed (or cavitied) adhesive felt pads around the at-risk site can be used to redistribute mechanical stress (compression, shear, torsion, friction, tension) over a wider surface area (Fig. 17.3). The advantage of an adhesive pad is that it will move around less than a replaceable pad, thus achieving its pur-

pose. If there is a risk of skin damage with an adhesive pad, then the pad can be applied onto tubigrip, tubegauze or other bandage and then strapped in place to minimize potential for movement. The skin can be protected to a certain extent by spraying with a plastic spray dressing (e.g. Opsite, S&N) or using a cyanoacrylate paint (e.g. Liquishield, Medlogic) before applying a pad. The skin may deform through the pad aperture, which may interfere with blood flow in macro- and microangiopathy, so a careful bevel can be used to introduce the pad to the skin. A foam cushioning pad can be helpful in absorbing shock (Rome 1998, Hampton & Collins 2002) with the contact surface and for insulation.

Replaceable padding of a similar nature can be used, with disadvantages of unwanted movement and attachment loops interfering with blood flow. Polymer gel pads (e.g. Silipos) are useful for absorbing friction and shear stresses, and hydrocolloid dressings (e.g. Compeed, Coloplast) will hydrate the skin optimally and provide reduction in friction stress and some shear (Springett et al 2002). (NB: This is contentious for use in neuropathy.) Silicone devices to protect skin sites or to realign toes can be beneficial longer term methods (Fig. 17.4). Realignment of foot structures often results in

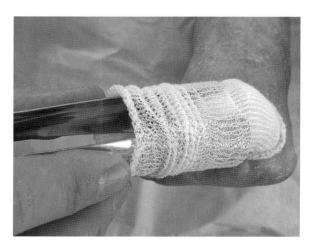

A   B

Figure 17.3   Padding can be applied around an ulcer as a method of off-loading mechanical stress.

reduction of any bony prominence and consequently less stress on the tissues.

Orthoses conformed to the foot contours to provide uniform tissue loading are invaluable. Selection of materials and covering material (Rome 1998, Hampton & Collins 2002) is also important. Footwear (see Box 17.3) that fits well and has sufficient girth and depth to accommodate deformity will often remove the need for digital devices. If orthoses are to be used, then footwear must be large enough to accommodate the devices, otherwise areas of ischaemia from shoe pressure will form, which could lead to ulceration.

Pressure ulcers (Fig. 17.5) can develop readily if the person does not move around periodically (Culley 2002, Stockton & Parker 2002). So advice to rest should be coupled with an explanation about not sitting or lying in one place for long but to move, transferring pressure from the contact surface to another tissue site, thus allowing resumption of blood flow. Raised legs should be supported along their length and not just rested on the heel (European Pressure Ulcer Advisory Panel 1998a,b, NICE 2001). Foam 'gutters' are available for chairs and beds (a useful contact source is the practice or district nurse) to raise the heel off the surface (Gebhardt et al 1996), oth-erwise a pillow placed longitudinally under the leg, finishing just proximal to the heel is a substitute; fleece heel covers are marginally helpful.

Some unfortunate people have both peripheral oedema (for which legs should be raised as often as practicable) and ischaemia (which is usually more painful when legs are raised: rest pain). This is an extraordinarily difficult situation to treat, and which may not be resolvable even following vascular intervention such as angioplasty (see Case study 17.1). In this instance, symptomatic management may be all that is possible, including pain relief (e.g. systemic analgesics, acupuncture, transcutaneous electrical nerve stimulation (TENS), cognitive distraction techniques, aromatherapy), referral to appropriate specialties (e.g. vascular department, pain clinic), ensuring the patient knows they are still being cared about, careful wound dressing (Box 17.4) and off-loading mechanical stress.

Controlling foot function in poor tissue viability

Managing, and perhaps altering, foot structure and function (i.e. managing the musculoskeletal, biomechanical function of the foot) is also central to managing the at-risk foot (Colagiuri et al 1995,

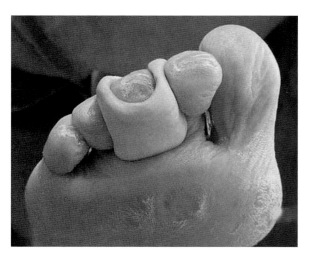

Figure 17.4 A silicone protective toe device aimed at reducing load on tissues.

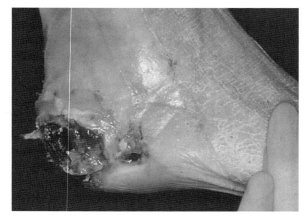

Figure 17.5 Where possible, an immobile patient should move around a little to minimize the potential for pressure ulcers, such as this on the heel.

Box 17.4 Principles of wound dressing

Selection of a wound dressing will depend on many variables, the major of which are noted below. Consider:

- Is the dressing to absorb low, moderate or high volumes of wound exudate?
- Is the wound infected or aseptic?
- If infected, is the pus thick (as usual with staphylococcal infections) or runny (e.g. haemolytic streptococcal infection)?
- Is the dressing to be passive, forming a covering over the wound site?
- Is the dressing to be active, creating a moist environment to optimize potential for healing?
- Is an interactive dressing suitable, promoting wound resolution through, for example, the provision of a biodegradable scaffold to encourage cell motility or growth factors to encourage cellular activity?
- How has the wound changed since the last redressing?
- Should another type of wound dressing be used?
- A wound dressing alone will not aid healing of a chronic foot ulcer, all relevant aspects of management need to be undertaken concurrently (e.g. off-loading mechanical stress).

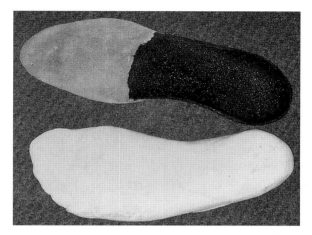

Figure 17.6 Functional orthosis with layered forefoot extension of PPT and a thermoplastic material (Plastazote). The aim is to control foot function and to provide redistribution of load as well as insulation. (The orthosis shown is not covered, for purposes of illustration.)

Frykberg 1998, Boulton et al 2000, Levin 2002). Accommodative and functional orthoses, providing they have been accurately prescribed and manufactured, are extremely valuable methods of off-loading mechanical stress from different sites on the foot and allow the patient to remain ambulant. Also, maintaining balance and functional ability is important, particularly in older people (Menz & Lord 2001) to minimize potential for falls and development of further tissue viability problems.

Base and padding materials, as well as pad shape, need to be selected with a view to function. Foams provide good thermal insulation, and different densities provide opportunity for differential distribution of load (Rome 1998). Layers of different materials and the covering material will affect orthotic function and, used imaginatively, can be very effective at providing long-term (years) relief from mechanical stress (Fig. 17.6), minimizing the chance of tissue breakdown. Heat moulding 10 mm light- or medium-density Plastazote directly to the patient's foot (possible as the Plastazote is an insulating material), then bevelling the shoe–contact side flat provides a quick method of distributing load uniformly over the surface of the foot as well as offering thermal insulation. If the patient's condition deteriorates, then a Scotchcast shoe or boot can be made (Fig. 17.7). To achieve a change in foot function, it may also be valuable to supplement orthotic management by a podiatrist with help from a physiotherapist, osteopath or chiropractor for mobilization or adjustment of a stiff joint, or to help muscle function (particularly of the intrinsic muscles for their effect on toe function).

Treatment of herald and preulcerative lesions

Specific lesions (Dawber et al 2001) need to be treated. (Information on tissue breakdown, necrosis and ulceration is covered later in this chapter.) Practitioners should recognize when conditions are minor or when they should be referred to the appropriate specialist (see Table 17.3).

Mechanically induced hyperkeratosis (callus and corns) can herald (be a predictor of) tissue breakdown in the at-risk foot (Murray et al 1996, Woodburn et al 2000, Sage et al 2001) and,

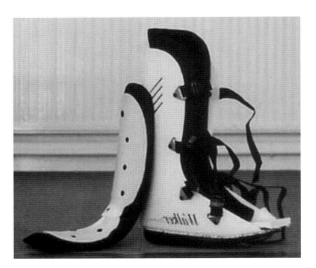

Figure 17.7 Scotch cast shoe can be used to shed load more uniformly over the plantar aspect of the foot, and away from the ulcer site. A boot may be more effective at off-loading but, having very reduced mobility, was not an option in this patient's life.

therefore, need treating. Scalpel debridement of these lesions by a podiatrist/chiropodist registered with HPC is usually the method of choice, with protection of lesion sites as described above. The frequency for this is difficult to advise as rate of callus formation varies with site (Potter 2000), but it appears to be around 4–8 weeks (Springett et al 2002). Patients with poor tissue viability should not use medicated corn plasters (Box 17.3), though use of caustic topical preparations (e.g. salicylic acid plaster 40%) by an experienced podiatrist, fully cogniscent of the adverse effects of caustics, is not necessarily always contraindicated. The structural and functional cause of these lesions should also be addressed.

Anhydrotic fissures may be debrided if there is marked associated hyperkeratosis and then closed using a skin closure or, more conveniently with a hydrocolloid dressing (e.g. Compeed, Coloplast), as this also has the effect of optimally hydrating the stratum corneum (Springett et al 2002) at the normal 10% water content (Potts et al 1985). It should be noted, however, there is contention over use of hydrocolloid dressings, especially in neuropathic feet (Lithner 1990) as

there is a history of these dressings being used inappropriately and being left on for too long. If there are signs of minor, localized infection, a topical antibacterial (antiseptic) cream (e.g. povidone iodine 10%, assuming no allergy to iodine) can be placed within the fissure. Cellulitis will need to be managed with systemic antibiotics.

There is some discussion over whether anhydrotic, atrophic, ischaemic lesions should be debrided or whether autolysis (unaided separation of dead from viable tissue) should be allowed to take its course. A guideline may be that any bulk of tissue should be removed if it could predispose to ulceration or inhibit healing (Bale 1997, Jones 1998a). Similar discussion arises over the use of emollients in this skin state. Overhydration (maceration; Cutting & White 2002) will make the skin weak, as does anhydrosis (Springett & Merriman 1995). The cause of any moist interdigital fissuring needs to be determined and treated with surgical spirit as an astringent, or antifungal preparation if appropriate (e.g. miconazole nitrate 2% or tolnaftate 1%). If the skin is very fragile, gauze placed (without creases) interdigitally will encourage air flow and transepidermal water loss, thus reducing potential for maceration.

Areas of blanching, cyanosis or hyperaemia need thermal insulation as well as protection from mechanical stress. Insulating insoles and hosiery (e.g. over-the-counter insole purchases, light- or medium-density Plastazote, fleecy shoe liners, 'double' socks) are all helpful providing there is sufficient space in any footwear worn. Avoiding extremes of temperature is beneficial, as is controlled, slow rewarming of tissues following exposure to cold. Footwear may need adapting or new shoes/slippers bought to accommodate changes.

PREVENTING RECURRENCE

As with preventing initial ulceration, preventing ulcer recurrence also requires anticipation of the event by both the patient and the practitioner.

- Is there space enough in footwear for feet and any orthotic devices?

- Does skin quality need treating?
- Are there specific lesions, e.g. scarring, that need attention?

For example, it should be anticipated that there will be reduction of space available inside any footwear when pads or insoles are used. This can cause ischaemia (often seen as reactive hyperaemia (Bliss 2000)) through increased pressure when the foot is squashed into the smaller space. Presence of oedema will make the situation worse, so all footwear should be checked for shape and space available, and adaptations made accordingly. Shoes, slippers and socks may be stretched, cut or insert added. Alternatively, extra-depth footwear can be bought, or bespoke footwear made.

Ulcer recurrence and footwear

There is a strong indication that diabetic foot ulceration recurs at the same site (Boulton 1996, Frykberg 1998) and it is reasonable to assume this is the case for all causes of at-risk feet, given the reduced robustness of scar compared with normal tissue. One strong influencing factor appears to be footwear (Mantey et al 1999) and the patient needs to receive, and act on, advice accordingly (see Box 17.3).

Management of scarring and skin quality

In addition to deterioration in the underlying cause of foot problems, recurrence of lesions, and particularly ulceration, is also likely to be associated with soft tissue biomechanical alteration. Altered foot structure and function in rheumatoid arthritis (Kerry et al 1994) can lead to ulceration and scarring on healing. Peripheral vascular disease, with poor arterial supply and venous drainage also can result in ulceration and scarring on healing. Non-enzymatic glycation of tissues in diabetes (Murray et al 1996, Hashmi 2000) will change tissue biomechanics and load-transfer capacity, as will scarring.

Scarring from past injury means the skin in that site is mechanically weaker than normal and less able to transfer mechanical stress; applied external stresses may be beyond its integral strength (Vincent 1990, Baden & Bouten 2000). Further tissue breakdown ensues, complicated by the relatively avascular nature of scar tissue.

Management of scarring (Eissenbeiss et al 1998) to optimize strength and minimize soft tissue adhesions and fibrosis is, therefore, valuable, involving the skills of a number of health professionals, podiatrist, acupuncturist, physiotherapist and aromatherapist (Baker 1998, Field et al 1998), assuming access to these professions is available. Low-level laser therapy (660 nm and 820 nm wavelengths) (Stadler et al 2001, Lagan et al 2002) and therapeutic ultrasound (3 MHz) (Hart 1998, Low & Reed 2000) can be helpful in cutaneous scar treatment, orientating collagen fibres in line with strain and controlling fibroblast activity. Systematic review of the effects of low-level laser therapy is less enthusiastic (Lucas et al 2000), but nevertheless clinicians continue its use, responding to patients' positive comments. Massage of tissues in burns is beneficial (Field et al 1998) and it is likely this approach is transferable to all states resulting in scarring. However, massage load applied to the tissues will need to be adjusted according to the stage of inflammation and repair, and the site of application will change as the wound progresses. Practitioners skilled in massage techniques will need to be involved and will need to amend their practice procedures according to healing stage.

Silicone sheeting has proved to be a valuable method of managing scarring (Eissenbeiss et al 1998), and anecdotal information suggests that the silicone should be cut to the size of the wound/scar for best effect. Corns that form at sites of scars, when carefully enucleated, can be filled with an acrylic gel (e.g. Viscogel) or silicone plug, finished flush with the skin's surface to mimic normal tissue density. Anecdotally, patients report comfort and improvement. Hydrocolloid dressings (e.g. Compeed (Coloplast), Granuflex (ConvaTec)) can be used for optimal hydration of the stratum corneum over scar tissue and there seems to be some beneficial associated change in underlying tissues that can be detected by imaging in vivo using ultrasound (diagnostic imaging, ultrasonography).

Use of aromatherapy oils (e.g. rosemary oil, peppermint oil) and gentle, superficial massage may also be beneficial in reducing vertical soft tissue adhesions (fibrosis) and discomfort. There may be some beneficial effect with use of *Calendula officianalis* cream. Pain from scarring may also be helped by acupuncture.

Managing skin quality and hydration levels is also important both for symptom management and to minimize the potential for tissue breakdown and possible consequent bacterial infection.

TREATING ULCERATION IN THE FOOT

The treatment may be summarized as:

- aim to heal the ulcer in as fast a time as possible
- diagnose ulcer type and stage of healing
- monitor and record progress
- follow national and local management guidelines and adapt these to the individual as appropriate
- treat bacterial and fungal infection
- off-load mechanical stress (provide rest)
- debride as appropriate
- consider how the cause of chronic wound can be managed to allow the ulcer to heal
- provide symptom relief
- apply suitable dressing(s)
- refer promptly and appropriately (use skills of multidisciplinary team)
- prioritize management to meet need (e.g. patient's concerns about volume of exudate).

Aims of ulcer treatment

Tempting though it is to deal only with the ulcer (see Table 17.4, below), management must take into account the condition of the whole person and the state of the peripheral tissues (Edmonds & Foster 2001). Assessment will also need to record the characteristics of the ulcer: dimensions, pain, nature and estimate of volume of exudate, presence of infection, extent of inflammation, etc. Classifying the at-risk status of an

individual and the stage of the ulcer (e.g. Flanagan 1997, MacFarlane & Jeffcoate, 1999, Edmonds & Foster 2001, Russell 2002), as well as reviewing and recording the classifications, takes time and self-discipline. It also poses a particular problem as ulcers can change rapidly from one visit to another, sometimes necessitating review at each visit. National and local guidelines can provide a helpful indication of the frequency for review and the timing and route for referral.

The aims of treating a chronic wound (ulcer) include to have it heal as soon as possible and, in the meantime, for it to be as pain free as possible, free from infection and to be minimally disruptive to life (Thomas 1997). A chronic wound will need stimulating into a controlled acute inflammatory response for the normal, tightly controlled, sequential process of healing to occur (Yamaguchi & Yoishikawa 2001, Cullen 2002). These ideals take considerable effort on the part of the practitioner and patient and/or carer. Also, removing the cause of the chronic wound may not be possible, so treatment works towards minimizing its effects.

However, patients with chronic wounds may surprise the practitioner by having a realistic view on healing time and by having a different expectation of treatment (Mandy et al 2002), such as exudate and odour control to allow them to get out and about without social stigma. In an instance such as this, the management aim would need to be adapted following discussions with the patient so that exudate and odour control became the primary and initial aim. Pain (Hawthorne & Redmond 1998) exudate and smell (Dealey 1994) are the major causes of distress for someone with a chronic wound. To that individual, management of these symptoms is more important than healing the wound quickly. It is worthwhile considering the wide portfolio of management approaches available from the multidisciplinary team, for example TENS or acupuncture for pain management, pain clinic cognitive approaches (Nurmikko & Nash 1998), culture and sensitivity to identify antibiotic treatment for odour-producing microbes, exudate management and low-level laser therapy for its variable effect on wound healing (Stadler et al 2001). Some alternative therapy treatments may be beneficial, such as aromatherapy (Baker 1998, Hartman & Coetzee 2002) or massage well proximal to the wound site

It is helpful to diagnose the type of ulcer (ischaemic, venous, neuropathic, pressure, mixed aetiology, fungating) as well as stage of healing, as this will influence treatment selection (see Box 17.4). However, there is some suggestion that biochemical changes in a variety of chronic wounds are similar (Fig. 17.8) (Cullen 2002). Locally applied treatment for one ulcer type may, therefore, be transferable to another (and in practice all seem helpful to one degree or other), but chronic wound pathology is still

poorly understood and investigation continues. A notable exception to the concept that treatment methods may be transferable is that venous ulcers require some compression while this is contraindicated in ischaemic ulceration. Practice nurses and district nurses are experienced in applying the required compression (Guest et al 1999, Moore 2002) via bandaging techniques for venous ulcers.

Managing infection in chronic wounds

In bacterial infection, cleansing the lesion with potable (drinking) water (Griffiths et al 2001) or sterile normal saline is a valuable start to treat-

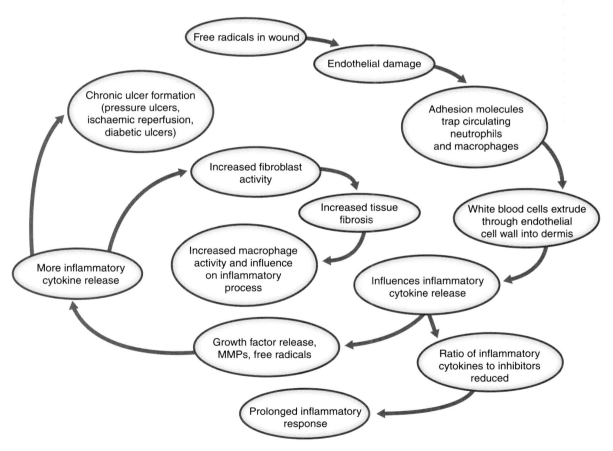

Figure 17.8 Diagramatic representation of biochemical changes in a chronic ulcer. MMP, matrix metalloproteases. (Adapted from Cullen (2001), with permission.)

ment. Washing away pathogens as well as chronic wound fluid, which can inhibit fibroblast activity (Phillips et al 1998), is helpful. Hypertonic saline footbaths (handful of cooking salt to a bowl full of warm water) have been used historically and the survival of this method suggests it is beneficial, though evidence is lacking.

Bacterial infection may be identified through all or some of the following:

- clinical signs of inflammation
- increased volume of exudate (in the wound and on the dressing; difficult to estimate)
- smell
- increased pain.

Small areas of infection (<2 cm) can be treated with topical antiseptics, which then avoids use of topical and systemic antibiotics (White et al 2002). Although information on their efficacy is lacking (O'Meara et al 2000), antiseptic use provides a first-line approach while awaiting antibiotic therapy for practitioners who do not have prescription rights. Depending upon the severity and vigour of the infection, antiseptic use may obviate the need for antibiotics. Some essential oils (Baker 1998, Hartman & Coetzee 2002) appear to have useful antimicrobial properties (e.g. tea tree oil, lavender oil). Manuka honey has been shown to have antimicrobial activity through its hydrogen peroxide content (Cooper et al 1999). Nevertheless, antibiotics remain the method of choice for managing severe infection (Kilmartin 2001).

Of the antiseptics, povidone iodine seems to be the least damaging to healing tissues (Brennan & Leaper 1985), but there are differing views over its use (Leelaporn et al 1994, Gilchrist 1997). There appears to be no information relating to toxicity of polynoxylin, a formaldehyde based product, to healing tissues, but its wide use does not seem to have resulted in recorded adverse effects. Choice of base vehicle is important to ensure the active ingredient reaches the target site and does not damage exposed tissues. An aqueous solution may appear suitable but may not track into the wound because of surface tension, while spirit-based solutions sting and can astringe overly damaging granulating tissue;

consequently, a cream base may be most suitable. Dry powder sprays may not target the required tissues but are easy to use and the potential for contamination is minimal. Antimicrobial impregnated gauzes (e.g. Inadine (J&J), Actisorb Silver (S&N) (Table 17.4) provide a convenient way of dealing with infection (Case study 17.4). Negative pressure application (Collier 1997) can be beneficial in deep-seated infection in pressure ulcers, but currently this is really only feasible with inpatient care.

An ulcer which is slow to heal may well be infected as confirmed by deep swabs or biopsy rather than superficial swabbing (White et al 2002), and will benefit from antibiotic therapy. Systemic antibiotics are useful in marked, extensive and/or deep-seated, or long-term infection, e.g. clindamycin, flucloxacillin, cephalexin (Therstrup-Petersen 1998).

Pain with infection may have been found during assessment to be a marked problem (Hawthorne & Redmond 1998) and the practitioner should consider this in the management regimen.

Management of ulcers that are slow to respond to treatment

As well as infection, there are a number of causes for slow, or no, ulcer response to treatment. One is malignancy. It is possible that some longstanding venous ulcers may show malignant changes on biopsy and the practitioner should be aware of cutaneous malignancy in general, including rodent ulcers (basal cell carcinoma). If malignancy is suspected, prompt referral is necessary to the patient's GP and/or specialist.

Healing can also be delayed by secondary or superimposed fungal infection (e.g. candidal infection), which will require treatment with an antifungal drug such as clotrimazole 1%; povidone iodine also has some antifungal activity. Occasionally, slow wound healing occurs because of an allergic reaction (delayed hypersensitivity) to the topical substances or dressings used; obviously the dressing should be changed to another (perhaps with prior patch testing on another skin site) and the immunology depart-

---

Case study 17.4 Management of an infected chronic wound

Miss E, admitted to hospital following a severe road traffic accident, had a cannula inserted via the dorsalis pedis, right foot. As her clinical condition improved, so the area on the dorsum of this foot deteriorated, showing signs of marked infection. She was started on flucloxacillin and amoxicillin; septicaemia was avoided but the dorsum of her foot ulcerated, exposing the extensor tendons (Fig. 17.9).

The tissue viability nurse involved in her care avoided using open weave gauze dressings (e.g. Bactigras) as capillary buds can grow up through the mesh. Removal of these types of dressing can result in removal of some of the newly developed capillaries (which in compromised tissue viability may be the only ones grown over those few days). Instead a low-adherent dressing with a capacity to absorb moderate volumes of exudate was used (e.g. Allevyn). Her nutrient intake was optimized (including trace minerals and vitamins) and she was moved frequently (Stockton and Parker 2002) to minimize the chances of pressure ulcer development. Pain was managed with systemic analgesics, and the moist environment aimed at promoting healing under the dressing also helped to reduce nerve ending irritation. Slough removal was promoted with biosurgical debridement (see Fig. 17.9) (Courtney 1999).

With continued antimicrobial management and wound dressing, the ulcer was kept free from infection. Granulation tissue developed enclosing the extensor tendons, and after around 10 weeks there were signs of reepithelialization from the wound margins. In view of this wound activity, autologous grafting, use of living skin equivalents (e.g. Dermagraft (S&N)) or the growth factor beclapermin (Regranex (Janssen-Cilag)) was considered unnecessary. Wound management continued at home following discharge from hospital (district nurse and podiatrist liased to optimize care and visits). Though scarring and soft tissue adhesion was marked, this was not treated owing to resource limitations.

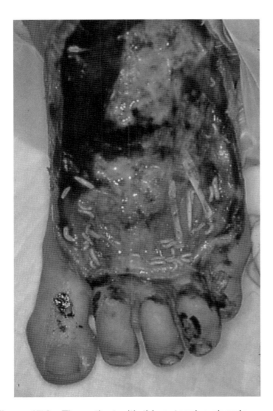

Figure 17.9 The patient with this extensive chronic wound was kept in hospital for wound management, including biosurgical debridement (larval therapy), following infection and necrosis after canalization through a dorsalis vein.

ment (e.g. an allergy clinic) may be a useful resource for help.

Poor nutrition and lack of trace minerals can delay healing (Shetty & McPherson 1997, Williams 2002). It is worthwhile enquiring about the patient's diet and their medical status, and commenting or referring as appropriate according to the practitioner's scope of practice.

Reducing mechanical stress at the ulcer site

As described earlier in this chapter, providing rest by off-loading mechanical stress is essential (Gebhardt et al 1996, Spencer 2000). Foot ulcers will not heal unless tissues are protected from compression, shear, torsion, friction and tensile stresses. (However, hypergranulation tissue, particularly that associated with venous ulceration, seems clinically to benefit from controlled compression.) Depending upon the severity of the ulcer, and complications such as infection, the patient may be admitted for hospital bed rest, take time off work to rest at home (true rest, not pottering around the house) or may be kept ambulant.

It can be difficult to determine when a patient should be admitted to hospital, but the following may be helpful guidelines (adapted from

Table 17.4 Ulcer types and exudate and example(s) of suitable wound dressings[a]

Type of ulcer and site	Nature and volume of exudate	Type of dressing suitable	Examples of wound dressings
Ischaemic			
Plus eschar (necrotic tissue), aseptic, any site	Ulcers often dry and painful (wounds have no/low exudates)	Passive, active dressing; benefit obtained will be dependent upon quality of blood flow	*Either* Leave eschar intact (see also 'necrosis') and cover with low adherent dressing (e.g. Melolin (S&N), Tiele (J&J)), polymer film (e.g. Opsite Flexigrid (S&N); NB: may be difficult to remove) or foam (e.g. Flexipore (Innovative Technologies)) *Or (less favoured; contention over best practice)* Hydrate to promote autolysis to debride necrotic eschar (e.g. Aqacel (ConvaTec), IntraSite gel (S&N))
No slough, aseptic	Often painful, minimal exudates (low-exudate wound)	Passive, active dressing, interactive dressing may be beneficial on the clean wound bed	Low-adherent dressing (e.g. Melolin (S&N), N-A dressing (J&J)), non-adherent dressing (e.g. Urgotul (Parema)) or absorbent and insulatory dressing (e.g. Allevyn (S&N)); hydrogel for pain management (e.g. Geliperm (Geistlich Pharma)) Consider use of dressing that interactively influences inflammatory process and promotes wound healing (e.g. Promogram (J&J), a collagen dressing), a bioactive dressing (e.g. Hyalofill (ConvaTec), a hyaluronic acid derivative) or skin replacements (e.g. Dermagraft (S&N), fibroblasts seeded on a biodegradable scaffold; Regranex (Janssen-Cilag), a growth factor). NB: Cost-benefit?
Neuropathic (usually over site of high magnitude of mechanical stress and/or long duration of loading)			
Dorsum/plantar	Often moderate exudate (low to moderate exudates wound)	Passive, active or interactive dressing (if wound bed clear of slough). Beware maceration of wound margins	NB: The absorption profile of dressing will change dorsum to plantar owing to differences in compression Foam dressing (e.g. Allevyn (S&N)); Mepilex Life (Molnlycke), a silicone contact dressing Hydrocolloid (controversial) (e.g. Granuflex (ConvaTec), Comfeel (Coloplast), Cutinova (S&N)) Alginate dressing (e.g. Kaltostat (ConvaTec) or Curasorb (Tyco Healthcare)) Non-adherent dressing (e.g. Urgotul (Parema)) Bioactive dressing (e.g. Hyalofill (ConvaTec), Promogram (J&J)) Skin replacements (e.g. Dermagraft (S&N)) Growth factors (e.g. Regranex (Janssen-Cilag))
Tracking ulcer	Low, moderate or high exudate	Active dressing, also to maintain drainage; role of interactive dressings not yet established in this context	Do not occlude; maintain drainage by lightly packing wound. Cavity wound dressings are usually too large for foot wounds. Check frequently, daily in diabetic ulceration. Intrasite gel (S&N), Sorbsan ribbon (Unomedical), Hyalofill R (ConvaTec)

Wound type	Exudate	Dressing type	Management
Venous Usually medial and/or lateral ankle	Often high volume of exudates, odour from contaminating microbes	Passive, active dressings; interactive dressing if wound bed free from slough. Beware maceration of wound margins	High-absorption, low-frequency of replacement dressings such as hydrocolloid wafer (e.g. Granuflex (ConvaTec), Comfeel (Coloplast), Cutinova (S&N)), odour absorption dressing (e.g. Sorbsan plus carbon (Unomedical), Actisorb Silver (S&N)), high-absorption foams (e.g. 3M foam (3M)), negative pressure therapy (e.g. vacuum-assisted closure (VAC, KCI)), skin replacements (e.g. Dermagraft (S&N)), growth factors (e.g. Regranex (Janssen-Cilag)); control biochemical activity (e.g. Promogram (J&J)); compression bandaging
Mixed aetiology	Variable exudate volumes	Passive, active dressing; interactive dressing if wound bed free from slough	Select dressing according to clinical features, wound site and exudate volume and nature
Pressure ulcer	Variable exudate volumes	Passive, active dressing; interactive dressing if wound bed free from slough	Off-loading pressure is an essential part of treatment. Moderate to high absorption such as hydrocolloid wafer (e.g. Granuflex (ConvaTec), Comfeel (Coloplast), Cutinove (S&N)), odour absorption dressing (e.g. Lyofoam C (Medlock), Actisorb Silver (S&N)), negative pressure therapy (e.g. vacuum-assisted closure (VAC, KCI)), skin replacements (e.g. Dermagraft (S&N)), growth factors (e.g. Regranex (Janssen-Cilag)); control biochemical activity (e.g. Promogram (J&J)); autologous skin graft
Infected	Odour, moderate to high volume exudate, discoloured. Beware of shiny surface, indicative of bacterial biofilm and reduction in antimicrobial efficacy	Passive, active dressing	Antimicrobial drugs (systemic, topical); negative pressure therapy (e.g. vacuum-assisted closure (VAC, KCI)); low- and non-adherent dressings containing an antimicrobial drug (e.g. Inadine (J&J), Acticoat (S&N), Anabact Gel (CHS) POM, Metrotop Gel (Medlock Medical) POM, both metronidazole); non-occlusive dressings with moderate-to-high exudate absorption profiles (e.g. Allevyn (S&N), 3M foam (3M))
Necrosis Dry eschar (black leathery)	No exudate	Passive, active dressing	Promote autolysis using hydrogel (e.g. Intrasite gel (S&N)) or saline irrigation. Debride (sharp or biosurgical) (e.g. LarvE (Biosurgical Research Unit, SMTL)). Low absorption foam (e.g. Mepiform (Molnlycke))
Wet slough (yellow-grey, stringy, sticky)	Low-moderate exudate, perhaps slight odour	Passive, active dressing	As above. Use of antimicrobial therapy in infection; beware of bacterial biofilm formation. Absorbent foam also for thermal insulation (e.g. Allevyn (S&N), Biatain (Coloplast)), honey (e.g. ApiNate (Apimed NZ); manuka, honey impregnated alginate)

[a]The general information given here will require adapting for each individual. Generally, the nature and volume of exudate will determine the dressing used. Most wounds on the foot are likely to require additional methods of minimizing mechanical stress and for providing thermal insulation; for clarity these are not included in the table.

Adapted from Dealey (1994), Thomas (1997), Bradley et al (1999), Moffat (2001), Ballard and Baxter (2002) and Cutting and White (2002), with permission.

Flanagan 1997, MacFarlane & Jeffcoate 1999, Edmonds & Foster 2001, NSF for Diabetes):

- cellulitis affecting the whole of the forefoot (or worse)
- severe pain
- general malaise
- foot ulceration greater than approximately 8 cm diameter
- foot ulceration plus extensive tracking (Fig. 17.10)
- suspected active osteomyelitis
- in a large ulcer after, say, 4 weeks of no improvement.

Padding to accommodate a deformity and ulcer is a very useful, short-term approach to providing rest, but footwear (see Box 17.3) must be suitable and large enough to accommodate these additions, otherwise ischaemia arising from tissue compression will cause deterioration or ulceration at a different site.

For longer-term use, orthoses need to be prescribed with a view to off-loading the ulcer site (see Fig. 17.6). This entails judicious selection of materials. Ideally a washable/ wipeable covering material that does not affect the function of the orthoses should be used and that also maintains a healthy microenvironment at the skin–contact interface (Bliss 1995, Hampton & Collins 2002). Often layers of foam with different physical characteristics (Rome 1998) provide simple, but effective, insulatory insoles (e.g. 3 mm light-density Plastazote adhesed to 2 or 3 mm PPT or Poron). Additions of felt or foam padding to the underside of these insoles can provide easily made, additional relief from mechanical stress. Newer materials, such as Memory Poron, can be useful as inserts into insoles and orthoses, creating a differential in density and shock absorption compared with adjacent materials.

Scotchcast shoes, boots and total contact casts and walkers (see Fig. 17.7) are a valuable method of reducing load at the ulcer site by transferring it more uniformly to other tissue sites, although studies to support this view are limited (Spencer 2000). With use of casts (Armstrong et al 1998, Cavenagh et al 2000, Frykberg & Armstrong 2002, Levin 2002) or adapted sandals/shoes,

exposed tissue still needs to be protected from changes in temperature and other trauma. Patients can wear large, soft socks over the toe of the cast, covering this with a plastic bag in wet weather. Some podiatrists and plaster technicians have developed the necessary skill in application of these devices, which need checking within the first week of application. However, referral may be necessary to the appropriate specialist centre. Casts of varying forms may be replaced and worn indefinitely until wound healing is achieved but may need changing following findings on review. Once the ulcer has healed, then prevention of recurrence is paramount.

With bed rest or sitting for prolonged periods, the microenvironment at the skin–contact sur-

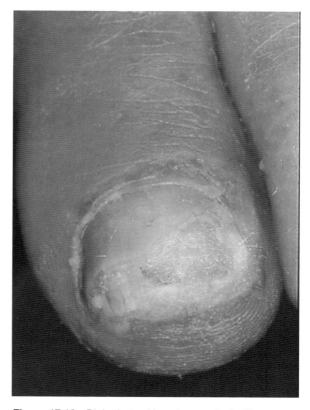

Figure 17.10 Diabetic tracking ulcer packed with a dressing (Hyalofill) to maintain drainage and to provide granulating tissue with a collagen support to promote cellular motility.

face interface needs controlling to minimize potential for overhydration (and consequent increase in friction and shear stresses and bacterial and/or candidal infection; Hampton & Collins 2002, Stockton & Parker 2002). If possible, the patient needs to move around a little, loading different tissue sites frequently to avoid the development of pressure ulcers (Stockton & Parker 2002). Occupational therapists with special skills in seating, tissue viability nurse specialists and diabetes nurse specialists are invaluable colleagues in managing people with these problems.

Debriding ulcers

There is some contention over whether dry, ischaemic necrosis (eschar) in the foot should be debrided or not. Many consider that reepithelialization (the final stage of the repair process) cannot occur satisfactorily until the necrotic eschar is removed through use of sharp (scalpel) debridement or autolysis following hydration on application of a hydrogel (e.g. Intrasite gel (S&N) or Aquacel (ConvaTec)) (Bale 1997, Jones 1998a). Others consider scalpel debridement or autolysis are inappropriate for use on ischaemic wounds, exposing uninfected tissue to the potential for bacterial and/or fungal invasion. Biosurgery (larval therapy, use of the green bottle fly larvae) to debride dry ischaemic necrosis seems to be helpful, though more effective on slough (Courtney 1999). Advice and evidence for good practice in the form of rigorous clinical studies are lacking (Bradley et al 1999, Smith & Thow 2001).

In diabetic foot ulceration, hyperkeratosis should be removed and the thickened macerated tissue surrounding a plantar neuropathic ulcer should also be sharp debrided by a podiatrist to remove the bulk of tissue, which can be a predisposing cause of ulceration (Murray et al 1996). If there are signs of epidermal emargination over a wound that is not granulating, then this too needs to be debrided. Otherwise, there will be an epidermal covering over a cavity, preventing loss of any exudate that builds up, which will then track in another direction. Although callus removal has been shown to have little effect on

pressure distribution in the rheumatoid foot (Woodburn et al 2000), hyperkeratotic tissue will need to be removed to minimize adjacent and subjacent tissue damage from this hard, bulky tissue (Springett et al 2002); a similar situation occurs in peripheral vascular disease.

Some practitioners choose to debride foot wound margins and/or bed enthusiastically, to bleeding point, to trigger a normal acute inflammatory response to override the chronic state and lead to resolution of the ulcer. Others consider this to be unnecessarily traumatic to tissues that, because of poor tissue viability, are struggling to produce granulation tissue, and that removal of tissue is counterproductive. It is possible that marked debriding may promote a demand for blood flow that cannot be met by the peripheral circulation. Currently advice on the level of debriding best for keratotic tissue in the foot is lacking (Bradley et al 1999, Smith & Thow 2001). The practitioner will need to keep up to date with national guidelines and consult with local colleagues as to local practice.

Moist necrotic tissue in a wound bed (slough) can be sharp debrided or removed through application of a hydrogel to promote autolysis (e.g. Intrasite gel (S&N) or Aquacel (ConvaTec)). Biosurgery, assuming the recipient can cope with the concept, is beneficial (Courtney 1999), and the periwound tissues need to be covered with a dressing such as hydrocolloid wafers to contain the larvae at the wound site until removal a few days later.

Dressing ulcers

Ulcers, regardless of type or cause, need dressing (Table 17.4) to reduce potential for infection, to provide pain relief and to give thermal and mechanical protection (Dealey 1994, Baker 1997, Thomas 1997). The benefits from reducing pain, optimizing fibroblast activity, promoting capillary angiogenesis and encouraging reepithelialization within a moist environment are well recorded (Eaglestein 1985, Centre for Medical Education 1992, Ballard & Baxter 2002), and many current wound dressings (active dressings) function using this concept.

A wound dressing alone will not aid healing of a chronic foot ulcer. All aspects of management need to be undertaken concurrently (see Box 17.4) (Jones 1998b), as described in earlier sections of this chapter. For example, if mechanical stress is not off-loaded, if infection is left untreated or if footwear is worn that is tight or has a rough lining, then use of expensive dressings is a waste of time and money for the patient, practitioner and service provider.

Wound dressings should be cost effective (Thomas 1997). There is concern that frequent redressing will disturb healing tissue, as well as lowering wound temperatures, inhibiting mitosis. Also materials for redressing ulcers and staff time for redressings add to the cost of chronic wound management (Williams 1999, Ballard & Baxter 2002, Cullen 2002). Many of the active wound dressings that aim to promote a moist environment to optimize healing may be left in place for a few days (3–8 days), whereas the traditional, passive dressings (e.g. gauze and low-adherent dressings, e.g. Melolin (S&N), Tiele (J&J)) may need to be replaced at least daily, depending upon wound exudate volumes, unless used with an additional, secondary dressing. The practitioner needs to be aware of the cost–benefit relation when selecting dressings for different purposes. For example, it is unnecessarily expensive to use a hydrocolloid wafer on a 1 mm diameter superficial wound when a low-adherent gauze would be more than suitable.

The wide range of wound dressings available can be confusing. Dressings may be passive (provide a covering for the wound, e.g. gauze), active (promote an optimum, moist environment for healing (Eaglestein 1985), e.g. hydrocolloids) or interactive/bioactive (work with the body's processes to promote healing (Ballard & Baxter 2002), e.g. growth factors). Also dressings are chosen for their different exudates-absorption capacities. Presence of infection will also affect the choice of dressing (see Box 17.4).

For all wounds, ideally a low- or non-adherent dressing should be used (see Table 17.4), though dressing availability varies throughout the world and suitable dressings range from clean cloth to gauze swabs to sterile, non-adherent dressings.

In some countries (e.g. USA) a wet–dry method is used for debriding the wound (as the wet dressing dries it adheres to the wound bed and when removed pulls away slough, with concurrent, often marked, pain and distress).

Wound dressings and volume of wound exudate

When selecting a wound dressing (see Table 17.4), a useful rule of thumb is to look at the nature and volume of the wound exudate, both in the wound and on the removed wound dressing (Baker 1997, Thomas 1997, Jones 1998b, Ballard & Baxter 2002).

If there is little exudate (e.g. in ischaemic ulceration), use a low-absorption wound dressing such as alginate (Bale et al 2001). Clinical reports indicate some people have discomfort when dressings with strong hygroscopic (tissue fluids absorbed enthusiastically into the dressing matrix) properties are used on ischaemic wounds.

Autolysis of a dry ischaemic eschar, promoted by use of a hydrogel (e.g. Intrasite gel (S&N), Aquacel (a carboxymethylcellulose gel; ConvaTec)), may expose a moist wound base. Then a dressing with low-to-moderate absorption (e.g. Allevyn (S&N)) may be helpful in removing excess chronic wound fluid (as this can have the effect of inhibiting fibroblast activity; Phillips et al 1998). It is worth noting that the absorption profile of dressings applied to the foot will be different from those on non-load bearing sites (Thomas 1997).

A wound with a dry but non-necrotic wound bed may benefit from controlled hydration (e.g. a hydrogel, such as Geliperm (Geistlich Pharma)). Also hydration of nerve endings may help to reduce pain. It is essential to prevent maceration (Cutting & White 2002) of periwound tissues, as this creates an environment for bacterial and fungal colonization as well as eroding the ulcer margins further.

Venous ulcers traditionally produce copious quantities of exudate and a high-absorption dressing is required to minimize potential for periwound maceration (Cutting & White 2002).

These dressings should be coupled with compression therapy after ensuring there is no concurrent ischaemia (European Pressure Ulcer Advisory Panel 1998b, Guest et al 1999, Moore 2002). Tissue viability nurses and practice nurses have skills in applying the appropriate, graded compression through bandaging and/or compression hosiery.

Neuropathic ulcers, particularly those associated with diabetes, produce moderate volumes of exudate and a dressing should be selected accordingly (Baker 1997, Sherman & Kerr 2000, Edmonds & Foster 2001), for example a foam (e.g. Alleyvn (S&N)). There are conflicting views over how appropriate hydrocolloid wafer dressings are in diabetic neuropathic ulceration (Lithner 1990), which may be related to their inappropriate use.

High exudate volumes and odour are frequent problems with fungating wounds but can also occur with venous and diabetic ulceration. Control of bacterial infection (Bowler et al 1999) involved in odour production in these wounds, through use of antimicrobial drugs, can help. Charcoal-based, odour-absorbing dressings (e.g. Actisorb Silver (S&N), Sorbsan plus carbon (Unomedical)) are also helpful.

Wound dressings and infection

Infection will change the nature (and smell; Bowler et al 1999) of the exudate, for example staphylococcal infection induces thick yellow pus and haemolytic streptococcal infection has a thin watery exudate; the dressing may be changed to incorporate an antimicrobial drug (topical antibiotic, e.g. Anabact Gel (CHS) pom, but be aware of problems with resistance) or antiseptic (O'Meara et al 2000, Swartz 2004). A topical antiseptic can be used in conjunction with a suitable dressing, though this may not be included in the named and regulated uses noted by the producer, and the practitioner should be aware of indemnity issues. With infection, the volume of exudate usually also increases and a dressing with higher absorption (see Table 17.4) may be needed until the infection clears and exudate production reduces. Topical antiseptic

dressings frequently used include those with povidone iodine or silver as an active ingredient.

If partial or totally occlusive dressings (e.g. hydrocolloid wafers or films) have been used but infection develops, then the dressing type should be changed to a non-occlusive dressing (see Table 17.4), for example to an alginate, which forms a hydrogel at the wound interface, or a foam dressing, which removes excess fluid into its matrix. Wound progress should be monitored frequently (daily or more frequently in diabetic wounds) and antibiotic therapy started if required (Bowler et al 1999, Swartz 2004).

Dressings for different stages of chronic wound healing and interactive dressings

Chronic ulceration often features the different stages of wound healing all within the same wound (Ballard & Baxter 2002) (see Case study 17.4). Wet, dead tissue (slough) may be seen with areas of black–grey dry necrosis/gangrene. Necrosis may be present alongside reepithelialization (Fig. 17.11). To add a further variable to be considered in wound management and dressing selection, wounds change over time (Flanagan 1997, Moffat 2001). Different dressings will need to be applied in these differing clinical situations. The wound will accordingly need to be reassessed at each visit and the appropriate dressing selected (see Table 17.4). A dressing will need to be used that is suitable for all the stages clinically evident within the wound. The options are to select from the range of passive, active and interactive dressings, while also bearing in mind the volume of exudate production and whether infection is present.

Tracking wounds, or those with a sinus, will require a dressing that allows exudate drainage and can be introduced into the length of the wound. Alginate rope/gauze (e.g. Sorbsan (Unomedical)) is a helpful foot cavity wound dressing. Hydrating this dressing on removal makes it an easier and less-uncomfortable process. Hyalofill (ConvaTec), a biopolymeric fleece or ribbon composed of an ester of hyaluronic acid, is also a helpful dressing, promoting wound healing in part through its

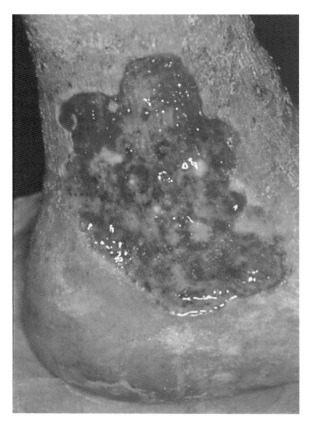

Figure 17.11 All stages of healing are evident in this chronic venous ulcer. Epithelialization is evident, alongside necrosis and granulation tissue with slough.

antioxidant properties as well as providing a framework for macrophages and fibroblasts. These dressings will need a secondary covering low/non-adherent dressing (see Table 17.4). Sterile gauze can be used to pack wounds if no other product is available; this will need soaking before it can be removed (unless the intention is to remove slough in a wet–dry dressing). Proprietary cavity wound dressings are rarely used in managing foot ulceration as they often will not fit into a tracking foot wound; if used, they can be difficult to remove.

Grafting of slow healing, or large wounds is undertaken using autologous grafts (the patient's own skin), usually by a surgeon. The result is that two wound sites (donor site and wound) need managing. Synthetic skin substitutes (skin equivalents, e.g. Dermagraft (S&N); Grey et al 1998, McColgan et al 1998) provide a good solution to this problem as well as, theoretically, providing all that a wound needs to heal. For example, Dermagraft consists of cryopreserved neonatal fibroblasts seeded onto a biodegradable three-dimensional scaffold (Newton et al 2002) to provide the wound with growth factors required for healing and a framework to promote cell motility. Other dressings (e.g. Oasis (Cook)), which provide a collagen-matrix structural support for the wound as well as a moist microenvironment for cellular activity, are also helpful in promoting wound healing. In all instances, an adequate blood supply is invaluable, and referral to a vascular surgeon is worthwhile.

Investigation of the biochemical phases of, and growth factors within, chronic wounds continues promisingly (Yamaguchi & Yoishikawa 2001). Promogram (J&J) is a collagen and oxidized regenerated cellulose product (Veves et al 2002) that deactivates and binds matrix metalloproteinases, which inhibit local growth factors (Cullen 2002).

Research into the effects of growth factors (Cox 1993) in chronic wounds has been applied clinically and is becoming more effective (Graham 1998). For example, becalpermin (Regranex 0.01% gel (Janssen-Cilag) pom), a topically applied growth factor (similar to indigenous platelet derived growth factor), has been shown to be beneficial in diabetic ulceration (Wiemann et al 1998) through promoting the chemotactic recruitment and cell proliferation involved in wound repair.

When to start using these more expensive, interactive dressings is a vexing question. Ideally the sooner started the sooner they can exert a beneficial effect, but they are costly. A suggestion is that obvious causes should be treated and excluded during a period of, say, 4 weeks. Then a more advanced regimen is started that controls all extrinsic factors which may be influential in wound development and that manages intrinsic factors closely. After a further arbitrary period of a further 4 weeks, if there is no sign of resolution, then start with the interactive dressings. The

NSF for Diabetes provides diabetes-specific guidelines.

To date, interactive dressings have had a variable uptake by the different professions involved in wound care in the foot; this may be related to their cost, ease of use (instructions for use need following precisely), frequency of reapplication and the activity the patient can undertake in the meantime. Although all these developments, and others not noted, represent remarkable achievements in chronic wound care, as yet the panacea is still awaited. Also, many clinical studies reporting on methods of wound management have small sample sizes and some lack rigour; the special interest groups could liaise to address this issue.

Ulcer treatment with physical therapies

A different approach to chronic wound management is that of vacuum-assisted closure (Collier 1997, Armstrong et al 2002). Although this system is available in a portable form, it is usually only readily applied as inpatient treatment. A specific, cavity foam-based wound dressing adhered to the wound margins forms an end point through which a gentle vacuum is drawn, having the effect of pulling granulating tissues nearer to the surface. It also appears to have a beneficial effect in increasing capillary angiogenesis and removing chronic wound fluid (Phillips 1998).

Hyperbaric oxygen therapy can be helpful in providing the wound interface with high pressures of oxygen to improve tissue viability, and hence potential for healing. This modality waxes and wanes in popularity.

Low-level laser therapy has value in scar management and also in promoting wound healing (Lagan et al 2002) through stimulating macrophage and fibroblast mitochondrial activity with a 660 nm wavelength laser and a range of pulse frequencies and duration of application (Lucas et al 2000). Ultrasound, 3 MHz pulsed, has a similar end result, though the site of stimulation appears to be more the tissue cell membranes. Treatments need to be repeated twice a week for the first 2 weeks decreasing to one irradiation per week. However, this dosimetry may change as information available progresses.

SUMMARY

This chapter has described the management of skin or soft tissue injuries in the foot and its modification for those at-risk of chronic problems such as ulceration. Assessment of the whole patient, assessment and diagnosis of the wound type and management processes are outlined (see Box 17.5). The prevention of ulceration and of ulcer recurrence is also discussed.

Box 17.5 A sequence for treating a small (<5 cm diameter) chronic wound (ulcer) on the foot

Assessment of the whole patient, assessment and diagnosis of the wound type and management processes will have been carried out.

1. Check national and local wound management guidelines
2. Cleanse wound (potable water, sterile normal saline – non-touch technique)
3. Debride slough, hyperkeratosis
4. Measure and record wound status (margins and wound bed)
5. Treat any infection (e.g. systemic antibiotics, topical antiseptics or antifungal drugs)
6. Select and apply wound dressing according to wound site and dressing function (i.e. insulation, exudate absorption capacity; apply with bandage rather than strapping if necessary)
7. Provide method of reducing mechanical stress (e.g. padding, orthosis, total contact cast)
8. Provide patient with information on wound care and footwear advice
9. Check footwear for fit, rough linings and advise accordingly

Continued

> **Box 17.5** (contd)
>
> 10. Manage cause of ulceration, referring as necessary
> 11. Involve patient, carer and practice nurse, district nurse (or clinical nurse specialist) in dressing regimen
> 12. Ensure patient knows who, when and how to access health care professionals as necessary
> 13. Arrange follow-up appointment (which will vary according to wound state, and arrangements made for patient self-care).

REFERENCES

Armstrong D, Lavery L, Harkless L 1998 Who is at risk for diabetic foot ulceration? Clinics in Podiatric Medicine and Surgery 15: 11–19

Armstrong D G, Lavery L A, Abu-Rumman P et al 2002 Outcomes of subatmospheric pressure dressing therapy on wounds of the diabetic foot. Ostomy and Wound Management 48: 64–68

Bader D, Bouten C 2000 Clinical biomechanics. In: Zeevi Drir (ed) Biomechanics of soft tissues. Churchill Livingstone, New York, p 35–64

Baker J 1998 Essential oils: a complementary therapy in wound management. Journal of Wound Care 7: 355–357

Baker N 1997 Foot ulcer management. Journal of Wound Care 6: resource file supplement

Bale S 1997 A guide to wound debridement. Journal of Wound Care 6: 179–184

Bale S, Baker N, Crock H, Rayman G, Harding K 2001 Exploring the use of an alginate dressing for diabetic foot ulcers. Journal of Wound Care 10: 81–84

Ballard K, Baxter H 2002 Developments in wound care for difficult to manage wounds. In: White R (ed) Trends in wound care. British Journal of Nursing monograph. Quay Books Division, Mark Allen, Dinton, UK

Bennett P, Patterson C 1998 The Foot Health Status Questionnaire (FHSQ): a new instrument for measuring outcomes of footcare. Australasian Journal of Podiatric Medicine 32: 87–92

Blenkharn J 1985 Biological activity of polynoxylin – an insoluble urea–formaldehyde condensation product. Journal of Clinical and Hospital Pharmacy 10(4): 367–372

Bliss M R 1995 Preventing sores in elderly patients: a comparison of seven mattress overlays. Age and Ageing 24: 297–302

Bliss M 2000 Pressure sores: demographic perspectives. Journal of Tissue Viability 10: 106

Boulton A J M 1996 The pathogenesis of diabetic foot problems. Diabetic Medicine 13(suppl 1): S12–S16

Boulton A, Connor H, Cavanagh P 2000 The foot in diabetes, 3rd edn. Wiley, New York

Bowler P, Davies B, Jones S 1999 Microbial involvement in chronic wound malodour. Journal of Wound Care 8: 216–218

Bowman C 1998 Clinical gerontology: evidence based multidisciplinary integrated geriatric care. Reviews in Clinical Gerontology 8: 275–277

Bradley M, Cullum N, Sheldon T 1999 The debridement of chronic wounds: a systematic review. Health Technology Assessment 3: 1–2

Bradshaw T 1999 Multiprofessional care of the diabetic foot: the role of the podiatrist. British Journal of Therapy and Rehabilitation 6: 8–13

Brennan S S, Leaper D J 1985 The effect of antiseptics on the healing wound: a study using the rabbit ear chamber. British Journal of Surgery 72: 780–782

Brennan S, Foster M, Leaper D 1986 Antiseptic toxicity in wounds healing by secondary intention. Journal of Hospital Medicine 8: 263–267

Budiman-Mak E, Conrad K J, Roach K E 1991 The foot function index; a measure of foot pain and disability Journal of Clinical Epidemiology 44: 561–570

Cavenagh P, Ulbrecht J S, Caputo G 2000 New developments in the biomechanics of the diabetic foot. Diabetes/Metabolism Research Reviews 16(suppl 1): S6–S10

Centre for Medical Education 1992 The Wound Programme. Centre for Medical Education, Dundee, UK

Colagiuri S, Marsden L, Naidu V, Taylor I 1995 The use of orthotic devices to correct plantar callus in people with diabetes. Diabetic Clinical Research and Practice 28: 29–34

Collier M 1997 Know how: vacuum assisted closure (VAC). Nursing Times 93: 32–33

Cooper R A, Molan P C, Harding K G. 1999 Antibacterial activity of honey against strains of *Staphylococcus aureus* from infected wounds. Journal of the Royal Society of Medicine 92: 283–285

Cox D 1993 Growth factors in wound healing. Journal of Wound Care 6: 339–342

Courtney M 1999 The use of larval therapy in wound management in the UK. Journal of Wound Care 8: 177–179

Cullen B 2001 Chronic wound healing. Wound care device expert meeting, summary report. Diabetic Foot 4(3): S4–S5

Culley F 2002 Nursing aspects of pressure ulcer prevention and therapy. In: White R (ed) Trends in wound care. British Journal of Nursing monograph. Quay Books Division, Mark Allen, Dinton, UK

Cutting K, White R 2002 Maceration of the skin and wound bed I: its nature and causes. Journal of Wound Care 11: 275–278

Dawber R, Bristow I, Turner W 2001 Text atlas of podiatric dermatology. Martin Dunitz, London

Dealey C 1994 The care of wounds. Blackwell Scientific, Oxford

Eaglestein W H 1985 The effect of occlusive dressings on collagen synthesis and re-epithelialisation in superficial wounds. In: Ryan TJ (ed) An environment for healing: the role of occlusion. International Congress and Symposium Series 88. Royal Society of Medicine, London, p 31–38

Edmonds M, Foster A 2001 Managing the diabetic foot. Blackwell Science, London

Eissenbeiss W, Peter F, Bakhtiari C, Frenz C 1998

Hypertrophic scars and keloids. Journal of Wound Care 7: 255–257

European Pressure Ulcer Advisory Panel 1998a Pressure ulcer prevention guidelines. Available at: http://www.epuap.org

European Pressure Ulcer Advisory Panel 1998b Pressure ulcer treatment guidelines. Available at: http://www.epuap.org

Field T, Peck M, Krugman S et al 1998 Burn injuries benefit from massage therapy. Journal of Burn Care and Rehabilitation 19: 241–244

Flanagan M 1997 A practical framework for wound assessment. 2: Methods. British Journal of Nursing 6: 6–11

Foster A 2002 Is there an evidence base for diabetic foot care? Journal of Tissue Viability 12: 113–117

Frykberg R 1997 Team approach toward lower extremity amputation prevention in diabetes. Journal of the American Podiatric Medical Association 87: 305–312

Frykberg R G 1998 Diabetic foot ulcers: Current concepts. Journal of Foot and Ankle Surgery 37: 441–446

Frykberg R G, Armstrong D G 2002 The diabetic foot 2001. A summary of the proceedings of the American Diabetes Association's 61st Scientific Symposium. Journal of the American Podiatric Medical Association 92: 2–6

Gebhardt K S, Bliss M R, Winwright P L, Thomas J M 1996 Pressure-relieving supports in an ICU. Journal of Wound Care 5: 116–121

Gilchrist B 1997 Should iodine be reconsidered in wound management? Journal of Wound Care 6: 148–150

Graham A 1998 The use of growth factors in clinical practice. Journal of Wound Care 7: 464–466

Grey J, Bale S, Harding K 1998 The use of cultured dermis in the treatment of diabetic foot ulcers. Journal of Wound Care 7: 324–325

Griffiths R D, Fernandez R S, Ussia C 2001 Is tap water a safe alternative to normal saline for wound irrigation in the community setting? Journal of Wound Care 10: 407–411

Gripton J 2002 Development and validation of the foot health and activities questionnaire. A podiatric outcome measure. PhD Thesis, University of Brighton, UK

Guest M, Smith J, Sira M, Madden P, Greenhalg R, Davies A 1999 Venous ulcer healing by four-layer compression-bandaging is not influenced by the pattern of venous incompetence. British Journal of Surgery and Endovascular Surgery 18: 540–541

Hampton S, Collins F 2002 Tissue viability: a comprehensive guide to pressure ulcer management and wound care. Whurr, London

Hardy S 2002 Human microbiology. Lifelines. Taylor & Francis, London

Hart J 1998 The use of ultraso.und therapy in wound healing. Journal of Wound Care 7: 25–28

Hart J 2002 Inflammation: its role in the healing of chronic wounds. Journal of Wound Care 11: 205–209, 245–249

Hartman D, Coetzee J 2002 Two US practitioners' experience of using essential oils for wound care. Journal of Wound Care 11: 317–320

Hashmi F 2000 Non-enzymatic glycation and the development of plantar callus. British Journal of Podiatry 3: 91–94

Hawthorne J, Redmond K 1998 Pain. Causes and management. Blackwell Science, Oxford

Humphreys W 1999 The red, painful fool: inflammation or ischaemia. British Medical Journal 318: 925–926

International Working Group on the Diabetic Foot 1999 International Consensus on the Diabetic Foot, Amsterdam, the Netherlands

Jones V 1998a Debridement of diabetic foot lesions. Diabetic Foot 1: 99–94

Jones V 1998b Selecting a dressing for the diabetic foot: factors to consider. Diabetic Foot 1: 48–52

Jude E, Boulton A 1998 Foot problems in diabetes mellitus. British Journal of Podiatry 1: 117–120

Kerry R M, Holt G M, Stockley I 1994 The foot in chronic rheumatoid arthritis; a continuing problem The Foot 4: 201–203

Kilmartin T 2001 The use of antimicrobials in podiatric practice. British Journal of Podiatry 4: 8–14

Lagan K M, McKenna T, Witherow A, Johns J, McDonough S M, Baxter G D 2002 Low-intensity laser therapy/combined phototherapy in the management of chronic venous ulceration: a placebo-controlled study. Journal of Clinical Laser Medicine and Surgery 20: 109–116

Leelaporn A, Pualsen I, Tennent J, Littlejohn T, Skurray R 1994 Multidrug resistance to antiseptics and disinfection in coagulase negative staphylococci. Journal of Medicine and Biology 40: 214–230

Levin M 2002 Management of the diabetic foot: preventing amputation. Southern Medical Association 95: 10–20

Lithner F 1990 Adverse effects on diabetic foot ulcers of highly adhesive hydrocolloid adhesive dressings. Diabetes Care 13: 814–815

Lorimer D, French G, O'Donnell M, Burrow JG 2001 Neale's disorders of the foot: diagnosis and management. Churchill Livingstone, Edinburgh

Low A, Reed J 2000 Electrotherapy explained. Butterworth-Heinemann, London

Lucas C, Stanborough R, Freeman C, de Haan R 2000 Efficacy of low level laser therapy on wound healing in human subjects: a systematic review. Lasers in Medical Science 15: 84–93

MacFarlane R, Jeffcoate W (1999) Classification of diabetic foot ulcers: The S(AD) SAD system. Diabetic Foot 2: 123–126

Mandy A, McInnes J, Lucas K 2002 Psychosocial aspects to podiatry. Harcourt, London

Mantey I, Foster A, Spencer S, Edmonds M 1999 Why do foot ulcers recur in diabetic patients? Diabetic Medicine 16: 245–249

McColgan M, Foster A, Edmonds M 1998 Dermagraft in the treatment of diabetic foot ulcers. Diabetic Foot 1: 75–78

Menz H, Lord S 2001 Foot pain impairs balance and functional ability in community-dwelling older people. Journal of American Podiatric Medicine Assocation 91: 222–229

Merriman L, Tollafield D (eds) 1995 Assessment of the lower limb. Edinburgh, Churchill Livingstone

Moffat C 2001 Leg ulcers. In: Murray S (ed) Vascular disease: nursing and management. Whurr, London, p 200–237

Molan P 1999 The role of honey in the management of wounds. Journal of Wound Care 8: 415–453

Moore P, Foster L 2002 Acute surgical wound care 1 and 2. In: White R (ed) Trends in wound care. British Journal of Nursing monograph. Quay Books Division, Mark Allen, Dinton, UK, p 77–84, 85–92

Moore Z 2002 Compression bandaging: are practitioners

achieving the ideal sub-bandage pressures? Journal of Wound Care 11: 265–268

Morgan D 2004 Formulary of wound management products. Euromed Communications, Haslemere, Surrey

Murray H, Young M, Hollis S, Boulton A 1996 Plantar callus is highly predictive of diabetic ulceration. Diabetic Medicine 13: 979–982

National Institute for Clinical Excellence (NICE). Available at: http://www.nice.org.uk

National Institute for Clinical Excellence 2001 Pressure ulcer risk assessment and prevention. Inherited clinical guideline B. NICE, London. Available at: http://www.nice.org.uk

Newton D, Khan F, Belch J, Mitcel M, Leese G 2002 Blood flow changes in diabetic foot ulcers treated with a dermal replacement. Journal of Foot and Ankle Surgery 41: 283–287

NICE Clinical guidelines for type 2 diabetes: prevention and management of foot problems. Available at: http://www.nice.org.uk/pdf/CG10fullguideline.pdf (last accessed November 2004)

Nurmikko T, Nash T 1998 Control of chronic pain. British Medical Journal 317: 1438–1441

O'Meara S O, Cullum N, Majid M, Sheldon T 2000 Systematic reviews of wound care management: 3. Antimicrobial agents. Health Technology Assessment 4: 1–237

Oxford Centre for Evidence Based Medicine: http://www.jr2.ox.ac.uk/bandolier/

Philips T, Al-Amoudi H, Leverkus M, Park H-Y 1998 Effect of chronic wound fluid on fibroblasts. Journal of Wound Care 7: 527–532

Potter J 2000 Regrowth patterns of plantar callus. The Foot 10: 144–148

Potts R O, Guzek D B, Harris R R, McKie J E 1985 A non-invasive, in vitro technique to quantitatively measure water content of the stratum corneum using attenuated total reflectance infrared spectroscopy. Archives of Dermatology Research 277: 489–495

Rome K 1998 Orthotic materials: a review of the selection process. Diabetic Foot 1: 14–19

Ryan T 1998 Evidence based medicine: a critique. Journal of Tissue Viability 8: 7–8

Russell L 2002 The importance of wound documentation and classification. In: White R (ed) Trends in wound care. British Journal of Nursing monograph. Quay Books Division, Mark Allen, Dinton, UK, p 65–98

Sage R, Webster J, Fisher S 2001 Outpatient care and morbidity reduction in diabetic foot ulcers associated with chronic pressure callus. Journal of the American Podiatric Medicine Association 91: 275–279

Scottish Intercollegiate Guidelines Network 1998 The care of patients with chronic leg ulcers: a National Clinical Guideline. Royal College of Physicians, Edinburgh

Sherman D, Kerr D 2000 Practical management of neuropathic diabetic foot ulcers. The Diabetic Foot 3(2): 49–54

Shetty P, McPherson K 1997 Diet, nutrition and chronic disease: lessons from contrasting worlds. Wiley, Chichester, UK

Smith J, Thow J 2001 Is debridement effective for diabetic foot ulcers? Diabetic Foot 4: 10–12, 77–80, 165–172

Spencer S 2000 Pressure relieving interventions for preventing and treating diabetic foot ulcers (Cochrane review). The Cochrane Library Issue 4, Update Software, Oxford

Springett K 2002a An introduction to some common cutaneous foot conditions and their management. Journal of Tissue Viability 12: 100–107

Springett K 2002b Ulceration in the diabetic foot. Home Health Care Consultant (USA) 9: 10–17

Springett K, Merriman L 1995 Dermatological assessment of the lower limb. In: Merriman L, Tollafield D (eds) Assessment of the lower limb. Edinburgh, Churchill Livingstone, p 213–244

Springett K, Deane M, Dancaster P 1997 Treatment of corns, calluses and heel fissures with a hydrocolloid dressing. British Journal of Podiatric Medicine 52: 102–104

Springett K, Parsons S, Young M, Cheek E 2002 The effect and safety of three corn care products. British Journal of Podiatry 5: 82–86

Stadler I, Lanzafame R, Evans R et al 2001 830 nm irradiation increases wound tensile strength in a diabetic murine model. Lasers in Surgery and Medicine 28: 220–226

Stephens P, Thomas D W 2002 The cellular proliferative phase of the wound repair process. Journal of Wound Care 11: 253–261

Stockton L, Parker D 2002 Pressure relief behaviour and the prevention of pressure ulcers in wheelchair users in the community. Journal of Tissue Viability 12: 84–99

Swartz M 2004 Cellulitis. A review. New England Journal of Medicine 350: 904–912

Therstrup-Petersen K 1998 Bacterial infection and the skin: clinical practice and therapy update. British Journal of Dermatology 139(suppl 53): 1–3

Thomas S 1997 Wound management and dressings. Assessment and management of wound exudate. Journal of Wound Care 6: 327–330

Veves A, Sheehan P, Pham H 2002 A randomised controlled trial of Promogran (a collagen/oxidised regenerated cellulose dressing) vs standard treatment in the management of diabetic foot ulcers. Archives of Surgery 137: 822–827

Vincent J 1990 Structural biomaterials. Princeton University Press, Princeton, NJ

Waterlow J 1985 Pressure sores: a risk assessment card. Nursing Times 81: 49–55

White R, Cooper R, Kingsley A 2002 A topical issue: the use of antibacterials in wound pathogen control. In: White R (ed) Trends in wound care. British Journal of Nursing monograph. Quay Books Division, Mark Allen, Dinton, UK, p 110–123

Wieman T, Smeill J, Su Y 1998 Efficacy and safety of a topical gel formulation of recombinant human platelet-derived growth factor-BB (Becalpermin) in patients with chronic neuropathic diabetic ulcers. Diabetes Care 21: 822–827

Williams D R R 1999 The size of the problem: epidemiology and economic aspects of foot problems in diabetes. In: Boulton A J M, Connor H, Cavanagh P R (eds) The foot in diabetes. Wiley, Chichester, UK

Williams L 2002 Assessing patients' nutritional needs in the wound-healing process. Journal of Wound Care 11: 225–228

Woodburn J, Stableford Z, Helliwell P 2000 Preliminary investigation of debridement of plantar callosities in rheumatoid arthritis. Rheumatology 39: 652–654

Yamaguchi Y, Yoishikawa K 2001 Cutaneous wound healing: an update. Journal of Dermatology 28: 521–534

Appendices

Appendix 1

Management of exudation in ulcers

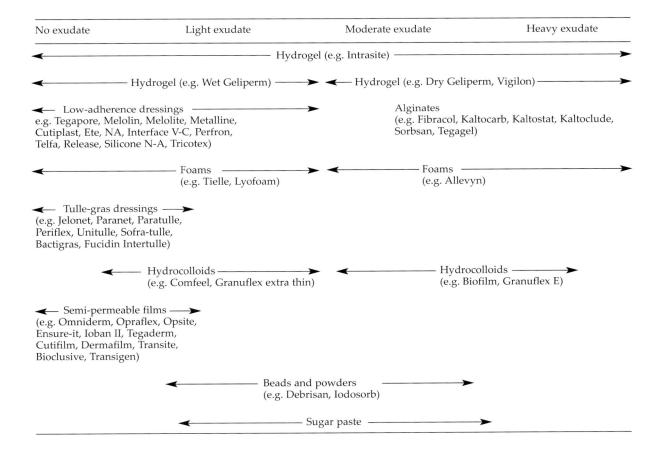

| No exudate | Light exudate | Moderate exudate | Heavy exudate |

Hydrogel (e.g. Intrasite)

Hydrogel (e.g. Wet Geliperm)   Hydrogel (e.g. Dry Geliperm, Vigilon)

Low-adherence dressings
e.g. Tegapore, Melolin, Melolite, Metalline,
Cutiplast, Ete, NA, Interface V-C, Perfron,
Telfa, Release, Silicone N-A, Tricotex)

Alginates
(e.g. Fibracol, Kaltocarb, Kaltostat, Kaltoclude,
Sorbsan, Tegagel)

Foams
(e.g. Tielle, Lyofoam)

Foams
(e.g. Allevyn)

Tulle-gras dressings
(e.g. Jelonet, Paranet, Paratulle,
Periflex, Unitulle, Sofra-tulle,
Bactigras, Fucidin Intertulle)

Hydrocolloids
(e.g. Comfeel, Granuflex extra thin)

Hydrocolloids
(e.g. Biofilm, Granuflex E)

Semi-permeable films
(e.g. Omniderm, Opraflex, Opsite,
Ensure-it, Ioban II, Tegaderm,
Cutifilm, Dermafilm, Transite,
Bioclusive, Transigen)

Beads and powders
(e.g. Debrisan, Iodosorb)

Sugar paste

465

Appendix 2

Foot care advice for people with diabetes

Diabetes can affect the circulation to your feet and make them go numb. This means that you must take particular care of them. In order to avoid infection and prevent foot ulcers from forming check your feet daily.

1. Wash your feet carefully every day. Use warm water and mild soap. Do not soak your feet. Dry gently and thoroughly. Dab surgical spirit between the toes. Rub moisturizing cream onto the rest of the foot, especially the heel areas.

2. Wear clean socks/stockings every day. Make sure that there are no holes in them, and wear them inside out if the seams are prominent. Socks/stockings should be made of cotton mixture, and should fit your feet – try to avoid stretch-fit socks, and never use those made from artificial fibres.

3. Ask the fitter to measure your feet whenever you buy new shoes. Try to shop for them in the afternoon, as feet tend to swell during the day. Choose a pair made with soft leather uppers, and check that the lining is smooth. Make sure that the shoe is wide enough, deep enough and long enough, and avoid high heels. If you have insoles, check there is room for them in the shoe before you make a purchase. Try to get a pair with some form of fastening, such as laces or T-bar, and avoid slip-on or court shoe styles.

4. Consult a state registered chiropodist regularly (the practitioner will have the letters 'SRCh' after their name). They will examine and treat your feet and advise you on how best to look after them. Use clippers to carefully cut your toenails after a bath, keeping the end of the nail level with the top of the toe. Do not cut down the sides. Do not cut away hard skin and never use corn plasters.

5. Check your feet every day for any signs of skin problems, such as blisters, cuts, abrasions or infection. Any blistered, broken or inflamed skin should be washed with warm water, dried gently and covered with an antiseptic cream such as Savlon and clean gauze. Consult your state registered chiropodist if it does not heal within a few days.

6. Do your best to control your blood sugar levels. Poorly controlled diabetics are much more likely to develop serious foot problems. STOP smoking.

Appendix 3

Using crutches

Crutches offer a useful method of immobilizing the foot and ankle, while allowing the patient the benefit of movement. However, crutches should not be used indefinitely without good reason. Disuse of the limb may cause atrophy of muscle and demineralization of bone. The following information may be useful when guiding patients in the use of elbow crutches, probably the most common type of crutch issued today. Such instructions should always be issued with a visual demonstration before the crutches are dispensed to the patient.

Crutches are available in a number of designs. Remember, not all patients will be able to use them, and alternative methods such as wheelchairs may have to be used instead. The instructions given below have been assumed for patients who will be using such aids for short periods only. Patients with disability and chronic conditions should seek the advice of a state registered physiotherapist.

Patients using the aluminium elbow style crutch would be expected to be able to manoeuvre without difficulty, compared with other designs. This type of crutch is, therefore, to be used as an aid, using the good side for additional stability. Patients with poor balance coordination and weak muscles affecting the contralateral side often progress poorly with the aluminium elbow crutch. Negotiating stairs and inclines should be discouraged until the foot has undergone some recovery. The hollow aluminium crutches are popular because they are economical, light, strong and adjustable. Tall, heavy patients can bend the aluminium stem and each crutch must be checked for such damage before being dispensed. Other styles of crutches do exist – these are discussed briefly.

Gutter crutches provide more support for those patients with wrist and shoulder problems. The gutter forms the arm support and does not require the same amount of wrist strength as other crutches.

Where patients obviously would be unstable using crutches, *Zimmer frames* are very beneficial. These provide four stable supportive legs, reducing the likelihood of falling over.

Axillary crutches may be beneficial for younger stable patients where the body can be lifted up. These crutches need greater energy than elbow crutches and can cause discomfort to the shoulder or axillary region.

Elbow crutches – information for patients

Crutches are adjustable for your arm length and leg height. While the crutches provided are made of hollow aluminium, they can be abused and will bend if used incorrectly. Follow these instructions to help you move about safely:

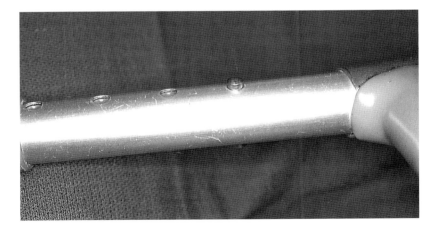

Figure A.1

1. Always adjust the arm length to coincide with a comfortable wrist position. The length of the upper section should be adjusted between the elbow and wrist, using the press-in stud/buttons (Fig. A.1) to shorten or lengthen the stem.

2. The lower section is similarly adjusted so that the hand support comfortably drops beside the thigh. The wrist should be extended and rested on the handle without strain (Fig. A.2).

3. The hand support is best used facing forwards. The point just below the elbow sits in a shaped rest, designed to support the lower arm.

4. Never attempt to take long steps or try to move quickly. If you have no existing heel pain, the use of heel contact will assist stability while keeping pressure off the forefoot.

5. Crutches may not suit you if you have weak arms or painful shoulders. An alternative system may have to be arranged. It is often better to use a walking stick than a single crutch.

6. If you cannot get on with your crutches, contact your practitioner.

7. Do not allow anyone to play with your crutches.

8. Stop using your crutches if you notice that they are damaged or bent.

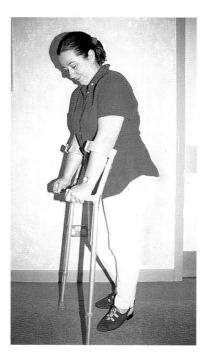

Figure A.2

Index